INTELLIGENT SYSTEMS AND TECHNOLOGIES IN REHABILITATION ENGINEERING

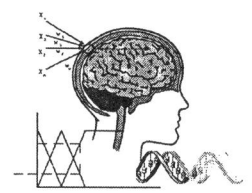

The CRC Press
International Series on Computational Intelligence

Series Editor
L.C. Jain, Ph.D., M.E., B.E. (Hons), Fellow I.E. (Australia)

L.C. Jain, R.P. Johnson, Y. Takefuji, and L.A. Zadeh
Knowledge-Based Intelligent Techniques in Industry

L.C. Jain and C.W. de Silva
**Intelligent Adaptive Control: Industrial Applications in the
Applied Computational Intelligence Set**

L.C. Jain and N.M. Martin
**Fusion of Neural Networks, Fuzzy Systems, and Genetic Algorithms:
Industrial Applications**

H.-N. Teodorescu, A. Kandel, and L.C. Jain
Fuzzy and Neuro-Fuzzy Systems in Medicine

C.L. Karr and L.M. Freeman
Industrial Applications of Genetic Algorithms

L.C. Jain and B. Lazzerini
Knowledge-Based Intelligent Techniques in Character Recognition

L.C. Jain and V. Vemuri
Industrial Applications of Neural Networks

H.-N. Teodorescu, A. Kandel, and L.C. Jain
Soft Computing in Human-Related Sciences

B. Lazzerini, D. Dumitrescu, L.C. Jain, and A. Dumitrescu
Evolutionary Computing and Applications

B. Lazzerini, D. Dumitrescu, and L.C. Jain
Fuzzy Sets and Their Application to Clustering and Training

L.C. Jain, U. Halici, I. Hayashi, S.B. Lee, and S. Tsutsui
Intelligent Biometric Techniques in Fingerprint and Face Recognition

Z. Chen
Computational Intelligence for Decision Support

L.C. Jain
Evolution of Engineering and Information Systems and Their Applications

H.-N. Teodorescu and A. Kandel
Dynamic Fuzzy Systems and Chaos Applications

L. Medsker and L.C. Jain
Recurrent Neural Networks: Design and Applications

L.C. Jain and A.M. Fanelli
Recent Advances in Artifical Neural Networks: Design and Applications

M. Russo and L.C. Jain
Fuzzy Learning and Applications

J. Liu
Multiagent Robotic Systems

M. Kennedy, R. Rovatti, and G. Setti
Chaotic Electronics in Telecommunications

H.-N. Teodorescu and L.C. Jain
Intelligent Systems and Technologies in Rehabilitation Engineering

I. Baturone, A. Barriga, C. Jimenez-Fernandez, D. Lopez, and S. Sanchez-Solano
Microelectronics Design of Fuzzy Logic-Based Systems

T. Nishida
Dynamic Knowledge Interaction

C.L. Karr
Practical Applications of Computational Intelligence for Adaptive Control

INTELLIGENT SYSTEMS AND TECHNOLOGIES IN REHABILITATION ENGINEERING

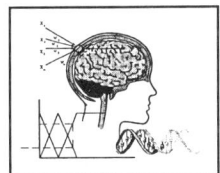

Edited by
Horia-Nicolai L. Teodorescu
Lakhmi C. Jain

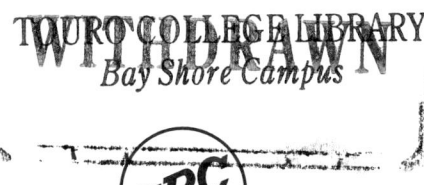

CRC Press
Boca Raton   London   New York   Washington, D.C.

The information in this volume is believed to be reliable and correct. The contributors are scientists active in the field in which they contributed chapters. However, the information provided in this volume reflects the scientific opinions of the contributors and is not intended to be used as a recommendation to users of the various designs or products presented in the volume. Under no circumstances can the information provided in this book be considered as medical recommendation to patients or persons seeking medical advice. By no means should this volume or any part of it replace advice of a qualified physician or expert caregiver.

The critical opinions expressed on different products or designs reflect the respective chapter contributors' opinions and represent "researcher opinions" intended to contrast with various technical solutions for the purpose of improving existing technologies, for the benefit of mankind. These opinions refer only to research, design, and application concepts, and should not be considered critical to commercial products.

The editors have made an effort to offer a high level scientific text aimed at scientists and designers. However, advances in the field may invalidate or make outdated the information included in this volume. Accuracy of the information cannot be guaranteed. The editors, the publisher, and the contributors assume no responsibility for how the public uses the information contained in this volume, make no warranties about the information in this volume, and assume no legal liability or responsibility with respect to this information or its use.

Library of Congress Cataloging-in-Publication Data

Intelligent systems and technologies in rehabilitation engineering / Horia-Nicolai L. Teodorescu and Lakhmi C. Jain (editors).
    p. cm.— (CRC Press international series on computational intelligence)
    Includes bibliographical references and index.
    ISBN 0-8493-0140-8 (alk. paper)
    1. Rehabilitation technology. 2. Self-help devices for the disabled. 3. Artificial intelligence. I. Teodorescu, Horia-Nicolai. II. Jain, L.C. III. Series.

RM950 .I56 2000
617'.03—dc21   00-051893

This book contains information obtained from authentic and highly regarded sources. Reprinted material is quoted with permission, and sources are indicated. A wide variety of references are listed. Reasonable efforts have been made to publish reliable data and information, but the author and the publisher cannot assume responsibility for the validity of all materials or for the consequences of their use.

Neither this book nor any part may be reproduced or transmitted in any form or by any means, electronic or mechanical, including photocopying, microfilming, and recording, or by any information storage or retrieval system, without prior permission in writing from the publisher.

All rights reserved. Authorization to photocopy items for internal or personal use, or the personal or internal use of specific clients, may be granted by CRC Press LLC, provided that $.50 per page photocopied is paid directly to Copyright Clearance Center, 222 Rosewood Drive, Danvers, MA 01923 USA. The fee code for users of the Transactional Reporting Service is ISBN 0-8493-0140-8/01/$0.00+$.50. The fee is subject to change without notice. For organizations that have been granted a photocopy license by the CCC, a separate system of payment has been arranged.

The consent of CRC Press LLC does not extend to copying for general distribution, for promotion, for creating new works, or for resale. Specific permission must be obtained in writing from CRC Press LLC for such copying.

Direct all inquiries to CRC Press LLC, 2000 N.W. Corporate Blvd., Boca Raton, Florida 33431, or visit our Web site at www.crcpress.com

Trademark Notice: Product or corporate names may be trademarks or registered trademarks, and are used only for identification and explanation, without intent to infringe.

© 2001 by CRC Press LLC

No claim to original U.S. Government works
International Standard Book Number 0-8493-0140-8
Library of Congress Card Number 00-051893
Printed in the United States of America 1 2 3 4 5 6 7 8 9 0
Printed on acid-free paper

My work to this volume is dedicated to the memory of the late ORL Professor **Leonid Teodorescu**, *who healed patients from around the world in an effort to alleviate the suffering and to limit the effect of disabilities.*

Horia-Nicolai Teodorescu

Acknowledgments

The editors thank the contributors for their vision, commitment, hard work, and patience during the preparation of the chapters. Without the considerable efforts of the authors and of the reviewers, this volume could not have come to fulfillment.

The editors thank Suzanne Lassandro, production manager, Naomi Lynch, and Elizabeth Spangenberger, from CRC Press, for their kind support and professional advice during the preparation of this volume and for their commitment to the project.

The editors are grateful to the following peer reviewers for their help in reviewing this volume: Dr. Dragos Arotaritei (Romanian Academy, Computer Science Institute), Dr. L. Boiculese (University of Medicine, Iasi, Romania), Dr. Cristian Bonciu (Technical University of Iasi), Dr. Adrian Brezulianu (Technical University of Iasi), Dr. Mircea Chelaru (Duke University), Dr. Dorian Cojocaru (University of Craiova, Romania), Dan Marius Dobre (Technical University of Iasi), R.K. Jain (University of South Australia, Adelaide, Australia), Dr. Florin Grigoras (Institute for Computer Science, Romanian Academy), Doron Leca (Tel Aviv, Israel), Prof. Daniel Mlynek (Swiss Federal Institute of Technology, Lausanne), Xavier Peillon (Swiss Federal Institute of Technology, Lausanne, Switzerland), and Dennis W. Siemsen, OD, MHPE (Department of Ophthalmology, Mayo Clinic, Rochester, MN).

Virtually all contributors to this volume helped with the cross-referring process. Their invaluable help is heartily acknowledged. Moreover, Dr. Van der Loos provided advice and comments on the Table of Contents of the volume. His comments helped improve the volume.

October 1999

Horia-Nicolai Teodorescu *Lakhmi C. Jain*
Tampa, Florida Adelaide, South Australia

Preface

This volume represents a comprehensive overview of a dynamic field that has evolved tremendously over the last three decades, namely the application of intelligent technologies in rehabilitation. Prostheses, assistive systems, and rehabilitation systems are essential components in increasing the well-being of people with disabling conditions around the world. The focus is on state-of-the-art information related to innovative technologies and their applications aiming to better the lives of people with disabling conditions. The contributors present various topics related to prostheses and assistive systems, ranging from the underlying principles of the "intelligent" systems, design, practical applications, and assessment of results. The emphasis is on the main principles and applications of intelligent technologies in prosthetics and rehabilitation. Both applications and technology are extensively covered. In addition to offering original scientific thought and surveying recent and current research, all chapters provide pointers to future developments.

The volume is organized into five parts. The first part is introductory and consists of a single chapter summarizing some major trends in the field. The second part of the volume is devoted to sensorial prostheses and includes two chapters that present the state-of-the-art in visual (retinal) prostheses, hearing aids, and implanted hearing (cochlear) prostheses. While cochlear prostheses are in common use, retinal prostheses are still in the research phase.

Part 3 is devoted to locomotor prostheses. The first chapter in this section makes a connection between the second and the third parts of the volume by presenting sensory feedback to the users of lower limb prostheses. The advances in the field of myoelectric and neural prostheses are presented in Chapters 5 to 7. The problem of interfacing in neuronal and myoelectric control is the primary focus in these chapters. The requirements of selective and graded, yet stable and reliable activation of specific groups of neurons with fully implantable electrodes, to provide adequate function, is the main topic in Chapter 6. Myoelectric control is analyzed in Chapter 5 and a detailed application in the control of upper limb prostheses is presented in Chapter 7.

The fourth part of the book covers pacemakers and life-sustaining devices. In Chapter 8, the authors present a computer-aided support technique for artificial heart control and new methods for hemodynamic measurements for use in conjunction with artificial hearts. Chapter 9 is devoted to diaphragm pacing for chronic respiratory insufficiency – an emerging and less known field. An application of intelligent systems in heart pacemakers is presented in Chapter 10.

The fifth part of the volume is devoted to robotic systems and advanced mechanics for prostheses. Service robots for rehabilitation and assistance are presented in Chapter 11, while computerized aids for the blind and visually impaired are presented in Chapter 12. The emphasis in the last chapter is on improving mechanical design of limb prostheses to increase the efficiency and complexity of movements – a goal that current designs only partly fulfill.

The chapters are comprehensive and the information presented is up to date. Extensive bibliographies help the researcher to find original sources and provide an ample overview of the literature. A detailed *Index of terms* and an *Index of acronyms and abbreviations* further assist the reader.

We are confident that this volume covers a significant part of the field and will satisfy a large readership. Graduate and postgraduate students and researchers involved in the design, manufacture, and use of technology for rehabilitation will benefit from this volume. The "reader profile" of this volume includes:

- Scientists and engineers in biomedical engineering and medical technology.
- Computer scientists applying intelligent technologies, including fuzzy systems, neural networks, and robotics in the field of medicine.
- Engineers working in the areas of electronics, microtechnology, robotics for medicine, as well as technology managers and consultants in health care and medical engineering.
- Bioengineering or biomedical engineering students at the graduate level.
- Consultants and managers in rehabilitation.

The book may be used as a text or as supplementary reading for courses in biomedical engineering and in advanced courses in computer science – artificial intelligence.

This volume follows two volumes recently published by CRC Press, namely:

- H.N. Teodorescu, A. Kandel, and L.C. Jain (Eds.): *Fuzzy and Neuro-Fuzzy Systems in Medicine*. CRC Press, Boca Raton, Florida, USA, 394 p.+ *xxviii*, 1998 (ISBN: 0-8493-9806-1)

and

- H.N. Teodorescu, A. Kandel, and L.C. Jain (Eds.): *Soft-Computing in Human-Related Sciences*. CRC Press, Boca Raton, Florida, USA May 1999 (ISBN: 0-8493-1635-9)

Several chapters in these two volumes provide background to this book and are complementary. The following chapters are of particular note:

In the volume: H.N. Teodorescu, A. Kandel, and L.C. Jain (Eds.), *Soft Computing in Human-Related Sciences*, CRC Press, 1999

Chapter 1. Fuzzy control methodology: basics and state of the art, by *T. Fukuda and N. Kubota*

Chapter 2. Learning eye-arm coordination using neural and fuzzy neural techniques, by *A. Stoica*

Chapter 3. Learning stiffness characteristics of the human hand using a neuro-fuzzy system, by *A. Iliesh and A. Kandel*

In the volume: H.N. Teodorescu, A. Kandel, and L.C. Jain (Eds.), *Fuzzy and Neuro-Fuzzy Systems in Medicine*, CRC Press, 1998

Chapter 1. Fuzzy logic and neuro-fuzzy systems in medicine and bio-medical engineering. A historical perspective, by *H.N. Teodorescu, A. Kandel, and L.C. Jain*

Chapter 11. Fuzzy control and decision making in drug delivery, by *J.W. Huang, C.M. Held, and R.J. Roy*

Chapter 12B. Neural networks and fuzzy-based integrated circuit and system solutions applied to the biomedical field, by *A. Schmid and D. Mlynek*

Material supplementing this volume to assist teaching may soon be available from the first editor, on request.
The editors invite comments from readers of this volume.

Horia-Nicolai L. Teodorescu *Lakhmi C. Jain*
Tampa, Florida *Adelaide, South Australia*

About the Editors

Horia-Nicolai L. Teodorescu served as a professor in several universities, currently being charged with courses at the University of South Florida and Technical University of Iasi, Iasi, Romania. Dr. Teodorescu received an M.S. degree and a Doctoral degree in Electronics, in 1975 and 1981, respectively. He has served as a founding director of the Center for Fuzzy Systems and Approximate Reasoning at Technical University of Iasi, Iasi, Romania, since 1990, and as a professor at the same university. He was an invited or visiting professor in Japan (1992, 1993, 1994), Switzerland (1994, 1995, 1996, 1997, 1999) and Spain (1993, 1996). Dr. Teodorescu has written about 250 papers, authored, co-authored, edited or co-edited more than 20 volumes, and holds 21 patents. He won several gold and silver medals for his inventions in various invention exhibitions. He authored many papers on biomedical engineering and applications of fuzzy and neuro-fuzzy systems to medical engineering and holds 11 patents in the field of biomedical engineering. He won several grants for research on applying fuzzy systems in biomedical applications. He is a Senior Member of the IEEE and holds several honorific titles, including "Eminent scientist" of Fuzzy Logic Systems Institute, Japan, and he was awarded the Honorary Medal of the Higher Economic School in Barcelona, Spain. He has been *correspondent member* of the Romanian Academy since 1993. Dr. Teodorescu is a founding Chief Editor of *Fuzzy Systems & A.I.– Reports and Letters, International Journal for Chaos Theory and Applications, Iasi Polytechnic Magazine* and *Magazine for Fuzzy Systems* and he was a founding Co-Director of *Fuzzy Economic Review* (Spain). He is currently an Associate Editor to IEEE Transactions on Cybernetic and Systems – C. He is a member of the editorial boards of *Fuzzy Sets and Systems, The Journal of Grey Systems, BUSEFAL – Bulletin for Studies and Exchange of Fuzziness and its Applications, Journal of Information Sciences of Moldavia, Review for Inventions, Romanian Journal of Information Science and Technology*, and *Journal of AEDEM*. He served as a chairman or co-chairman of the scientific committees of several international conferences and was a member of the scientific committees of more than 40 international conferences.

Address: University of South Florida, Computer Science and Engineering (CSEE), ENB 340, 4202 E. Fowler Ave., Tampa, Fl 33620-5399 USA. Phone: (813) 974-9036. Fax: 813-974-5456. E-mail: teodores@csee.usf.edu

Lakhmi C. Jain is Director/Founder of the Knowledge-Based Intelligent Engineering Systems (KES) Centre, located in the Division of Information Technology, Engineering and the Environment. He is a fellow of the Institution of Engineers Australia. He has initiated a postgraduate stream by research in the Knowledge-Based Intelligent Engineering systems area. He is the Founding Editor-in-Chief of the International Journal of Knowledge-Based Intelligent Engineering Systems and served as an Associate Editor of the IEEE Transactions on Industrial Electronics. Dr. Jain was the Technical Chair of the ETD2000 International Conference in 1995 and Publications Chair of the Australian and New Zealand Conference on Intelligent Information Systems in 1996. He also initiated the first International Conference on Knowledge-Based Intelligent Electronic Systems in 1997. This is now an annual event. He served as the Vice-President by the Electronics Association of South Australia in 1997. He is the Editor-in-Chief of the International Book Series on Computational Intelligence, CRC Press, USA. His interests focus on the use of novel techniques such as knowledge-based systems, artificial neural networks, fuzzy systems, and genetic algorithms and the application of these techniques.

Address: Knowledge-Based Intelligent Engineering Systems Center, Division of Information Technology, Engineering and the Environment, University of South Australia, Mawson Lakes, Adelaide, South Australia, 5095. Phone: 61883023315. Fax: 61883023384. E-mail: http://www.unisa.edu.au/pes/kes.htm

Contributors

Harish Aiyar received a B.S. degree in biomedical engineering from Rensselaer Polytechnic Institute, Troy, NY, in 1991. He is currently pursuing a Ph.D. degree in biomedical engineering from Case Western Reserve University, Cleveland, OH. His research interests include neural prostheses for the restoration of lost or impaired function and minimally invasive surgical techniques.
> *Address: Applied Neural Control Laboratory, Department of Biomedical Engineering, Case Western Reserve University, Charles B. Bolton Building, Rm. 3480, Cleveland, OH 44106-4912. Phone: (216) 368-3884. E-mail: hxa14@po.cwru.edu*

W. Anthony Alford was born in 1971 in Lafayette, LA. He received a B.S. degree in electrical engineering (1993) from Louisiana Tech University and the M.S. degree in electrical engineering (1995) from the University of Tennessee Space Institute. He is currently enrolled in the Ph.D. program at Vanderbilt University.
> *Address: Center for Intelligent Systems (CIS), Electrical Engineering and Computer Science Department, Box 131 Station B, Vanderbilt University, Nashville, TN 37235. Phone: 615-322-2735/343-0697. Fax: 615-322-7062. E-mail: alford@vuse.vanderbilt.edu*

Ken'ichi Asami has been a research associate in the Department of Mechanical System Engineering at Kyushu Institute of Technology since 1997. He received B.E. and M.E. degrees in information engineering in 1992 and 1994, respectively, and the Dr. Eng. in information science in 1997, all from Kyushu Institute of Technology. His current research interests include knowledge engineering and intelligent human interface.
> *Address: Kyushu Institute of Technology, Department of Mechanical System Engineering, 680-4, Kawazu, Iizuka, Fukuoka 820-8502, Japan. Phone: +81-948-29-7785. Fax: +81-948-29-7751. E-mail: asami@mse.kyutech.ac.jp*

Jeffrey R. Basford, M.D., Ph.D., has a diverse background in science and medicine. Doctor Basford received a Bachelor of Physics degree in 1963. He next taught university level physics as a Peace Corps Volunteer and then served as an officer in the U.S. Army. Following the award of a Ph.D. degree in Physics and Mathematics in 1974, he worked as a research and development consultant and attended medical school at the University of Miami. He completed residency training in Physical Medicine and Rehabilitation in 1981. Doctor Basford has been a member of the Department of Physical Medicine and Rehabilitation at the Mayo Clinic since 1982 where his clinical responsibilities have emphasized neurological rehabilitation and musculoskeletal pain. Doctor Basford's research has emphasized the physiological effects of the physical agents on the body with particular interest in biomechanics and electromagnetic forces.

Address: Department of Physical Medicine and Rehabilitation, Mayo Clinic and Foundation, 200 Second Street SW, Rochester, MN 55902. Phone: (+)507-255-8972. Fax: (+) 507-255-4641

Christian Berger-Vachon is a Professor at the University of Lyon, France, Department of Medical Physics. Prof. Berger-Vachon was born in Lyon (France) in 1944. He graduated as an Electrical Engineer, Ph.D. and M.D. His research interests are in Signal Processing applied to hearing and voice impairment in the laboratory, "Perception & Hearing Mechanisms," affiliated with the French CNRS (Research Council) with the number UPRESA 5020. In addition, Prof. Christian Breger-Vachon's research interest lies in applying new technologies, including neural networks and fuzzy systems, to medicine. Dr. Berger-Vachon is also General Secretary of the AMSE Society and Editor-in-Chief of the AMSE periodicals, France.

Address: Pavillon U (ORL), Hopital Edouard-Herriot, 69437 Lyon-CEDEX 03, France. Phone: 33 4 72 11 05 03. Fax: 33-4-72-11 05 04. E-mail: cbv@univ-lyon1.fr

Johann Borenstein (M'88) received B.Sc., M.Sc., and D.Sc. degrees in Mechanical Engineering in 1981, 1983, and 1987, respectively, from the Technion - Israel Institute of Technology, Haifa, Israel. Since 1987, he has been with the Robotics Systems Division at the University of Michigan, Ann Arbor, where he is currently a Research Scientist and Head of the MEAM Mobile Robotics Lab. His research interests include mobile robot navigation, obstacle avoidance, kinematic design of mobile robots, real-time control, sensors for robotic applications, multisensor integration, and robotics for the handicapped. In 1998 Dr. Borenstein received the Discover Magazine Award for Technological Innovation, Robotics Category, for his invention of the GuideCane.

Address: The University of Michigan, Advanced Technologies Lab, 1101 Beal Avenue, Ann Arbor, MI 48109-2110. Phone: (734) 763-1560. Fax: (209) 879-5169. E-mail: johannb@umich.edu

Claudio Bonivento was born in 1941 in Bologna, Italy. He graduated *cum laude* in Electrical Engineering from the University of Bologna in 1964. Since

1975, he has been Professor of Automatic Control in that university. He has held visiting positions at various academic institutions, including the University of California at Berkeley, the University of Florida at Gainesville, and MIT in Boston. He served as President of GRIS – Italian Group of Researchers on Computer and Systems, 1981-1982, and as President of CIRA –Italian Inter-University Center of Research on Automatics, 1989-1992. From 1993 to 1996, he was a coordinator of ERNET (European Robotics Research Network). Since 1994, he has been a member of the Italian delegation at the IFAC. His main research interests are in control systems theory and robotics. He is author or co-author of five books on applied mathematics, digital control systems, and system identification and simulation, as well as of many other technical and scientific publications. Professor Bonivento is a senior member of IEEE and an elected member of the Administrative Council of EUCA (European Union Control Association) for the term 1997-2001.

Address: University of Bologna, Department of Electronics Computer and Systems, Viale Risorgimento, 2, 40139 Bologna, Italy. Phone: +39 051 644 3045. Fax: +39 051 644 3073. E-mail: cbonivento@ deis.unibo.it

Edward E. Brown, Jr. was born in 1970 in Gary, IN. He received a B.S. degree in Electrical Engineering (1992) from the University of Pennsylvania and afterwards worked for IBM Federal Systems Company in Owego, NY for 3 years. He received an M.S. degree in Electrical Engineering (1999) from Vanderbilt University and is currently enrolled in the Ph.D. program at Vanderbilt University.

Address: Center for Intelligent Systems (CIS), Electrical Engineering and Computer Science Department, Box 131 Station B, Vanderbilt University, Nashville TN 37235. Phone: 615-322-2735/343-0697. Fax: 615-322-7062. E-mail: maverick@vuse.vanderbilt.edu

Angelo Davalli was born in 1962 in Budrio, Italy. He received an M.Sc. degree in Electronic Engineering (1988) from the University of Bologna, Italy. Now he is the referent of research area in the INAIL Prosthetic Center in Bologna.

Address: INAIL Prosthetic Center, Via Rabbuina, 16, 40054 Budrio (BO), Italy. Phone: +39 051 6936610. Fax: +39 051 802232. E-mail: a.davalli@inail.it

Kevin Englehart received a Ph.D. degree from the University of New Brunswick (UNB) in 1998. His doctoral research integrated emerging methods in pattern recognition, time-frequency transforms, and signal projection to develop an improved means of controlling artificial limbs. He has an extensive background in the design and implementation of real-time embedded DSP systems in biomedical engineering, telephony, and acoustic applications. He is currently an Assistant Professor in the Department of Electrical and Computer Engineering at UNB.

> *Address: University of New Brunswick, Department of Electrical and Computer Engineering, P.O. Box 4400, Fredericton, New Brunswick E3B 5A3 Canada. Fax:(506) 453-3589. E-mail: kengleha@unb.ca*

Warren M. Grill, Jr. received a B.S. degree in biomedical engineering with honors in 1989 from Boston University, Boston, MA. He earned an M.S. degree in 1992 and a Ph.D. degree in 1995, both in biomedical engineering, from Case Western Reserve University, Cleveland, OH. Dr. Grill is presently Elmer L. Lindseth Assistant Professor of Biomedical Engineering at Case Western Reserve University and a Principal Investigator of the Cleveland FES Center. His research interests are in neural engineering and include neural prostheses, the electrical properties of tissues and cells, computational neuroscience, and neural control.

> *Address: Department of Biomedical Engineering, Applied Neural Control Lab, Case Western Reserve University, C.B. Bolton Building, Rm 3480, Cleveland OH 44106-4912. Phone (216) 368-8625. Fax (216) 368-4872. E-mail: wmg@po.cwru.edu*

Bernard Hudgins received a Ph.D. degree from UNB in 1991. His doctoral research helped define a new approach to multifunction myoelectric control. He is currently a Senior Research Associate with the Institute of Biomedical Engineering at UNB in Fredericton, NB. His primary research interests are in the area of myoelectric signal processing for control of artificial limbs. He was a recipient of a Whitaker Investigator award and recently spent 2 years on a NATO workgroup assessing alternative technologies for cockpit applications.

> *Address: Institute of Biomedical Engineering, University of New Brunswick, P.O. Box 4400, Fredericton, New Brunswick E3B 5A3 Canada. Phone (506) 453-4966. Fax: (506) 453-4827. E-mail: hudgins@unb.ca*

Steven E. Irby received his B.S. degree in Bioengineering from the University of California, San Diego, in 1985. He earned an M.S. degree in Mechanical Engineering from San Diego State University in 1994. From 1987-1997, he worked as an engineer in the Motion Analysis Laboratory of Children's Hospital and Health Center San Diego. In 1995 he was awarded the first place award in the Master's Level Student Design Competition of the ASME International Conference, Bioengineering Division, for his presentation entitled "A Digital Logic Controlled Electromechanical Free Knee Brace." From 1997-1999 he has worked in the Biomechanics Laboratory of the Mayo Clinic, Rochester, MN. His research interests are human motion measurement and biomechanics of the knee.

Address: Biomechanics Laboratory, Division of Orthopedic Research, Mayo Clinic and Mayo Foundation, Rochester, MN 55905. Phone: 507/ 284-2262. Fax: 507/ 284-5392

Kenton R. Kaufman, Ph.D., P.E., received his Ph.D. degree in biomechanical engineering from North Dakota State University in 1988. He is a registered professional engineer. He was employed as an Assistant Professor at North Dakota State University from 1976 to 1986. From 1986 to 1989, he worked as a Visiting Scientist and then as a Research Fellow in the Biomechanics Laboratory at the Mayo Clinic. From 1989 to 1996, he served as the Director of Orthopedic Research in the Motion Analysis Laboratory at Children's Hospital, San Diego, and as an Adjunct Associate Professor at the University of California, San Diego. Currently, he is the Co-Director of the Biomechanics Laboratory, Associate Professor of Bioengineering, and Consultant in the Department of Orthopedic Surgery at the Mayo Clinic. Dr. Kaufman's research focuses on the biomechanics of human movement. He currently holds several grants from NIH, with projects aimed at improving the mobility of disabled individuals. He has also conducted research to decrease overuse injuries in military recruits. He has won several awards for his research efforts. His awards include the American Society of Biomechanics Young Investigator Award in 1989, the Excellence in Research Award in 1989 and the O'Donoghue Sports Injury Research Award in 1993 from the American Orthopedic Society for Sports Medicine, the Clinical Research Award from the American Academy of Orthopedic Surgeons in 1996, and the Best Scientific Paper Award from the Gait and Clinical Movement Analysis Society in 1999. Dr. Kaufman has served the biomechanics research community in several forms. He has served as an ad-hoc grant reviewer for NIH since 1993 and for the National Institute on Disability and Rehabilitation Research in 1998. He was on the Working Group on Injury Prevention of the Armed Forces Epidemiological Board from 1994-1995. He is currently the Conference Chairperson and serves on the Accreditation Committee for the Gait and Clinical Movement Analysis Society. He is a member of the American Society of Biomechanics Graduate Student Grant-In-Aid Committee. He serves on the Commission for Motion Laboratory Accreditation. He is also on the editorial board of *Gait and Posture*.

Address: Biomechanics Laboratory, Department of Orthopedic Surgery, 128 Guggenheim Building, Mayo Clinic, 200 First Street SW, Rochester, MN 55905. Phone: (507)-284-2262. Fax: (507)-284-5392. E-mail: kaufman.kenton@mayo.edu

Kazuhiko Kawamura, Ph.D. was born in Nagoya, Japan and is a naturalized U.S. Citizen. He received his Ph.D. degree in 1971 in electrical engineering from the University of Michigan, Ann Arbor. He also holds a B.E. degree from

Waseda University, Tokyo, and an M.S. degree from the University of California, Berkeley. Dr. Kawamura is Professor of Electrical Engineering and Computer Engineering and Management of Technology at Vanderbilt University School of Engineering. He is also Director of the Center for Intelligent Systems, the U.S.-Japan Center for Technology Management, and Interim Director of the Management of Technology Program. He also serves as a board member of A-CIMS (Academic Coalition for Intelligent Manufacturing Systems), and currently serves as Chair of Technical Committee on Service Robots for the IEEE Robotics and Automation Society. He has published over 120 research papers and technical reports, a book, and book chapters in the fields of technology management, intelligent systems, intelligent robotics and control, intelligent manufacturing, and environmentally sound manufacturing.

> *Address: Center for Intelligent Systems (CIS), Electrical Engineering and Computer Science Department, Box 131 Station B, Vanderbilt University, Nashville, TN 37235. Phone: 615-322-2735/343-0697, Fax: 615-322-7062. E-mail: Kawamura@vuse.vanderbilt.edu kawamura@mailhost.vuse.vanderbilt.edu*

Tadashi Kitamura received a B.S. degree from Department of Mechanical Engineering at Waseda University, 1973, and M.S. and Dr. Eng. degrees from the Graduate School of Engineering at Kyoto University, 1975 and 1981, respectively. He was Assistant Professor of the EE Department from 1984 to 1987 at the University of Houston, University Park, joined the faculty at Kyushu Institute of Technology in 1987, and is Professor of Department of Mechanical System Engineering there since 1988. His current research interest is design of intelligent mechatronic systems including artificial hearts, biorobots, and superconducting actuators. Since 1997, he is the Editor-in-Chief of the *Bio-Medical Soft Computing and Human Sciences Journal*, published by the Biomedical Fuzzy Systems Association. He published over 100 academic papers, edited three books, and co-authored nine books. He is a member of IEEE, ISAO, JSAO, BMFSA, JSME, and JSICE.

> *Address: Dept. of Mechanical System Engineering, College of Computer Science and System Engineering, Kyushu Institute of Technology, 680-4 Kawazu, Iizuka-City, Fukuoka 820-8502, Japan. Fax: +81-948-29-7751. E-mail: kita@mse.kyutech.ac.jp*

Claudio Lamberti was born in 1948 in Bologna, Italy. He received an M.Sc. degree in mechanical engineering from the University of Bologna in 1974. In 1978, he received a post-graduate degree in biomedical technology from the University of Bologna School of Medicine. He is currently a Research Associate at the Department of Electronics, Computer Science and Systems of the University of Bologna. Since 1991, he has been charge at University of Bologna of the course Computer and Systems Science in Health Care. His

research activity is focused on biomedical signal and image processing and biomedical technology assessment.
Address: University of Bologna, Department of Electronics Computer and Systems, Viale Risorgimento, 2, 40139 Bologna, Italy. Phone: +39 051 6443098. Fax: +39 51 6443073. E-mail: clamberti@deis.unibo.it

Wentai Liu is a Professor of Electrical and Computer Engineering (ECE), Department of Electrical and Computer Engineering (ECE), Electronics Research Laboratory (ERL), North Carolina State University. He is an Associate Editor, *IEEE Transactions on Circuits and Systems*, Part II (IEEE), an Associate Editor, *Journal of Solid-State Circuits and Devices*, Tutorial Co-Chair for ISCAS96, General Chair for 1997 Solid-State Circuits Society Workshop on Clock Network Design and Distribution Representative, IEEE Circuits and Systems Society and Solid-State Circuits Society. He supervises several research projects on prostheses, interactive learning, microcircuits, etc. and has designed many integrated circuits related to these topics.
Address: Room 442, Engineering Graduate Research Center, Centennial Campus, North Carolina State University, Raleigh, NC 27695-7914. Phone: 919-515-7347. Fax: 919-515-2285. E-mail: wentai@eos.ncsu.edu

J. Thomas Mortimer is a native of Texas. He received a B.S.E.E. degree from Texas Technological College, Lubbock, TX; an M.S. degree from Case Institute of Technology, Cleveland, OH; and a Ph.D. degree from Case Western Reserve University, Cleveland, OH. His mentors during his graduate studies were J.B. Reswick and C.N. Shealy. From 1968 to 1969, he was a Visiting Research Associate at Chalmers Tekniska Hogskola, Gteborg, Sweden. He then joined the Department of Biomedical Engineering at Case Western Reserve University where he is currently a Professor. He is also the Director of the Applied Neural Control Laboratory. In 1977-1978 he was a Visiting Professor at the Institut für Biokybernetik und Biomedizinische Technik, Universitèt Karlsruhe, Karlsruhe, West Germany. In 1992, he was a Visiting Scholar at Tohoko University, Sendai, Japan. He is President of Axon Engineering, Inc., Willoughby, OH, a company providing electrodes and consulting services to parties interested in developing new products in the neural prosthesis area. His research interests concern electrically activating the nervous system. He holds nine patents in this area and has over 70 publications dealing with neural prostheses and related pain suppression, motor prostheses for restoration of limb function and respiration, bladder and bowel assist, electrodes, tissue damage, and methods of selective activation. Dr. Mortimer was the recipient of the 1996 United Cerebral Palsy Research and Education Foundation's Isabelle and Leonard H. Goldenson Technology Award. In 1976, he was awarded the Humboldt-Preis by the Alexander von Humboldt

Foundation, Federal Republic of Germany. He is a fellow of the American Institute for Medical and Biological Engineering.
> *Address: Applied Neural Control Laboratory, Case Western Reserve University, C.B. Bolton Building, Rm. 3480, Cleveland, OH. Phone: (216)368-3973. Fax: (216)368-4872. E-mail: jtm3@po.cwru.edu*

Todd Pack received his Bachelor's degree from Cornell University in 1992. He received an M.S. degree in 1994 and a Ph.D. degree in 1997, both in Electrical Engineering, from Vanderbilt University. He is currently employed at Real World Interfaces, Inc.
> *Address: Center for Intelligent Systems (CIS), Electrical Engineering and Computer Science Department, Box 131 Station B, Vanderbilt University, Nashville, TN 37235. Phone: 615-322-2735/343-0697. Fax: 615-322-7062. E-mail: todd@rwii.com*

Philip A. Parker received a B.Sc. degree in electrical engineering from UNB in 1964, an M.Sc. degree from the University of St. Andrews (Scotland) in 1966, and a Ph.D. degree from UNB in 1975. In 1966, he joined the National Research Council of Canada as a Communications Officer and the following year he joined the Institute of Biomedical Engineering, UNB, as a Research Associate. In 1976, he was appointed to the Department of Electrical Engineering, UNB, and currently holds the rank of Professor in that department. He is also a Research Consultant to the Institute of Biomedical Engineering, UNB. His research interests are primarily in the area of biological signal processing.
> *Address: Institute of Biomedical Engineering, University of New Brunswick, Fredericton, New Brunswick E3B 5A3 Canada. Phone: (506) 453-4966. Fax: (506) 453-4827. E-mail: pap@unb.ca*

Richard Alan Peters II was born in Warren, PA in 1956. He is a Phi Beta Kappa graduate of Oberlin College (Oberlin, OH) where he received an A.B. degree in Mathematics (May 1979). He attended the University of Arizona (Tucson) where he was a fellow of the American Electronics Association. He received an M.S. degree in Electrical Engineering in 1985. Peters received a Ph.D. degree. in Electrical Engineering from the University of Arizona in August 1988. Currently, he is an Associate Professor of Electrical Engineering in the School of Engineering at Vanderbilt University in Nashville, TN.
> *Address: Center for Intelligent Systems (CIS), Electrical Engineering and Computer Science Department, Box 131 Station B, Vanderbilt University, Nashville TN 37235. Phone: 615-322-2735/343-0697. Fax: 615-322-7062. E-mail: rap2@vuse.vanderbilt.edu*

Stefan Popescu, Ph.D., is a Professor at Polytechnic University Bucharest, Department of Biomedical Engineering. He was born in 1960 in Calafat, Romania. He received an M.S. degree "Magna cum laude" in Electronics (1985) from the University of Timisoara, and a Ph.D. degree in Electronic Engineering (1994) from the University of Bucharest. Until 1989 he was with the Medical Institute of Timisoara and the Electronic Research Institute in Bucharest. In 1990, he joined the University of Bucharest teaching lessons on biomedical engineering and medical imaging. Since 1995, he has been a scientist partner at Siemens Medical Group in Erlangen-Germany, working in the field of computer tomography.
Address: "Politehnica" University of Bucharest, Department of Electronics and Telecommunications, Romania. Phone: +40-1-230 2818. Fax: +40-1-223 2284. E-mail: popescus@elmed.pub.ro, Popescu Stefan Stefan.Popescu@med.siemens.de

Tamara E. Rogers was born in 1971 in Nashville, TN. She received a B.S. degree in Electrical Engineering (1993) and an M.S. degree in Electrical Engineering (1995) from Vanderbilt University. She is currently enrolled in the Ph.D. program at Vanderbilt University.
Address: Center for Intelligent Systems (CIS), Electrical Engineering and Computer Science Department, Box 131 Station B, Vanderbilt University, Nashville TN 37235. Phone: 615-322-2735/343-0697. Fax: 615-322-7062. E-mail: tamarar@vuse.vanderbilt.edu

Rinaldo Sacchetti was born in 1958 in Italy. He received an M.Sc. degree in Mechanic Engineering (1982) from the University in Genova. He is currently the head of upper limbs prosthesis line in the INAIL Prosthetic Center in Bologna (Italy).
Address: INAIL Prosthetic Center, Via Rabbuina, 16, 40054 Budrio (BO), Italy. Phone: +39 051 6936505. Fax: +39 051 802232. E-mail: r.sacchetti@inail.it

Micaela Schmid was born in 1971 in Milano, Italy. She received the *laurea* degree in Informatics Engineering (1997) from the University of Pavia. She is at present a Ph.D. student in Bioengineering and Medical Informatics at the University of Pavia. Her main research topic is the analysis of gait and balance in lower limb amputee subjects.
Address: University of Pavia, Department of Computer and System Sciences, via Ferrata 1, 27100 Pavia, Italy. Phone: +39-0382505370. Fax: +39-0382505373. E-mail: miki@linus2.unipv.it

Shraga Shoval received B.Sc. and M.Sc. degrees in Mechanical Engineering from the Technion - Israel Institute of Technology, Haifa, in 1985 and 1987, respectively. He received his Ph.D. degree in Mechanical Engineering from the University of Michigan in 1994. From 1987-1990, he worked as a scientist with the DCIRO, Division of Manufacturing Technologies, Sydney, Australia, where he developed an automatic system for gemstone processing. He is currently a research fellow at the Faculty of Industrial Engineering and Management, Technion, Haifa, where he manages the Computer Integrated Manufacturing and Robotics laboratory. His research interests include mobile robot navigation, kinematic design of multilegged spider-like mechanisms, steering control of autonomous passenger vehicles, analysis of robot motion performance, and integration of robots in manufacturing systems.

Address: Faculty of Industrial Engineering & Management, Technion Israel Institute of Technology, Haifa 32000, Israel. Phone: 972-4-8292040. Fax: 972-4-8235194. E-mail: shraga@hitech.technion.ac.il

Rodica Strungaru is a Professor at Faculty of Electronics and Telecommunication, Polytechnic University of Bucharest, Bucharest, Romania. She was born in 1942 in Chisinau, Romania. She received an M.Sc. degree in Physics Engineering (1965) on "Liner Accelerator with Built-In Power Supply" from the "Politehnica" University of Bucharest in Romania, and a Ph.D. degree in Electronic Engineering (1973) from the same university.

Address: Faculty of Electronics and Telecommunications, Polytechnic University of Bucharest, 77202 Bucharest, Romania. Phone: + 40- 1 312 24 52. Fax: + 40- 1 312 24 52. E-mail: strungar@elmed.pub.ro

David H. Sutherland received his B.S. degree from the University of Washington, Seattle, in 1944 and graduated from Marquette University School of Medicine, Milwaukee, WI in 1946. He completed his orthopedic residency at the Veteran's Affairs Hospital, San Francisco, in 1955. During this time, he was inspired by V. Inman, M.D., to enter into the field of gait analysis. He went on to establish the first gait laboratory in the Shriners System of Hospitals at the San Francisco Shriners Hospital, CA in 1956. In 1972, he accepted an academic appointment at the University of California, San Diego, and in 1974 founded the Motion Analysis Laboratory at San Diego Children's Hospital. He has authored two textbooks: *The Development of Mature Walking* and *Gait Disorders in Childhood and Adolescence*. He is currently a Pediatric Orthopedic Surgeon who has devoted much of his professional life to developing and applying clinical motion analysis. His publications on normal and pathologic gait can be found in many journals. He currently holds the title of Emeritus Professor, Department of Orthopedics, University of California, San Diego, and the position of Medical Director, Motion Analysis Laboratory, Children's Hospital, San Diego. Dr. Sutherland has received the Weinstein-Goldenson Award for outstanding scientific contributions from the United

Cerebral Palsy Association. He also received the Pioneer Award from the Pediatric Orthopedic Society of North America for "pioneering work in the development of gait analysis in children and for major contributions to the orthopedic management of children with cerebral palsy and congenital hip dysplasia." He is past-President of the American Academy for Cerebral Palsy and Developmental Medicine.
Address: Motion Analysis Laboratory, Children's Hospital, 3020 Children's Way, San Diego, CA 92123. Phone: 619/ 576-5807. Fax: 619/ 576-7134

Andrea Tura was born in 1970 in Bologna, Italy. He received an M.Sc. degree in Electronic Engineering (1995) with a thesis on a sensory control system for an upper limb myoelectric prosthesis, from University of Bologna, and his Ph.D. in Bioengineering (1999), from University of Bologna as well. Besides the sensorially controlled prosthesis, his current interests are related to the study of arterial hemodynamics assessed by numerical simulation. He co-authored several papers on rehabilitation.
Address: LADSEB-CNR, Corso Stati Uniti, 4, 35100 Padova, Italy. Phone: +39 049 829 5786. Fax: +39 049 829 5763. E-mail: tura@ladseb.pd.cnr.it

Iwan Ulrich received the title of Engineer in Microengineering from the Swiss Federal Institute of Technology at Lausanne (EPFL) in 1995. He received an M.Sc. degree in Mechanical Engineering and Applied Mechanics from the University of Michigan at Ann Arbor in 1997. During his two years at the University of Michigan Mobile Robotics Laboratory, he built the GuideCane, the topic of his Master's thesis. Since 1997, he has been a Ph.D. student in Robotics at Carnegie Mellon University. His research interests are in mobile robotics, including topics such as localization, mapping, path planning, obstacle detection, obstacle avoidance, computer vision, sensors, artificial intelligence, machine learning, and robotics for the disabled.
Address: Robotics Institute, Carnegie Mellon University, 5000 Forbes Avenue, Pittsburgh, PA 15213. Phone: 412-268-6568. Fax: 412-268-5571. E-mail: iwan@ri.cmu.edu

Gennaro Verni was born in 1952 in Bari, Italy. He received the *laurea* degree in Mechanical Engineering (1980) from the University of Bari. He is at present technical manager at the Centro Protesi INAIL and he is in charge of research and development in the field of lower limb prostheses.
Address: Centro Protesi INAIL, via Rabuina 14, 40054 Vigorso di Budrio (Bologna), Italy. Phone: +39-0516936500. Fax: +39-051802232. E-mail: g.verni@inail.it

D. Mitchell Wilkes received a B.S.E.E. degree from Florida Atlantic University, and M.S.E.E. and Ph.D. degrees from the Georgia Institute of Technology, in 1981, 1984, and 1987, respectively. From 1983 to 1984, he was a graduate teaching assistant at Georgia Tech and from 1984 to 1987 he was a graduate research assistant. From August 1987 to June 1994, he was an Assistant Professor of Electrical Engineering and from June 1994 to the present he has been an Associate Professor of Electrical Engineering at Vanderbilt University. He is a member of the Institute of Electrical and Electronic Engineers and Phi Kappa Phi. His research interests include intelligent service robotics, image processing and computer vision, digital signal processing, sensor array processing, signal modeling, spectrum estimation, and adaptive systems.

Address: Center for Intelligent Systems (CIS), Electrical Engineering and Computer Science Department, Box 131 Station B, Vanderbilt University, Nashville, TN 37235. Phone: 615-322-2735/343-0697. Fax: 615-322-7062. E-mail: wilkes@vuse.vanderbilt.edu

Daniela Zambarbieri was born in 1954 in Milano, Italy. She received the *laurea* degree in Electronic Engineering (1978) from the Polytechnic of Milano, Italy. She was a researcher at the University of Pavia from 1978 until 1992. Since 1992, she has been an Associate Professor of Biomedical Instrumentation at the University of Pavia. Her main research interests are oculomotor control system, eye-head coordination, mathematical models of biological systems, and upper and lower limb prostheses.

Address: University of Pavia, Department of Computer and System Sciences, via Ferrata 1, 27100 Pavia, Italy. Phone: +39-0382505353. Fax: +39-0382505353. E-mail: dani@unipv.it

Contents

Preface
About the Editors
Contributors
Acknowledgments
Disclaimer

Part 1.
Introduction

Chapter 1
  New technologies in rehabilitation. General trends   3
  Horia-Nicolai Teodorescu

1. Introduction *4*
    1.1. Generalities *4*
    1.2. Techniques *5*
    1.3. Global challenges *6*
2. Factors of development *6*
    2.1. General factors *6*
    2.2. The impact of the population age pattern changes *8*
    2.3. Technology and medical-related factors *9*
    2.4. Other factors favoring the use of new technologies in rehabilitation *9*
3. On terminology: moving borders between terms *10*
    3.1. Terms: rehabilitation, assistive devices, and prostheses *10*
    3.2. Levels of "intelligence" in new technologies *12*
4. Literature overview *14*
    4.1. Medical-oriented journal papers *14*
    4.2. Overview of the patent literature *19*
5. A brief discussion of patent literature *22*
6. Other examples of advanced techniques used in rehabilitation *24*
7. Conclusions *25*
References *27*

Part 2.
Sensorial prostheses

Chapter 2
A retinal prosthesis to benefit the visually impaired   31
Wentai Liu, Elliot McGucken, Ralph Cavin, Mark Clements, Kasin Vichienchom, Chris Demarco, Mark Humayun, Eugene de Juan, James Weiland, and Robert Greenberg

1. Introduction *32*
   1.1. Clinical research and motivation for a visual prosthesis *32*
   1.2. A retinal prosthesis: engineering solution to biological problem *36*
2. The Multiple unit artificial retina chip (MARC) prosthesis *38*
   2.1. Clinical and engineering overview *38*
      2.1.1 Foundational clinical research *38*
      2.1.2 Engineering overview: feasibility and significance of the MARC *42*
   2.2. Prior art and related research *43*
   2.3. Evolution of the MARC prosthesis *45*
3. Current engineering research *46*
   3.1. Early generation chip *46*
   3.2. Overall system functionality of advanced generations *49*
      3.2.1 Advantages of the MARC system *50*
      3.2.2 Advanced generation retina telemetric processing chips *51*
   3.3. Implantable retinal chip *53*
      3.3.1 Chip functionality *53*
      3.3.2 Chip operation *61*
      3.3.3 Measurement results *63*
      3.3.4 Design enhancement *69*
   3.4. Video camera and processing board *70*
      3.4.1 Extraocular CMOS camera and video processing *70*
   3.5. MARC RF telemetry *72*
   3.6. Electrode array design *78*
      3.6.1 The electrode array *78*
      3.6.2 Current electrode array *79*
      3.6.3 Substrate for electrode array *79*
      3.6.4 Electrode materials and geometry *81*
      3.6.5 Electrochemical evaluation of stimulating electrode arrays *84*
   3.7. Bonding and packaging *84*
4. Conclusions *87*
References *87*

Chapter 3
Intelligent techniques in hearing rehabilitation   93
Christian Berger-Vachon

1. Introduction *94*
    1.1. Understanding models *94*
    1.2. Influence of the pathology *95*
2. Auditory system *96*
    2.1. Voice production *96*
    2.2. Auditory system *98*
    2.3. Auditory pathways *99*
    2.4. Brain stage *100*
3. Normal (external) aids *100*
    3.1. General principles *100*
    3.2. Normal hearing aids *100*
    3.3. Bone-integrated vibrator *103*
    3.4. Middle ear aids *104*
    3.5. Numeric revolution *104*
4. Cochlear implants *105*
    4.1. General principles *105*
    4.2. Australian *Nucleus*® *108*
    4.3. French *Digisonic*® *110*
    4.4. American *Clarion*® *112*
    4.5. Other systems *114*
    4.6. Surrounding facilities *115*
    4.7. New trends in research *116*
5. Future prospects *120*
    5.1. Simulation of the pathology *120*
    5.2. Classical simulations *121*
    5.3. Discussion *122*
6. Conclusions *123*
References *124*

Part 3.
Locomotor prostheses

Chapter 4
Sensory feedback for lower limb prostheses   129
Daniela Zambarbieri, Micaela Schmid, and Gennaro Verni

1. Introduction *129*
2. Theories of movement control *130*
    2.1. Coordination between posture and movement *131*
    2.2. The internal model *132*
3. Natural feedback *133*
    3.1. Tactile sensation *134*
    3.2. Proprioceptive sensation *134*
4. Artificial feedback *135*
5. Center of pressure *136*
    5.1. Instrumentation for center of pressure (CP) evaluation *136*
        5.1.1 Forceplates *137*
        5.1.2 Sensorized insoles *137*
        5.1.3 Telemetric acquisition of CP *138*
    5.2. Normal trajectory of CP during walking *139*
6. Visual and auditory feedback *142*
    6.1. Visual feedback *142*
    6.2. Acoustic biofeedback *142*
7. Tactile and proprioceptive biofeedback *143*
8. A portable device for tactile stimulation *144*
    8.1. The system *144*
    8.2. Rehabilitation protocol *146*
9. Conclusions *148*
References *149*

Chapter 5
Multifunction control of prostheses using the myoelectric signal   **153**
Kevin Englehart, Bernard Hudgins, and Philip Parker

1. Introduction *153*
    1.1. Externally powered prostheses *153*
    1.2. Clinical impact *155*
2. Myoelectric control *158*
    2.1. An overview *158*
    2.2. Multifunction control research *161*
        2.1.1 Control based on myoelectric statistical pattern recognition techniques: Temple University *161*
        2.2.2 Control based on myoelectric statistical pattern recognition techniques: Swedish research *163*
        2.2.3 Control based on myoelectric statistical pattern recognition techniques: UCLA research *163*
        2.2.4 Endpoint control *164*
        2.2.5 Extended physiological proprioception *169*
        2.2.6 Modeling of musculo-skeletal dynamics *170*
        2.2.7 Statistical features for control *173*

   2.2.8 Autoregressive models *176*
   2.2.9 Equilibrium-point control *179*
   2.2.10 Pattern recognition-based control using the transient myoelectric signal *181*
  2.3. Significant contributions of previous work *186*
3. Research directions *188*
  3.1. Sequential control *188*
   3.1.1 Signal acquisition *189*
   3.1.2 Feature extraction *190*
   3.1.3 Classifiers *190*
  3.2. Simultaneous, coordinated control *191*
   3.2.1 Trajectory generation *192*
   3.2.2 Motion control *195*
  3.3. Discussion *198*
References *200*

Chapter 6
Selective activation of the nervous system for motor system neural prostheses   209
Warren M. Grill

1. Introduction *209*
2. Fundamental considerations for neural prosthesis electrodes *211*
3. Approaches to the nervous system *212*
  3.1. Muscle-based electrodes *212*
  3.2. Nerve-based electrodes *214*
  3.3. Anatomy of peripheral nerves *216*
  3.4. Intraneural electrodes *217*
  3.5. Epineural electrodes *218*
  3.6. Cuff electrodes *219*
4. Conclusions and future prospects in motor system neural prostheses *230*
References *231*

Chapter 7
Upper limb myoelectric prostheses: sensory control system and automatic tuning of parameters   243
Andrea Tura, Angelo Davalli, Rinaldo Sacchetti, Claudio Lamberti, and Claudio Bonivento

1. The sensory control in upper limb prostheses *243*
2. A sensory control system for the Otto Bock prosthesis *246*
  2.1. Involuntary feedback in a sensory control system *246*
  2.2. The microcontroller card for the sensory control system *247*
  2.3. The FSR sensors *250*
  2.4. The "intelligent" hand: automatic touch *251*

    2.5. The slipping problem: an optical sensor for motion detection *252*
    2.6. Tests on the sensory control system *256*
    2.7. Development of new sensors *260*
3. Automatic tuning of prosthesis parameters *262*
    3.1. A fuzzy expert system for tuning parameters *262*
    3.2. Parameters involved in the automatic tuning procedure *263*
    3.3. Examples of rules of the fuzzy expert system *264*
    3.4. The tele-assistance project *267*
4. Conclusions *268*
References *269*

Part 4.
Pacemakers and life-sustaining devices

Chapter 8
Computer-aided support technologies for artificial heart control. Diagnosis and hemodynamic measurements   **273**
Tadashi Kitamura and Ken'ichi Asami

1. Introduction *274*
2. Method *276*
    2.1. Model reduction *276*
    2.2. Interpretive structural modeling (ISM) *278*
3. System description *280*
    3.1. Structure of the system *280*
    3.2. *Human* model *281*
4. Indirect measurement technique *283*
    4.1. Model identification *283*
    4.2. Estimation technique *286*
5. Results and discussion *287*
    5.1. Diagnostic aids *287*
    5.2. Analytical and modeling aids *290*
    5.3. Indirect measurement *294*
6. Conclusions *297*
References *298*

Chapter 9
Diaphragm pacing for chronic respiratory insufficiency   **301**
Harish Aiyar and J. Thomas Mortimer

1. Respiratory insufficiency *302*
    1.1. Spinal cord injury *303*
    1.2. Central hypoventilation syndrome *305*
2. Respiration *306*

2.1. Primary muscles *308*
   2.2. Accessory muscles *313*
   2.3. Inspiration and expiration *315*
3. Diaphragm pacing systems *316*
   3.1. Prerequisites for diaphragm pacing *317*
   3.2. Nerve electrodes *318*
   3.3. Intramuscular electrodes *326*
   3.4. Epimysial electrodes *327*
4. Alternatives to diaphragm pacing systems *328*
   4.1. Mechanical ventilation *329*
   4.2. Pharmacologic *332*
   4.3. Rehabilitative *332*
   4.4. Surgical intervention *333*
   4.5. Magnetic stimulation *334*
   4.6. Electrical stimulation of the intercostal muscles *334*
5. Conclusions and future direction *335*
References *337*

Chapter 10
Intelligent systems in heart pacemakers   **347**
Rodica Strungaru and Stefan Popescu

1. Pacemakers *347*
   1.1. Introduction *347*
   1.2. Classification of pacemakers *349*
   1.3. Methods of adaptations to the demands of the body activity *353*
2. System requirements and design consideration for implementation of intelligent cardiac pacemakers *356*
   2.1. Short introduction to fuzzy logic *356*
   2.2. Hardware and software for fuzzy logic in medical applications *358*
      2.2.1 Generalities *358*
      2.2.2 A fuzzy microcontroller *359*
      2.2.3 The fuzzy logic language *360*
   2.3. Implementing a fuzzy controller for pacemakers *360*
   2.4. Simulation of a fuzzy pacemaker *365*
   2.5. Experimental results *366*
   2.6. Conclusions *369*
3. Discussion *370*
Appendix – Fu.L.L. program for the heart controller *372*
References *374*

Part 5.
Robotic systems and advanced mechanics

Chapter 11
Service robots for rehabilitation and assistance 381
Mitch Wilkes, Anthony Alford, Todd Pack, Tamara Rogers, Edward Brown, Jr., Alan Peters, II, and Kazuhiko Kawamura

1. Introduction *381*
   - 1.1. Service robotics *382*
   - 1.2. Human-machine interfacing and system integration *382*
   - 1.3. System integration using agents *383*
   - 1.4. Software architectures *384*
   - 1.5. Intelligent machine architecture (IMA) *385*
   - 1.6. Human directed local autonomy (HuDL) *385*
2. Historical background: software architectures in the IRL *388*
   - 2.1. The previous architecture *388*
   - 2.2. Shortcomings of the previous approach *389*
     - 2.2.1 Motivations *389*
     - 2.2.2 Pitfalls of the past *389*
     - 2.2.3 The problem of interfaces *389*
     - 2.2.4 The problem of streams *390*
     - 2.2.5 The problem of the blackboard *390*
     - 2.2.6 Desirable properties of a new architecture *391*
3. A new architecture *392*
4. Intelligent agents for human-robot interaction *394*
   - 4.1. HuDL, humans and robots working together *394*
     - 4.1.1 Speech *397*
     - 4.1.2 Gesture *397*
     - 4.1.3 Human detection and localization *398*
     - 4.1.4 Face detection and tracking *398*
     - 4.1.5 Skin detection and tracking *398*
     - 4.1.6 Sound localization *399*
     - 4.1.7 Identification of users *399*
     - 4.1.8 Physical interaction *399*
   - 4.2. The human agent *399*
   - 4.3. The self agent *403*
5. Results *405*
6. Conclusions and future work *407*
References *408*

Chapter 12
Computerized obstacle avoidance systems for the blind and visually impaired 413
Shraga Shoval, Iwan Ulrich, and Johann Borenstein

1. Introduction *414*
2. Conventional electronic travel aids *414*

3. Mobile robotics technologies for the visually impaired *416*
   3.1. Mobile robot obstacle avoidance sensors *416*
   3.2. Mobile robot obstacle avoidance *418*
      3.2.1 The vector field histogram method for obstacle avoidance *418*
      3.2.2 Limitations of mobile robots as guides for the blind *422*
4. The NavBelt *422*
   4.1. Concept *422*
   4.2. Implementation of the guidance mode *428*
   4.3. Implementation of the image mode *428*
   4.4. Experimental results *432*
      4.4.1 Experiments with real obstacles *432*
      4.4.2 Experiments with different walking patterns *432*
   4.5. Conclusions on the NavBelt *433*
5. The GuideCane *434*
   5.1. Functional description *434*
   5.2. Guidance signals versus obstacle information *437*
   5.3. Information transfer *437*
   5.4. Hardware implementation *438*
      5.4.1 Mechanical hardware *438*
      5.4.2 Electronic hardware *440*
   5.5. Software implementation *441*
   5.6. Experimental results *443*
6. Discussion *445*
References *446*

Chapter 13
Advanced design concepts for a knee-ankle-foot orthosis   **449**
Kenton R. Kaufmann, Steven E. Irby, Jeffrey Basford, and David H. Sutherland

1. Introduction *450*
2. History *452*
3. Current knee-ankle-foot orthosis design *452*
4. Advanced concepts in orthosis design *453*
   4.1. Logic-controlled electromechanical free-knee orthosis *453*
   4.2. UTX®—swing orthosis *461*
   4.3. Selectively lockable knee brace *464*
5. Design critique *468*
References *468*

Index of acronyms and abbreviations   471
Index of terms   473

Part 1.

Introduction

Chapter 1

New technologies in rehabilitation. General trends

Horia-Nicolai Teodorescu

Some of the major developments in rehabilitation and prosthesis technology are expected to come from the use of such diverse fields as neural networks, fuzzy systems, virtual reality, robotics, nonlinear system theory, microtechnology, and mechatronics. Several progresses in applying these "intelligent technologies" in rehabilitation and prosthesis technology are briefly discussed, along with the background of the field.

The progresses in rehabilitation and prosthesis technology are reflected, at different levels, by conference papers, journal papers, patents, and commercial products. In this chapter, we balance the discussion of the research having potentially important consequences in the field, and currently existing higher end technology. A special emphasis is on advanced technologies in rehabilitation as echoed in the journal and patent literature. A balance in reporting on various sub-fields of rehabilitation, as reflected in the journal and patent literatures, is observed. We address only some of the trends in using intelligent technologies in rehabilitation, namely those we believe important by their potential.

1. Introduction

1.1. Generalities

In the last decades, the assistive devices have evolved far beyond the traditional walking sticks, canes, crutches, walkers, and wheelchairs. New technologies aim to ease the use of traditional assistive devices, to extend their capabilities, moreover to provide new types of aids, and to improve the overall rehabilitation process. In an epoch when the third-age population becomes increasingly numerous and relatively large as a percentage of the population, the assistive devices and their increased intelligence are needed to cope with new demands. The population of the US above 65 years old, in 2005, is expected to be 24% – about five times that percentage 100 years ago [1]. This population's specific needs have to be satisfied. The needs range from more assistance to improved and increased medical care and help in the home.

The field is extremely dynamic, benefiting from new cognitive technologies, robotics, advanced materials, intelligent systems, and sensors – pushing at the same time the progress in these fields. The field is also very demanding. When an assistive device is designed, the designer has to take into account that several disabilities may occur in a single subject. The design should be flexible, possibly self-adaptive, and intelligent. The extent of requirements is frequently huge and often difficult to predict by the designer.

Hopefully, the advances in fundamental medicine, namely genetics and gene manipulation and "treatment," will make many of these inventions and technologies obsolete. However, genetic science and treatment cannot help in injuries due to accidents and probably will not eliminate all the impairments / disabilities due to aging. Therefore, the development of the field is a necessity in the predictable future; moreover, a fast development in the near future can be foreseen, due to the increase of intelligence in assistive systems and devices, progresses in material science, and progresses in medicine.

The analysis performed in this chapter uses statistical facts to derive conclusions on the state of the art in research and development in rehabilitation technology. Statistics of the number of journal papers, conference papers, and patents are contrasted to reveal the level attained by "intelligent technologies" in rehabilitation and to derive conclusions on the state of the art, the trends, the existing limits and constraints, and the future requirements. In the subsequent sections, we discuss several trends in the rehabilitation technology. The discussion is not meant to be exhaustive.

In Section 2, we briefly discuss the main factors of development in the rehabilitation field. In Section 3, we present a brief analysis of the terms "rehabilitation," "prosthesis," and "assistive device." In Section 4, we analyze the tendencies in the journal and patent literatures, as related to the topic of this chapter, and we discuss their statistical characteristics. In Section 5, the patent literature related to the main novel technologies used in rehabilitation systems is briefly discussed. In Section 6, other novel techniques are considered. In Section 7, we present several conclusions on the state of the art and predictable trends.

1.2. Techniques

What "intelligent" and "advanced" technologies represent is a matter of debate. These are continually evolving concepts. A list of the main technologies to be considered and briefly discussed in relation to rehabilitation and prostheses includes:
- Fuzzy logic
- Neural networks (NN)
- Genetic algorithms (GA)
- Nonlinear system theory and chaos
- Pattern recognition
- Expert systems (ES)
- Intelligent agents
- Virtual reality (VR)
- Robots
- Micro-sensors and fused sensors
- Mechatronic devices
- Microtechnology

A graphical overview of part of the constellation of novel, "intelligent technologies" that are used in rehabilitation and prostheses is sketched in Figure 1. The superposition of the domains is only partly shown in this planar representation.

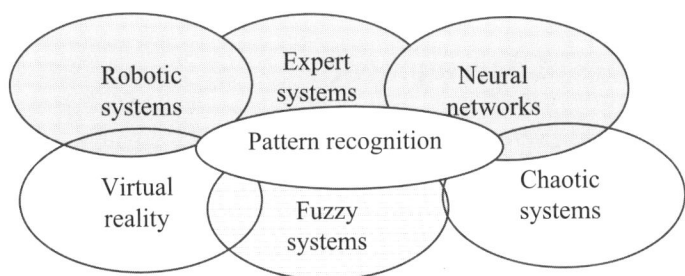

Figure 1. Various "intelligent" technologies and partial overlapping.

1.3. Global challenges

The major changes in the population age pattern require structural changes of the society, too, including changes in the economic structure, medical system, and specialized assistance system. Although there is no doubt of the importance of the field, essential progresses in the infrastructure are slow to develop, and there is a significant delay between the needs and the adaptation. In a document of the Association for the Advancement of Assistive Technology in Europe, it was recently stated: "Rehabilitation strategies/ assistive technologies (AT) have clearly demonstrated their usefulness towards attaining this goal, i.e. providing better quality of life to the disabled or older individual, as well as having positive consequences for relatives, social networks, service provide – in other words the society at large" [2]. The challenge seen in the quoted document is that: "There is also a need to stimulate industrial developments in the field of technology for disabled and elderly and to strengthen SMEs [Small and Medium Enterprises] – thereby promoting competitiveness – as well as to qualify the professional actors in this important field." This shows that the society becomes aware of the problem; however, the solutions are still lacking, and it is uncertain that only a strengthening of the SMEs will help solve the problem.

It is probably the first time in history that a specific[1] linking is created between global demographics and economics, and the two are conflicting on a long term in the future. National and international communities have not addressed in advance this issue; moreover, they seem to be only partly aware of it. The change in the social behavioral pattern, namely the change in the traditional family patterns, with a much larger percentage of older people living alone, outside the traditional, inter-generation family, has amplified the social and economic pressures. So far, the only available way that has seen progresses in alleviating this disparity is the emergence and development of new technologies.

2. Factors of development

2.1. General factors

The global importance of the rehabilitation field is continuously increasing, in the first place, because the population in need of assistive devices and prostheses is increasing everywhere in the world. The increase is a tremendous one despite medicine being able to solve more cases than solved in

---

[1] By "specific," we mean here "related to a basic population segment." Links between the population as a whole and the economic infrastructure, at national or regional levels, are not new.

the past. The increase is due to several unrelated factors, such as wars, transport accidents, and aging. Wars worldwide create an increasingly large number of disabled people (the land mines alone generate a huge number of motor disabilities), the number of casualties due to transport accidents is higher than decades ago, and, more important for the statistics, the overall population of the world is aging, on average.

In industrialized countries, the elderly population growth rate significantly exceeds the overall population growth rate [1]. The important increase of the elderly population in the USA is sketched in Figure 2. In addition, in industrialized countries such as the USA, "The oldest old is the fastest growing segment of the population," while the disability rate for the segment 85 years and over is 84.2%, and for the segment 65 to 74 years old it is only 44.6% [1]. This means that the disability rate is fast increasing, at a rate higher than the increase rate of the elderly segment of the population.

The oldest old (persons 85 years old and over) group comprised 3.5 million persons in 1994, increasing about 2.7 times over the period 1960 to 1994, and about 28 times over the period 1900 to 1994. Now, this population segment represents about 1% of the American population. Consequently, the need for assistive devices and rehabilitation technology is increasing about at the same rate. At stated in the quoted report [1], "The elderly need increasing help in everyday activities as they age" (p. 5). The segment populations in the USA are shown in Figure 3a, with an emphasis on the elderly population, while the probability of a disabling condition, as a function of age, is sketched in Figure 3b. (The probability is estimated based on present situation and may change with progresses in medical science.)

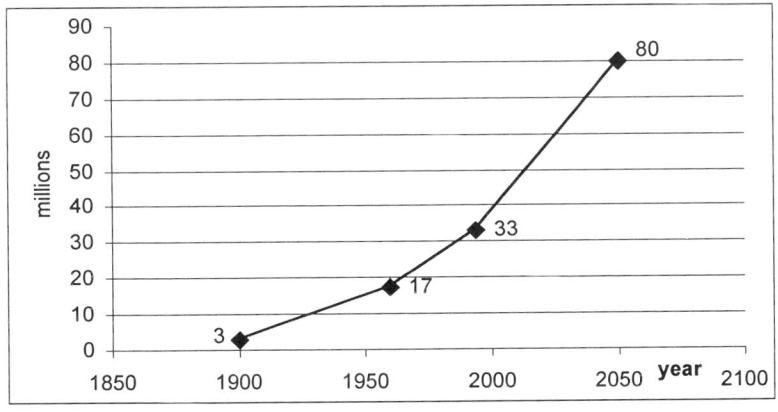

Figure 2. Elderly population increase in the USA (based on [1]).

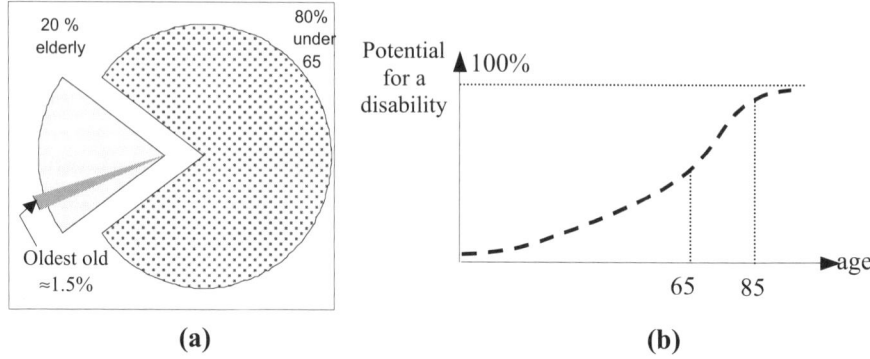

Figure 3. (a) Age groups in the USA, and (b) potential for acquiring a disabling condition [3]. (Oldest old segment includes people 85 years old and older.)

2.2. The impact of the population age pattern changes

According to the document [1], "In 1991 and 1992, about 49 million Americans had a disability, of whom 24 million had a severe disability."[2] Related to age, several disabilities are more frequent, due to an increase in probability specific diseases manifest. Sensorial disabilities and the disabilities related to locomotion constitute well-known examples. Musculoskeletal impairments are considered a major concern in elderly people. The impact of these impairments is growing with the age, mainly due to osteoporosis- and arthritis-related problems. To these, neurologic impairments are added, many due to stroke that may create severe movement disabilities.

The challenges are tremendous and the pressure on the society could be difficult to bear in the near future if these problems are not addressed in due time and with due effort. Unfortunately, no country seems to be completely prepared today to face the needs of the aged population in the new millenium. To be prepared for the happy event of an increase of the elderly population segment, the society and the world as a whole should immediately do a huge effort. The solution can come from technological advances.

---

[2] Other statistics slightly disagree, suggesting that the rate of increase of the elderly population will be higher. According to http://guide.stanford.edu/Projects/Proj.html, "Individuals older than 65 represented just 4% of the US population 100 years ago. Now they represent 13% and in 30 years will represent 22% of the population."

2.3. Technology and medical-related factors

The development of artificial intelligence tools, including neural networks, fuzzy logic, genetic algorithms, powerful algorithms to perform image processing, guiding and path searching, robotic technology, new materials, new sensors, and micromachining, helped develop more effective systems for rehabilitation, and moreover promise a fast development in the near future. On the other hand, development of knowledge in the medical field and new surgery techniques have allowed the engineers to find new applications and to invent new types of prostheses. Some of these developments are illustrated in various applications in the chapters in this volume.

2.4. Other factors favoring the use of new technologies in rehabilitation

The research in the field is influenced by several factors related to the research community, to the general public awareness of the problems related to disabilities, and to the feedback from the groups representing the interested segments in the population. The research community-related factors include professional societies, foundations involved in research supporting, national and international organizations, and research communication media, including the research journals. All these factors have seen a fast growth in recent decades, and the awareness of the population at large has significantly grown too. Some of these general factors are successfully acting for increased performance and efficiency, and for lower prices of the related products.

There are two major organizations devoted to rehabilitation engineering: RESNA (Rehabilitation Engineering Society of North America), in the United States [4], and the European AAATE (Association for the Advancement of Assistive Technology in Europe, created in 1995, see [2]). Several other national associations also exist, for example, the Australian Rehabilitation & Assistive Technology Association (see [5]), and the Italian Society of Physical Medicine and Rehabilitation, SIMFER, founded in 1958 [6]. All these societies aim to develop new technologies and to transfer the technology to marketable devices.

Another factor playing an essential role is constituted by foundations and by a large number of associations of interested peoples. However, such groups were not always favorable to the development of an advanced technology (see chapter by Berger-Vachon, in this volume). For more information on different professional, governmental, and non-profit or for-profit organizations in the field, the reader can access several Web pages with links to such organizations, for example, the Web page of RESNA [4], the Web page of WebABLE, www.yuri.org/webable/index.html, the addresses at www.disabiltynet.co.uk/classified/addressuk.html, or the Web page "Assistive Technology Internet Links," www.ucpa.org/html/innovative/atfsc/link.html.

3. On terminology: moving borders between terms

3.1. Terms: rehabilitation, assistive devices, and prostheses

There are vague, continuously moving borders between the fields of rehabilitation, assistive devices, and prostheses today; these boundaries tend to become even thinner, as the fields tend to merge.

Traditionally, *rehabilitation* refers to methods and means aimed to recover some abilities lost due to an accident or severe illness: "*Rehabilitation:* treatment for an injury or illness aimed at restoring physical abilities" [7]; "*rehabilitation:* The return of function after illness or injury, often with the assistance of specialised medical professionals" [8]. *Webster On-Line Dictionary* [9] defines *rehabilitate* as "1*a*: to restore to a former capacity; 2*a*: to restore to a former state (as of efficiency) *b*: to restore or bring to a condition of health or useful and constructive activity." And, for more details: "Rehabilitation: The restoration of skills by a person who has suffered an illness or injury so they regain maximum self-sufficiency. After a stroke, rehabilitation may be important to walk again and speak clearly again" [9]. Similar definitions can be found in other sources, e.g., [10].

One of the major limits in the above definitions is that rehabilitation is restricted to physical abilities, while cognitive, emotional, and even social abilities are not addressed. Although this limit makes sense in the frame of traditional medical applications, it cannot be supported nowadays, when intelligent technologies are already able to improve cognitive abilities and beyond them, emotional and social abilities as well (at least in the frame of family life). Another limit that should be removed from the definition is included in the "return of function after illness or injury." Rehabilitation, or maybe "habilitation technologies," may address endowment with a function that has not existed at birth, due to a natural error or birth-related problem.

"Rehabilitation" may have two meanings; the narrower, related to restoring the function of a natural organ, and the wider, restoring a function by any means, including the use of prostheses, organ-replacing or organ function enhancing devices, or assistive devices.

Related to *assistive technology*, the Medical Glossary of the AMA (American Medical Association) does not provide any explanation (terms starting with "assist" are missing). The "On-line Medical Dictionary" [8] defines "*assistive device:* Any device that is designed, made, or adapted to assist a person performing a particular task. For example, canes, crutches, walkers, wheel chairs, and shower chairs are all assistive devices (12 Dec 1998)." An identical definition is provided by [10].

Regarding the term "prosthesis," references [7], [8], [9], and [10] provide similar definitions: "Prosthesis: an artificial replacement for a missing part of the body" [7]; "*prosthesis:* An artificial substitute for a missing body part, such as an arm or leg, eye or tooth, used for functional or cosmetic reasons or both (18 Nov 1997)" [8]; "Prosthesis: An artificial replacement of a part of the body, such as a tooth, a facial bone, the palate, or a joint" [10]. Also, Webster On Line [9] defines *prosthesis* as "an artificial device to replace a missing part of the body," which is an unsuitable definition for the current state of the art.

The term *prosthesis* has to be expanded in scope, because some part of the body may still exist, but *malfunction*. Moreover, the prosthesis should be incorporated into the body. For example, the demand pacemaker is in our understanding a prosthesis, as it *functionally* replaces the natural heart pacemaker, yet it is not a total replacement because the natural pacemaker still exists; moreover, only in specific time windows it is replaced by the artificial one. An electrolarynx is not totally replacing an organ in the physical sense (it is not in the place of the larynx). Moreover, it is not performing a complete function by itself, as it just produces a non-speech, humming sound to help laryngectomees talk and it stands for part of the function of the vocal cords and larynx; still it is considered here a prosthesis.

The boundaries between the meanings of these terms and the corresponding fields are not well defined; a prosthesis may be seen as an assistive device and may help rehabilitation, and assistive devices at least partly perform the role of and can be seen as a kind of prosthesis in many cases. One may consider that rehabilitation also includes treatment aimed to restore cognitive or emotional or even social abilities. In addition, a departure from the quoted definitions, we consider rehabilitation may address a disability that is born with, innate, not only *acquired* disability through illness or accident. On the other side, we see the need to restrict the definition in [7]-[10] by eliminating purely surgical restoration of the function. Cataract surgery, for example, may not be considered a rehabilitation procedure, although it is aimed to rehabilitate the eye function. Of course, we are interested here in rehabilitation means using in a significant manner advanced technical methods and devices, and the discussion in this chapter will be focused on this topic only.

With these limits expanded, rehabilitation could be defined as any "treatment, possibly including prosthesis use and temporally or permanent assistive devices, with the purpose of restoring functions and physical, emotional, cognitive, or social skills."

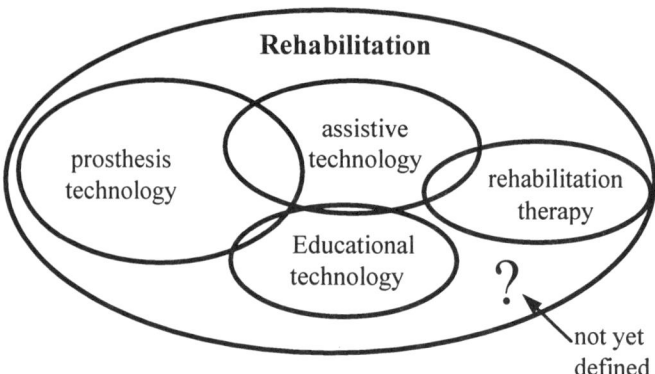

Figure 4. The overlapping fields inside the rehabilitation domain.

These are the borders inside which this volume is conceived. Assistive devices, prostheses, and technology aimed to support the rehabilitation process – either on the patient side or the physician side – are contained between these borders. Aids and appliances, for people with a reduced ability, range today from dedicated, specific home appliances to simple home aid robots to guidance systems to education services to various sensorial prostheses to life-sustaining devices.

The term "disability" will not be discussed here, because its definition has still to be given by the medical community; moreover, its boundaries are continuously moving. We prefer to use the expression "disabling condition" instead of "disability." We emphasize that the number of disabling conditions the medical community understands and diagnoses is continuously increasing. Sleep disorders, for example, can be seen as a disability, because they reduce the normal abilities of a person for long periods of his life. As a consequence, sleep apnea may be seen as a perturbing, even disabling disorder, which causes and consequences are not yet fully understood and which affects about two to ten million people in US alone.

Only an extended discussion of the terminology in the medical and bio-medical engineering community could establish a meaningful terminology suitable to represent basic concepts related to rehabilitation.

3.2. Levels of "intelligence" in new technologies

In this volume, the contributors address the use of "intelligent technologies" in rehabilitation. "Intelligent systems" and "intelligent technologies" are not satisfactorily defined terms, and as it goes with many new fields, the meaning of the terms and the coverage of the field are continuously evolving. The degrees of intelligence at the system level are summarized in Figure 5. In this chapter, we assume for a minimal level of "intelligence" the existence of at least an adaptive system for the prosthesis or assistive device to be considered "intelligent." Moreover, we require the adaptability to be performed through a knowledge-based system, neural network, or similar new, essentially non-linear technique (see Figure 5).

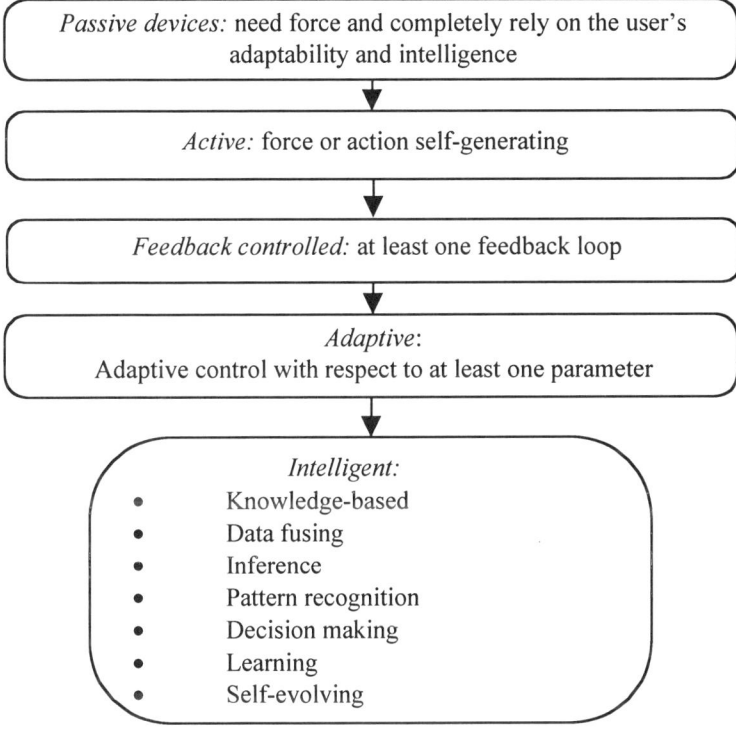

Figure 5. Levels of "intelligence."

We do not discuss the definitions of various "intelligent" technologies here. For each of these technologies, the meaning is continuously changing and no consensus exists on the terminology. For example, the definition of the "robots" is under dispute. Reportedly, at the ICORR'97 Conference, this question was specifically addressed, without a definite answer found. The "inclusive" definition accepts, among others, powered feeders as robots. As a matter of fact, voices arose asking that the term "robots" be completely abandoned as no longer suitable, while other voices asked for a new, intermediate category – not named as yet – between robots and simpler devices (see the discussion in [11]).

4. Literature overview

4.1. Medical-oriented journal papers

The literature on prostheses and rehabilitation is huge. A search on the PubMed [12] database (provided by U.S. National Library of Medicine (NLM); see www.nlm.nih.gov/) shows that the literature on prostheses includes more than 170,000 citations (in June 1999), and similarly for rehabilitation (about 141,000 items, as per June 1999), while "assistive device" retrieves about 3600 documents.

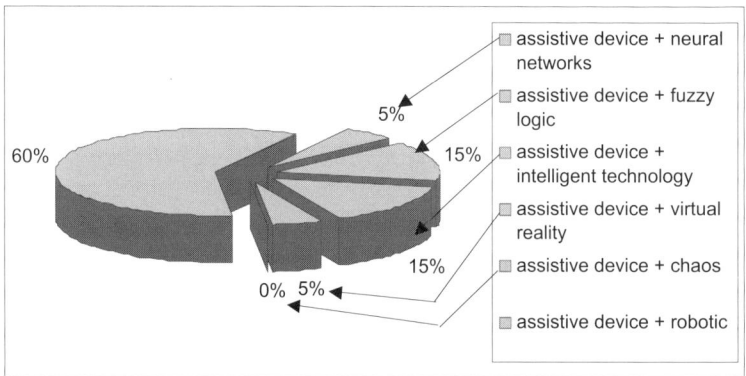

Figure 6. Assistive devices technologies: journal paper distribution.

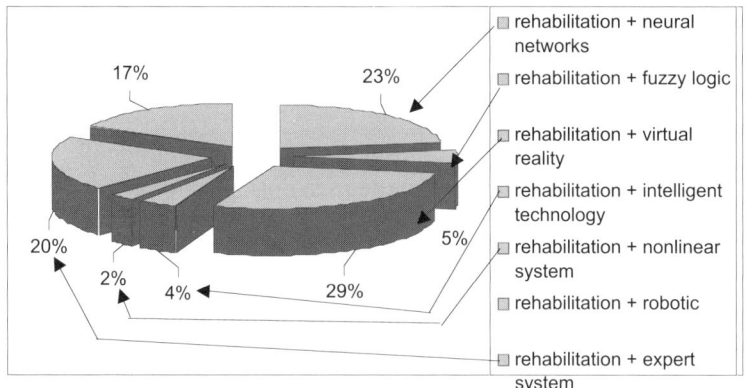

Figure 7. Rehabilitation-related technologies: journal paper distribution.

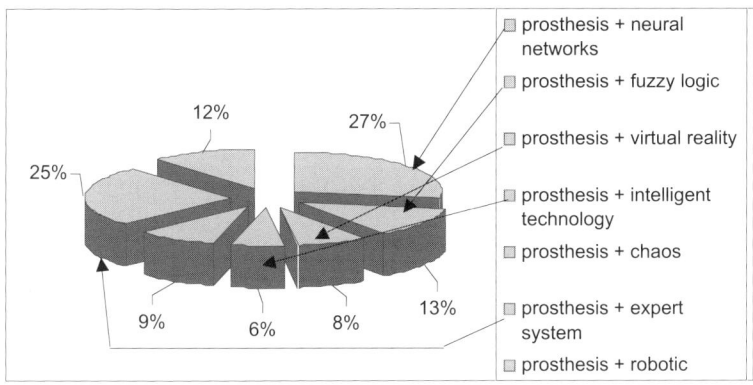

Figure 8. Prosthesis technologies: journal paper distribution.

A synthesis of the number of papers related to major new technologies in rehabilitation, prosthesis technology and assistive device technology is presented in Table 1. The distribution of the journal papers is presented in the Figures 6, 7, and 8.

Table 1. Number of journal papers, per field and technology
(Based on PubMed database)

	Rehabilitation	Prosthesis	Assistive device	Total
Neural networks	38	28	1	77
Fuzzy logic	8	13	3	24
Virtual reality	48	8	1	57
Chaos / nonlinear system	9	9	3	21
Robot	34	12	12	58
Expert system	29	26	2	57
Genetic algorithm	0	0	0	0
Artificial intelligence[3]	120	100	34	255

We stress that the database used for this statistic (PubMed®) is not complete. It includes references to medical journals and a few major engineering journals. Many papers and review articles in several significant engineering journals are not included, not to refer to proceedings of engineering conferences, including IEEE, or to journals not included in the list used by PubMed. The primary reason we use this specific database is that it

---

[3] Includes NN and fuzzy logic; approximate number.

reflects the medical community point of view. This perspective is essential to assess the degree to which a technology was successful in penetrating the target population.

There are several trends in the literature deserving a special mention. First, there are some fields making significant progresses in a consistent manner. For example, the field of virtual reality applications to rehabilitation has seen a typical exponential increase between 1993 and 1998 (Figure 9). The number of papers in this field almost doubled every year.

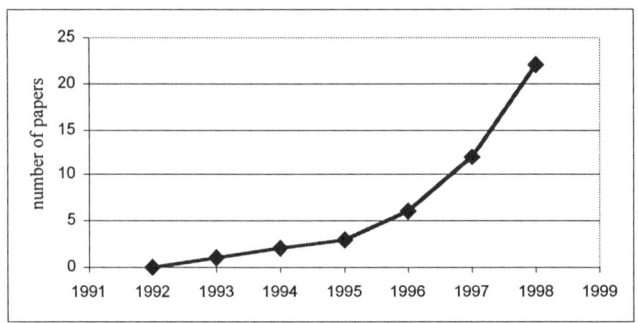

Figure 9. Number of journal papers on applications of virtual reality to rehabilitation. (Based on data in the PubMed® database.)

On the other side, the number of papers referring to neural network in the field of prostheses has seen a surge during the period 1993-1995, and a decline in 1996-1998 (see Figure 10). There is no specific trend over the period 1990-1998 in the corresponding time series. In contrast, the number of papers referring to neural networks in rehabilitation seems to show a more consistent increase, close to the exponential one (Figure 11). The doubling period is about 4 years, which is somewhat slow for a new field, taking into account the maturity of the neural network domain. This may show that the field is still to take off, or that the technology (neural networks) has been seen inadequate to prostheses. Yet, caution should be exercised in deriving conclusions. Most probably, neural networks will be soon embedded in specific niches of the prosthesis field.

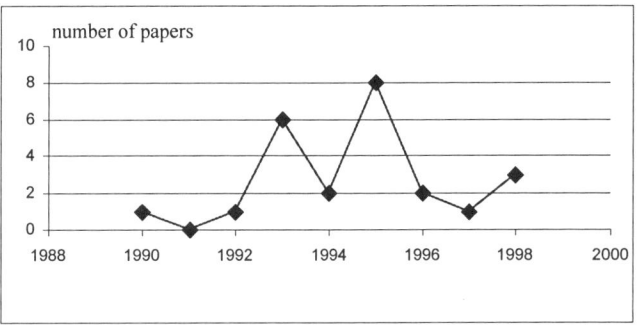

Figure 10. Number of papers referring to neural network in the field of prostheses (based on database PubMed®).

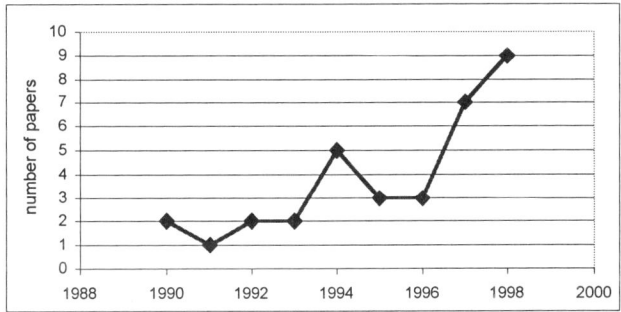

Figure 11. Number of papers referring to neural network in the field of rehabilitation (based on database PubMed®).

The evolution of the number of medicine-related journal papers referring to robots in rehabilitation is disappointing (Figure 12). The trend over more than 10 years is constant, showing probably a limited progress in the field, which should be considered not yet started on the way of progress. A synthesis of the data discussed above is shown in Table 2.

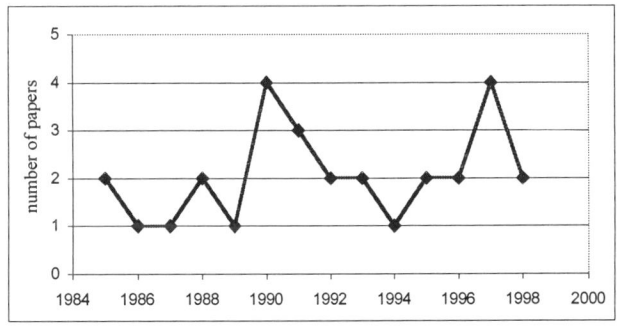

Figure 12. Evolution of the number of journal papers on robots and rehabilitation. (Data after PubMed.)

Table 2. Number of journal papers in different fields, per year
(Based on PubMed database)

	Rehabilitation + robotic	Rehabilitation + VR	Rehabilitation + NN	Rehabilitation + expert system	Prosthesis + NN	Prosthesis + expert system
1998	2	22	9	4	3	2
1997	4	12	7	1	1	2
1996	2	6	3	1	2	2
1995	2	3	3	4	8	2
1994	1	2	5	2	2	0
1993	2	1	2	1	6	2
1992	2	0	2	2	1	1
1991	3	-	1	4	0	5
1990	4	-	2	2	1	2
1989	1	-	-	4	-	3
1988	2	-	-	1	-	1
1987	1	-	-	1	-	2
1986	1	-	-	0	-	0
1985	2	-	-	0	-	1

A similar pattern is encountered in the evolution of the number of papers on robots and assistive technology. We also note that many references on robotics and assistive devices or prostheses are older than 5 years and many of them refer to robotic surgery (some of them in relation to rehabilitation or prostheses implantation), rather than to robotic assistive devices or prostheses. Despite the great progresses in robotics, their use in prostheses has yet a limited extent, due to the difficulty of generating complex movements. We believe that the advances we have seen in recent years may reverse the trend of slow extension of such applications.

Robots and manipulators offer a good example of the state of the art of "intelligent technologies" in rehabilitation. No doubt, robots are an obvious direction for research in assistive devices and rehabilitation. The direct application could result in help in several ways, to various disabling condition cases. The robots will become at some time in the future a home appliance and people with neuro-motor disabilities will benefit in the first place from them. The research in the field already has a long history. In addition, a significant number of journal papers are devoted to workstations aimed to help people with severe neuro-motor disabilities. Nevertheless, as pointed out in [13], "rehabilitation robotics is penetrating the market very slowly and still seen a future technology by many people, at least in Europe." The same disappointing state of the art is seen in the USA [14].

Finally, the annual number of research papers on applications of expert systems in rehabilitation shows a pattern of fluctuations around the average (Figure 13).

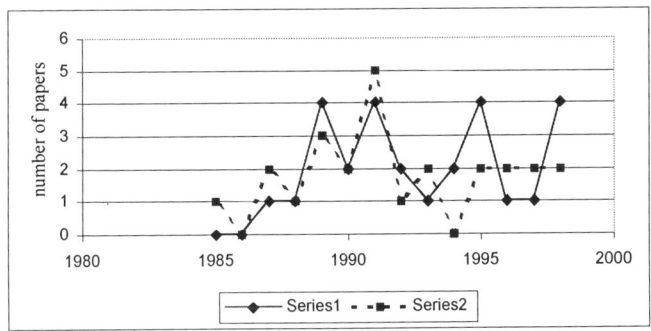

Figure 13. Number of journal papers on expert systems in rehabilitation (Series 1) and in prosthesis (Series 2) vs. year of publication (based on PubMed database).

In this section, we reviewed only the literature as in major journals related to medical sciences. The number of conference papers is at least double that of journal papers. Moreover, there is a lag of two to three years between conference papers and journal papers, meaning that a conference paper may become a journal paper and be published in about two or three years. This delay has to be considered when discussing specific recent topics. For example, the number of journal papers on robotic applications may be expected to increase in a significant manner in the next few years, taking into account a similar trend in conference papers.

4.2. Overview of the patent literature

The patent literature provides a different viewpoint than the journal and conference papers. It highlights the technical solutions that gained credibility for commercial applications and has increased support from companies potentially interested in manufacturing devices based on the patented solution. The patent literature is also much more selective. For example, there are almost 200,000 journal papers on prostheses, but only about 10,000 patents worldwide – a ratio of about 1/20. A much lower ratio, of about 1/200, is between papers on rehabilitation and patents related to rehabilitation. This is a dramatic figure, pointing to the incipiency of the industrial development in the field of rehabilitation. Not surprisingly, a large number of patents in rehabilitation refer to mechanical or conventional electronic technology – the only technology mature enough to be extensively used in this domain.

A summary of the number of patents related to the keywords "rehabilitation," "assistive device/system," and "prosthesis" is presented in Table 3. Notice that this is not a "brute force" search; a simple search does not guarantee that the patent including these keywords refers to rehabilitation or assistive devices as seen in medicine, and may produces large errors.[4] The data used in this section were obtained by search over the databases "*Esp@cenet*" [Espacenet] of the European Patent Office [15], the search being performed for European and worldwide (PCT) patents; moreover, the search was performed on the US Patent Office database, to double-check for US patents.

Table 3. Patents worldwide by main classes in the field

Keyword(s)	Approximate number of matching patents (worldwide)	Approximate number of matching patents (USA)
Prosthesis	9800	3450
Rehabilitation	900	700
Assistive and device / system	20	20

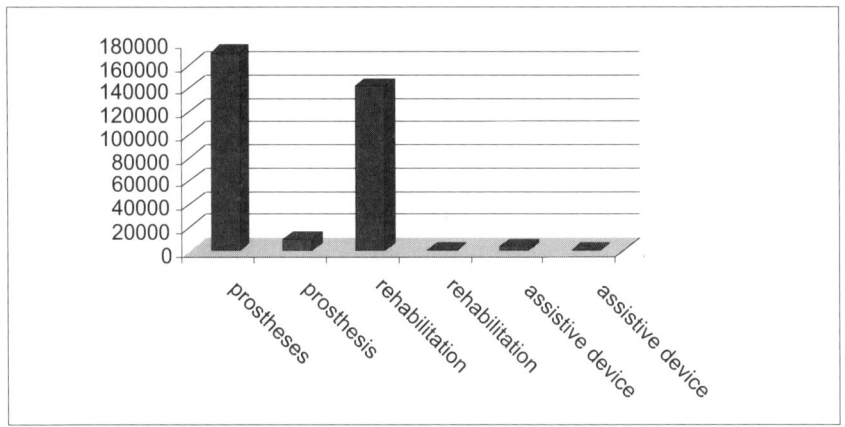

Figure 14. Comparison of the journal paper and patent literatures.
Light gray textured: journal papers; solid color: patents.
Based on PubMed and PCT databases (1999).

Beyond the figures and the statistics, what is more disappointing is the extremely low penetration until now of the high level technologies in the field of prostheses and rehabilitation. There is a large unevenness between the

---

[4] For example, about half of the patents including the "assistive device" keyword refer to steering assistive devices, while "rehabilitation" may refer, for example, to rehabilitation of the asphalt cover of the roads. Table data are during the period May-July 1999.

number of research papers and the number of patents describing intelligent systems in rehabilitation and prostheses. We can but conclude that the penetration of intelligent technologies in the commercial products is still in its infancy. This is not to be considered a pessimistic perspective. On the other hand, this shows that a higher priority should be given by project leaders and project managers to patenting. In addition, a reconsideration of the founding policy in projects is advisable, to turn the results toward more patents, possibly with the corresponding reduction of journal papers.

Table 4. Number of patents, per field and technology
(Based on European Patent Office database)

	Rehabilitation	Prostheses	Assistive devices	Total
Neural networks	0	1	0	1
Fuzzy logic	0	1^5	0	1
Virtual reality	4^6 (3)	0	0	4
Chaos / nonlinear system	0	0	1^7 (0)	1
Robot	1^8	4^9 (0)	0	1
Expert system	0	0	0	0
Genetic algorithm	0	0	0	0

Table 4 deserves some comments. Not included are couples of more general terms, such as "prosthesis" + "artificial intelligence." However, in this rather general class, there is no patent directly including the terms in the title or abstract. Moreover, surprisingly, no patent includes in the title or abstract the couple of terms "intelligent" + "prosthesis." Instead, there are 12 patents referring to robotic surgery ("robots" + "surgery"), showing that the interest of the companies relies rather with hospital use than with individual, end users of robotics in rehabilitation. This fact may have a simple interpretation: hospitals can afford the high price of present robots, while individual end users cannot. Moreover, surgery robots may be less complex (and hence easier to manufacture) than an advanced home-appliance robot devoted to help in a large range of manners people with disabilities.

---

[5] This patent is the same one recorded at the neural networks category and deals with neuro-fuzzy systems.

[6] Actually, three different patents; one of the four is repeated in another country coverage.

[7] The patent included here does not directly mention the use of chaos theory, yet it makes use of it in an assistive device (implantable defibrillator). The patent is discussed in a subsequent section of this chapter.

[8] According to the description, the system is an actuator rather than a robot.

[9] All four patents are on robots in surgery for rehabilitation purposes, none in rehabilitation devices.

The comparison we performed between the number of journal papers and the number of papers – not necessarily on advanced technologies – in rehabilitation may be extended to papers and patents involving at least one "intelligent technology." Table 5 summarizes this comparison.

Table 5. Number of journal papers and number of patents involving "intelligent technologies" in rehabilitation,[10] per type of technology

	Patents	Journal papers	Ratio patents vs. papers %
Neural networks	1	77	1.2
Fuzzy logic	1	24	4.2
Virtual reality	4	57	7.0
Chaos / nonlinear systems	1	21	4.7
Robot	1	58	1.7
Expert system	0	57	1.7

For comparison, a typical value for the ratio of patents vs. journal papers, in a mature, but still significantly growing field, is about 5%, while in a mature, but aging field the ratio may be 20%. Because of the low number of patents in the fields analyzed, the data in Table 5 are not statistically significant. The only conclusion one can derive is that the new technologies have a high growing potential in rehabilitation, yet to be demonstrated.

5. A brief discussion of patent literature

In this section, we briefly discuss the few patents in the field. The relevance of the discussion is limited because of the low number of existing patents. As the domain matures, the number of patents on intelligent technologies in rehabilitation applications is expected to fast increase in this first decade of the new millenium.

The only patent using either fuzzy logic or neural networks in rehabilitation is a PCT (WO) patent (the acronym PCT stands for Patent Cooperation Treatise; WO stands for "World patent" as issued according to PCT). The patent (WO-9919779) discloses "A neuro-fuzzy based device for programmable hearing aids" [16].

According to the published abstract, the patent application refers to "*A neurofuzzy device that provides a fuzzy logic based user-machine interface for optimal fitting of programmable hearing prosthesis using a neural network that*

---

[10] Including prostheses and assistive devices.

generates targets to be matched by the hearing prosthesis based on individual audiometric and other relevant data." The NN will learn during the prosthesis matching process and improve its ability to matching. To achieve this goal, the prosthesis fitting results are assessed using a user interface, which applies fuzzy logic to determine relevant information on fitting quality. Fuzzy logic is used to improve the interface with a human user that is not knowledgeable in medicine and to adapt to the imprecision in the responses of the user. Fuzzy rules constitute a knowledge base that performs a processing of the information provided by the user.

The solution proposed in this patent is sound and one may expect it imposing in the field. The ability of the neural network to learn and to perform adaptation (i.e., acquire nonlinear mappings) of systems like human-prosthesis is widely recognized. Moreover, the use of fuzzy logic to the interface and data interpretation is a natural choice. Also, notice that similar applications of fuzzy logic to various rehabilitation systems are presented in the chapters by Tura *et al.*, Berger-Vachon, and Strungaru and Popescu, in this volume.

A classification and quality assessment of the pronunciation, marginally based on fuzzy methods, in a rehabilitation system for children with a speech disability was claimed in an older patent [17]; moreover, marginal use of neuro-fuzzy systems in classification and recognition tasks in a system that may be used as assistive system for elderly and the newborn as well was claimed in a patent application [18].

Although a search based on "chaos" does not produce any match together with "prosthesis" or "rehabilitation," there are 5 patents that are related to prostheses/assistive devices using chaos analysis. These patents refer to diagnosis methods, however all are oriented toward preventing fibrillation and use in pacemakers/defibrillators. Namely, a defibrillator is activated based on the analysis of chaotic behavior of the cardiac electric potential (EKG signals). The chaos analysis is backed by the classic method of Fourier analysis. This set of related patents [19] probably represents the first breakthrough in using chaos analysis in prostheses and assistive devices.

There are several patents related to arm and foot prostheses that may be considered for use in robotic technologies, yet not emphasizing on this aspect. For example, the NTU-Hand, Patent no. 107115, Taiwan, R.O.C., refers to a hand prosthesis which has 5 fingers with 17 degrees of freedom and that can be considered a robotic arm, although it rather falls in the actuator category. Other robotic systems were patented for general applications, but may have found applications as assistive devices as well.

The patents related to the use of virtual reality in rehabilitation are aimed to enhance the sensorial environment of the subject during rehabilitation exercises. The virtual environment either enhances the information presented by visual [20], audio, force [21], or tactile means, or provides a "sense-conversion" to subjects with a sense-related disability, as in [22]. The methods presented in these patents are not departing from the general technology used in virtual reality, except the adaptation to the disability and the training exercises assumed in the patent. Some patents, while not declaring the use of virtual reality methods and continuing a trend existent in the last four decades of the previous century, use sensorial conversion, i.e., transmission of information normally received by one sense through another sense, when the first sense is impaired. Such visual-to-audio or audio-to-tactile conversions are frequently seen in older patents, before the advent of virtual reality technology. An example of such conversion is the NavBelt, presented by Shoval *et al.* in a chapter in this volume. Also, the patent titled "Artificial sensitivity" [23] is an example of skillful use of sensorial conversion, performing a conversion from tactile sensation to auditive sensation for rehabilitating subjects. The invention starts from the idea that "Loss or absence of sensibility in the hand, foot or other part of the body can constitute a severe handicap after injury or in disease. Also when hand prostheses are used following amputation, injuries lack of sensibility in the prostheses constitutes a major problem." Consequently, the tactile sensation is replaced by sounds, aimed to provide the subject with some sort of equivalent information. The results are not reported, but the idea might be improved to enhance the feedback a rehabilitating person needs. A similar concept is presented in the chapter by Zambarbieri *et al.* in this volume and in the patent [22].

6. Other examples of advanced techniques used in rehabilitation

There are many systems proposed for rehabilitation or prosthesis purposes that do not fit into the categories discussed above, but still match the "intelligent technology" or "advanced technology" classes. Prosthetic or assistive systems to help people that cannot produce speech in a normal way, systems to produce alternate sensing, when a sense is lost, or systems that use optical fibers and photonic excitation to contact to neurons [24] are some of these applications. Several electromyographic control procedures for speech prostheses have been proposed [25], [26] (for coverage of the early research see [27]). Recently, in a potentially seminal research, a hybrid syntactic-statistic word prediction system for helping people with a speech disability was proposed [28]. The proposed augmentative and alternative communication system is based on an enhanced prediction combining statistical and syntactical methods. The system predicts the utterances intended to be communicated by subjects with a speech disabling condition and generates sentence-completion sequences. The reported results significantly enhance the syntactic-only and statistic-only methods.

The traditional development has seen the *device* as the only objective. However, significant progress has already been made in the *assistive systems*. The assistive systems are aimed to offer a large pallet of services to people with disabilities, and moreover, will be able to adapt to the specific disability and requirement of the subject. Many subjects will be able to access at the same time the assistive service and several of them may use in cooperation the system. One example of such a system is telephony for disabled. A system of this type is described in the invention registered by AT&T on a telephone device for the deaf (TDD) and an assistive call center. The center is able to "automatically identifying the expertise needed, including the language being used, selecting a communication assistant (CA) capable of speaking in the language and other expertise, routing the call to the selected CA, and connecting the call." The system may help in using the telephone by a large segment of the population [29].

7. Conclusions

The need for extensive supply of advanced rehabilitation technology is acute and may become dramatic for industrialized nations, where the age expectation is believed to increase to 90 years in the next four decades. The international community, the industrialized nations, the industry, and the research community worldwide should become aware of this necessity before it produces an extended economic and social crisis with a significant gap between the welfare and the well-being of the elderly population and the other population groups. Not recognizing this gap on the long term would be to disregard the needs of a large population group and would be unpardonable.

The pressure over the society is increasingly high to adapt to the needs of a fast growth of the elderly population segment. The whole population should face the problems of the aging population, and provide for and meet its expectation for a decent life. New technologies represent the only available tool so far, but it cannot succeed without a large effort at national and international levels. Economic and infrastructure means should be developed.

In what regards the state of the art, there is a significant gap between the medical-oriented literature and the engineering-oriented literature in reflecting the recent advances and the state of the art in using "intelligent" technologies in rehabilitation and prosthesis technology. This gap is partly due and reflects the present stage of development in the field, corresponding to incipient research, not yet arrived in the development phase.

There is a definite lack of medical-oriented analysis and assessment of the benefits of the intelligent technologies in rehabilitation. The few number of studies reported so far provide rather mixed results, and the absence of commercial products and of a large market shows a low acceptance by the users, until now. These facts point to an initial phase of development, when technology is still at its infancy.

However, engineers are advancing the domain and several trends can be expected to manifest:

- Robotic systems are on the verge of becoming – and should become – a major field in rehabilitation technology.
- Neural networks may become a common way to deal in an efficient manner with pattern recognition functions, control, and advanced signal processing in prostheses and rehabilitation systems.
- Fuzzy logic and fuzzy systems show promise as a developing tool, and when combined with neural networks and various algorithms for training will help in the tuning and adaptation of prostheses and rehabilitation systems.

The new rehabilitation technologies, like robot technology, face several hurdles before they are accepted and widely deployed in hospitals and then in homes, where the highest need is. A serious potential problem is that if the medical community and medical assistance providers are not prepared – technically and financially – to correctly support the new technology, users won't be able to use it in a significant manner and quantity. There is still a long way to go, from technical solutions to manufacturing to medical assessment to standardization to user education to financial viability and affordability.

No doubt, some of the most important progresses are done in the less glorious, "small," but essential technological advances aimed for a large population of persons with disabilities. These advances play an important role and should not be neglected.

Acknowledgments. A significant part of this chapter is reproduced with permission from the report:

H.N. Teodorescu: *New Technologies in Rehabilitation and Prosthetics: State of the Art.* Techniques & Technologies Ltd., 1999. The support of Techniques & Technologies Ltd. is acknowledged. A research grant offered by Swiss National Funds (SNF, 1997-1998) is also acknowledged for the support of an earlier literature review used in this chapter.

References

[1] *Population Profile of the United State 1995. Current Population Reports* – Special Studies Series 23-289, US Department of Commerce – Bureau of the Census, July 1995, http://www.census.gov/population/pop-profile/p23-189.pdf.
[2] AATE document *"Empowering older and disabled people in the EU,"* 3rd March 1997, www.fernuni-hagen.de/FTB/aaate/position.htm.
[3] Teodorescu, H.N.: *New Technologies in Rehabilitation and Prosthetics: State of the Art*, Techniques & Technologies Ltd., 1999.
[4] RESNA, http://www.resna.org/wwwrsour_web.html.
[5] Australian Rehabilitation & Assistive Technology Association web site: http://www.iinet.net.au/~sharono/arata/index.html. For Australian Disability Information also see: http://www.vicnet.net.au/disability/.
[6] SIMFER web site: www.simfer.it/.
[7] Medical Glossary on AMA (American Medical Association) web site: http://www.ama-assn.org/insight/gen_hlth/glossary/glos_nq.htm.
[8] The On-line Medical Dictionary web site: http://www.graylab.ac.uk/omd/.
[9] Webster-On-line: http://www.m-w.com/cgi-bin/dictionary.
[10] Dictionary, MedicineNet.com, http://www.medicinenet.com/
[11] ICORR page on http://www.bath.ac.uk/Centres/BIME/icorr97.htm.
[12] U.S. National Library of Medicine (NLM) web site: http://www.nlm.nih.gov/. PubMed http://www.ncbi.nlm.nih.gov/pubmed/.
[13] Buhler, C.: Robotics for rehabilitation – A European (?) perspective? *Int. Conf. Rehab Robotics*, ICORR'97, 14-15 April 1997, Bath, U.K., http://www.bath.ac.uk/Centres/BIME/proceed.htm.
[14] Mahoney, R.M.: Robotics products for rehabilitation: status and strategy. *Int. Conf. Rehab Robotics*, ICORR'97, 14-15 April 1997, Bath, U.K., http://www.bath.ac.uk/Centres/BIME/proceed.htm
[15] *"Esp@cenet"* [Espacenet] of the European Patent Office (http://ep.dips.org/dips/ep/en/dips.htm). Recently changed to http://ep.espacenet.com/.
[16] Basseas Stavros Photios: *A neurofuzzy based device for programmable hearing aids*. WO9919779. Publication date: 1999-04-22. Application no. Wo98US21701 19981014, Priority nos. US-970062354P 19971015. Equivalents: AU1086099.
[17] Teodorescu, H.N., Posa, C., and Teodorescu, L.: Biofeedback Method. Patent RO no. 4396/03.28.1984.
[18] Teodorescu, H.N. and Mlynek, D.: Respiratory Monitoring System. Patent Application, USA, January 7, 1998, International Application WO99/04691, 21 July 1999.
[19] Khan, S.S., Evans, S., Denton, T.A., Diamond, G.A., and Karagueuzian, H.S.: Defibrillator with Shock Energy Based on EKG Transform. Patent no. US5643325, Publication date: 1997-07-01. Application no. US960590546 19960124, Related patents: WO9809226, Methods for Detecting Propensity for Fibrillation Using an Electrical Restitution Curve; US5678561, Methods for Detecting Propensity for Fibrillation; US5643325, Defibrillator with Shock

Energy Based on EKG Transform; US5555889, Methods for Detecting Propensity Fibrillation; US5201321, Method and Apparatus for Diagnosing Vulnerability to Lethal Cardiac Arrhythmias.
[20] Hitoshi, M., Shinya, I., and Hisashi, U., Rehabilitation Device Incorporating Virtual Reality Function. Patent no. Jp9313552, Publication date: 97-12-09.
[21] Burdea, G.C., and Langrana, N.A.: Integrated Virtual Reality Rehabilitation System. Patent no. US 5,429,140, Publication date: 1995-07-04.
[22] Teodorescu, H.N., Talmaciu, M., and Teodorescu, L.: Hearing-Disabled Aid. Patent RO no. 84641/04.10.1984.
[23] Lundborg, G.: Artificial sensibility. Patent no. WO9848740, Publication date: 1998-11-05, Equivalents: AU7355498, SE9701595.
[24] Houri, H., Ostrowski, D., and De Michelli, M.: Opto-Electronic Prosthesis for the Rehabilitation of the Neuromotorically or Neurosensorially Handicapped Using at Least One Light Source and Optical Fibers. Patent FR 2643561, European patent request EP 0377547, Publication 1990.
[25] Teodorescu, H.N., Teodorescu, L., and Buchholtzer, L.: Command Device for Laryngeal Prostheses. Patent RO no. 84397/03.28.1984.
[26] Teodorescu, H.N., Buchholtzer, L., Chelaru, M., and Teodorescu, L.: A laryngeal prosthesis based on perilaryngean reflexes, Proc. 9th Int. EMBS Conf. IEEE, Boston, 4 (IEEE), pp. 2114-2115, 1987.
[27] Teodorescu, H.N. et al.: Neurological control of laryngeal prosthesis, in Progress Report in Electronic in Medicine and Biology, IERE Press, London, 1986, 269-275.
[28] Wood, M. and Lewis, E.: Pace–grammatical recognition in computer aided conversation, Technical report ACRC-93:SP-01, Department of Computer Science, University of Bristol, U.K., September 1993.
[29] Eisdorfer, J., Schulz, D.E., and Kasday, L.: Multiple Accommodated Message Relaying for Hearing Impaired Callers. Patent no. US5745550, Publication date: 1998-04-28, Applicant(s): AT&T (US), Application no. US950476811 19950607.

Part 2.

Sensorial prostheses

Chapter 2

A retinal prosthesis to benefit the visually impaired

Wentai Liu, Elliot McGucken, Ralph Cavin,
Mark Clements, Kasin Vichienchom, Chris Demarco,
Mark Humayun, Eugene de Juan, James Weiland,
and Robert Greenberg

The development of a retinal prosthesis, from early through advanced generations, is presented, along with characterizations of the hurdles and breakthroughs encountered in the wide array of clinical and engineering disciplines which the project spans. The rehabilitative device replaces the functionality of defective photoreceptors within patients suffering from degenerative retinal diseases such as Age-related Macular Degeneration (AMD) and Retinitis Pigmentosa (RP). The clinical experiments and components and functionality of the prosthesis are characterized, from the extraocular unit including a video camera, video processing chip, and RF telemetry unit and primary coil, to the intraocular unit, including a secondary coil, rectifier and regulator, processing and demultiplexing chips, and the electrode array.

1. Introduction

1.1. Clinical research and motivation for a visual prosthesis

Progress relating to the engineering of a visual prosthesis is presented, along with characterizations of the major hurdles and breakthroughs from the wide array of scientific and engineering disciplines that are called upon in the pursuit of an electronic device to aid the visually impaired. The heart and soul of this project is centered about replacing defective retinal cells with an electronic device, or solving the biological problem of blindness with an engineering solution. This retinal prosthesis project has consisted of a collaboration between researchers at the Johns Hopkins University (JHU) Wilmer Eye Institute and the College of Engineering at North Carolina State University (NCSU) for more than a decade. The team has maintained steady progress in clinical and engineering research directed toward an implantable retinal prosthetic device. Our group has identified and overcome many medical and technological hurdles, which are characterized throughout this chapter.

Over 10,000,000 people worldwide are blind because of photoreceptor loss due to degenerative retinal diseases such as Age-related Macular Degeneration (AMD) and Retinitis Pigmentosa (RP). The NCSU/JHU retinal prosthesis currently undergoing research and development is based on the concept of replacing photoreceptor functionality with an electronic device. Researchers at JHU have pioneered non-intrusive stimulation of the retina, while engineers at NCSU have been incorporating the evolving clinical data into the designs of the prototype Multiple Unit Artificial Retina Chipset (MARC) prostheses.

The photoreceptors in a healthy retina, which manifest themselves as rods and cones, initiate a neural signal in response to light. Along the visual pathway, this neural signal is processed by bipolar cells and ganglion cells, before being sent along the surface of the retina towards the optic nerve. Photoreceptors are almost completely absent in the retina of end-stage Retinitis Pigmentosa (RP) and Age-related Macular Degeneration (AMD) patients, while the bipolar cells and ganglion cells, through which the photoreceptors normally synapse, survive at high rates [1]. The ganglion and bipolar cells remain intact, and due to the anatomy of the retina, they are in a position where they may respond to electrical stimulation. Ganglion cells, which are further on down the signal-processing line, reside upon the retinal surface. The reason for the retina's seemingly inverted architecture (light must first pass through the ganglion cells and bipolar cells en route to the photoreceptors) is that the photoreceptors require a continuous supply of oxygen. As a consequence, the retina evolved with the rods and cones positioned close to the robust blood flow which is found at the very back of the retina. The placement of the retina in close proximity to a robust blood supply aids greatly in the constant temperature control of the retina. Silicon photonic devices can be fabricated to respond to the visible spectrum, and electrodes can be designed to stimulate nerve cells. Thus, the basic task in creating a retinal prosthesis is to engineer an artificial intermediary device, which resides in-between the material picture which the silicon photonic device can perceive and the operative neurons which the electrodes can interface with and stimulate. In addition to benefiting the visually impaired, restoring vision to a large subset of blind patients also promises to have a positive impact on government health care spending. Furthermore, by pioneering new techniques for interfacing chronically-implanted electronic devices with neural tissue, it is hoped that this project will provide new insight into methods and means for engineering electronic biomedical monitoring and rehabilitative devices.

Over the past thirty years, many different electronic devices designed to convey visual information to blind patients have been proposed. Some devices are designed to convert visual information and present it in an auditory or tactile manner (i.e. sensory substitution devices) [2]. Others strive to restore vision by electrically stimulating the visual cortex or optic tract [3], [4], [5], [6]. However, each device had its limitations from medical and/or engineering perspectives, preventing the development of a visual prosthesis that could help a large subset of blind patients.

Motivated by recent clinical research demonstrating electrical stimulation of partially-degenerated retinal tissue in visually impaired patients, several research groups have taken a new approach [7], [8], [9], [10], [11], [12]. This approach consists of the development of an electronic device that stimulates remaining retinal neurons of patients who are blind from end-stage photoreceptor degenerative diseases such as Retinitis Pigmentosa (RP) and Age-related Macular Degeneration (AMD) [13].

Post-mortem RP eyes with bare or no light perception prior to death were analyzed morphometrically [14], [15]. This analysis showed that only 4% or less of the nuclei were left remaining in the outer nuclear layer. In contrast, the ganglion cell layer contained 30% and the inner nuclear layer contained 80% of its nuclei. Given this limited transneuronal degeneration, a retinal implant could conceivably electrically stimulate the remaining retinal neurons, thus potentially providing useful vision.

Even though photoreceptors are almost completely absent in the retina of end-stage RP and AMD patients, the cells to which photoreceptors normally synapse (i.e., the next neuron in the signal path) survive at high rates [1]. Clinical studies have shown that controlled electrical signals applied to a small area of the retina with a microelectrode can be used to initiate a local neural response in the remaining retinal cells [1], [16], [17], [18]. The neural response was perceived by otherwise completely blind patients as a small spot of light. When multiple electrodes were activated in a two-dimensional electrode array, a number of small spots of light were perceived by the patient(s), which when viewed together formed an image representative of the pattern of active electrodes. In the experiments reported by Humayun *et al.* [1], simple forms such as an English character or a matchbox have been perceived by human subjects when the retina receives electrical stimulation corresponding to the original pattern. Thus, similar to how an image is formed by a dot-matrix printer, when controlled pattern electrical stimulation of the remaining retinal neurons is coupled with an extraocular image acquisition and transmission system, it could allow blind patients to regain form vision. This suggests that a retinal implant could electrically stimulate the remaining retinal neurons and provide useful vision. The system is conceptually illustrated in Figure 1. The clinically determined requisite waveform of the electrical stimulus is characteristerized by four parameters and is shown in Figure 2. A desirable waveform could be either an anodic pulse first, followed by a cathodic pulse, or vice versa.

The Multiple-unit Artificial Retinal Chipset (MARC) prosthesis is designed to provide useful vision to over 10,000,000 people blind because of photoreceptor loss due to partial retinal degeneration from diseases such as Age-related Macular Degeneration (AMD) and Retinitis Pigmentosa (RP). The retinal prosthesis is based on the fundamental concept of replacing photoreceptor function with an electronic device, which has been developed by Humayun *et al.* [16], [17], [18]. A discrete percept was elicited in fourteen out of fifteen patients tested, thirteen with their vision impaired by RP, and two with end-stage AMD. The patients were able to identify the stimulated retinal quadrant by the change in position of the visual sensation.

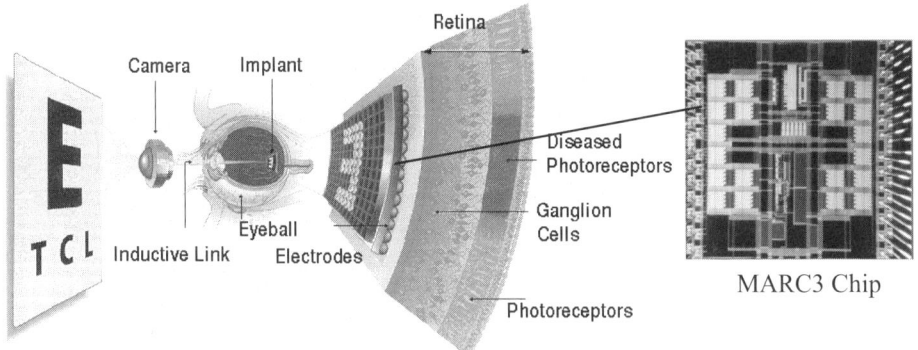

Figure 1. Conceptual design of MARC retinal prosthesis.

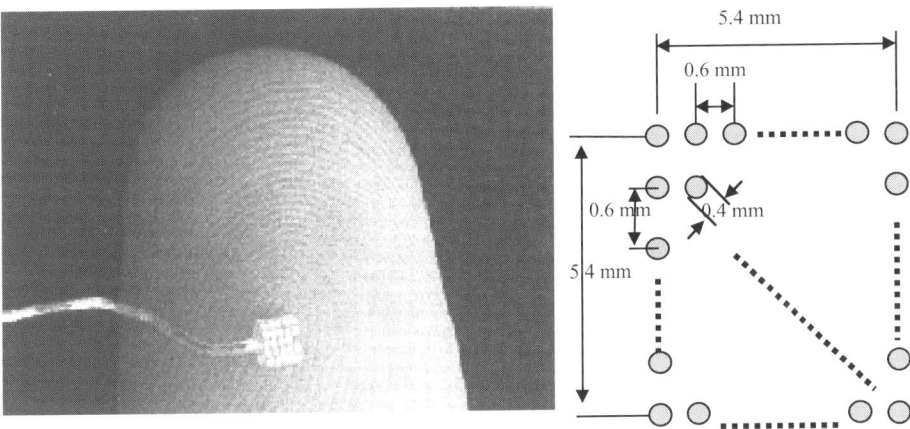

Figure 2. RF coil configuration of the MARC system. A secondary coil may also be implanted intraocularly.

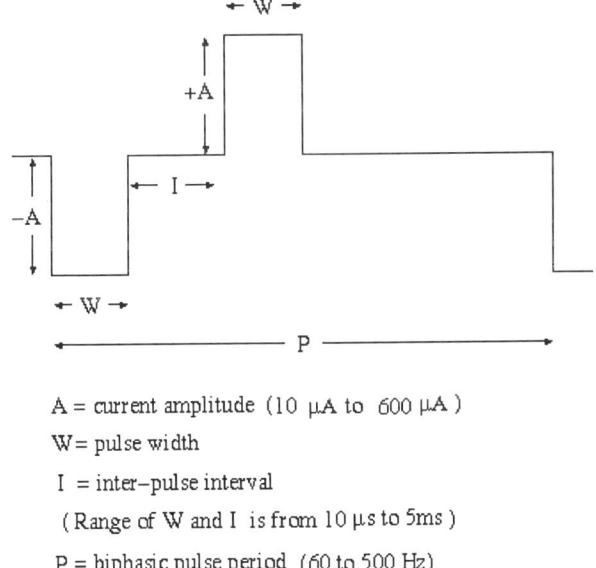

A = current amplitude (10 μA to 600 μA)
W = pulse width
I = inter-pulse interval
(Range of W and I is from 10 μs to 5ms)
P = biphasic pulse period (60 to 500 Hz)

Figure 3. Bipolar waveform for electrical retinal stimulation.

1.2. A retinal prosthesis: engineering solution to biological problem

The basic task in creating a retinal prosthesis is to create an artificial intermediary device which resides in-between the silicon photonic device (camera) which can transduce an image of a visual scene and the operative neurons which the electrodes interface with and stimulate the retina. As shown in Figure 1, our visual prosthesis is implemented as an extraocular and an intraocular unit. The implantable intraocular unit receives power and signal via a telemetric inductive link with the extraocular unit. The extraocular unit consists of a video camera and video processing board, a telemetry protocol encoder chip, and an RF amplifier and primary coil, while the intraocular unit consists of a secondary receiving coil mounted in close proximity to the cornea, a power and signal transceiver and processing chip, a stimulation-current driver, and a proposed electrode array fabricated on a material such as silicone rubber [3], [14], thin silicon [19], or polyimide [25] with ribbon cables connecting the devices. The bio-compatibility of polyimide [20], [21] is being studied, and its thin, lightweight consistency suggests its possible use as a non-intrusive material for an electrode array. Titanium tacks [22] or cyanoacrylate glue [23] may be used to hold the electrode array in place.

The stimulating electrode array, an example of which is given in Figure 2, is mounted on the retina, as shown in Figure 4, while the power and signal transceiver is mounted in close proximity to the cornea. An external miniature low-power CMOS camera worn in an eyeglass frame will capture an image and transfer the visual information and power to the intraocular components via RF telemetry. The intraocular prosthesis will decode the signal and electrically stimulate the retinal neurons through the electrodes in a manner that corresponds to the image acquired by the CMOS camera.

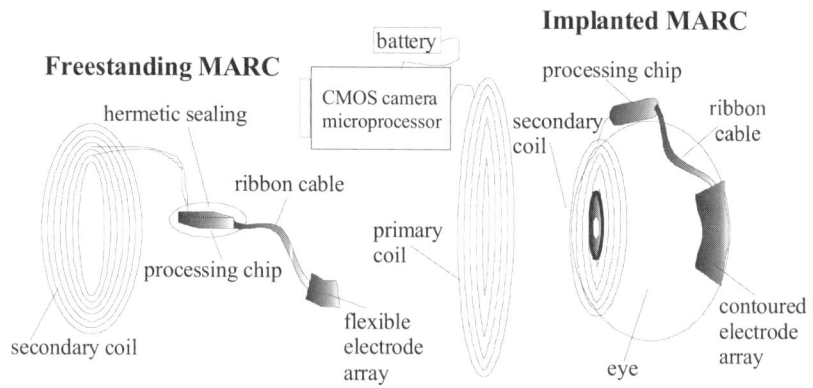

Figure 4. RF coil configuration of the MARC system. A secondary coil may also be implanted intraocularly.

Due to the size of the intraocular cavity (2.5 cm in diameter), the delicate tissue-paper like thickness of the retina (100-300 µm), and the fact that the eye is mobile, a retinal implant poses difficult engineering challenges. Over the past several years, all of these factors and constraints have been taken into consideration in the engineering research of our implantable MARC device. Encouraging results from clinical studies and the testing of engineered devices have inspired our efforts to produce a prototype human retinal implant. These results include: 1) Tests in blind volunteers have demonstrated that controlled-pattern electrical stimulation of the remaining retinal neurons using hand-held electrode arrays wired to a PC-controlled signal generator results in vision compatible with mobility and recognizing large-letter forms [3], [24], [25]. 2) Preliminary bio-compatibility tests in animals performed by researchers at Johns Hopkins University have shown that the eye can tolerate the proposed materials as well as the surgical implantation [26]. 3) Technology exists for the transmission of power and data using RF telemetry [27]. 4) Standard semiconductor technology can be used to fabricate a power and signal-receiving chip, which would then drive current through an electrode array and stimulate the retinal neurons [4], [5]. 5) The first three generations of MARC chips have been designed, fabricated, and tested at North Carolina State University.

This in addition to the demonstration that simultaneous electrical stimulation less than 300 µm apart resulted in two distinct percepts suggested that multi-focal electrical stimulation of the retina might be a viable approach to providing visual input to patients who have profound visual loss due to outer retinal degeneration. A stimulating current of 600 µA, passed through an electrode 400 µm in diameter, elicited a visual percept [3]. Humayun et al. were able to demonstrate that a 2×2 mm^2 5×5 silicone rubber and platinum or iridium [1], [28], [29] electrode array could be used to stimulate simple images upon the patient's retina [14]. Pattern electrical stimulation of the retina was tested in 2 patients. The first patient was able to perceive an activated 'U'-shaped electrode pattern as an 'H.' The second patient correctly identified a square electrode pattern as a 'match box.' Building upon these medical results, our team [30], [31], [32] of medical doctors, physicists, and engineers have worked towards developing MARC prototypes based on the clinical stimulation data [1], [3], and conceptually illustrated in Figure 1. For retinal stimulation in blind patients, it was determined that the biphasic current pulse amplitude (**A**) should be 100-600 µA, the current pulse duration (**W**) should be 0.1-2 ms, and the period between biphasic pulses (**I**) should be 8-100 ms, corresponding to a stimulating frequency of 10-125 Hz.

The chips are all designed in accordance with the biological constraints determined by our group [33], as well as the technological constraints imposed by the standard 2 µm and 1.2 µm CMOS technology available at MOSIS.

Calculations concerning the requisite power for the dual-unit retina chip are as follows: Humayun *et al.*'s experiments have shown that a 600 µA with 2 ms bipolar pulse is required for initial retinal stimulation. The equivalent retinal impedance seen by the electrode is 10 KΩ. To prevent flicker perception, a 60 Hz image presentation rate is required, which means that the 600 µA must be generated 60 times a second per driver, or once every 16.6 ms.

In recent tests, the 600 µA stimulation seemed to be saturating the retina. It was also found that an array of negative (cathodic) microsecond pulses followed by an array of positive (anodic) microsecond pulses would give better results, allowing for a stimulation with 100 µA, implying that lower currents will be enough to stimulate the retina [1]. These are the basic biological parameters about which any functioning prosthesis must be designed, and they are elaborated on in the following section.

2. The multiple unit artificial retina chip (MARC) prosthesis

2.1. Clinical and engineering overview

2.1.1. Foundational clinical research

This project is founded upon the clinical research, which has demonstrated the possibility of inducing visual perception by electrical stimulation of the retina. In 1990, Humayun *et al.* first demonstrated that retinal ganglion cells could be electrically stimulated without penetrating the retinal surface [34]. A patent has been issued for this concept, the main drawing of which is illustrated in Figure 5. The importance of this was that a patient with a dysfunctional retina could be made to perceive a point of light when a current flowed between two electrodes positioned in close proximity to the retina, ensuring that the delicate retina remained intact. Prior work [1], [35] had concentrated on demonstrating that the retina could be stimulated with electrodes which penetrated the retinal membrane. In Humayun's Ph.D. thesis [36], it was demonstrated that a visually impaired person could be made to "see" a point of light at different positions corresponding to the different selected positions where the retina was electrically stimulated by a probe inserted into the ocular cavity. A discrete percept was elicited in five out of the six patients tested, four with their vision impaired by RP, and two with end-stage AMD. The patients were able to identify the stimulated retinal quadrant by the change in position of the visual sensation. This in addition to the demonstration that simultaneous electrical stimulation less than 1 mm apart resulted in 2 distinct percepts suggested that multi-focal electrical stimulation of the retina might be a viable approach to providing visual input to patients who have profound visual loss due to outer retinal degeneration. A stimulating current of 600 µA passed through an electrode 400 µm in diameter elicited a visual percept. Humayun has discovered that after twenty minutes in the operating room, the patient could "learn" to see with 300 µA, and the most recent tests have demonstrated that percepts can be elicited at currents as low as 100 µA. The electrodes were composed of platinum disks mounted on silicone rubber. The disks are fabricated by an Australian company, which manufactures electrodes for the Clarion artificial cochlear implant.

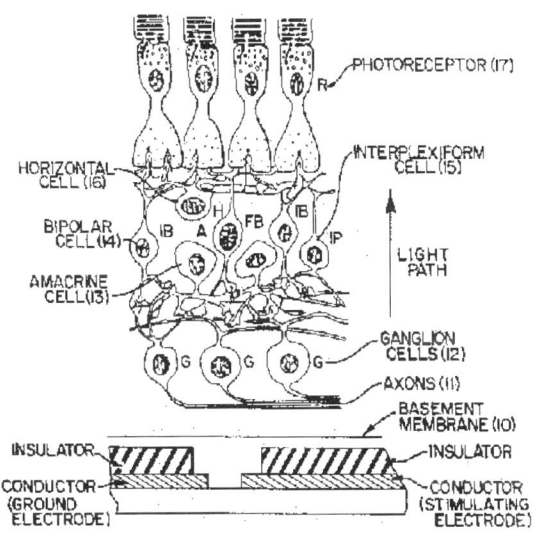

Figure 5. Main drawing from Humayun *et al.*'s U.S. Patent #5109844, for non-intrusive retinal microstimulation.

Humayun *et al.* have pursued this research [1], [2] more extensively, and they recently demonstrated that more complex patterns, originating from a 5×5 electrode array with an area of 2×2 mm^2, as pictured in Figure 2, could be stimulated on a patient's retina. When five neighboring electrodes were fired simultaneously, the patient perceived a line, and patients were recently able to recognize the letters 'H' and 'U.' Humayun *et al.*'s research has delineated specific numbers concerning the size and duration of current pulses that are necessary to elicit a percept upon a visually impaired patient's retina. In the second generation MARC design, with a 10×10 pixel array, the patient will be able to perceive simple shapes and outlines of windows and doors. A 250×250 electrode array on a 2×2 mm^2 chip would approach a 1 electrode to 1 ganglion cell ratio, and thus it would approach maximum resolution. Because the original electrodes were fabricated by flattening tiny platinum balls on a silicone substrate by hand, achieving resolutions of greater than 5×5 may prove to be difficult and costly. Whereas the artificial cochlear only requires six electrodes, the artificial retina will require over 100 if it is to provide useful vision. Future electrodes will be fabricated either upon polyimide or silicon substrates.

Recent studies demonstrated that 15 human subjects were able to perceive phosphenes with pattern electrical stimulation. All but one of these patients were able to localize the position of the stimulating electrode and could track the stimulus as it moved along the retina. Most of the subjects reported seeing a white or yellow flashing light, though some of the subjects saw a black dot surrounded by a white or yellow ring. The results included a 61-year-old male with RP (no light perception vision) who described the phosphene to be as small as the head of a match, indicating that electrical stimulation can be very focal. He also discriminated between two points 435 μm apart, corresponding to 4/200 (crude ambulatory) vision [1]. The experimental result can be summarized in the Tables 1 and 2.

Tests conducted by Humayun *et al.* at Johns Hopkins Hospital with a 5×5 array yielded the following results: a) when electrodes were stimulated in rows or columns, the patient saw horizontal and vertical lines, respectively, b) when electrodes in a 'U' like pattern were activated, the patient saw the letter 'H' [2]. Although the patient's responses were not always correct, this result is very encouraging for a number of reasons. First, the experimental conditions were not ideal, as the stimulating electrode is hand-held and the eye is fully mobile, resulting in movement of the electrodes relative to the retina, which in turn lead to electrical fields which were neither spatially nor temporally constant. Second, the tests were conducted for periods of less than one hour, which is a very short period to get accustomed to a new mode of visual input. In the cochlear implant experience, it usually takes weeks for the patient to "learn" how to respond to the artificial auditory input. Third, the choice of the letter 'U' was not optimal as it is frequently confused with the letter 'H.' This may have been especially true in the test, since the electrodes created a straight horizontal bottom for the letter 'U' rather than the slightly curved shape we are accustomed to seeing.

Table 1. Electrode specification

Probe Type	Number of Electrode	Diameter of Disk Electrodes (μm)	Electrode Spacing Edge-to-Edge (μm)
(1) 3×3 Array	9	400	200
(2) 5×5 Array	25	400	200
(3) Wire	3	125	250

Table 2. Humayun et al.'s [1] clinical results from testing ten human subjects

Subject	Diagnosis	Flash Threshold (dB)	ERG (μV)	Stimulating Probe Type	Percept Shape	Percept Color	Threshold Charge (μC)
HC	RP	NLP*	N/A	(2)	LETTER H	White	0.4
BC	RP	-12	NR	(3)	PIN	Yellow	1.6
RJ	RP	-28	NR	(3)	PIN	Yellow	1.8
BH	RP	+11	NR	(3)	PIN	White	1.1
AB	AMD	20/400	NR	(3)	PIN	White	0.3
CS	RP	-28	NR	(3)	PIN	Blue	2.4
VO	RP	-30	1.0	(3)	PIN	Yellow	1.0
HW	RP	-18	NR	(3)	DOT	White	0.4
JT	RP	+18	NR	(3),(1)	DOT, BOX**	White	0.6
JL	RP	-14	NR	(3)	FIREFLY	White	0.2

For another patient, the doctors at Johns Hopkins University Hospital selected a more distinct pattern than the letter 'U.' A 73-year-old female with RP (bare light perception vision) saw lights that outlined the shape of a 'matchbox' when pattern stimulation was applied through electrodes positioned on the perimeter of a square-shaped electrode array. Every electrode on the perimeter of a 3×3 electrode array was activated to form this perception. The combination of electrodes that formed the box covered a square area of retina 1.2 mm on a side. The electrode in the eye as viewed through the surgical microscope is shown in Figure 6.

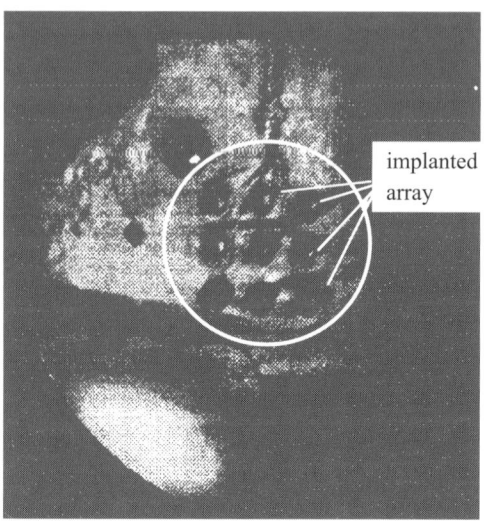

Figure 6. Retinal photography showing implanted array.

A 52-year-old female with RP (bare light perception vision) described the perception as a firefly; again indicating that the perception produced by electrical stimulation is focused on a small part of the visual field. Medical doctors at JHU were able to map out her visual function by moving the stimulating electrode over the surface of the retina (i.e., akin to dynamic perimeter testing). Stimulation thresholds were lower for macular regions. The phosphene seen by the subject would disappear as the probe was moved peripherally, and then reappear as the probe was moved back into the macula. We believe that this difference in the threshold to elicit visual perceptions indicates more damage in the extramacular region, which has extensive bone-spicule change [2].

2.1.2. Engineering overview: feasibility and significance of the MARC

Before embarking on the chip design, it was necessary to assess how useful a limited-resolution view would be to the blind. Simple visual feasibility experiments have been conducted at NCSU to determine how well sight could be restored with a 15×15 array of pixels, each of them able of four-bit stimulation, or sixteen gray levels. A picture from a video camera was projected onto a television screen at the low resolution of 15×15 pixels. When subjects who wore glasses removed their glasses, or when those with good sight intentionally blurred their vision, the natural spatial-temporal processing of the brain allowed them to actually distinguish features and recognize people. When the subject focused on the screen, it appeared as a 15×15 array of gray blocks, but when the subject "trained" themselves to defocus their vision, they were able to "learn" to see definitive edges and details such as beards, teeth, and opened or closed eyes. These results are reminiscent of the experiences with the artificial cochlear implant. When the artificial cochlear was originally being designed, it was believed that over 2,400 electrodes would be needed to stimulate the nerves in a manner that would be conducive to hearing. Today, however, within a few weeks of receiving an implant, a patient can understand telephone conversations with an artificial cochlear that has only six electrodes. One of the advantages of this project is that the MARC device will be interfaced with the world's greatest computer – the brain. The MARC won't be duplicating the exact functioning of the retina, but rather the device will be an entity that the brain will "learn" to use. A good analogy to think of is that in attempting flight, the Wright brothers did not attempt to imitate nature by building a plane which flapped its wings, but rather they did it in a way that had not yet appeared in the natural world. Thus, we believe that a 15×15 pixel array will facilitate a level of sight which will be of significant value to the patient.

2.2. Prior art and related research

In the Artificial Retina Device developed by Chow [37], an array of photodiodes is to be implanted in-between the inner and outer retinal layers. The violation of human retinal tissue necessary to perform such an implantation renders the introduction of a chronic device a difficult procedure, and it increases the risk of subsequent retinal detachment. Furthermore, Chow suggests the use of an external power supply or an internal battery connected to the chip to provide power. Batteries would necessitate the existence of wires that are not free to rotate with the eye, increasing the chances of irritation, especially during periods of REM or while the patient is blinking.

In Michelson's patent [38], a visual prosthesis for blindness due to retinal malfunction includes a compact device having a close-packed array of photosensitive devices on one surface thereof. A plurality of electrodes extends from the opposed surface of the device and is connected to the outputs of the photosensitive devices. The device is adapted to be inserted in the posterior chamber of the eye, generally disposed at the focal plane of the optical pathway and impinging on the retina. There exist anchoring means to secure the device with the electrodes operatively connected to the neuron array at the surface of the retina to stimulate the neurons in a pattern corresponding to the illumination pattern of the photosensitive array. The device is powered by externally induced electromagnetic or radio frequency energy and is encased in a biologically inert housing. An amplifier array may be interposed between the sensing elements and the electrodes to amplify, shape, and temporally process the visual signals. It would be difficult to transmit power to a device located so far back in the ocular cavity, "in the posterior chamber of the eye." In addition, the processing amplification circuitry required in-between the array of photosensors and the array of electrodes would necessitate non-standard, difficult, and thus expensive processing. The weight of the entire device upon the retina may be disadvantageous. Furthermore, one could not send a custom test signal to such a device, and there is no diagnostic circuitry which would be capable of sensing malfunctions and transmitting diagnostic signals to an external device. Having all the power signal transceiving and processing circuitry in a single location close to the retina would also serve to concentrate the locale of heat dissipation next to the retina.

MIT's work [39] consists of pioneering research advancing towards the fabrication of an implantable artificial retina chip designed to provide electrical stimulation. Their device employs a laser for providing power to the chip, and the chip is designed to be mounted on the surface of the retina and to stimulate the ganglion cells by the current induced in-between pairs of electrodes positioned in close proximity to the retinal surface. However, MIT takes a different approach from us, as their entire device, which comprises a chip designed to decode variations in the intensity of the incident laser light and an electrode array, sits entirely upon the retina. MIT's design will require a CCD camera/microprocessing unit, which would exist external to the eye, as well as the existence of a microprocessor upon the implanted chip. The CCD camera picks up a picture of the patient's environment and uses the information to modulate an external laser beam, which is shone through the cornea, incident upon the chip. Their chip decodes the laser modulations, and the picture of the environment stimulated upon the retina. There are a few disadvantages to this design. It would be difficult to keep a laser focused upon a chip sitting at the back of the retina, and by shining a laser into the eye, one heats the retina. Furthermore, the weight of the entire device on the retina may be harmful to the retina.

A Japanese team [40] is currently working on a retinal prosthesis which will use a novel technique to interface between the retina and the electrode array. They will grow a culture of live nerve cells on a silicon array, and then attempt to graft those cells to the living retinal tissue. However, at present even if live cultured neurons can be grown in silicon wells, it remains unclear how the processes of these neurons would be directed to exact small areas of host neurons in order to ensure localized effects. The grafting of foreign tissue and electronic devices is an emerging field, and if it is proven feasible, it will definitely serve as an enhancement to future design.

A German team is also working on an approach [41] to an implantable retinal prosthesis similar to ours. They too are utilizing RF telemetry with an intraocular coil mounted in close proximity to the cornea, connected to a chipset with processing circuitry, which in turn is connected to a polyimide electrode array. As there are a finite number of ways in which to configure the project, it is expected that there should be overlap between the various approaches. The German team comprises a formidable consortium, with over 40 scientists and ample funding from the German government. However, to our best knowledge, our team has been the only one as of yet to successfully stimulate a visual percept within a human being and to fabricate a chip which is capable of delivering the requisite signals.

2.3. Evolution of the MARC prosthesis

As we approach a functioning retinal MARC prosthesis, the design will continue to evolve, as the refinement of any one parameter affects all the rest. For instance, should the main intraocular chip be subdivided into smaller individually-sealed chips so as to reduce the risk of realizing a complete system failure if one chip should malfunction, the basic chip design, as well as the hermetic packaging, will have to be altered. An alteration in the hermetic packaging will affect where the chip may be mounted. A different chip design will require a different power source and thus telemetry configuration. Moreover, a different telemetry configuration may alter the coil designs, which would affect the size of the external battery. Thus, an alteration in any one aspect of the design resounds throughout the entire system. The spirit of this chapter is to offer an overview of all the parameters affecting the design of the MARC, elaborate on all the clinical testing and engineering progress that has been made, anticipate design and engineering hurdles, and suggest approaches for future research.

The design of a retinal prosthesis prototype has been a gradually evolving process over the past several years. Many design iterations have been conducted, and valuable insights have been obtained concerning the optimum design. Our early device design consisted of a single-unit intraocularly implanted chip with a full integration of photosensors, image processing, current drivers, and an electrode array. This design required the photosensors to reside on the opposite side of the chip from the electrode array, thus creating a significant engineering challenge for fabrication. Over time, it became apparent that it would be better to have the photosensing or video capture performed extraocularly, allowing for enhanced video processing and more custom control over the video signal, and also minimizing the amount of hardware that has to be implanted into the eye. Currently, we are developing the prosthesis system, which is conceptually illustrated in Figures 1, 4, and 7. Section 3.2 provides an in-depth discussion of the advantage of this current system for a retinal prosthesis.

The system is composed of two units, an extraocular one and an intraocular one. The two units are connected by a telemetric inductive link, allowing the intraocular unit to receive both power and a data signal from the extraocular unit. The extraocular unit includes a video camera and video processing board, a telemetry protocol encoder chip, and an RF amplifier and primary coil. The intraocular unit consists of an intraocular secondary coil, a rectifier and regulator, a retinal chip with a telemetry protocol decoder and stimulus signal generator, and an electrode array.

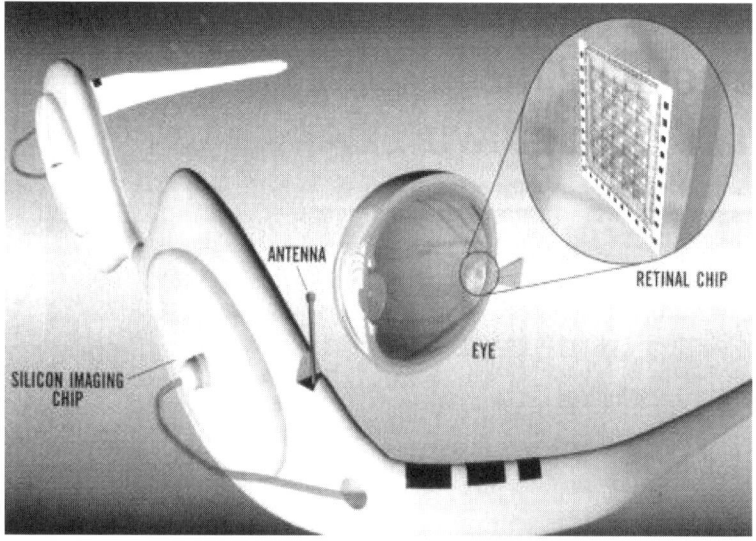

Figure 7. Conceptual drawing of the retinal prosthesis system.

3. Current engineering research

3.1. Early generation chip

Early versions of the Multiple Unit Artificial Retina Chipset (MARC) [4], [5] consisted of a photosensing, processing, and stimulating chip fabricated in 2.0 μm CMOS, which is endowed with a 5×5 phototransistor array. Measuring 2×2 mm^2 in dimension, it has been used to demonstrate that current stimulation patterns corresponding to simple images, such as the letter "E" presented optically to the chip, can be generated and used to drive the 5×5 array of electrodes. The chip delivered the requisite power for stimulation, as was determined by our clinical studies conducted on visually impaired patients with RP and AMD. For each of the 25 individual photosensing pixels, we were able to adjust the VDD, the clock frequency, the sensitivity to light, and the current output. The chip is fully packaged in a standard 40 pin DIP package, and a ribbon cable may facilitate a connection between the chip and the stimulating electrode array.

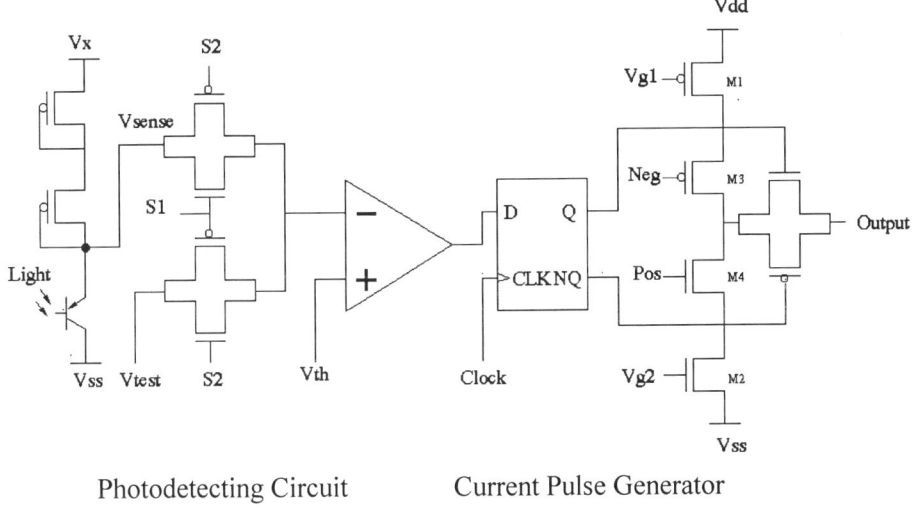

Photodetecting Circuit   Current Pulse Generator

Figure 8. MARC1 Photodetecting and stimulating circuit at pixel level.

Each pixel on this version of the MARC is divided into two parts, the photoreceptor and the current pulse generator, as shown in Figure 8. The photoreceptor converts light intensity into a voltage level. This voltage level is then compared to the threshold voltage (V_{th}) in the comparator, which controls the current pulse driver circuit. If light intensity is stronger than the threshold value, a biphasic stimulating signal is generated by that pixel. Timing of the current pulse is controlled by external pulses and a clock signal. The chip has been designed with the biological stimulating constraints determined in clinical studies conducted on patients with RP and AMD. It successfully delivered the 600 µA current in 1 ms bipolar pulses, which were required for retinal stimulation. Test results are shown in Figure 9.

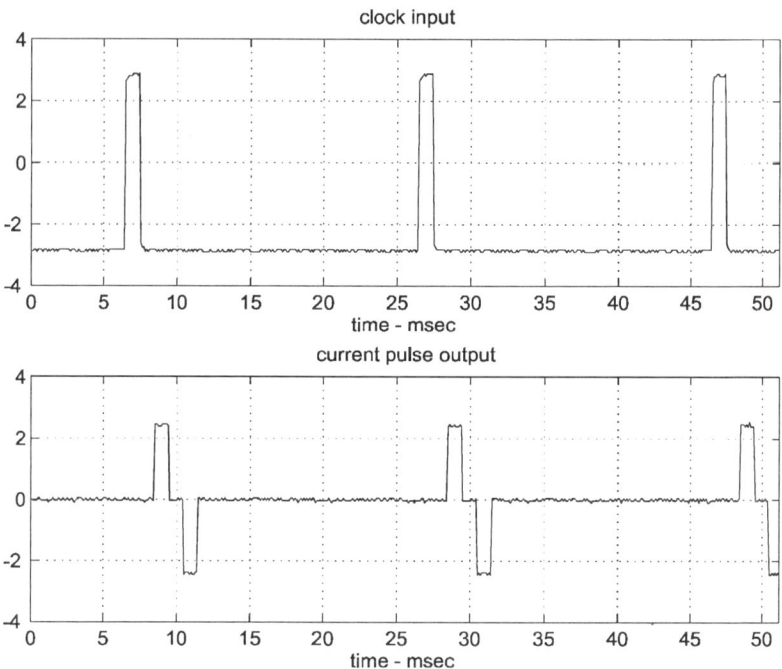

Figure 9. Waveform from MARC1 testing: the output from the "on" pixels, which resulted in 250 µA, 2 ms pulses at a 50 Hz clock rate, are shown beneath the external clock signal.

By successfully fabricating and testing a chip which receives an image and delivers the requisite currents for human retinal stimulation to a 5×5 electrode array, we gained the necessary insight and expertise which is allowing us to design the second and third generation chips which will drive 10×10 and 25×25 photosensing arrays. The design of MARC1 includes enhanced holed CMOS phototransistors [6]. This chip was designed before it was suggested that we split the components into two pieces, so as to facilitate the transmission of energy into the eye. As RF powering became feasible, so did telemetry and the transmission of visual information from an exterior camera. Thus, it was decided that all the video would be processed exterior to the eye.

3.2. Overall system functionality of advanced generations

Advanced generations of the MARC were designed about the principle of transmitting both power and signal into the eye, thus enabling the video capture to be performed extraocularly, as pictured in Figures 10 and 11. This method provides several advantages, including a greater control of the video signal, the ability to process the visual information, the ability to substitute computer enhanced or generated video for the image carried by ambient light, and reduced hardware in the eye, allowing for a less-intrusive implant and reduced heating. An external camera will acquire an image, whereupon it will be encoded into a data stream that will be transmitted via RF telemetry to an intraocular transceiver. The data signal will be transmitted by modulating the amplitude of a higher frequency carrier signal. The signal will be rectified and filtered, and the MARC will be capable of extracting power, data, and a clock signal. The generated image will then be stimulated upon the patient's retina.

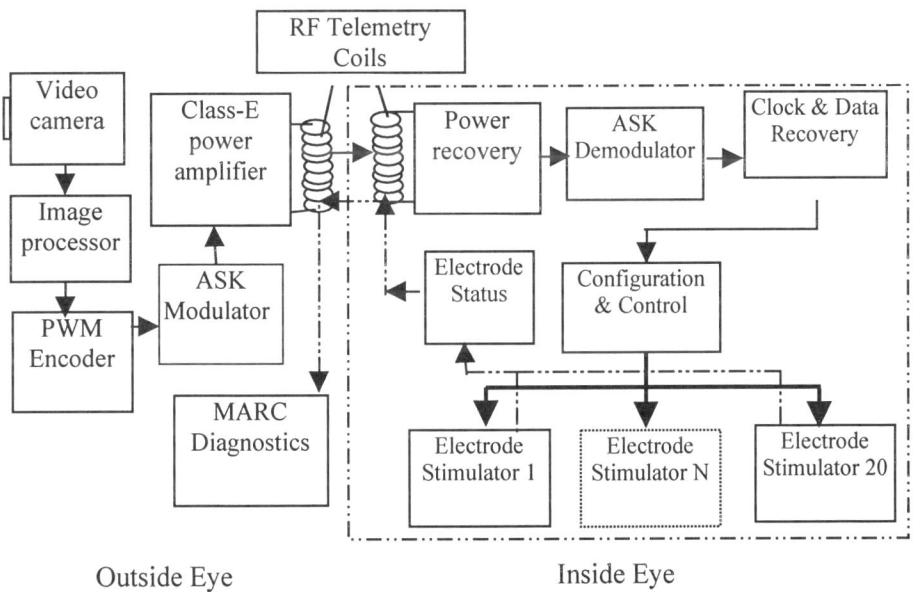

Figure 10. MARC system functionality.

As shown in Figures 1, 7, 8, and 10, the MARC system consists of two separate parts, which reside exterior to and within the eyeball. Each part is equipped with both a transmitter and a receiver. The primary coil can be driven with a 0.5-10 MHz carrier signal, accompanied by a 10 kHz amplitude modulated (AM/ASK) signal, which provides data for setting the configuration of the stimulating electrodes. A DC power supply is obtained by the rectification of the incoming RF signal. The receiver on the secondary side extracts four bits of data for each pixel from the incoming RF signal and provides filtering, demodulation, and amplification. The extracted data is interpreted by the electrode signal driver, which finally generates appropriate currents for the stimulating electrodes in terms of magnitude, pulse width, and frequency.

3.2.1. Advantages of the MARC system

Several limitations of previous approaches [25], [42], [43], [44], [45], [46], [47] to visual prostheses are overcome by the designs of the MARC1-4 systems:

i) *Component Size:*
The novel multiple-unit intraocular transceiver processing and electrode array-processing visual prosthesis allows for larger processing chips (6×6 mm), and thus more complex circuitry. Also, by splitting the chips up into smaller components, and utilizing techniques such as solder bumping to connect the chips with flexible electrode substrates, we keep the sizes to a minimum.

ii) *Heat Dissipation:*
The power transfer and rectification in the MARC2 and MARC3 designs are primary sources of heat generation, and they occur near the corneal surface, or at least remotely from the retina, rather than in close proximity to the more delicate retina.

iii) *Powering:*
The multiple-unit intraocular transceiver-processing and electrode array-processing visual prosthesis provides a more direct means for power and signal transfer, as the transceiver-processing unit is placed in close proximity to the cornea, making it more accessible to electromagnetic radiation in either the visible wavelength range or radio waves. Solar powering and especially RF powering are made more feasible.

iv) *Diagnostic Capability:*
The transceiver unit is positioned close to the cornea, and thus it can send and receive radio waves, granting it the capability of being programmed to perform different functions as well as giving diagnostic feedback to an external control system. Diagnostic feedback would be much more difficult with the solar powering.

v) *Physiological Functionality:*
The MARC was designed in conformance with the physiological data gained during tests on blind patients. We are the only group who has yet created a visual percept (with electrical stimulation) in a patient. Therefore, we have the unique advantage of designing around parameters, which are guaranteed to work.

vi)   Video Processing and Control:

As the video camera exists extraocularly, enhanced video processing may be conducted, and the video signal may be controlled.

vii)   Reduction of Stress Upon The Retina:

Our device would reduce the stress upon the retina, as it would only necessitate the mounting of the electrode array upon the delicate surface, while the signal processing and power transfer could be performed off the retina. Also, buoyancy could be added to the electrode array, to give it the same average density as the surrounding fluid.

3.2.2. Advanced generation retina telemetric processing chips

It became apparent that it is to our advantage to have the video capture performed extraocularly for reasons enumerated above, thus necessitating a chip capable of decoding a video signal and driving a large number of electrodes. Currently, we are developing the multiple-unit prosthesis system, which is conceptually illustrated in Figures 1, 7, and 8. The implantable intraocular unit receives power and video signal via a telemetric inductive link with the extraocular unit. The extraocular unit includes a video camera and video processing board, a telemetry protocol encoder chip, and an RF amplifier and primary coil. The intraocular unit consists of an intraocular secondary coil, a rectifier and regulator, a retinal chip with a telemetry protocol decoder and stimulus signal generator, and an electrode array. The system block diagram is shown in Figure 11.

The extraocular unit captures an external picture with a video camera and provides additional image processing whose output is further encoded with a specific data transmission protocol which is described in Section 3.3. Two types of data, image and configuration, are distinguished by bit patterns in the transmission protocol. The data are further processed by a pulse width modulation (PWM) circuit with an amplitude shift key (ASK) modulation. At this stage, the image/configuration data has been mixed with the power carrier frequency of 1-10 MHz. The modulated signal is then inductively transmitted over to the intraocular unit. A PWM data signal and power carrier of the received signal are then separated by the filter in the intraocular unit. The filter design dictates the ratio of carrier frequency to the data rate. In our design, the data rate can be 25-250 kbits/s. DC power is obtained from the carrier by rectifier and regulation and must be independent of the data stream. Our PWM scheme is designed to achieve such a stringent power requirement. Either image or configuration data is extracted through the reversal process of the extraocular unit. In other words, the digital signal is extracted from the PWM data signal and protocol decoder and is used as a specification for the generation of the current pulses. These current pulses drive the electrode array.

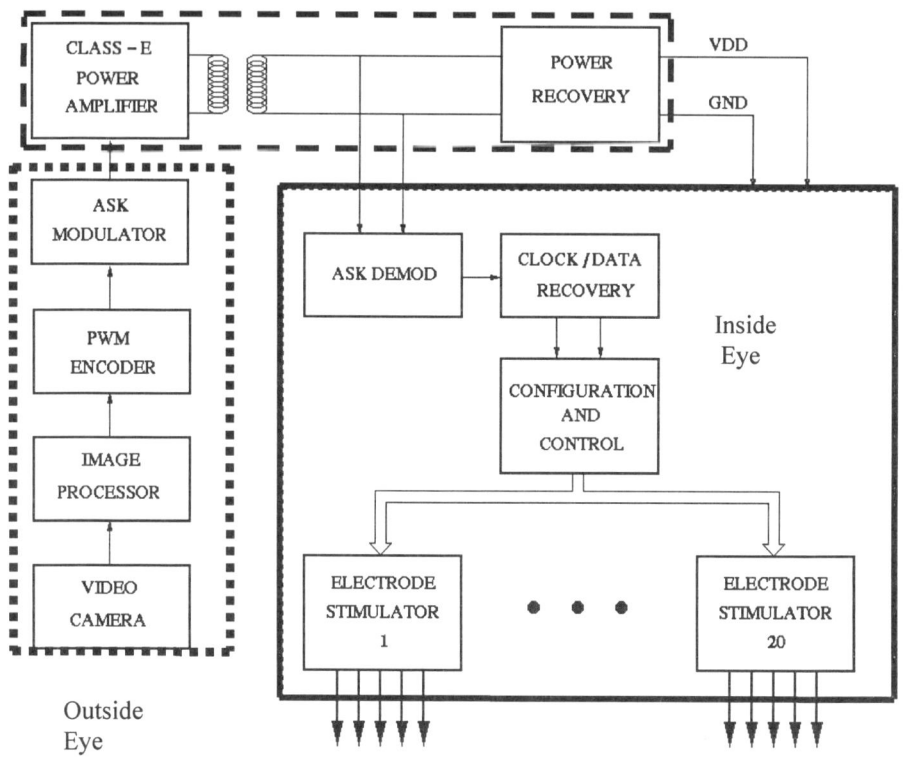

Figure 11. System block diagram for the proposed retinal prosthestic device.

Research pertaining to all of the component blocks in Figure 11 is underway. In this chapter, we describe the design and testing of the component chip enclosed by the solid rectangle. The chip accommodates the telemetry function, protocol receiver, and current driver. It serves as a flexible current waveform generator and could potentially obtain the optimization of stimulus waveforms via implant experiments. It supports the charge-balanced current with a biphasic waveform (annode phase first followed by a cathode phase) as shown in Figure 3. It is also capable of providing the wireless transfer of power and data to the implanted stimulator.

3.3. Implantable retinal chip

3.3.1. Chip functionality

Figure 12 shows the functional block diagram of a prototype implantable telemtric chip. The chip operates in two modes, configuration and run modes. The Amplitude Shift Key (ASK) demodulator receives the ASK envelope from the rectifier output, and generates the digital pulse width modulated (PWM) signal for the clock and data recovery block. Data and clock signals are then recovered by a Delay Locked Loop (DLL) and a decoder circuit. The chip enters the configuration mode after the detection of a synchronization word in the protocol by the synchronization circuit. As shown in Section 2.1.4, a configuration protocol frame has 400 bits and is made of two fields, "synchword" and "configuration data" fields. In this mode, according to the configuration data, the timing generator circuit specifies the timing of the stimulus waveform such as duration (W), dead time (I), and period (P). The current control circuit specifies the full-scale amplitude (A) of biphasic current pulses. This specification is then applied to each of the 20 current stimulation drivers, each drives five electrodes through demultiplexing. Once the configuration process is completed, the chip automatically enters the run mode. By multiplexing, the 20 electrode stimulators drive the desired biphasic current pulses to the 10×10 electrode array.

ASK Demodulator

The prototype implantable device receives both power and data via an inductive link. Amplitude modulation instead of frequency modulation is chosen in order to reduce the circuit complexity and power consumption and is able to sustain the data rate of the requisite functions. The amplitude shift keying modulation scheme regulates the amplitude of the carrier signal with the desired digital data. Because the recovered power is derived from this amplitude, the average transferred power could depend on the transmitted digital data pattern. To avoid this data dependency, we first encode the transmitted data using the alternate mark inversion pulse width modulation and then modulate the data with the carrier frequency, as shown in Figure 13. The system is designed for PWM data ranging from 25 to 250 kbps with a carrier frequency ranging from 1 to 10 MHz.

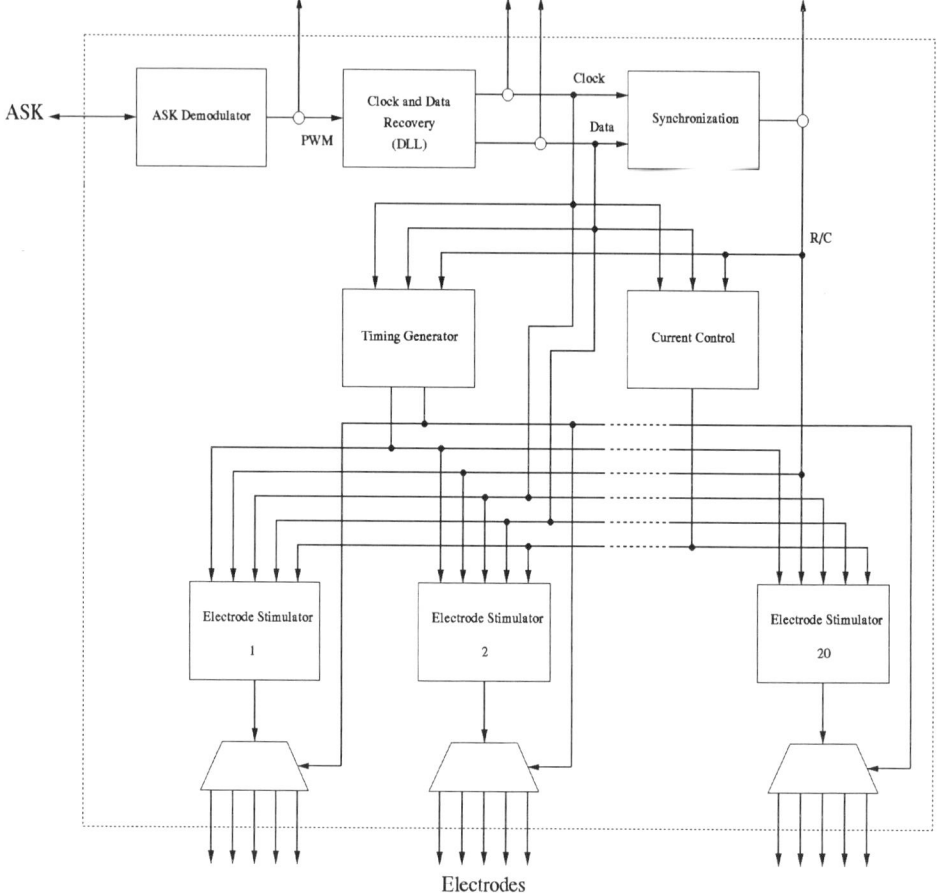

Figure 12. Chip functionality block diagram.

On the receiver side, the ASK signal is rectified and filtered out and a baseband PWM envelope is obtained. This signal is further filtered in order to provide a well-regulated DC voltage for the chip power supply. The unfiltered ASK envelope is fed into the ASK demodulator circuit, as shown in Figure 14, to extract the PWM waveform.

With a predefined amount of hysteresis, the demodulator is a comparator in which one input is from the modulated signal (the DC envelope) and another input is from the average of that signal [6], [7]. Transistors M0 and M1 provide a level shift of the input signal to the common mode range of the differential amplifier. Transistor M2 with the 10 pF capacitor C0 serves as a low pass filter and provides the average of an input signal. Both signals are applied to the differential amplifier with the cross-connected active load of M3-M6. The hysteresis is achieved via positive feedback. The demodulator is designed to process a DC envelope with a ripple between 6.5 and 7.5 V. It has a hysteresis of 500 mV, so as to ensure that the likelihood of an extra transition in the output waveform due to noise is minimized. The output waveform of the demodulator is the digital PWM with voltage swing between 0 and 7 V.

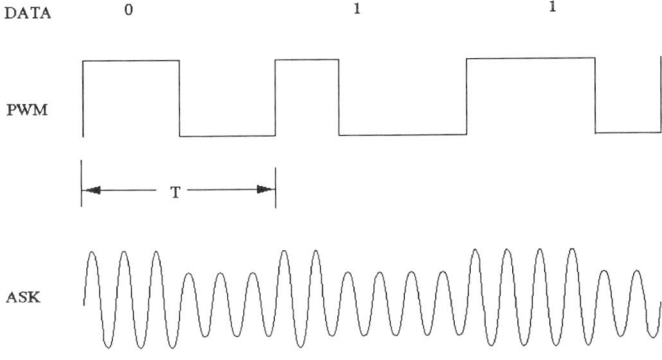

Figure 13. ASK and PWM waveforms.

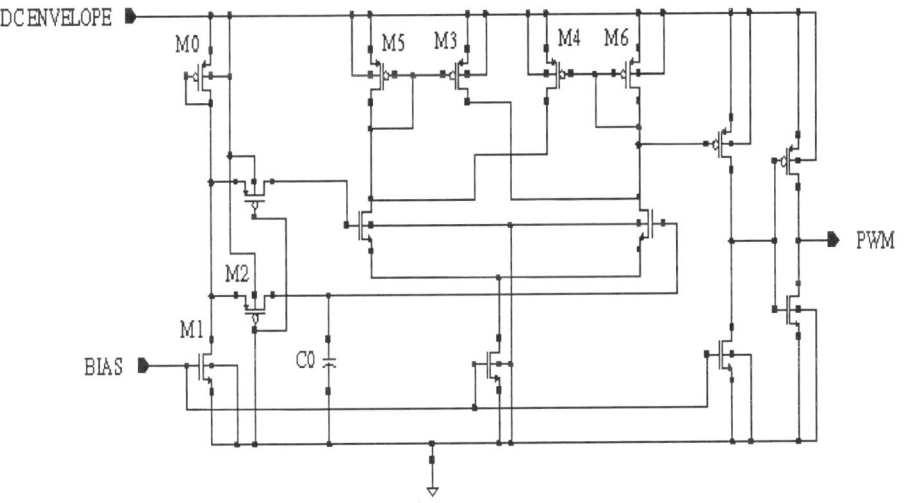

Figure 14. Demodulator circuit.

Clock and data recovery circuit

The rising edge of the PWM pulse generated by the demodulator is fixed in time periodically and serves as a reference in the derivation of an explicit clock signal. On the other hand, the data is encoded by the position of the falling transition at each pulse. In an alternate mark inversion encoding scheme, a zero is encoded as a 50 percent duty cycle pulse, and ones are alternately encoded by 40 or 60 percent duty cycle pulses. This eliminates the need for a local clock oscillator and the clock and data recovery circuit is simplified, and it also provides an average coupled power, which is essentially independent of the data.

The diagram of the clock and data recovery unit is shown in Figure 15. It consists of a delay locked loop (DLL) and decoder logic. The DLL consists of a phase-frequency detector (PFD), a charge-pump, a loop filter, and a voltage-controlled delay line. The 36-stage delay line is locked to one period of the PWM waveform. The waveform is decoded by an XNOR gate whose inputs are the tapped out signals at the 15th and the 21st stages, respectively. If the pulse encodes data "0," the tapped signals will be different, and the decoder logic will give data "0." On the other hand, both signals will be the same for a pulse that encodes a "1." The positions for tapped signals have to correspond to the percent of duty cycles used in the PWM.

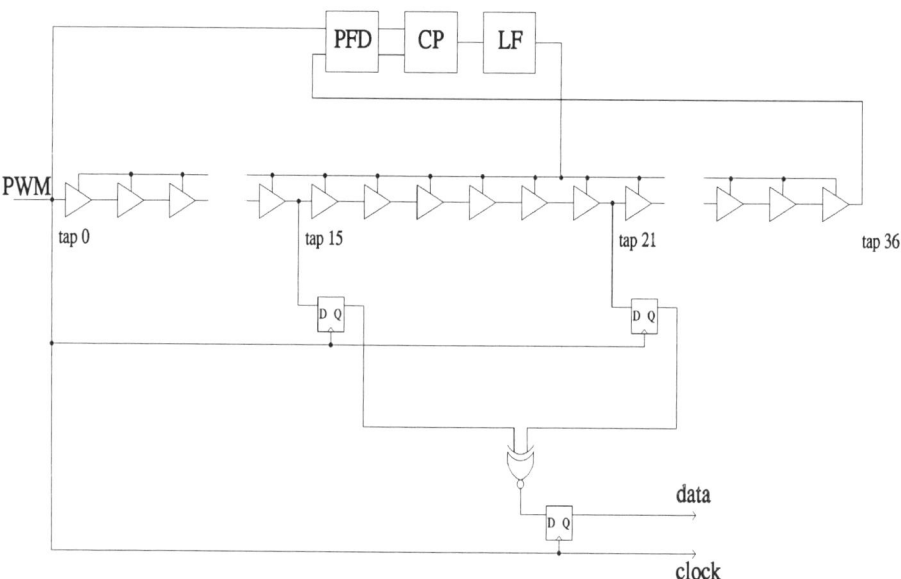

Figure 15. Chip functionality block diagram.

A challenge for the DLL design is to make the locked frequency as low as 25 kHz without consuming a large chip area. The schematic of the DLL circuit is shown in Figure 16. A three-state PFD is used with the additional delay at the reset path to reduce the dead zone effect. The voltage-controlled delay line is based on current-starved inverters made of low W/L transistors. The charge pump current is 3.5 µA provided by matched wide-swing current sources. A unity gain amplifier is included to prevent the ripple distortion of the control voltage due to charge sharing. The 200 pF loop filter capacitor is integrated on the chip. The initial condition of the DLL must be set up correctly to guarantee a correct locking. The very first input to the PFD after reset must be the rising edge of the PWM from the delay line. This can be accomplished by using a simple pulse swallow circuit, which would only ignore the very first pulse of the incoming PWM waveform before going to PFD. The loop filter capacitor is initialized to full charge when power is on. Consequently, the delay line starts with the smallest delay. The loop then initiates the discharge of the capacitor resulting in a decrease of the control voltage and an increase of the delay. This process continues until the delay is exactly equal to one period of the incoming PWM waveform. In this way, locking to a subharmonic of the PWM waveform is prevented. The DLL is always stable since it is a first order system.

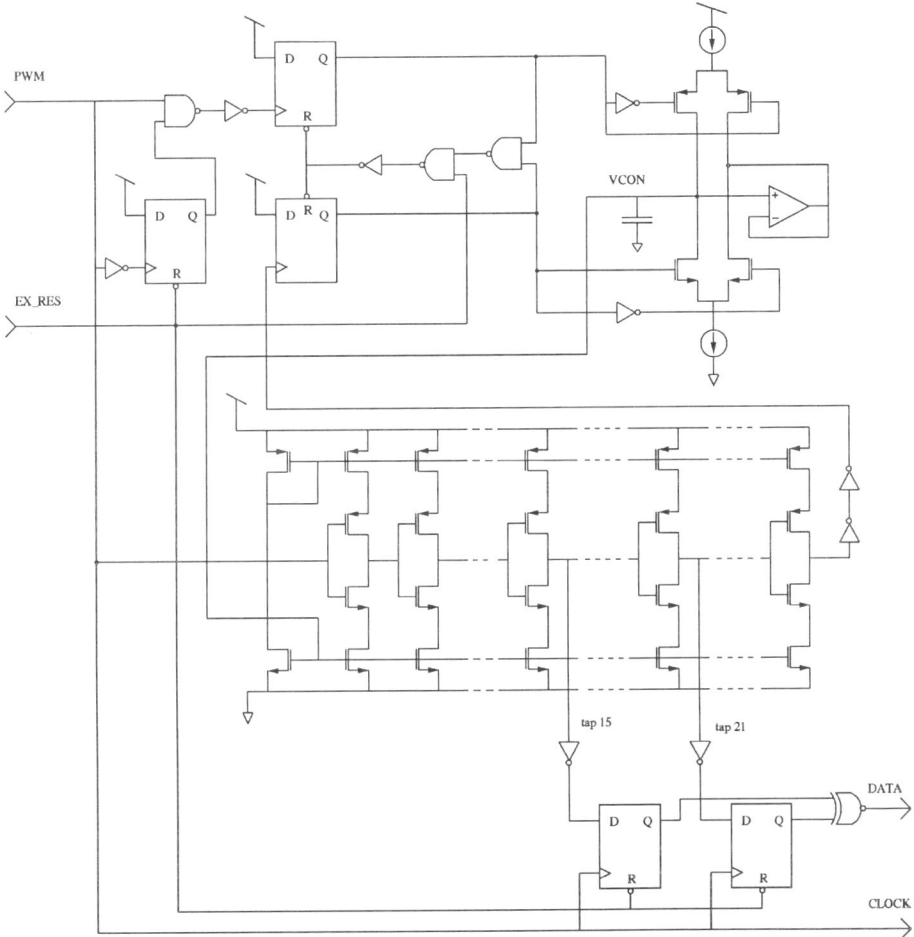

Figure 16. The schematic of the DLL circuit.

Synchronization circuit

The synchronization circuit implements the transitions of the device from the *power on state* through the *configuration state* to the *stimulus state*. It contains an eight-bit synhronization word detector circuit and an eight-bit counter as shown in Figure 17. Once the DLL begins producing the clock and data signals, the synchronization circuit examines the data until it detects the predefined eight-bit sync word that defines the beginning of the configuration state. This state lasts for 256 clocks periods. After 256 clocks, the synchronization circuit activates the R/C signal and the chip enters the stimulus state.

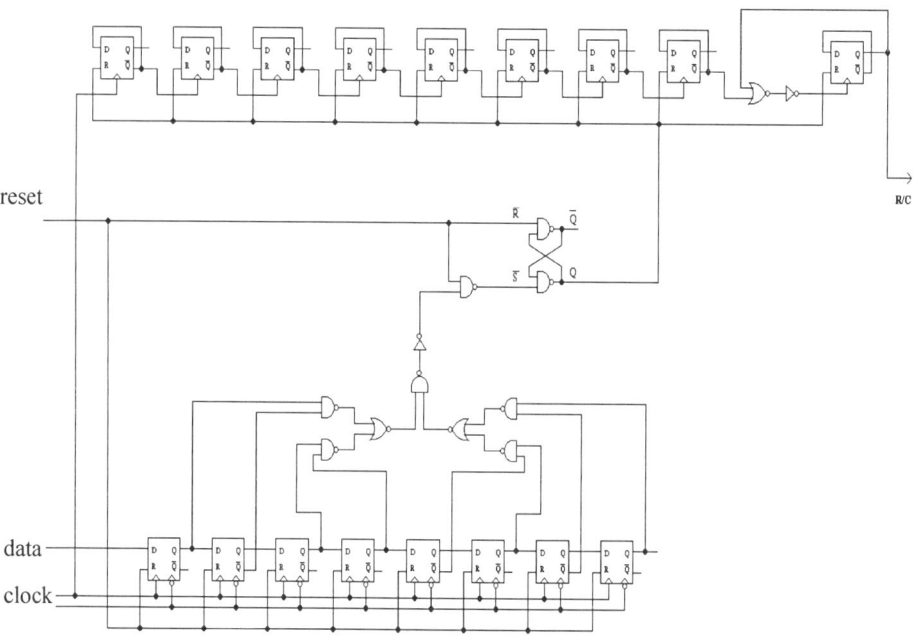

Figure 17. Synchronization circuit.

Timing generator and current control circuit

The timing of the stimulus pulse for all of the current drivers is centrally controlled and is specified in integer multiples of the master clock period. The timing control circuit contains 20 5-bit control FIFOs, an 80-bit timing FIFO, and combinational logic. The current control circuit is a two-bit current reference register and a bias generator circuit. The overall circuit diagram is shown in Figures 17 and 18. When the synchronization circuit detects the synchronization word and activates the R/C signal for the configuration mode, all the switches in Figure 18 are set to the C (configure) position. The 20 5-stage ring counters, the 80-stage ring counter, and the 2-bit reference current register are connected together as a single 182-stage FIFO. Being controlled by the recovery master clock for 256 clock periods, the FIFO serially shifts in 182 bits of configuration data by discarding the first 74 bits. The 182-bit data contains three fields. The first two bits define the bias voltage for controlling the reference current. The next 80 bits define the current pulse timing (A), and the last 100 bits define the firing sequences of the electrodes driven by each current demultiplexer. Each current driver controls a group of five electrodes, and the firing sequence for the group is specified by a five-stage ring counter When the counts of 256 clock periods are reached by the synchronization circuit, the R/C signal sets the switches at the R (run) position. The 182-bit FIFO is then regrouped as 20 5-bit control FIFOs, an 80-bit timing ring counter, and a 2-bit bias register. The chip is then ready to activate the stimulation mode. The image data is loaded into 20 4-bit data FIFOs (overall, it has 80 bits). The amplitude of each current driver is controlled by the 4-bit data FIFO, repesectively.

According to the 2-bit reference current register, a maximum current amplitude of 200, 400, or 600 µA for the wide-swing current source [9] is selected. A finer resolution could be obtained by the specification of the 4-bit data FIFO. The 80-bit ring counter is loaded with two blocks of consecutive ones which specify the width of the *anodic* and *cathodic* pulses and also the interpulse interval (dead time). During the stimulus state, the two blocks cycle through the counter five times per frame. The times that the block sweep past five particular counter tabs define the timing of the anodic and cathodic current pulse through the UP and DN signal generated by the combination logic. This provides the resolution for controlling the pulse width timing to be 1/400 frame. The associated logic produces COL_CLK for the 20 5-bit ring counters that no longer use the master clock after entering the stimulus state and PULSE_CLK used together with the image data to switch current sources between the bias voltage and GND in the stimulator circuits. Each 5-bit ring counter is loaded with a single one, and each controls the current demultiplexor by cycling through the five electrodes once per frame. Each counter can be configured so that any of the five electrodes is the first of each frame.

Current pulse stimulator circuit

There are 20 pulse stimulator circuits in the chip, and each of them supports a full-scale current value of 200, 400, or 600 µA. The current magnitude can be refined by a 4-bit linear amplitude control, achieving a resolution of 12.5, 15, and 37.5 µA. In our implementation, the selected current value is applicable all twenty stimulators during the configuration. The stimulator circuit is illustrated in Figure 19. Each stimulator consists of 15 parallel current drivers. Thus the resepective source of strength 8, 4, 2, and 1 is controlled by the corresponding four data bits in each protocol frame. Each source is controlled by the bit which specifies the connection of its gate to the bias voltage or ground. This method avoids the voltage overhead of series switching, thereby increasing the output voltage range. Due to the 10 kΩ tissue impedance, the current output experiences a voltage swing as large as 6 V. The current and cascode biases for the selected current range are created by a wide-swing cascode bias circuit and the required supply voltage overhead is minimized. The stimulus circuit can produce the 6 V output range with a 7 V supply. Cascode devices also improve the output impedance and linearity of control.

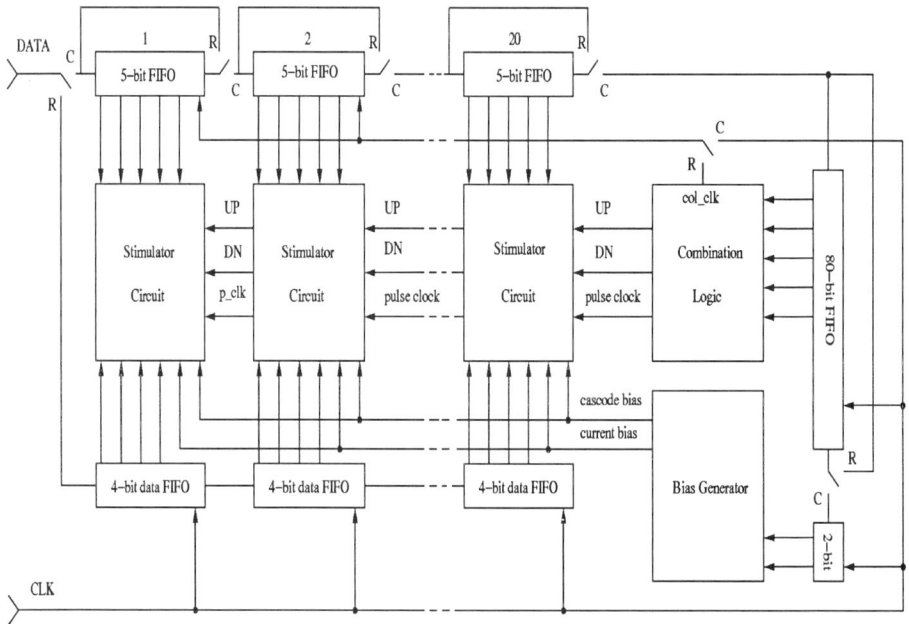

Figure 18. Stimulator generator circuit.

Directly creating biphasic current pulses requires dual supply rails spanning 14 V, as well as positive and negative current sources. A switch bridge circuit was designed to create a biphasic current pulse by only using a single current source with a 7 V supply voltage. It is implemented as part of the output demultiplexor and allows the electrodes to be connected to the stimulator with either polarity. Each demultiplexor is controlled by a 5-stage ring counter which sequentially activates the firing of the five electrodes per frame. To create a biphasic current pulse at E5, for example, the fifth tap of the ring counter would be activated. The UP signal turns on M1, M4 while M2, M3 remain off, allowing current to flow from A to B as an anodic pulse. Then the DN signal turns on M2, M3 while M1, M4 are off, and current flows reversely from B to A, creating a cathodic pulse. The other four non-selected electrodes are connected to the current return path through weak transmission gates to prevent the buildup of local charge in the retinal tissue.

Biasing circuit

The biasing circuit is shown in Figure 20. It is a threshold voltage referenced, self-biased circuit [6], [8]. The voltage reference is established from the interception point of the linear voltage-current relationship of R1 (50k resistance) and the quadratic voltage-current relationship of NMOS transistor M1. This gives a voltage reference independent from the supply voltage variation, which is mainly caused by the fluctuation of inductive coupling due to the movement of the eyeballs. Although the threshold voltage of the NMOS transistor is temperature dependent, it would not significantly affect the circuit, since the chip temperature is kept relatively constant and close to the body temperature. The drawback of this circuit, however, lies in the difficulty of fabricating precise resistances in CMOS technology.

The current of the biasing circuit is mirrored to six identical cascode transistors to form a reference current. The 2-bit bias voltage registers control switches on either two, four, or six cascode transistors, resulting in three reference current levels. The reference current flows through wide-swing biasing transistors, creating bias voltages for current sources in stimulator circuits.

3.3.2. Chip operation

The chip operates in three states: power-up, configuration, and stimulus. The operation is described subsequently.

Power-up

The power-up state is the initial state of the chip when a carrier signal is first applied to the primary side of the transformer. In the first phase, the carrier is applied without modulation for a few hundred milliseconds to allow the chip power rails to stabilize. An on-chip power on reset circuit provides a reset signal to ensure that the chip is always at a predefined state after power is applied.

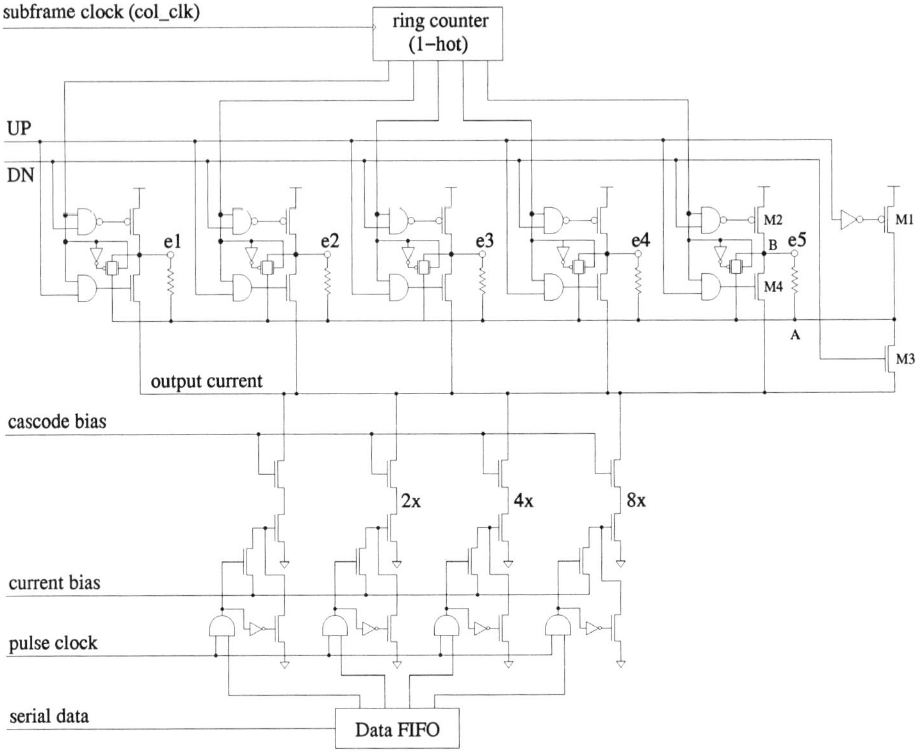

Figure 19. Stimulator circuit.

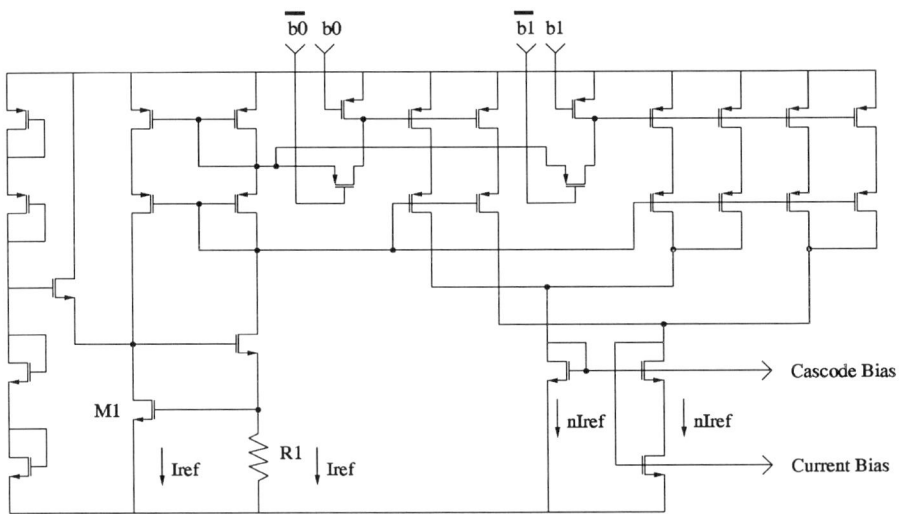

Figure 20. Bias generator circuit.

In the second phase, modulation of the carrier commences with at least a few hundred zeros. This phase ensures the stabilization of the demodulator and the lock of the DLL to the data clock. After the demodulator and DLL are running, the eight-bit synchronization word is checked so that the configuration state may be initiated.

Configuration

In this state, the timing generator and the current control circuit are configured such that the reference current, pulse timing, and firing sequence by a demultiplexer are defined by the 182-configuration bit as explained previously. This state lasts 256 clock periods.

Stimulus

After the power-up and configuration states, the chip is ready to stimulate the retinal electrodes. The image data is serially fed into the data FIFO at a constant clock rate. The data is grouped into 80-bit blocks that represent one fifth of a frame. The four data bits for each electrode are grouped consecutively with the most significant bit first. The order of the electrode data is determined by both the connection of the chip pins to the electrodes and the initial selection of the 20 demultiplexers. The chip remains in the stimulus state until an external reset is applied, or power is removed.

3.3.3. Measurement results

The prototype device was implemented in 1.2 μm CMOS technology. The die size is 4.7 mm × 4.6 mm. The minimum size is determined by the large number of bonding pads rather than the area of the circuits. The chip is designed such that it can be tested as a complete system or as separate subsystems.

Communication circuit

The chip is designed for one-way communication as a receiver. Although it is designed for a data rate ranging from 25 to 250 kbps, our measurements show that both the ASK and PWM demodulator circuits can operate up to more than 1 Mbps. At the very fast data rate, however, the modulation index needs to be increased up to 30%. It also shows that as long as the ratio of carrier frequency to the data rate is more than 40, they can be independent of one another. Figure 21 shows the measured communication waveforms, Ch1 is the DC envelope, Ch2 is the PWM output from the demodulator, and Ch3 is the recovered NRZ data. Note that there are two clock periods of latency between the NRZ output and the PWM input.

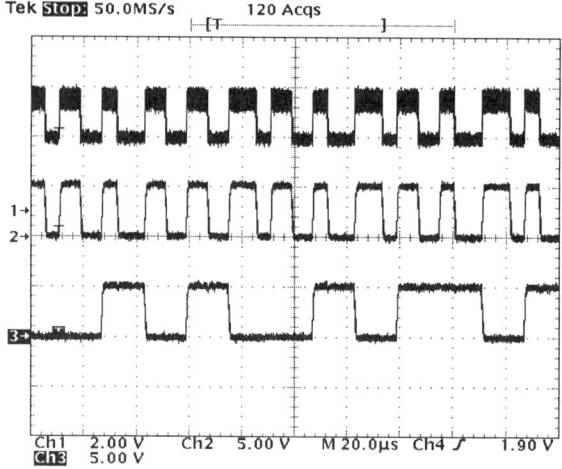

Figure 21. Measured communication waveforms.

Stimulator circuit

As described before, the stimulator circuit is capable of producing three full ranges of current amplitudes, namely 200, 400, and 600 µA through a 10 kΩ resistive load. In each range, there is 4-bit linear resolution or 16 different levels. Consequently, the current amplitude can be selected appropriately for individual patients in clinical testing. The ability to create the accurate charge-balanced, biphasic current pulse is the major concern. We characterize the performance of the stimulator circuit in terms of accuracy, linearity, and power supply sensitivity or the sensitivity to random variations in the inductive link, due to relative motion between the coils.

Accuracy

We measured the current output at the nominal supply voltage 7 V with a resistive load of 10 kΩ. The results show that both anodic and cathodic amplitudes are smaller than the nominal value in all three full scales. This apparently results from the smaller reference current. The reference current is the mirror of the biasing current, which depends on the resistor in a bias generator circuit. In this case, process variation makes resistance greater than design value. The matching between anodic and cathodic amplitudes is acceptable, as the mismatch error is less than 5%. With the built-in charge neutralizer switches at every electrode, the excess charge on the electrode can be neutralized quickly. Figure 22 shows example stimulus waveforms. It is composed of 15 stimulus waveforms from 3 stimulators, which stimulate 5 different amplitudes each.

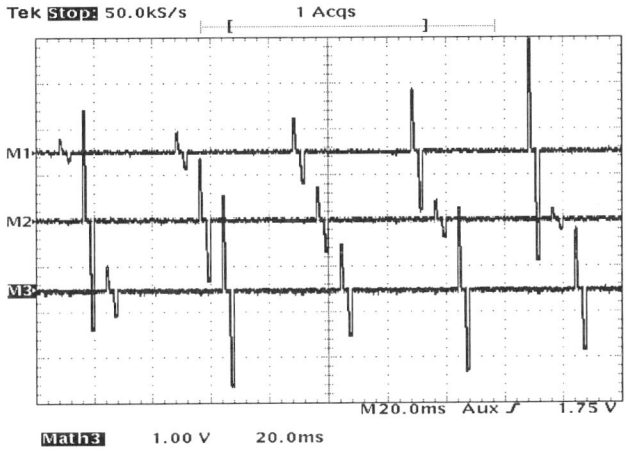

Figure 22. Measured stimulus waveform.

Linearity

In Figure 23, we plot the output current amplitude increasing by one LSB per step for all scales. Although the amplitude is smaller than the designed value, the DAC shows the linearity in all scales.

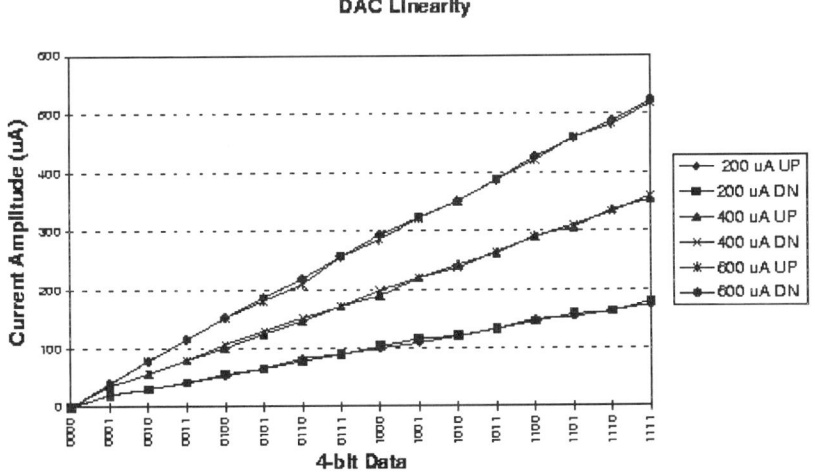

Figure 23. Linearity of DAC.

Power supply sensitivity

The variation of inductive coupling can affect the stimulator circuit in two different ways. One is the direct change of the power supply voltage, where the drain and source voltage (V_{ds}) of the current source is changed. This effect contributes the same result as the variation of the load (retinal tissue) from one patient to another patient. It may be alleviated by designing the current source with a high output impedance. In our design, we use a wide-swing cascode current source that gives the output impedance more than 2 MΩ.

The other effect comes indirectly through the bias generator circuit. The change of supply voltage can cause bias voltage variation which changes the gate-source voltage (V_{gs}) of the current source. The solution of eliminating this fluctuation is to use a biasing circuit that is less sensitive to supply variation. This is verified by varying the supply voltage from 6 to 9 V and measuring the output current. The plot of three full-scale output currents as a function of operating voltage is shown in Figure 24. The current amplitude is almost independent from supply voltage. The variation of amplitude over the range is less than 10%. Clearly, the circuit is able to maintain the acceptable current amplitude.

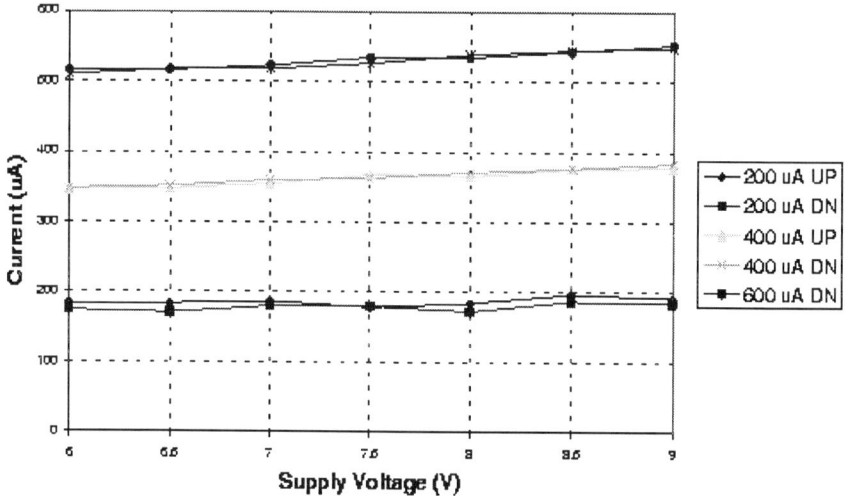

Figure 24. Full-scale output current as a function of operation voltage.

Power consumption

The total power consumption of the device comes from two parts, namely the power consumption of the stimulus chip itself, and the power dissipated into the load (retinal tissue). The power consumption in the stimulus chip depends on the image frame rate. In our application of retinal prosthesis, the frame rate is greater than 60 frames per second [1]. The power dissipation at 100 frames per second, corresponding to a data rate of 40 kbps, would be approximately 3 mW.

Depending on the pulse amplitude and the ratio of a pulse width to a frame period, the average power dissipation at the load impedance is calculated as an average power of a biphasic pulse period by the following equation:

$$P = NRI_{avg}^2 = NRA^2 \left(\frac{W}{400}\right)^2$$

where
N = number of driven electrodes
R = tissue equivalent impedance
$Iavg$ = average current for each electrode during the observation period
A = pulse amplitude
W = pulse width in clock periods
400 = number of clock periods per frame.

For the worst case scenario, all 100 electrodes are driven with the full 600 µA amplitude and a 25 clock-period pulse width (corresponding to one eighth of a stimulation period for counting both anode and cathode phases together, it is a realistic figure in our electrical stimulation experiment) to 100 of 10 kΩ loads, the average power is

$$P = 100(600\mu A)^2 (10k) \left(\frac{50}{400}\right)^2$$

This is equal to 5.6 mW. In this case, the highest power is dissipated by the chip, although it is unrealistic that all electrodes would be simultaneously fired. Based on a statistical assumption that an electrode is applied with a stimulus current by half of the observation period, a typical value is about one quarter of the worst case value, which is 1.8 mW. Combining both parts together could result in a total power dissipation of up to 5 mW.

The prototype device characteristics are summarized in Table 3. The die micrograph is shown in Figure 25.

Table 3. Chip performance specification and the measurement result

Technology	MOSIS's CMOS 1.2 µm
Die Size	4.7 × 4.6 mm
Carrier Frequency	1 – 10 MHz
Number of Current Generator	20
Number of Electrode	10 × 10
Data Rate	25 kbps – 250 bps[1]
Maximum Frame Rate	600 frame/sec
Amplitude Resolution	4-bit, 3 full-scale
Timing Resolution	1/400 of frame period
Power Consumption	5 mW @ 7 V and 100 frame/sec
Frame Size (image and configuration data)	400 bits

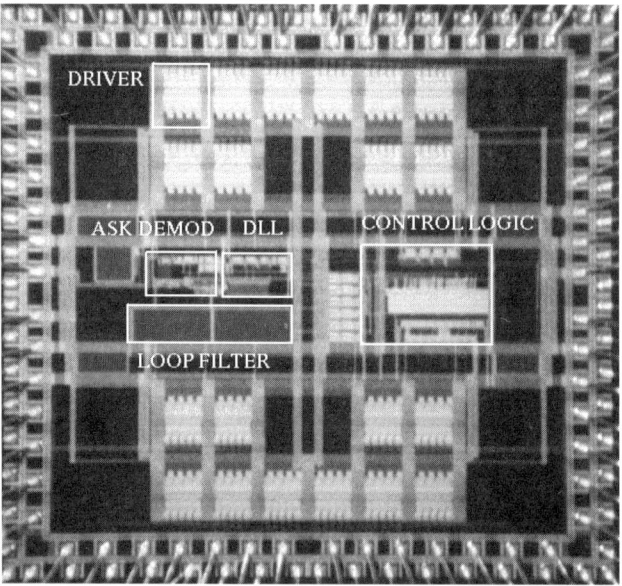

Figure 25. Die micrograph.

---

[1] Measurement results show that it works at 1 Mbps.

3.3.4. Design enhancement

The prototype chip behaved according to its design specifications, except for a small degradation of the current amplititude due to process variations. The communication circuit operates in a wide range of data rates up to 1 Mbps. This data rate is capable of supporting a 64×64 electrode array at 60 frames per second. In practice, however, it would be limited by the number of the I/O pads available at a specific chip area. Nevertheless, the ability to support a wide range of data rates allows for clinical testing with biphasic stimulating pulses at different frequencies and amplitudes, leading to a more detailed characterization of the relationship between visual perception and stimulation waveforms.

The current amplitude is smaller than the designed value, because there is a mismatch between the fabricated and simulated resistance values in the bias generator circuit as previously described. This kind of biasing circuit is susceptible to resistance values due to process variation, and it is useful for our application. In our case, rather than the absolute value, it is more critical to have the ability of generating a voltage reference which is less sensitive to supply voltage variation. In general, there is a 20% variation of the resistance value due to process variation. However, in practice there are two ways to correct this if the variation is beyond the tolerance. One is by trimming the resistors after the fabrication by the Focus Ion Beam (FIB) technique. The other is to design a set of resistors that can be externally programmed. Both methods may provide the desired resistor value.

This chip uses a simple synchronous protocol and timing control. After the chip is configured and enters the run mode, it continues to stimulate until it receives an external reset. This scheme requires only digital circuits with a small number of registers, making the chip less complicated and power consumptive. With more complicated digital circuits and on-chip memory, additional features may be included such as real-time reconfiguration, arbitrary pulse mode, and two-way communication.

Real-time reconfiguration
This allows the chip to change the configuration such as the timing, frame rate, and pulse amplitude while it is in the stimulus mode. One benefit is that patients will be able to tell the difference of each stimulus in a real-time manner.

Arbitrary pulse mode
Currently, the anodic pulse and cathodic pulse of a biphasic pulse are equal in both pulse width and current amplitude. However, with an arbitrary pulse mode, both anodic and cathodic pulses can be different in both amplitude and width as long as they both carry the same amount of charge if charge

balance is of concern. Also, it is possible to produce different types of pulse shapes other than a square wave.

Two-way communication

In clinical testing, the patient can directly provide verbal feedback regarding the stimulation. However, it is possible that the device itself can provide additional diagnostic information such as electrode status and retinal impedance by measuring the electrical signal at the electrodes and sending the information back as serial data to the primary side. Because this upstream data is a very small amount, the transmission can be a simple impedance modulating scheme. The impedance modulating scheme is based on the principle that a change in the impedance on the secondary side of the coil can change the effective impedance of the primary side.

3.4. Video camera and processing board

3.4.1. Extraocular CMOS camera and video processing

Standard technology can provide that which is needed for an image acquisition setup for a retinal implant. Usually, flicker fusion of individual frames of a movie appear continuous at a rate of 30 frames per second. This would lead one to believe that similar frame rates would be necessary for a retinal implant. However, because electrical stimulation bypasses phototransduction performed by the photoreceptors and stimulates the remaining retinal neurons directly, the flicker fusion rates are higher. In our group's tests in blind humans we have found the rate to be between 40 and 60 Hz [3], [12]. We will modify our camera input to accommodate this requirement, as a flickering strobe image is not appealing, let alone useful. Although color is not essential to be able to navigate or read, it is appealing and is missed by blind patients. We are in the process of gaining further understanding as to how different stimulus parameters elicit various colors, and we hope to convey the color information that our imaging system will be capable of delivering.

The CMOS image sensor offers the cost benefits of integrated device functionality and low power and volume production, and due to its compact size, it may be easily mounted on a pair of glasses. The extraocular video processor [48] will be implemented discretely using SRAM frame-buffers, an ADC, and a FPGA/EPLD. Reconfigurable FPGAs afford the flexibility of investigating the impact of various image-processing algorithms (including artificial neural networks) on image perception. This system will process the analog video signal from an off-chip monochrome CMOS mini-camera. Color mapping and indicial mapping provide further image data processing. An integrated, full-duplex RS232 asynchronous, serial communications port within the video processor will link the retinal prosthesis to a PC or workstation for configuration and monitoring. The video system will be endowed with an alternate test mode of operation, in which image input can be taken from the communications port instead of the camera. This will permit a selected still image to be transmitted from the PC to the video buffer for fixed pattern stimulation and biological monitoring in the early stages of development. A block diagram of the video processor is shown in Figure 26. All digital signals (Tx, Rx, and serial_data) are one bit wide.

Since the CMOS camera's spatial resolution is 320×240 and the retinal electrode-array dimension is far less at 10×10 to 25×25 (in the second to fourth generation MARC prototypes), the video signal will be subsampled to a 10×10 or 25×25 array using indicial mapping [30]. This is a lookup-based technique that can provide for complex spatial transformations of the image data, such as rotation about arbitrary angles, zooming in/out, translations, X/Y, U/V flipping (mirroring), masking, blanking, etc.

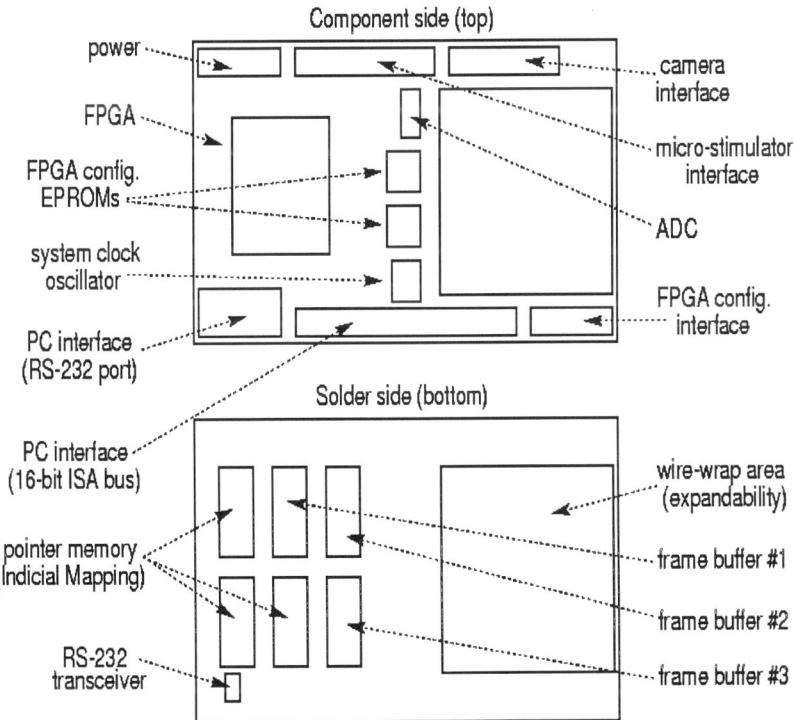

Figure 26. Block diagram of front-end MARC image acquisition system.

These transformations would be computed on a PC and then delivered to the video processor over the RS232 link. The novelty of this approach is that host intervention is required only when the mapping function is altered. Otherwise, the current transformation manifested in the map can be used via lookup. The initial imaging system need not have this feature, but as we gain more understanding on how to elicit more complex visual perceptions in conjunction with the doctors, future generations of the imaging system may include this feature as well.

These integrated features will provide the means for processing the visual information in a manner that will be meaningful to the MARC, and in later stages of testing the information will be transmitted via telemetry to the MARC. The specifications consist of a marriage between standard video protocols and the custom biological protocols required for effective retinal stimulation. The integrated circuitry in the preceding subsections has been designed and tested at NCSU, including the A/D converter and video buffer RAMs. The front and back of the recently fabricated video board is shown in Figure 27.

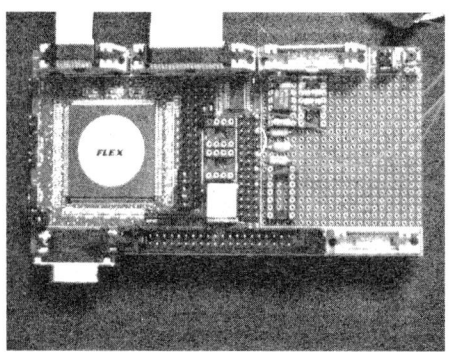
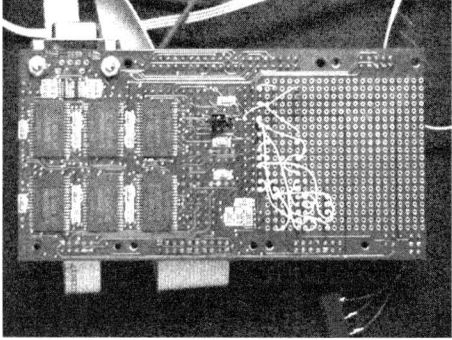

Figure 27. Front and back of video board. Block diagram is shown in Figure 11.

3.5. MARC RF telemetry

An inductive link consists of two resonant circuits, an external transmitter and an implanted receiver. The mutual inductance M is an important factor in the design of telemetric devices, as it characterizes how much of the original power can be recovered in the secondary coil. The MARC coil configurations are shown in Figure 28. As it is in our interests to make both the internal and external devices as small as possible, as light as possible, and as efficient as possible, it is also in our interests to maximize the mutual inductance between the coils. Efficient power transfer means smaller external batteries and less overall heat dissipation, as coil resistance generally rises with heat, further lowering the efficiency.

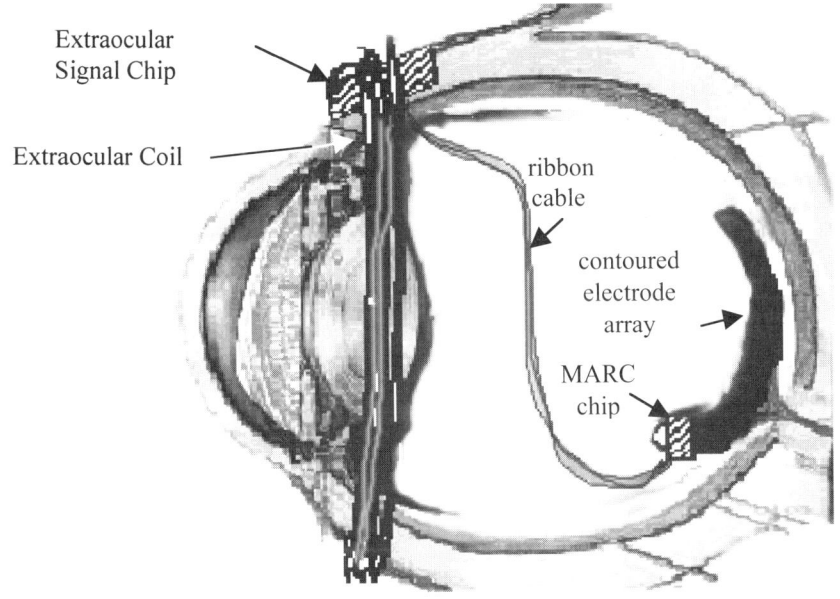

Figure 28. MARC surgical configuration. Secondary coils may also be implanted intraocularly for chronic devices.

The PWM-ASK telemetric information transmission protocol requires that the MARCs be designed to be sensitive to changes ranging from 10-20% of the post-rectified VDD. Thus, fluctuations greater than 10-20% in the coupling may be interpreted as intentional amplitude modulations sent from the external coil. For this reason, an important concern is how the coupling coefficient varies with small misalignments. As the MARC transmits information via amplitude modulation, fluctuations in the coupling constant could potentially be perceived as information by the processing chips. For these reasons preliminary studies [8] concerning the effects of random angular, lateral, and axial displacements have been conducted, and they have been found to be minimal when compared to the 10-20% fluctuations, which will mark the data. The patients will retain the freedom to adjust their glasses to maximize the performance of the device. For the MARC3, the external primary coil can be made as large or larger than the lens on a pair of glasses, but the secondary intraocular coil will be limited from 6×6 to 8×8 mm^2. For the MARC2, the secondary coil is implanted exterior to the eyeball, and it can thus be 2.5 cm in diameter, as it was for our feasibility experiments.

There have been numerous analyses and approaches to the design and fabrication of magnetic transcutaneous links [49], [50], [51], [52]. These studies have attempted to both accurately characterize and maximize the coupling efficiency and displacement tolerance in the design of the transmitting and receiving coil circuits. Because axial, lateral, and angular misalignment of the two coils leads to changes in the coupling efficiency, efforts have been made so as to make the transmission of energy via RF less sensitive to coupling displacements. Both power and data may be unexpectedly affected by random displacements, and thus minimizing the change in coupling coefficients resulting from random displacements also minimizes the chance that power or data will be interrupted.

MARC RF displacement tolerance experiments

For the MARC device, angular misalignment will occur for rotations of the eye, whereas lateral and axial displacements will occur for slight displacements of the pair of glasses. A study of these displacements is presented in Figures 29a-29c. As angular misalignment will be more common than either axial or lateral misalignment, we were encouraged to see that for small typical angular misalignments, from five to ten degrees, the post-rectification voltage (VR) across a 1 kΩ resistor varied by less than 1%, as shown in Figure 29a. Because the primary coil on the glasses is larger than the secondary coil within the eye, small lateral displacements result in small depreciations of VR. A lateral movement of 0.5 cm resulted in about an 8% drop, as seen in Figure 29c, which would be compatible with a functioning system, as we would consider a lateral displacement of 0.5 cm to be rather large. The lateral movement would result from a random movement of the glasses relative to the patient. A 0.5 cm movement will be unlikely to occur without the patient noticing it, and thus the patient will understand that any unexpected alterations in the perception quality were incurred by the motion.

Several different wire gauges, sizes of coils, and coils with different numbers of turns were used. The following graphs depict the data from the experiments where the primary coil was 5 cm in diameter while its inductance was L = 17 µH. It was made from twelve turns of #18 AWG wire. The secondary coil was 3 cm in diameter with an inductance of L = 15 µH, made from ten turns of copper #26 AWG bell wire. The primary coil was mounted on a pair of sunglasses and driven by a standard signal generator. Both the primary and secondary coils were subject to parallel resonance, and both circuits were tuned to 450 kHz. On the y axis is plotted the voltage across a 1 kΩ resistor after rectification, while upon the z axis is plotted the displacement or angle of rotation. The angular and lateral displacement experiments were conducted with a distance of 2 cm between the primary and secondary coils. This is the approximate distance between the primary and secondary coils of the MARC. For the MARC3, the secondary coil may be intraocular or extraocular, and thus it can be from 2-3 cm in diameter.

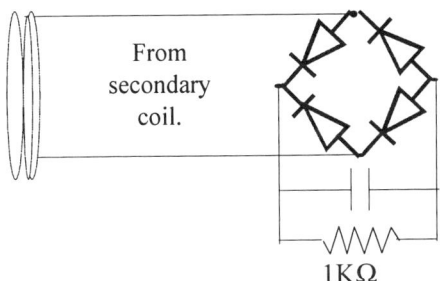

Figure 29a. Full-wave rectification of MARC2 telemetry signal. VR is measured across a 1 KΩ resistor.

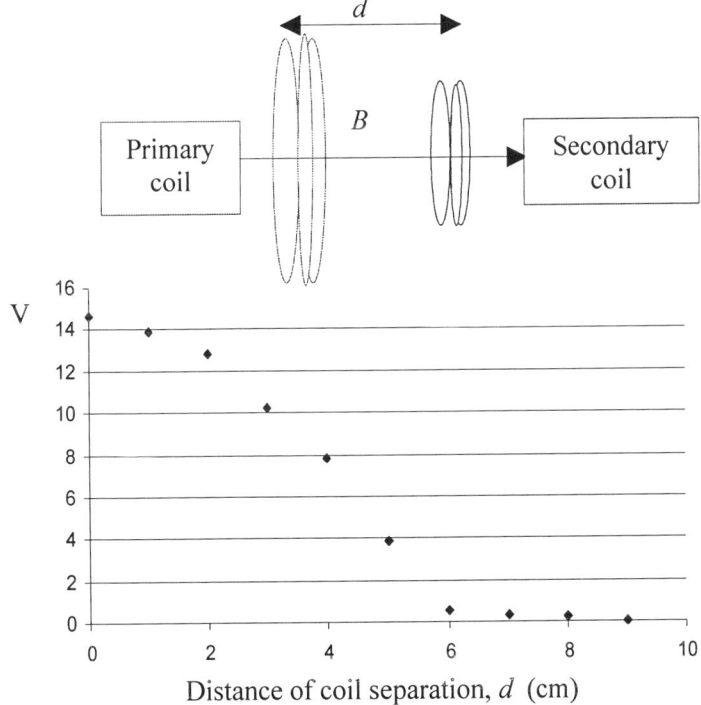

Figure 29b. Voltage vs. axial coil displacement, d.

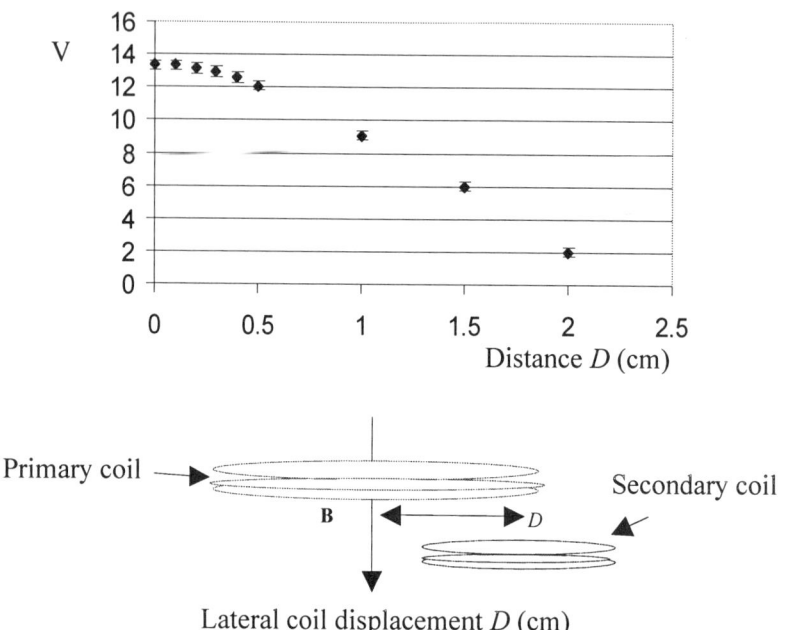

Figure 29c. Voltage vs. lateral coil displacement.

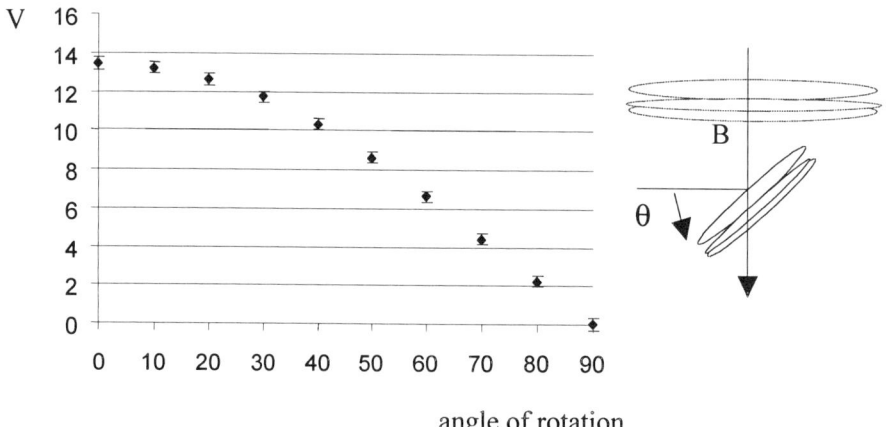

Figure 29d. Voltage vs. angular displacement.

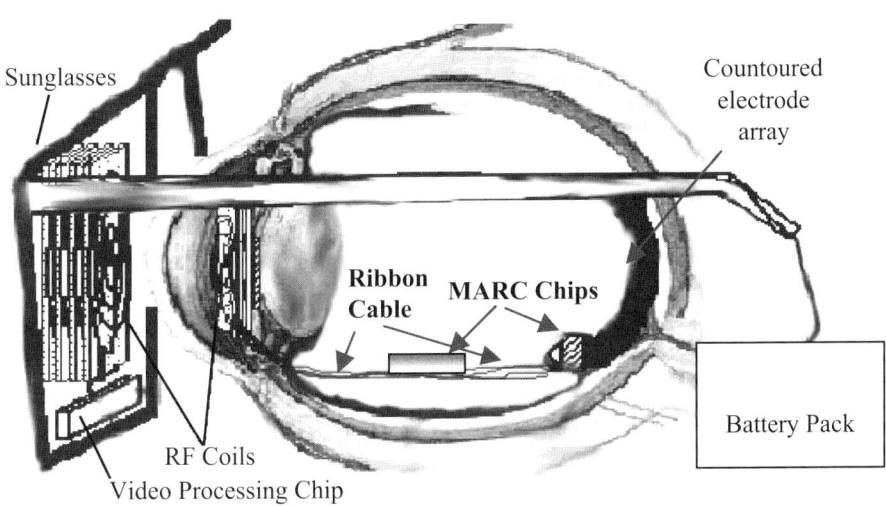

Figure 30. Third generation MARC system with intraocular secondary coils.

The primary coil will be driven by a Class E driver, similar to that which was developed by Troyk [53] and Schwan [54]. The Class E driver uses a multi-frequency load network, takes advantage of the impedance transformation inherent to the network, and is a switched-mode resonant driver; with the active device acting as a switch. The Class E point, or Class E mode, is characterized by voltage and current waveforms which are 180 degrees out of phase, and thus power dissipation, $P = I \cdot V$, in the primary coil is kept to a minimum. This results in nearly zero power loss in the switch. The Class E amplifier would be less taxing on an external battery, which could be made smaller.

Our preliminary experiments have demonstrated that ample, consistent power can be transmitted. The telemetry unit for the retinal prosthesis project is different from many other biomedical applications due to the eye structure, which severely limits the device size and power dissipation, as the retina cannot endure temperature fluctuations greater than 8°C. Simple heating and heat conduction calculations demonstrated that the maximum temperature rise from a continuous input of 80 mW into a 3×3×3 mm³ volume of water, surrounded on all sides by an infinite heat reservoir, would be less than 20°C [8]. Heat is conducted at a much faster rate than usual within the head, and the retina especially hosts a robust blood supply, implying that heat will be readily dissipated. The final telemetry unit must be hermetically sealed to avoid any interaction with the saline fluid within the vitreous humors, and methods of accomplishing the hermetic-sealing task have been presented in the design of the MARC4.

3.6. Electrode array design

The final design of the MARC device is largely contingent upon the material chosen for the electrode array. If the electrode array is fabricated upon a polyimide material, then the possibility for creating connecting ribbon cables upon the polyimide exists. One may also solder-bump chips or chip carriers to the polyimide, and one could fabricate an RF coil upon the polyimide. On the other hand, if the electrode array is fabricated upon a silicon or silicone gel substrate, then interconnecting ribbon cables will have to be wirebonded to the processing chips and the electrode arrays. The final design depends upon currently evolving technologies and methods of packaging chronic implants. Due to the contingency of the final MARC's design, in addition to offering solutions for the packaging and bonding, this chapter also serves to summarize the work performed so far, evaluate the options, and present a plan for future research.

3.6.1. The electrode array

From the chip engineering standpoint, the voltages required to drive the electrodes are an important factor, as they determine both how much power the chip may consume, and also what the minimum breakdown voltage on the chip can be.

Extensive research has been conducted by Humayun, Greenburg, Weiland, and colleagues concerning the optimization of the stimulating electrode array [55], [56], [57]. To determine the optimal current pulse width, height, and frequency targets for electrical stimulation of the retina, electrically elicited thresholds were measured in patients blind from photoreceptor loss as well as in normal and synaptically blocked frog retinas. Single-unit frog retinal ganglion cell (RGC) response latencies were observed to shorten while exhibiting a distinct discontinuity with increases in current, demonstrating the presence of another more sensitive cell. The observed strength-duration curves demonstrated that in contrast with other neural systems, different retinal cells have statistically different time-constraints. By exploiting these different retinal time-constants, long pulse duration can select deeper retinal cells and avoid the excitation of superficial RGC axons, permitting focal retinal stimulation. Currently, the optimal stimulating frequencies are being actively characterized.

Others have also evaluated electrode arrays [58], [59] for chronic neural stimulation in the cochlea as well as the central nervous system. The three materials most commonly utilized as the substrate upon which the metal for electrode sites is deposited are silicone rubber, thin 15-µm silicon, and thin

12-μm polyimide/Kapton. As for the metal from which electrode sites are constructed, the two most tested and used have been platinum and iridium oxide.

3.6.2. Current electrode array

The current electrode array utilized is hand-manufactured in Australia. It consists of platinum balls, which are flattened onto a piece of silicone rubber. The flattened platinum electrodes are each 400 μm in diameter, and the piece of silicone rubber is 0.5 μm in diameter. In recent discussions with Dr. Mark Humayun it was suggested that the current design is too heavy, as retinal area within a dog's eye directly beneath the electrode array began to degenerate within three months of being implanted. The electrodes will be housed in a silicon matrix, which is FDA approved. The entire electrode array will be fixed to the retina utilizing FDA titanium retinal tacks, which were designed by de Juan [22]. We have suggested introducing buoyancy so as to make the electrode array the same density as the surrounding fluid; moreover, our group is also contemplating utilizing a 5-10 μm Kapton/polyimide electrode array. Holes can be made in the non-conducting parts of the electrode array, to facilitate the ventilation of the retina beneath the electrode array. Patterning an electrode array onto Kapton seems far more feasible, but only the silicone rubber/platinum device has an established record of bio-compatibility at the moment.

3.6.3. Substrate for electrode array

We have focused our efforts on polyimide/Kapton substrates for several reasons. As already mentioned, the retina is very delicate and does not withstand mechanical trauma well. The silicone rubber substrate was the first choice because silicone is tolerated well in the eye, as demonstrated by our tests, but recent bio-compatibility studies in dogs suggests that the weight of the substrate may be a source of too much stress. A German team [60] has created different test structures on 15 μm light-weight polyimide, with oxide insulation layers and platinum as an electrode and interconnect metallization layer. This is much thinner and lighter than the 100-500 μm thick silicone rubber arrays. Another positive feature for RTV or polyimide is that foldable lens implants made out of silicone are FDA approved for intraocular use. Silicone arrays are also used in cochlear implants and have proven to be well tolerated. However, because the silicone electrode arrays are handmade and created by flattening balls of platinum or iridium upon slabs of silicone rubber, they are thicker and bulkier than the micromachined Kapton arrays. While the hand-fabricated arrays work fine for the cochlear implants, which only require six stimulating electrodes, it becomes impossible to develop or mass-produce handmade electrode arrays for even 12×12 pixel resolutions. Large arrays can be easily fabricated upon the Kapton utilizing standard photo-lithographic techniques. A one-piece Kapton design would allow for the following configuration, which would minimize the number of wirebonds, as the ribbon cables would be a part of the Kapton.

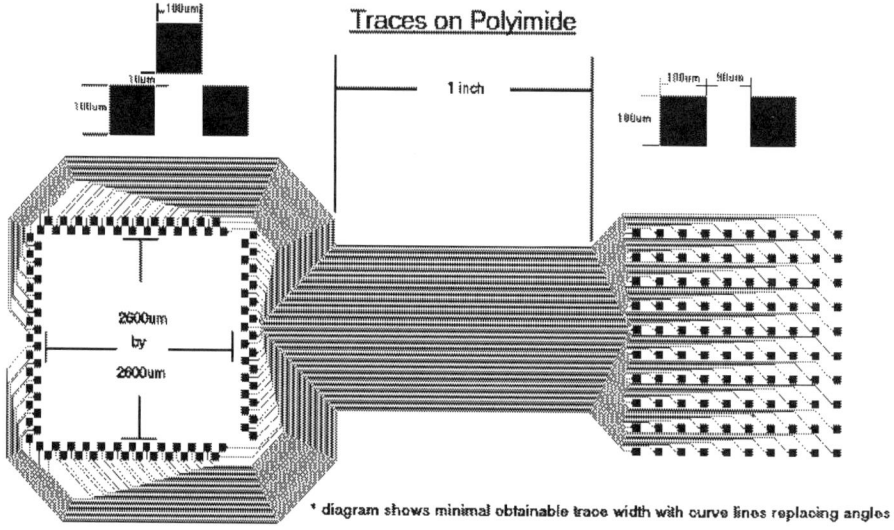

Figure 31. One piece polyimide chip mount, ribbon cable, and electrode array. A chip "landing pad" for flip-chip bonding is on the left, while a 10×10 electrode array is on the right.

Another benefit of using Kapton-polyimide is that much research has been conducted demonstrating its bio-compatibility and durability [61], even when implanted over a beating heart. Recently, there have been reports on the analytical performances of microelectronically fabricated ion sensors based on a flexible polyimide substrate (Kapton™, Du Pont). New sensor designs were tested using pH-sensitive PVC (polyvinyl chloride) membranes, cast from conventional and different modified PVCs, and incorporating various ionophores and plasticizers. In addition, these membranes have been subjected to bio-compatibility studies [62]. Membrane optimization has been carried out with macroelectrodes with a massive internal solution contact.

One final advantage of Kapton is that it allows for solder-bumping as opposed to wirebonding, which serves to minimize the overall chip area, as well as the surrounding Kapton substrate upon which it will be bumped to. Wirebonding requires more area for both the pads on the chip's border and the landing pads on the substrate. The currently proposed design, pictured in Figure 31, is a one-piece Kapton electrode array/Kapton cable/chip mount. We hope to marry the ongoing clinical successes with the Kapton electrode arrays with our research on the optimal electrode designs for retinal stimulation [63].

3.6.4. Electrode materials and geometry

Any material to be used for neural stimulation electrodes must meet several criteria [64]. It must be bio-compatible, it must be able to pass a large amount of current without producing harmful reactants due to the interface electrochemistry, and it must be durable enough not to dissolve. Two metals that meet these demands are platinum and iridium oxide.

The electrolytic and biological properties of electrodes of varying materials, sizes, and geometries have been studied by our team [65], [66], and we are currently considering either platinum or iridium oxide electrodes fabricated upon silicon, silicone rubber, or a polyimide such as Dupont's Kapton. To determine the retinal target of electrical stimulation, electrically elicited thresholds were measured in patients blind from photoreceptor loss and in normal and synaptically blocked frog retinas. Single-unit frog retinal ganglion cell (RGC) response latencies shortened and exhibited a distinct discontinuity with increases in current, demonstrating the presence of another more sensitive cell. Strength-duration curves demonstrated that in contrast with other neural systems, different retinal cells have statistically different time-constraints. By exploiting these different retinal time-constants, long pulse duration can select deeper retinal cells and avoid excitation of superficial RGC axons, permitting focal retinal stimulation. Similar results have also been noted in the human retina, meaning that the electrodes may be driven to selectively fire either the bipolar or the ganglion cells. These experiments will impact the MARC chip design in determining the minimum current, which may elicit a percept.

Greenburg *et al.* demonstrated that in practice dipole resolution is not significantly better than monopolar resolution in the configurations tested [66], [67]. When oriented parallel to the axon, dipole resolution was much worse. The human intraocular experiments did not show any difference in threshold or percept for monopolar vs. bipolar stimulation. These results suggest that the initial implant should employ monopolar electrodes. For maximum resolution the electrodes should be made as small as possible, but there is a limit imposed by the required amount of current for stimulation. Smaller electrodes imply higher current and charge densities. As the biological tissue and electrodes can be damaged by electrolytic reactions, which occur when certain charge densities are surpassed, there exists a theoretical limit as to how small electrodes can be.

Others have also evaluated electrode arrays [68], [69] for chronic neural stimulation in the cochlea as well as the central nervous system. At present, the three materials most often used as the substrate upon which the metal for electrode sites is deposited are silicone rubber, thin 15-µm silicon, and thin 12-µm polyimide/Kapton. As for the metal from which electrode sites are constructed, the two most tested and used have been platinum and iridium oxide. Greenburg states that conservative charge injection limits for chronic simple waveform stimulation with platinum are 100 $\mu C/cm^2$ per phase. For activated iridium oxide electrodes, the limit is an order of magnitude greater, at 1 $\mu C/cm^2$. The reason for iridium oxide's superior performance [70] has to do with the fact that iridium oxide is formed by growing a porous hydrous oxide layer on its surface when it is electrochemically activated in an electrolyte. The porous oxide, which can assume several oxidation states [71], increases the effective surface area, endowing the iridium oxide with a very high charge capacity as well as the ability to deliver large amounts of charge to aqueous solution. The material is also resistant to dissolution and corrosion during *in vitro* and *in vivo* stimulation [72]. Activation can also be used to reduce the impedance of iridium sites for use in recording applications.

The maximum size based on a 1 µC requirement for threshold stimulation of RP patients would be 0.01 cm^2 for platinum or 0.001 cm^2 for activated iridium oxide. For disk electrodes, these values correspond to minimum disk radii of 0.56 mm for platinum and 0.18 mm for activated iridium oxide. Thus the diameters for the electrodes should be about 1.1 mm for platinum and about 0.4 mm for activated iridium oxide disks. Smaller sizes may be achieved with holed electrode geometries when the electrodes are fabricated with photolithographically-generated patterns. Such electrodes could be fabricated upon a silicon or polyimide substrate.

Results from human tests helped determine the size and spacing of the individual electrodes in the array. The sites will be sized to handle a current pulse of 600 µA for 1 ms, as this is just above the threshold typically seen for electrical stimulation of a diseased retina. Human tests also showed that monopolar stimulation required less current than a dipole or coaxial configuration, with no loss of acuity (i.e., the size of the spot of light was the same). Single-unit recordings of frog RGCs (in response to electrical stimulation) determined the amount of retinal area that could be stimulated with a single electrode. This result helped define the spacing of the electrodes.

The electrode array design will consist of platinum disks on a Kapton substrate. A tantalum adhesion layer may be necessary since platinum has been known to delaminate from Kapton [73], and recent tests performed by Weiland on Kapton electrodes made by Nagle at NCSU have demonstrated this to be so [74]. Platinum has been chosen as a stimulating material for a number of reasons. It is bio-compatible and it can deliver large amounts of charge (400 µC/cm^2) [75] before the onset of irreversible electrochemical reactions. Platinum has a proven track record given its use in the cochlear implant, where platinum electrodes are subject to high intensity current pulsing for years with no apparent performance decrease. The exact dimension and spacing of the electrodes is shown in Figure 32.

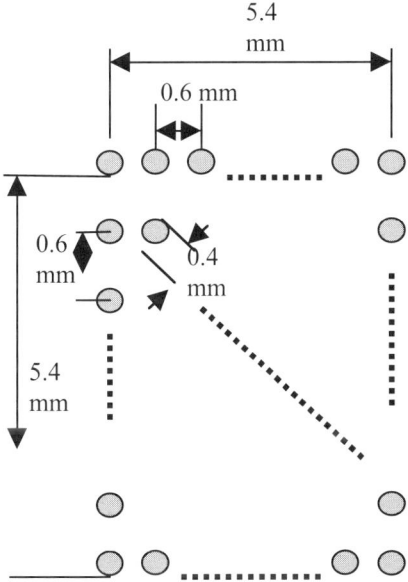

Figure 32. Weiland's dimensions and spacing of platinum disks in a 10×10 stimulation array. Iridium oxide will allow for smaller electrodes. Dimensions may be made smaller for holed geometries.

Iridium oxide [76] or possibly holed electrodes will be an alternative to platinum if higher charge injection limits are required, which will eventually be the case when the MARCs are fabricated to stimulate at higher resolutions. Iridium oxide has been shown to be bio-compatible in animals and to have a charge injection limit of 3 mC/cm^2, almost an order of magnitude higher than platinum. Iridium oxide [77], [78] electrodes could be formed in a number of ways. Iridium metal could be used in place of platinum in the electrode array fabrication process, and iridium oxide formed post-fabrication, by electro-chemically processing the individual electrodes. Iridium oxide can be electroplated to platinum electrodes if working iridium into the Kapton fabrication process proves troublesome. Alternatively, we could fabricate an array with protruding electrodes. This would bring the electrode surface closer to the target neuron, presumably lowering the current threshold. However, platinum disks remain our first choice for stimulating electrodes, since both iridium oxide and protruding electrodes require additional processing. In addition, iridium oxide doesn't have a proven track record of bio-compatibility in humans.

3.6.5. Electrochemical evaluation of stimulating electrode arrays

Electrochemical properties of electrodes are observed by using impedance spectroscopy and cyclic voltammetry [79], [80]. Impedance spectroscopy assesses various parts of the electrode tissue system by analyzing system impedance over a wide range of frequencies [81]. In this technique, small signal (<20 mV) sine waves are used to excite the test electrode. By studying the resulting current output, the impedance of the system at that specific frequency can be determined. Observing the impedance at several frequencies allows one to isolate the portions of the electrode-tissue system whose impedance is frequency dependent. Cyclic voltammetry (CV) measures electrode current while exciting the electrode over a large voltage range. CV data may be interpreted to provide details of the electrochemical reactions that may be occurring at the interface [82]. The two measurements can provide a complete assessment of the electrode's condition. Weiland states that if the structure of the electrode or ribbon cable is compromised in any way (e.g., leaks developing through the Kapton), it will most likely be accompanied by changes in the impedance and CV data. Thus, these two techniques will also be able to assess the implant's durability.

Kapton arrays with platinum electrodes will be fabricated for use as retinal stimulation electrodes. The devices will be tested *in vitro* and *in vivo* to ensure that they maintain stable electrical properties under conditions of chronic implantation and stimulation. Alternatives to both Kapton and platinum, including other polyimide materials and electrode arrays fabricated on silicon, will be explored further should Kapton or platinum not perform as expected.

3.7. Bonding and packaging

The final assembly of individual components discussed so far may be achieved within the double-sided MARC4, shown in Figures 33a-33c. This design satisfies the numerous engineering, packaging, and bio-compatibility requirements. The double-sided MARC4 provides a hermetically-sealed device with a minimum of feedthroughs. Only two AC feedthroughs are required for the secondary coil, and as the signal is AC, the feedthroughs are charge-balanced, and thus can be hermetically sealed with silicone gel.

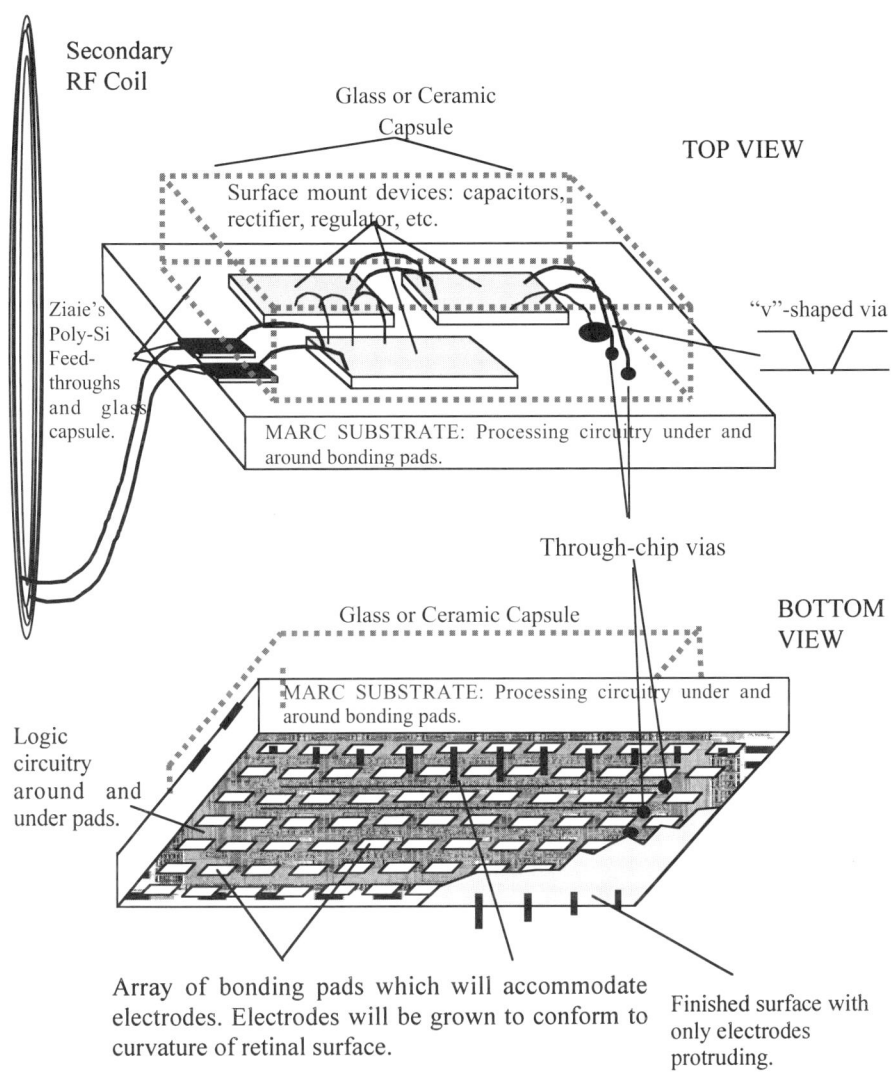

Figure 33a. Double-sided MARC4.

After rectification of the AC signal, the DC current is delivered to the other side of the chip by through-chip vias [83]. The through-chip vias can be far wider on the back of the chip, where the discrete rectification and regulation devices are mounted, than on the front, where the CMOS circuitry resides. Thus, depositing the through-chip via metalization should not be difficult in the "V"-shaped vias. A glass or ceramic [84] capsule is placed over the discreet-component surface mount devices and electrostatically bonded to the substrate and polysilicon feedthroughs Using Ziaie's [85] techniques. Electrodes will be grown to conform to the retinal surface.

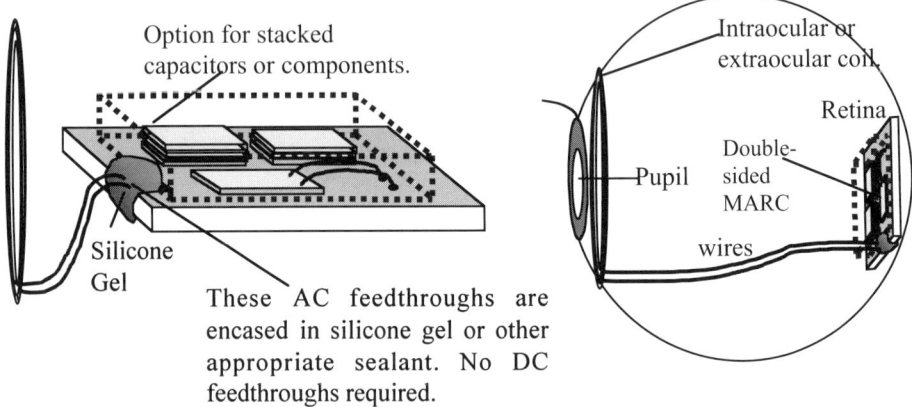

Figure 33b. Double-sided MARC4 hermetic sealing and positioning.

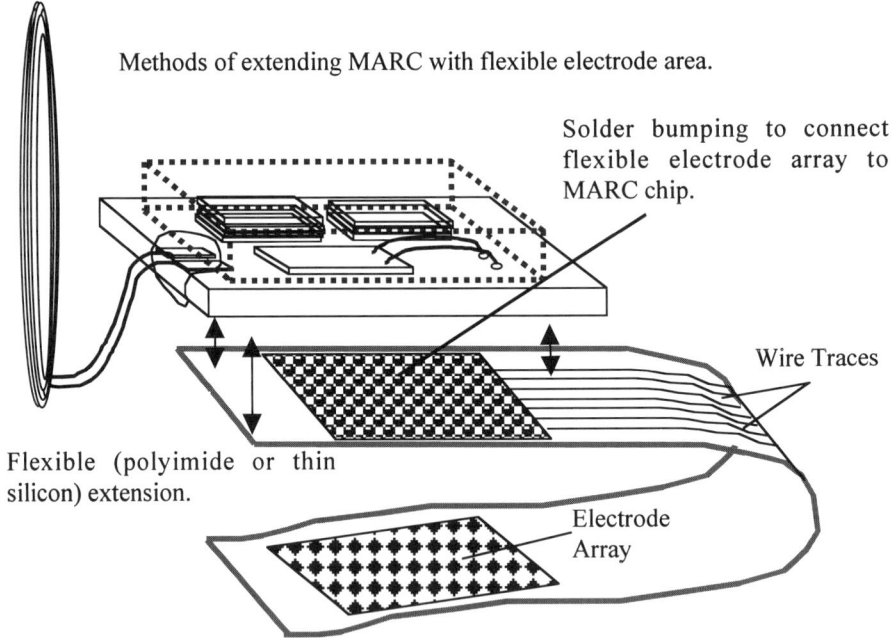

Figure 33c. Double-sided MARC4 connected to a flexible electrode array. Takes stress off retina and adds charge-balanced solder-bump connections, which may be hermetically sealed by silicone gel.

4. Conclusions

A retinal prosthesis system has been engineered in accordance with groundbreaking clinical data regarding retinal stimulation by electronic means. Its architecture contains two separat units: a front-end extraocular image-processing mounted on glasses, and the intraocular current stimulator device to be implanted within the eyeball. Data and power transfer between units are accomplished via inductive coupling. The prototype implantable device is capable of recovering data and power and generating a flexible stimulus waveform. The device has been fabricated in a 1.2 µm CMOS process. Test results show that the device performs as designed. The next step towards an artificial retinal prosthesis will be to develop the fourth generation MARCs which will be capable of driving 25×25 electrode arrays, and testing the devices for short periods within a human. The implications of this research may extend beyond this immediate project, as contributions are made to the overall field of chonically implanted prosthetic devices, telemetric monitoring and control, and hermetic packaging. The observations and clinical and engineering experiments performed should lend insight into the actual functioning of the human retina. The feedback gained by these studies should provide a vehicle for further understanding of the retinal perception process. A chronically-implanted retinal prosthesis is expected to be be realized in the near future.

Acknowledgments. This work was partially supported by the USA National Science Foundation under the Grants BES-9509758, BES-9808040.

References

[1] M. Humayun, E. de Juan, J. Weiland, G. Dagnelie, S. Katona, R. Greenberg, and S. Suzuki, "Pattern electrical stimulation of the human retina," *Vision Research*, 39:2569-2576, 1999.

[2] J. Brabyn, "Developments in electronic aids for the blind and visually impaired," *IEEE Engin. Medic. Biol.*, 4:33-37, 1986.

[3] G. S. Brindley and W. S. Lewin, "The sensations produced by electrical stimulation of the visual cortex," *J. Physiol.*, 196:479-493, 1968.

[4] D. A. Pollen, "Responses of single neurons to electrical stimulation of the surface of the visual cortex," *Brain Behav. Evol.*, 14:67-86, 1977.

[5] R. A. Normann, E. M. Maynard, K. S. Guillory, and D. J. Warren, "Cortical implants for the blind," *IEEE Spectrum*, 112:54-59, 1996.

[6] E. M. Schmidt, M. J. Bak, F. T. Hambrecht, C. V. Kufta, D.K. O'Rourke, and P. Vallabhnath, "Feasibility of a visual prosthesis for the blind based on intracortical microstimulation of the visual cortex," *Brain*, 119:507-522, 1996.

[7] W. Liu, E. McGucken, K. Vichiechom, M. Clements, E. De Juan, and M. Humayun, "Dual unit retinal prosthesis," *IEEE EMBS97* Conference, 1997.

[8] M. Humayun, E. de Juan, Jr., G. Dagnelie, R. J. Greenburg, R. H. Propst, and H. Phillips, "Visual perception elicited by electrical stimulation of retina in blind humans," *Arch. Ophthalmol.*, 114:40-46, 1996.

[9] E. Zrenner, K. Miliczek, V. Gabel, H. Graf, E. Guenther, H. Hammerle, B. Hoefflinger, K. Kohler, W. Nisch, M. Schubert, A. Stett, S. Weiss, "The development of subretinal microphotodiodes for replacement of degenerated photoreceptors," *Ophthalmic Res.*, 29:269-280, 1997.

[10] J. Wyatt and J. F. Rizzo, "Ocular implants for the blind," *IEEE Spectrum*, 112:47-53, 1996.

[11] R. Eckmiller, "Learning retina implants with epiretinal contact," *Ophthalmic Res.*, 29:281-289, 1997.

[12] A.Y. Chow and V.Y. Chow, "Subretinal electrical stimulation of the rabbit retina," *Neurosci. Lett.*, 225:13-16, 1997.

[13] J. Heckenlively, J. Boughman, and L. Friedman, "Diagnosis and classification of retinitis pigmentosa," in *Retinitis Pigmentosa*, J. R. Heckenlively (Ed.), Philadelphia, PA, JB Lippincott; 21, 1988.

[14] J.L. Stone, W.E. Barlow, M.S. Humayun, E. de Juan, Jr., and A.H. Milam, "Morphometric analysis of macular photoreceptors and ganglion cells in retinas with retinitis pigmentosa," *Arch. Ophthalmol.*, 110:1634-1639, 1992.

[15] A. Santos, M.S. Humayun, E. de Juan, R.J. Greenburg, M.J. Marsh, I.B. Klock, and A.H. Milam, "Preservation of the inner retina in retinitis pigmentosa," *Arch Ophthalmol.*, 115: 511-515, 1997.

[16] E.D. Juan, Jr., M. S. Humayun, and H. D. Phillips, "Retinal Microstimulation," US Patent #5,109,844, 1993.

[17] M. Humayun, "Is Surface Electrical Stimulation of the Retina a Feasible Approach Towards the Development of a Visual Prosthesis?" BME Ph.D. Dissertation, University of North Carolina at Chapel Hill, Chapel Hill, NC, 1992.

[18] M. S. Humayun, E. D. Juan, Jr., G. Dagnelie, R. J. Greenberg, R. H. Propst, and H. Phillips, "Visual perception elicited by electrical stimulation of retina in blind humans," *Arch. Ophthalmol*, 114: 40-46, January 1996.

[19] D.J. Anderson, K. Najafi, S.J. Tanghe, D.A. Evans, K.L. Levy, J.F. Hetke, X. Xue, J.J. Zappia, and K.D, Wise, "Batch-fabricated thin-film electrodes for stimulation of the central auditory system," *IEEE Trans. Biomed. Eng.*, 36 (7): July 1989.

[20] V.V. Cosofret, , M. Erdosy, T. Johnson, R.P. Buck, "Microfabricated sensor arrays sensitive to pH and K+ for ionic distribution measurements in the beating heart," *J. Biomed. Matter. Res.*, 1994.

[21] E. Linder, V.V. Cosofret, M. Erdosy, R.P. Buck, W.J. Kao, J.M. Anderson, E. Linder, and M.R. Neuman, *J. Biomed. Matter. Res.*, 1994.

[22] J. deJuan, B.W. McCuen, and R. Machemer, "The use of retina tacks in the repair of complicated retinal detachments," *Am. J. Ophthalmol.*, 102:20-24, 1986.

[23] J.F. Rizzo, M. Socha, D. Edell, B Antkowiak, andD. Brock, "Development of a silicon retinal implant: surgical methods and mechanical design," *Invest. Opthalmol. Vis. Sci.*, 34:1535, 1994.

[24] M.S. Humayun, E. De Juan, J.D. Weiland, S. Suzuki, G. Dagnelie, S.J. Katona, and R.J. Greenberg, "Visual Perceptions Elicited in Blind Patients by Retinal Electrical Stimulation: Understanding Artificial Vision," Program #4155, Session Title: Retinal Prosthesis II, *The Association for Research in Vision and Ophthalmology Conference*, May 1998.

[25] R.J. Greenberg, M.S. Humayun, and E. de Juan, "Different Cellular Time-Constants Allows Selective Electrical Stimulation of Retinal Neurons," Program #4159, Session Title: Retinal Prosthesis II, *The Association for Research in Vision and Ophthalmology Conference*, May 1998.

[26] S. Suzuki, M.S. Humayun, A.B. Majji, J.D. Weiland, S.A. D'anna, and E. de Juan, "Tolerance of Silicone/Platinum Electrodes Implanted for Long-Term in Dogs," Program #4157, Session Title: Retinal Prosthesis II, *The Association for Research in Vision and Ophthalmology Conference*, May 1998.

[27] P.R. Troyk and M.A. Schwan, "Closed-Loop Class E Transcutaneous Power and Data Link for Microimplants," *Transactions on Biomedical Engineering*, 39(6): 589-599, June 1992.

[28] S. J. Tanghe, K. Najafi, and K. D. Wise, "A planar IrOx multichannel stimulating electrode for use in neural prosthesis," *Sensors and Actuators*, B1:464-467, 1990.

[29] Weiland, J.D., "Electrochemical Properties of Iridium Oxide Stimulating Electrodes," Ph.D. Dissertation, University of Michigan, 1997.

[30] W. Liu, E. McGucken, K. Vichiechom, M. Clements, E. De Juan, and M. Humayun, "Dual unit retinal prosthesis," *IEEE EMBS97*.

[31] M. Clements, K. Vichiechom, C. Hughes, W. Liu, E. McGucken, C. Demarco, J. Mueller, M. Humayun, and E. de Juan, "An Implantable Neuro-stimulator Device for a Retinal Prosthesis," *1999 ISSCC*, San Francisco, February 15 - 17th, 1999.

[32] E. McGucken, "Multiple Unit Artificial Retina Chipset to Benefit the Visually Impaired and Enhanced CMOS Phototransistors," Physics Ph.D. Dissertation, University of North Carolina at Chapel Hill, North Carolina, 1998.

[33] M. S. Humayun, E. D. Juan, Jr., G. Dagnelie, R. J. Greenberg, R. H. Propst, and H. Phillips, "Visual perception elicited by electrical stimulation of retina in blind humans," *Arch. Ophthalmol*, 114: 40-46, January 1996.

[34] W. Dawson and N. Radtke, "Electrical stimulation of the retina by indwelling electrodes," *Invest. Opthalmol. Vis. Sci.*, 16:249-252, 1977.

[35] D. Crapper and W. Noell, retinal excitation and inhibition from direct electrical stimulation," *Journal Neurophysiology*, 26:924-927, 1963.

[36] M. Humayun, "Is Surface Electrical Stimulation of the Retina a Feasible Approach Towards the Development of a Visual Prosthesis?" Ph.D. Dissertation, UNCCH BME, 1992.

[37] A. Chow, "Subretinal Prosthesis Device," U.S. Patent no. 5,016,633.

[38] Michelson, "Retinal Prosthesis Device," U.S. Patent no. 4,628,933.

[39] J. Wyatt "*Silicon Retinal Implant to Aid Patients Suffering from Certain Forms of Blindness,*" MIT Progress Report, 1994.

[40] T. Yagi, *et al.*, "Development of Artificial Retina Using Cultured Neural Cells and Photoelectric Device: A Study on Electric Current with Membrane Model,"

Proceedings of The 4th International Conference on Neural Information Processing (ICONIP '97), 1997.
[41] T. Stieglitz, H. Beutel, R. Keller, and C. Blau, "Development of Flexible Stimulation Devices for a Retinal Implant System," Proc. IEEE EMBS Conf., 1997.
[42] A. Chow, "Subretinal Prosthesis Device," U.S. Patent no. 5,016,633.
[43] R. Michelson, "Retinal Prosthesis Device," U.S. Patent no. 4,628,933.
[44] J. Wyatt, "Silicon Retinal Implant to Aid Patients Suffering from Certain Forms of Blindness," *MIT Progress Report*, 1994.
[45] J. Rizzo and J.L. Wyatt, "Prospects for a visual prosthesis", *Neuroscientist*, 3: 251-262, July 1997.
[46] T. Yagi et al., "Development of Artificial Retina using Cultured Neural Cells and Photoelectric Device: A Study on Electric Current with Membrane Model," *Proceedings of the 4th International Conference on Neural Information Processing* (ICONIP'97), 1997.
[47] T. Stieglitz, H. Beutel, R. Keller, and C. Blau, "Development of Flexible Stimulation Devices for a Retinal Implant System," *IEEE EMBS*, 1997.
[48] S. Demarcos, "Video Processing for the MARC," *NCSU Technical Report*, NCSU, January 1998.
[49] W. Heetderks, "RF powering of millimeter- and submillimeter-sized neural prosthetic implants," *IEEE Trans. Biomed. Eng.*, BME-35:323-327, May 1998.
[50] N. Donaldson and T. Perkins, "Analyisis of resonant coupled coils in the design of radio frequency transcutaneous links," *Med. Biol. Eng. Comput.*, 21:612-627, September 1983.
[51] D. Aalbraith, M. Soma, and R. White, "A wide-band efficient inductive transdermal power and data link with coupling insensitive gain," *IEEE Trans. Biomed. Eng.*, BME-34:276-282, April 1987.
[52] M. Soma, D. Galbraith, and R. White, "Radio-frequency coils in implantible devices: misalignment analysis and design procedure," *IEEE Trans. Biomed. Eng.*, BME-34:276-282, April 1987.
[53] P. Troyk and M. Schwan, "Closed-loop class E transcutaneous power and data link for microimplants," *Trans. Biomed. Eng.* 39(6)589-599, June 1992.
[54] N. Sokal and A. Sokal, "Class E—a new class of high-efficiency tuned single-ended switching power amplifiers," *IEEE J. Solid-State Circ.*, 10:168-176, June 1975.
[55] R.Greenburg, M. Humayun, S. Mainigi, E. and de Juan, Jr., "*A Computational Model of Electrical Stimulation of the Retinal Ganglion Cell, Department of Biomedical Engineering*," Technical Report (Also: Greenburg's Ph.D. dissertation), Johns Hopkins University, Baltimore, MD.
[56] R. Greenburg, M. Humayun, S. Mainigi, E. and de Juan, Jr,. "*Selective Electrical Stimulation of Retinal Neurons by Varying Stimulus Pulse Duration, Department of Biomedical Engineering*," Technical Report (Also: Greenburg's Ph.D. dissertation), Johns Hopkins University, Baltimore, MD.
[57] J. Weiland, "*Electrochemical Properties of Iridium Oxide Stimulating Electrodes*," Ph.D. dissertation, University of Michigan, 1997.

[58] J. Ranck, "Which elements are excited in electrical stimulation of mammalian central nervous system: a review," *Brain Res.,* 98:417-440, 1975.

[59] M Humayun, R. Propst, E. de Juan, Jr., K. McCormick, and D. Hickinbotham, "Bipolar surface electrical stimulation of the vertebrate retina," *Arch. Opthalmol.,* 112:110-116, 1994.

[60] R. Greenburg, M. Humayun, N. Jafari, and E. de Juan, *"Electrode Geometry Design for a Retinal Prosthesis,"* Technical Report (Also: Greenburg R., Doctoral dissertation, The Wilmer Eye Institute, Johns Hopkins University), 1998.

[61] V. Cosofret, M. Erdosy, T. Johnson, and R. Buck, "Microfabricated sensor arrays sensitive to pH and K+ for ionic distribution measurements in the beating heart," *J. Biomed. Matter. Res.,* 1994.

[62] E. Linder, V.V. Cosofret, M. Erdosy, R.P. Buck, W.J. Kao, J.M. Anderson, E. Linder, and M.R. Neuman, *J. Biomed. Mater. Res.,* 1994

[63] R. J. Greenburg, M. S. Humayun, S. Mainigi, and E. de Juan, Jr., *"A Computational Model of Electrical Stimulation of the Retinal Ganglion Cell,"* research report, Department of Biomedical Engineering, The Johns Hopkins University, Baltimore, MD.

[64] S.B. Brummer, L.S. Robblee, F.T. Hambrecht, "Criteria for selecting electrodes for electrical stimulation: theoretical and practical considerations," *Ann. N.Y. Acad. Sci.,* 405:159-171, 1983.

[65] R. J. Greenburg, M. S. Humayun, S. Mainigi, E. and de Juan, Jr., *"A Computational Model of Electrical Stimulation of the Retinal Ganglion Cell,"* Research Report, Department of Biomedical Engineering, The Johns Hopkins University, Baltimore, MD.

[66] R. J. Greenburg, M.S. Humayun, S. Mainigi, and E. de Juan, Jr. *"Selective Electrical Stimulation of Retinal Neurons By Varying Stimulus Pulse Duration,"* Research Report, Department of Biomedical Engineering, The Johns Hopkins University, Baltimore, MD.

[67] T. Stieglitz, H. Beutel, R. Keller, and C. Blau, "Development of Flexible Stimulation Devices for a Retinal Implant System," *IEEE EMBS,* 1997.

[68] J.B. Ranck, "Which elements are excited in electrical stimulation of mammalian central nervous system: a review," *Brain Res.*, 98:417-440, 1975.

[69] M. Humayun, R. Propst, E. de Juan, Jr., K. McCormick, and D. Hickinbotham, "Bipolar surface electrical ztimulation of the vertebrate retina," *Arch. Opthalmol.,* 112:110-116, 1994.

[70] Center For Neural Communication Technology, University of Michigan, http://www.engin.umich.edu/facility/cnct/activ.html

[71] S Gottesfeld and J. McIntyre, "Electrochromism in anodic iridium oxide films," *J. Electrochem. Soc.,* 126:742-750, 1979.

[72] W.F. Agnew, T.G.H. Yuen, D.B. McCreery, and L.A. Bullara, "Histopathologic evaluation of prolonged intracortical electrical stimulation", *Exp. Neurol.* 92:162-185, 1986.

[73] S. Shamma-Donoghue, G. May, N. Cotter, R. White, and F. Simmons, "Thin-film multielectrode arrays for a cochlear prosthesis, " *IEEE Trans. Elec. Devices,* 29 (1), January 1982.

[74] J. Weiland and T. Nagle, *private communication,* 1999.
[75] S. Brummer, L.S. Robblee, and F.T. Hambrecht, "Criteria for selecting electrodes for electrical stimulation: theoretical and practical considerations," *Ann. N.Y. Acad. Sci.* 405:159-171, 1983.
[76] L. S. Robblee and T. L. Rose, "Electrochemical guidelines for selection of protocols and electrode materials for neural stimulation," in *Neural Prostheses, Fundamental Studies,* W. F. Agnew and D. B. McCreery (Eds.), New Jersey: Prentice Hall, 1990.
[77] L.S. Robblee, J.L. Lefko, and S.B. Brummer, "Activated Ir: an electrode suitable for reversible charge injection in saline solution," *J. Electrochem. Soc.*, 731-733, March 1983.
[78] S. J. Tanghe, K. Najafi, and K. D. Wise, "A planar irOx multichannel stimulating electrode for use in neural prosthesis," *Sensors and Actuators,* B1:464-467, 1990.
[79] Weiland, J.D., "Electrochemical Properties of Iridium Oxide Stimulating Electrodes," *Ph.D. dissertation,* University of Michigan, 1997.
[80] D.J. Anderson, K. Najafi, S.J. Tanghe, D.A. Evans, K.L. Levy, J.F. Hetke, X. Xue, J.J. Zappia, and K.D. Wise, "Batch-fabricated thin-film electrodes for stimulation of the central auditory system, " *IEEE Trans. Biomed. Eng.*, 36(7): July 1989.
[81] J.R. Macdonald, *Impedance Spectroscopy: Emphasizing Solid Materials and Systems,* John Wiley & Sons, New York, 1987.
[82] U.M. Twardoch, "Integrity of ultramicro-stimulation electrodes determined from electrochemical measurements, " *J. Applied Electrochem.*, 24: 1994
[83] O. Leistiko, The waffle: a new photovoltaic diode geometry having high efficiency and backside contacts, *First WCPEC,* Hawaii, December 5, 1994.
[84] P.R. Troyk, Multi-Channel Transcutaneous Cortical Stimulation System, *NIH Progress Report,* Contract # N01-NS-7-2365, 1998.
[85] B. Ziaie and J.A. Von Arx, "A hermetic glass-silicon micropackage with high-density on-chip feedthroughs for sensors and actuators," *J. Microelectromechanical Systems,* 5(3), September 1996.

Chapter 3

Intelligent techniques in hearing rehabilitation

Christian Berger-Vachon

"Intelligent techniques" in deafness rehabilitation is a concept not easy to introduce. Language belongs to the higher functions of Man, which are still very mysterious, despite recent dramatic advances. As much as we can, we must leave to humankind what belongs to humankind. In other words, intelligent techniques in deafness rehabilitation should be a compensation of deficiencies – provided we know them.

First, we will introduce some basic knowledge about the auditory system, in order to understand its working. We will focus on the peripheral auditory system; the central auditory system is classified in neurology and will not be addressed here. When the deficiency is considered to be "only" a loss of sensitivity, we will see what is offered to compensate this loss. Sometimes, the link between air vibrations and the physiological analysis made on the cochlea, before the transmission, is broken. Several devices have been developed to restore the link, beyond the developments in ear surgery.

A severe deficiency occurs when the cochlea is not functioning, as nothing can be passed on the auditory pathways. In that situation, a signal reconstruction is introduced; this is the field of cochlear implants. A number of signal reconstruction systems are available in the market, but unfortunately, they do not offer a fully satisfactory solution. We will go through these systems and describe the relevance of the signal reconstruction offered by the manufacturers. Finally, we will present a discussion on what could be available tomorrow. This is an open question and a lot of research is put on that subject throughout the world.

1. Introduction

An interesting way to see deafness rehabilitation is to take a model of the understanding chain. In the subsequent section, we deal with this topic.

1.1. Understanding models

Comprehension of a language belongs to a general behavior of all beings, which is the sensorial relation with the external world. Generally, two steps are considered:
- the sensorial input;
- the basic knowledge.

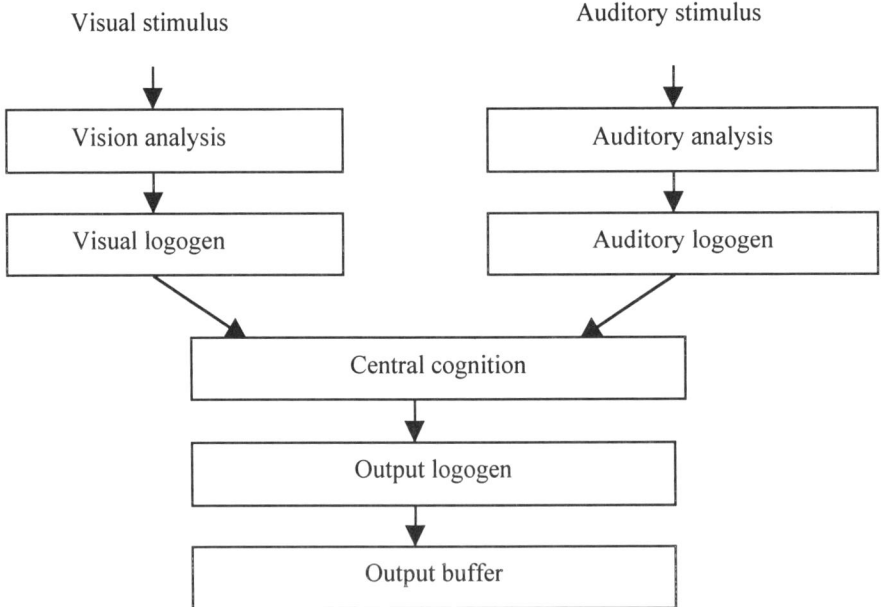

Figure 1. Organization of the information according to Morton's model.

When language is considered we must add "the fourth dimension," which is the time, because the information is sequentially delivered to the ear; this approach is different for the vision, where two dimensions (at least) are presented simultaneously. Several psychophysiological models have been introduced to give a formal frame, which is more or less intuitive. One of them is the Morton's model (Figure 1). A logogen is a virtual object suitable with the sensory information and with the cognitive expectation. There is a permanent exchange of information between the external stimuli and the brain interpretation.

Psychophysiological models play with these two elements [1]. At the beginning of a sentence, the choice is wide open for the coming words in the message. All the possibilities may be considered as a cohort. The logogens are fed by the sensory level and checked at the brain level. When the time flows, the set of words, suitable with the acoustic information and with the cognitive expectation, gets smaller and smaller, until the end of the sentence is reached with "one" meaning for the message.

1.2. Influence of the pathology

When pathology is considered, a lack of efficiency occurs at one level (or more). It could come from the brain (central) stage or from the periphery (ear and auditory pathways). Both domains are worthwhile to be considered, but we will focus, below, on peripheral handicaps.

At the brain stage [2], a lack of knowledge reducing the cohort of possible candidates will make the message difficult to understand: "You are talking about something which is not in my domain." In pathology, brain strokes may destroy information or cut off the links (associative fibbers) between the memory and the process "unit" in the brain. Other central nervous system diseases may block this function, which is generally called "Top-Down."

In psychoacoustical experiments, some unnatural situations are proposed to the listener, such as "how to milk a coat" [3], where the listener has to deal with the divergence between the acoustical message and the logical expectation. Listening in poor conditions can be obtained in a noisy signal [4] and, in this situation, high level assistance must be used, such as deep concentration, visual attention, and asking the speaker to talk as clearly as he/she can.

Poor conditions also can be seen in the case of hearing impairment [5]. In total cophosis, people with good training can follow a conversation using lip reading only. Complementation may come from sign language. Before this extreme situation, partial impairment is often seen and the person's performance can be severely affected. If we consider that the difference with a normal hearing subject can be represented by a smearing of the signal, represented by a function φ, a good hearing aid should provide the function φ^{-1}. However, the determination of φ is not easy, and several deficiencies can be listed as:

- loss on the auditory threshold;
- compression of the dynamics (the difference between the discomfort level and the auditory threshold is reduced);
- diminution of the frequency selectivity;
- lack of distinction in loudness.

This list is not exhaustive, and other deficiencies need to be considered. Furthermore, when noise is involved the performance of hearing impaired people is dramatically affected [6]. Clearly, the first two points indicated above can be corrected, provided the patient gets used to the new hearing conditions resulting from the use of a classical hearing aid. This is the task of audiologists. Nevertheless, to go further in adverse conditions, or when the disability is more severe, the use of signal reconstruction and a good rehabilitation are compulsory to reach an acceptable situation. Consequently, it is not absolutely safe to claim that intelligent techniques are used; it is more exact to say that "intelligent" machines rely on the patient's intelligence to improve his performances in speech understanding.

2. Auditory system

Voice production and hearing are coupled processes. Both processes should be considered for a successful development of technological means to help hearing impaired people. We will discuss in more detail the auditory system (situated between air and brain).

2.1. Voice production

It is not absolutely necessary to know how the voice is produced in order to understand the comprehension of speech. Nevertheless, considering the link between these two important functions in communication, some general information should be welcome [7]. Different steps (Figure 2) can be suggested.

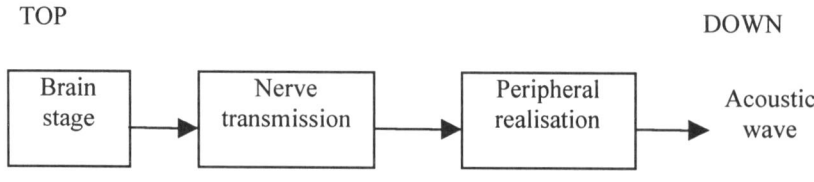

Figure 2. Main steps of the acoustic wave generation.

Brain stage

The upper level of language is subject to many hypotheses. The conception of a spoken message, backed by the subject's background, is then translated into a phoneme chain made of the adjunction of several words. Transitions are established to ensure the continuity between all the phonemes embedded in the message. Although everybody does not accept the idea of a smoothed juxtaposition, we will keep this assumption. Then, the order is forwarded to the brain nucleus in charge of the phonation, under the cerebellum control. In addition, the amplitude (loudness) depends on the auditory system through the auditory phonation loop [8], [9].

Nerve transmission

The order is forwarded to the different organs concerned by the phonation. This transmission is not direct, and some surrounding influence can play a decisive part in this mechanism.

Peripheral realization

The periphery, controlled by the higher level, is made of:
- a blowing system (the lungs);
- a vibrating device (the larynx).

In the larynx, the vocal folds can vibrate (voiced sound) or make a constriction leading to air turbulence considered as a noise source. In the case of a periodic vibration, air pulses excite the vocal tract and resonance frequencies occur.

Resonance function

The vocal tract can be represented (Figure 3) by an air pipe with a changing configuration. Some frequencies are reinforced, and they can be seen in the sonogram, which is a frequency-time representation of speech. This air pipe is made of the larynx, followed by the mouth. The tongue, which moves very quickly, has an important part to set up the characteristics of the air pipe. At the end of the mouth, the lips introduce a derivation of the signal, and the air stream leaves the mouth toward the auditory system of people nearby.

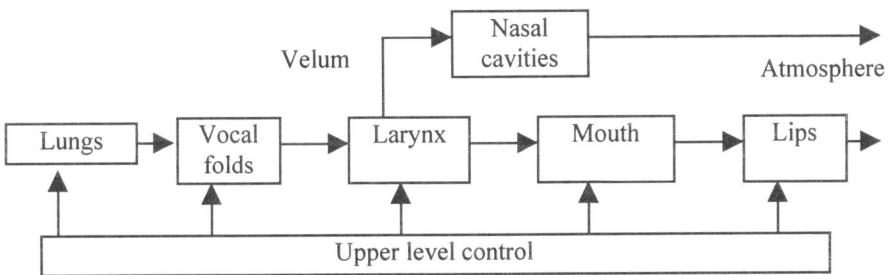

Figure 3. Block diagram of the voice production.

In parallel, the nasal track is opened or closed under the influence of the velum and it has its own resonance.

2.2. Auditory system

The auditory system is composed of two pathways, one ascending and one descending.

General structure
Models indicating the different stages of speech understanding are very numerous. A simple one is indicated in Figure 4.

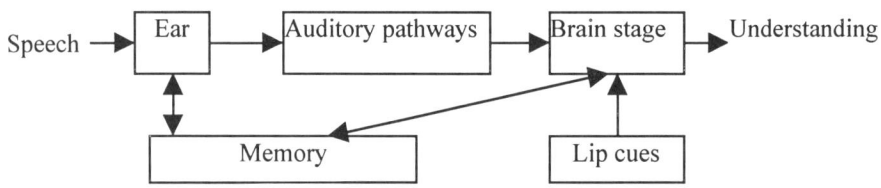

Figure 4. Some stages of hearing.

The hearing mechanisms are essentially interactive. Usually, and in adverse conditions, the auditory system can get some help from the vision. Gesture and lip cues are efficient means to assist the listener.

Ear
The ear is a complex system, which can be divided into several parts (see Figure 5).

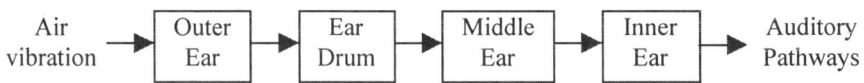

Figure 5. Main structures of the ear.

Pinna (external ear)
The *pinna* is composed of cartilage with adherent perichondrium and skin. Its main function is the reception of the air vibration and to direct it toward the external auditory meatus.

External auditory meatus (outer ear)
It is about 25 millimeters long and acts as a filter advantaging (by resonance) the vibration corresponding to speech. It ends on the tympanic membrane (also called "ear drum").

Tympanic cavity (middle ear)

It is an air containing space, which houses the ossicular chain of *malleus*, *incus*, and *stapes*. It is connected to the external ear by the eardrum (tympanic membrane) and to the nasopharynx by the Eustachian tube, in order to balance the pressures on both sides of the eardrum.

Its main functions are:
- impedance adaptation,
- transmission of vibrations,
- high pass filter,
- acoustic amplification.

Inner ear

The inner ear is composed of the cochlea situated in a duct filled with the endolymphatic fluid. Innovative developments would be needed to better understand its function. We can say that the acoustic wave is analyzed by filters (basilar membrane), which are reinforced by the efferent system and the tuning of the acoustic nerve fibbers (tonotopic and biological organization). Then, the information is forwarded toward the higher structures of the brain.

2.3. Auditory pathways

Auditory pathways are very complex, and we will make, once more, a dramatic simplification to show them. At each stage, the number of fibbers going toward the brain is multiplied by about 10, starting by 30,000 outside the cochlea and ending by 1,000,000 at the cortex.

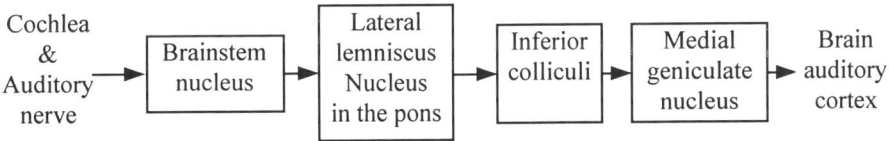

Figure 6. Main synapses on the auditory pathways.

The general organization is given on Figure 6. All the axons going to the brain interact on both sides (right and left pathways). Finally, they reach the cortex (primary cortex) with a frequency mapping. Then, the primary cortex is linked to other areas in the cortex, and many properties (including the memory) are concerned. The cranial nerve organization is very complex. Behavior and neurophysiology are important fields dealing with this sensory function.

2.4. Brain stage

For the listener, the objective in speech is to understand the talker's message. Many concepts have been introduced. The processing which takes place in the brain is rather inaccessible and obscure, and many attempts have been made in order to break into it. The melting pot includes linguistic theories, psychophysiology, linguistic models, and computer science, with other fields also concerned.

The following steps take place:
- extraction of neural cues (stop, rising, fall…in the signal);
- detection of acoustical features;
- elaboration of phonemes;
- construction of words;
- organization of meaningful sentences.

Memory and experience have a fundamental part and they are specific to each person; nevertheless, attempts are made to construct large groups of people, more or less homogeneous. It is admitted that a listener tries to find in the acoustical signal what is coherent to the message elaborated in his mind. The bottom up (acoustic cues to brain) and top-down (brain to acoustic cues) strategies gave birth to many models; each one bears a little part of the unknown truth.

3. Normal (external) aids

The basic function of normal (external) aids is to restore the auditory link by a selective amplification of the signal.

3.1. General principles

Classically, normal aids perform several functions [10]:
- signal amplification;
- transmission;
- frequency shift into the patient's auditory rests.

The so-called "numeric revolution" should be understood as a numeric evolution. The principles of the classical hearing aids are kept, but the correction is more precise as filters are more accurate and less distorting. This aspect will be discussed at the end of this section.

3.2. Normal hearing aids

Basic structure
The basic structure of a hearing aid is indicated in Figure 7.

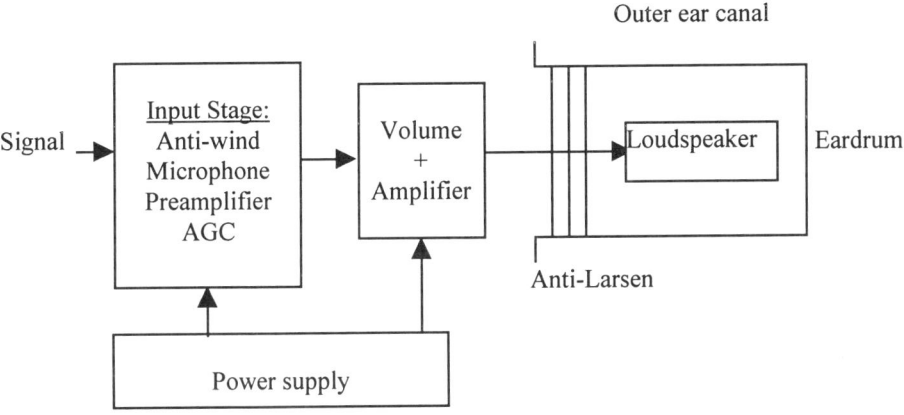

Figure 7. Block diagram of a normal hearing aid.

The idea is the correction of the hearing loss revealed by audiograms (such as the classical one indicated in Figure 8 [11]). The prosthesis is in charge of the selective amplification of the signal. The frequency-dependent amplification is adapted to the actual hearing loss. For the example shown in Figure 8, the amplification should be put essentially on the high frequencies. The correction [12] is merely amplification. The wind protector system is added to stop the whistling effect seen when an air draft occurs. The anti-Larsen system prevents the auto-oscillation of the system.

Improvements

Several improvements have been made on the basic principle described above. Several of them are worthwhile to mention.

Programmable prostheses

In this section, the spectrum is divided into three ranges and each range has a specific processing. The parameters of each processing are passed to the prosthesis by an interface connected to a computer (PC). The block diagram of a programmable hearing aid is illustrated in Figure 9.

It can be seen, in this structure, that each channel is processed independently. It allows the high, medium, or low frequencies to have a specific amplification and compression, more adapted to the patient's possibilities and to the signal properties. Then, the acoustic wave is reconstructed before the power stage (speaker). Similar to the classical systems, a general amplification and an automatic gain control (AGC) take place at the input of the system.

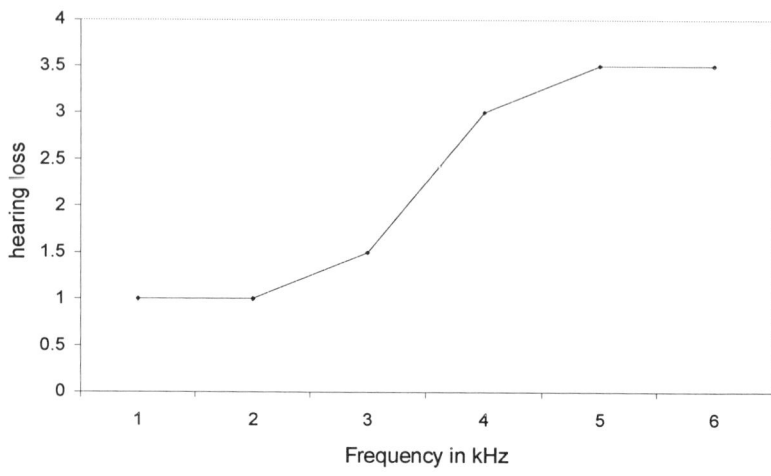

Figure 8. Classical representation of a presbyacousy (the hearing loss, given in bels, is on the high frequencies).

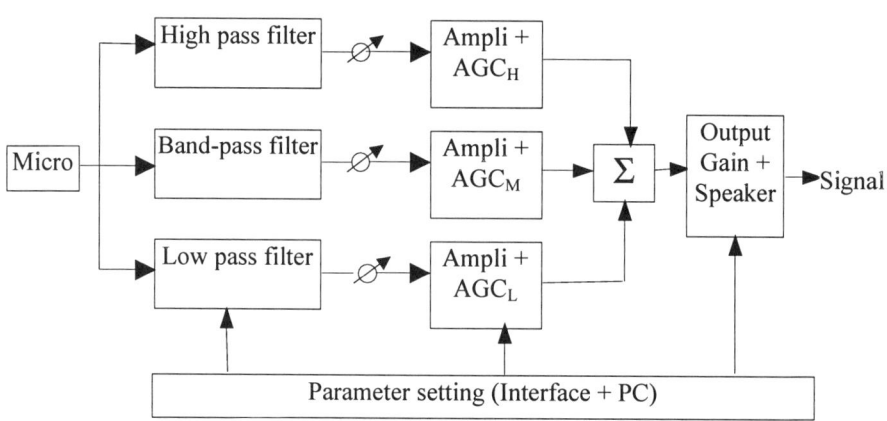

Figure 9. Block diagram of a programmable hearing aid.

Frequency shift

When the patient's hearing zone is on the low frequencies, it is possible to transfer some information coming from the high frequencies into the low frequencies. The principle is simple: the signal is multiplied by itself (Figure 10), and some information is transferred to the lower frequencies. The equation used in this circumstance is:

$$\sin(2\pi ft) \cdot \sin(2\pi f't) = [\cos(2\pi(f-f')t) - \cos(2\pi(f+f')t)]/2$$

The low frequency component $(f - f')$ is brought into the hearing zone of the subject, and the high frequency component $(f + f')$ is eliminated.

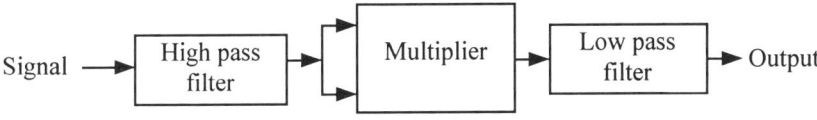

Figure 10. Multiplication by itself of a high frequency signal.

Other similar systems were elaborated by playing on the time (contraction or dilatation), and this is easily done by changing the sampling frequency. Nevertheless, a philosophical question is raised: can a normal brain cope with all these data, as the shifted information is added to the information normally present in the audible frequencies? The answer is Yes in some cases and No in others.

3.3. Bone-integrated vibrator

This type of system belongs to the category "transmission restoring" systems.

Principle
The acoustic wave is amplified and distributed into a coil, which stimulates, by induction, a "screw" (integrated device used as a vibrator) fixed to the patient's skull. The principle is indicated in Figure 11. The bone vibration transmits the signal to the inner ear, when the normal airway cannot be used.

Systems
Two main systems are currently on the market.
Audiant
In this device, the integrated screw is covered by the skin and the transmission is made by induction. There is a high loss of power, but the skin is respected and the infection risk is kept low.

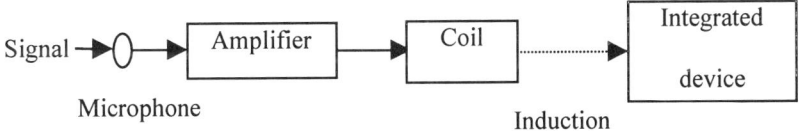

Figure 11. Block diagram of a bone-integrated vibrator.

BAHA (Bone anchored hearing aid)
In this system, the magnetic induction stimulates directly (mechanical transmission) a bone-integrated screw, which is open to the air. The transmission is more efficient, but the risk of infection cannot be neglected.

3.4. Middle ear aids

This system category provides another means to restore the transmission.

American system
A magnet is placed on one of the three middle ear bones (malleus, uncus, stapes). The coil is situated inside the outer ear canal, and the transmission is done by induction (similar to the system described in Figure 11).

Japanese system
The vibration is now transmitted by an electric field (situated inside a condenser, Figure 12). Two blades, with different piezoelectric coefficients, are joined together, and the deformation follows the variation of the electric field.

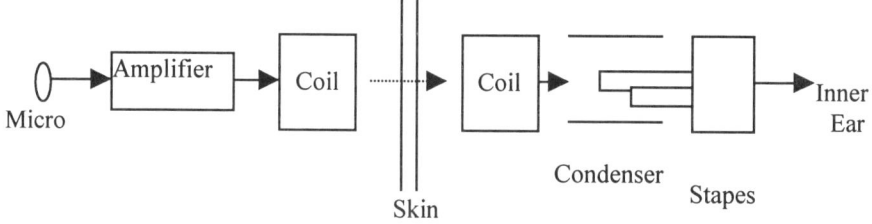

Figure 12. Transmission of the acoustic wave, using the Japanese system, which leads to the vibration of the middle ear bones.

The two-blade system is situated between the plates of a condenser and is bound to the stapes. The deformation of the two-blade system is passed to the inner ear. In this way, the acoustic signal is transmitted, by the inner ear, to the auditory pathways.

3.5. Numeric revolution

As it was indicated earlier, the numeric revolution [13] should be denoted more accurately as a numeric evolution. Most manufacturers have introduced, into their range of devices, a numeric system. Let us consider, in a few words, one of the earliest systems, the Digifocus® of Oticon™.

The signal (refer Figure 13) is split by a digital filter bank, such that the high and low frequencies can be processed differently. Then, the signal is reconstructed and the output is distributed to the patient's ears.

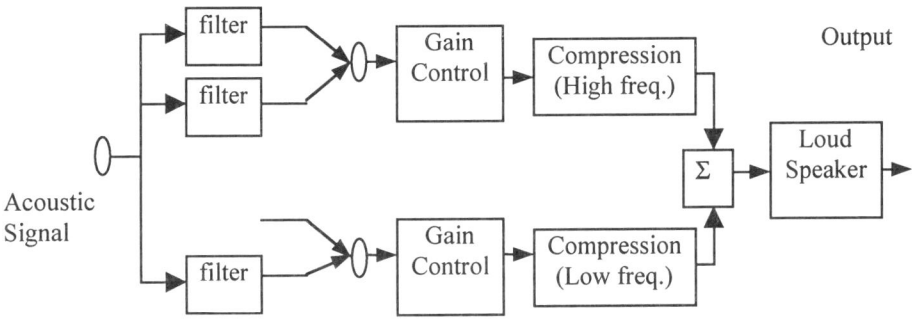

Figure 13. Main functions of a numeric hearing aid.

Consequently, we can see that the main improvements are:
- filters can be processed independently;
- technology is light (a simple microprocessor);
- band-pass filters have rather sharp edges, and the frequency bands are well separated;
- all the processing is done numerically, and the distortion rate is kept very low.

This organization brings us [14] close to the cochlear implant technology, which is developed in the next section.

4. Cochlear implants

4.1. General principles

History

Cochlear implants (CI) are devices designed to replace the Corti's organ when this organ is totally not functional [15]. Basically, the CI can be seen as an interface in charge of the transduction of the acoustical vibration into an electrical stimulus to be carried along the auditory pathways toward the brain.

The idea of CI is very old. Two centuries ago, Volta reported that an electrical stimulation between his two ears led to a noise sounding like "running water." Luckily (or unluckily), there was no ethical committees at this time, and now this experimentation would lead this author to a mental hospital as he used a 50-volt direct stimulation (quite enough to produce irreversible damage to his auditory system). Just after the turn of the 20th century, several other experiments indicated that deaf people can perceive auditory sensations when an electrical stimulation is used on their ears.

The reference paper came in 1957 in "La Presse Medicale Française" (The French Medical Journal) where Djourno and Eyries [16] reported their experience of this kind of stimulation. However, considering the poor results they obtained, their conclusion was that this technique had no future. William House in Los Angeles was told (by one of his deaf patients) about this article and he became very interested. He took again the idea and constructed the first wearable system able to produce this electrical stimulation. In 1973, in San Francisco, the first symposium on this topic gathered the pioneers of the technique. They were clinicians and scientists from all over the world.

Then systems blossomed on several continents with results less and less experimental. The way was open, and in the 1980s all the major hospitals in the world started to perform this implantation. Strong negative reactions from the deaf community slowed down the movement, but it was impossible to block this evolution which belongs to the progress of medicine.

Main functions of the system

The general organization of the system is given in Figure 14. The air vibrations are captured, sampled, and fed into a microprocessor system (DSP = Digital Speech Processor). Then, the signal is reconstructed and used to modulate a high frequency (HF) carrier which goes, through the skin, to a receiver surgically introduced and which is (strictly speaking) the cochlear implant (CI).

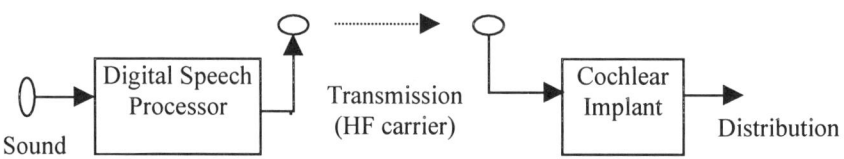

Figure 14. General organization of a cochlear implant system.

The cochlear implant takes the modulated signal and detects and reshapes the information, which is then distributed to electrodes situated inside the cochlea duct. Nowadays, mostly multielectrode systems are used. A multielectrode implant transmits the following information:
- Yes/No: presence or absence of sounds;
- Rhythm: this is an extension of the yes/no property (the "beat" is enhanced);
- Amplitude: sounds are more or less intense;

- Frequency: the "color" of the signal is distributed along the electrodes.

The organization of a multielectrode (multichannel) CI is indicated in Figure 15.

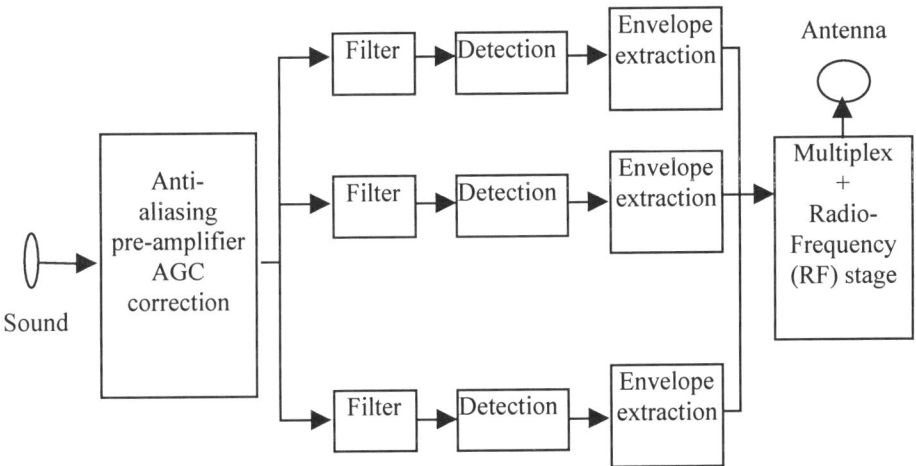

Figure 15. Block diagram showing the main functions of the DSP of a multichannel cochlear implant (MCI).

The stages indicated in Figure 15 are numerically performed:

- the signal is captured, pre-processed, sampled, and fed into buffers;
- a fast Fourier transform (FFT) calculates the spectrum lines;
- the lines are grouped into sets, according to the residual possibilities of the auditory pathways;
- the energy of each set is used to make an amplitude modulation of the HF carrier;
- the carrier is emitted from an aerial, situated against the scalp skin.

From the receiver point of view (Figure 16), several functions can be pointed out:

- the signal is demodulated and leads to a power supply and to the auditory information (amplitude and duration of the pulses);
- the pulses are distributed to the electrodes according to a system "address + content" or a "round-robin + content" system.

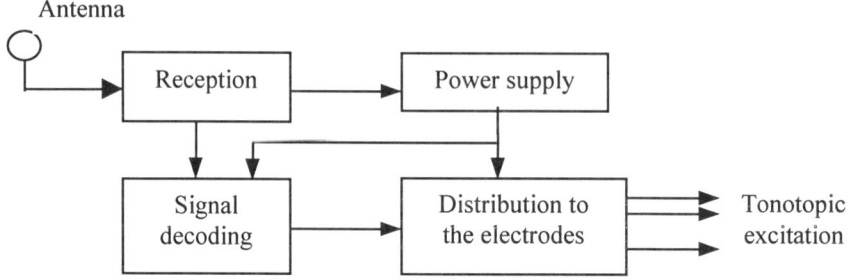

Figure 16. Block diagram of the main functions of the implanted part of a cochlear implant system.

4.2. Australian *Nucleus®*

History

Born from the giant power of Dunlop Pacific and from a simple but bright idea of Graeme Clark, the Nucleus CI (manufactured by Cochlear) has been the indisputable king of the 1980s and has been at the top in the 1990s, despite the efforts of its challengers [17], [18]. Graeme Clark's idea was based on some basic assumptions on the voice:
- information is embedded in the vowels;
- vowels can be recognized by the value of their first two formants ($F1$ and $F2$) [19];
- the voice fundamental frequency is important in the message.

Furthermore, this idea was not greedy in bit transmission rate and was well adapted to the limited speed of the 1980s processors [20].

Evolution of the strategies
- $F0/F2$: only the second formant is detected and the spikes are repeated at the $F0$ rate. The energy ($A2$) is delivered on the correct electrode.
- $F0/F1/F2$: spike energy ($A1$ for $F1$, and $A2$ for $F2$) is delivered on the electrodes corresponding to $F1$ and $F2$, at the $F0$ rate.
- *MPEAK (Multipeak)*: the signal is more complex as some energy is detected on the high frequencies (to describe the "whistling" consonants) and delivered to the more basal electrodes which indicate the high frequencies on the cochlea.
- *SMSP (Spectral Maxima Sound Processor)*: in each spectral analysis, only the six highest energy bands are kept and distributed to the electrodes, according to a fixed rate or to a rate proportional to $F0$.
- *SPEAK*: following the same idea, the frequency bands having their energy above a given level are kept. The number of selected bands

ranges from 4 to 10. The rhythm of delivery depends on the number of selected electrodes.
- *Advanced strategies*: several other strategies have been tested, such as a stimulation rhythm adapted to each electrode.

The explosion of ideas has been backed by the finding that each patient responds more or less to his own strategy [21], [22], [23]. The temptation is high to explore many possibilities; then, a strategy will have to be adapted to the implantee. One of the ideas of the selection "above a level (threshold)," Figure 17, is the elimination of the noise, as speech is considered to be "above" the noise. This conception can be discussed because it is not so easy to increase the signal to noise ratio (SNR).

Technological support
The basic strategy of the Nucleus system can be illustrated as shown in Figure 18. Nowadays, signal processing is numerically performed and the algorithms can be adapted to match efficiently the patient's abilities [24].

Evolution of coding
This important number of strategies indicates that no one is satisfactory. Obviously, there are still improvements to be done [25]. The percentage of star patients (patients who can communicate over the phone) increases permanently, thanks to the speech coding and to an efficient selection in potential subjects. Then, the assessment of patients is an interesting question to be raised [26].

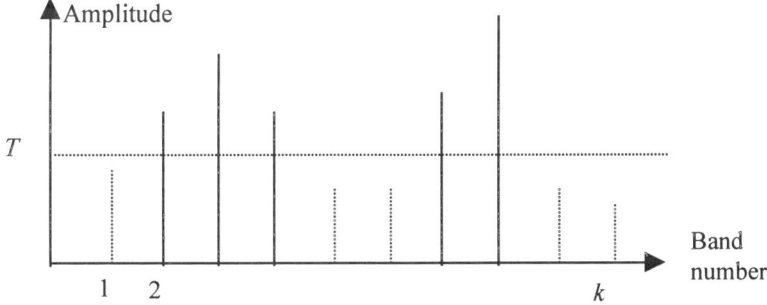

Figure 17. Band selection in the SPEAK strategy.
T is the threshold, and dotted bands are ignored.

Nevertheless, a question remains unanswered: what can be done for the poor performers? This debate is far from being closed, mostly when money is brought in, and when it is more or less officially admitted that some people may benefit less from some progresses. This consideration is difficult to be borne, but it must be taken into account when economical considerations step in.

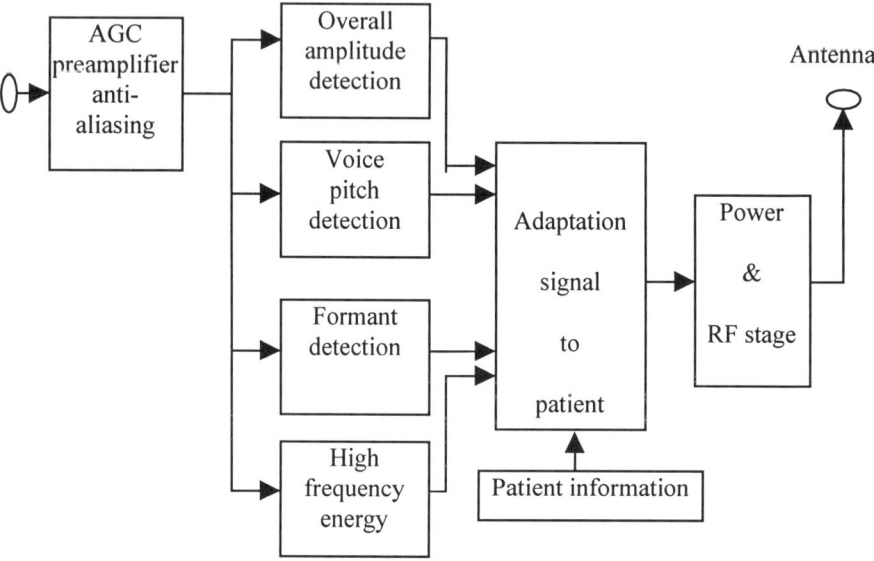

Figure 18. Block diagram of the speech processor of the Nucleus implant.

4.3. French *Digisonic®*

Basis of the system

Born out of the French technology, the MXM cochlear implant ("Digisonic") states that the spectrum contains all the information needed by the brain. Thus, there is no need to extract "more of less artificially" special features in the speech to enhance the performances. This is similar to the natural function of hearing. The idea [27] is to take directly the speech spectrum and to group the spectrum lines into frequency bands, which will be distributed to the cochlea. This strategy looks like SPEAK, but arouses earlier.

One of its characteristic is the "winner takes all" strategy. It means that if a frequency band has a much smaller energy than one of its neighbors it is switched off in the coding. The meaning of "much smaller" needs to be adapted to each situation. This "Xerox effect" enhances the bands with a high energy, in order to reduce the surrounding noise. Bands with a relatively small energy are eliminated. The principle is indicated in Figure 19.

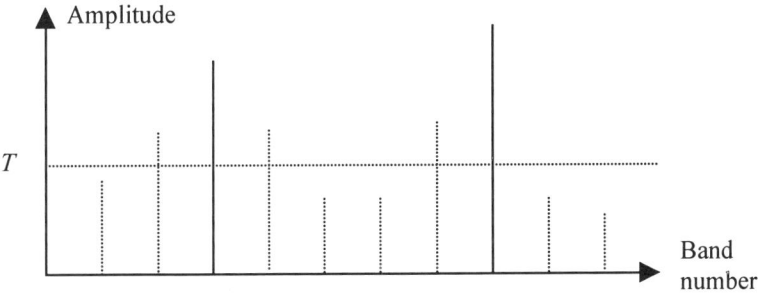

Figure 19. Band selection in the Digisonic strategy.
T is the threshold, and dotted spectrum lines are ignored.

Then, the selected bands are distributed to their associated electrode. The system can work with 15 bands. When the spectrum is obtained, many corrections are available, such as the amplification of high or low frequencies, and the signal is artificially manipulated. The ultimate goal is the satisfaction and the performance of the patient.

Technological support

The main functions embedded in the speech processor are illustrated in Figure 20. The first block is classical. The DSP is in charge of the FFT and of the frequency band construction according to the patient's physiological possibility (map). A cycle is associated to a sweep of the 15 bands, and the cycles can be delivered to the electrodes at a constant rate or according to a period linked to $F0$ (the voice fundamental frequency or voice pitch) when it is detected, or randomly for unvoiced sounds. As usual, the strategy must be adapted to the patient. The system has a high flexibility, and a trained staff is needed to handle properly the setting of the system.

The output logic is in charge of the conversion of the energy detected in each band into the size of the pulses in order to pass the information on the amplitude [28]. Finally, the RF (radio frequency) stage is rather classical. A feedback checks the voltage of the output signal and stops the system if the level is too low, due a failure in the system. The output control suppresses the pulses that are too small compared to their neighbors.

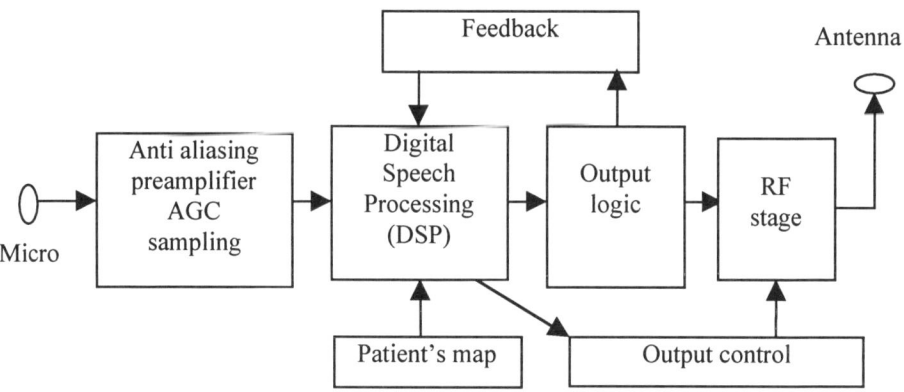

Figure 20. Main functions embedded in the French MXM cochlear implant.

Alternative strategies
Fast stimulation rate (FSR)

This strategy takes only five frequency bands to shorten the cycle period, in a continuous mode, and it should be more efficient with the transient segments of the signal. But, there is a lack of precision in the frequency coding. Overall, this strategy did not turn out to be better than the classical FFT analysis. Let us recall that a cycle corresponds to a scan of the CI's 15 channels.

Multirate stimulation (MRS)

In this situation, the sampling rate of the signal depends on the channel; it may be sensible to deliver more pulses (higher rate) on some channels. Once more, this coding did not lead to better results than the other strategies.

Music mode

In the normal mode (speech mode), a maximum of six pulses is delivered at each scan. Similar to the SPEAK strategy, only the energy "above the noise" is transmitted. In the music mode, in order "to enjoy" the wide spectrum of the sounds, all the 15 channels can be passed to the electrodes at each scan. This consideration is highly theoretical.

4.4. American *Clarion*®

General considerations

Born in the 1990s, the American implant Clarion (Los Angeles, California), manufactured by Advanced Bionics Corporation, has some attractive possibilities where one can find its "intelligence." The adaptability of the strategies offered by this system should benefit a large range of patients.

Large range of strategies

The speech coding includes many techniques. We briefly review the main ones.

Compressed analog (CA)

Each electrode permanently delivers sine waves to the cochlea. Each wave is reconstructed, using short duration segments, to make a sine amplitude. A frequency is associated to each electrode. The amplitude is regularly updated according to the energy detected in the corresponding channel. It is not necessary to make the amplitude refreshment at the same rate everywhere. Then the ends of the auditory nerve receive a sine excitation more natural than pulses. But is it important, considering the nature's plasticity [29]?

Continuous interleaved samples (CIS)

This widely used speech coding is offered, also, by the Clarion system. Pulses are delivered sequentially to the electrode with the system "address + content." As two pulses are not simultaneous, the interaction between two electrodes is limited.

Paired pulsatile samples (PPS)

In this strategy, two distant pulses are delivered, simultaneously, at the auditory nerve ends. Thus, more information comes to the ear, compared with the CIS strategy. But is this really an advantage if the patient cannot process all the information and even worse if this mixing destroys what could be understood separately?

Hybrid strategies

CA and CIS can be played at the same time on different electrodes. For instance, the lower half of the electrodes is on CA and the higher half on CIS. Every combination is possible; the "aim of the game" is to find which one is the more efficient for a given patient.

Electrodes configuration

The normal configuration of the electrodes is indicated in Figure 21.

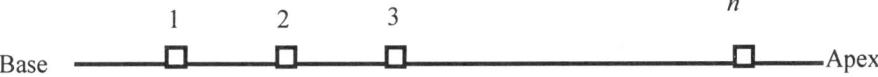

Figure 21. Electrode repartition along the cochlea.

The usual excitation mode is common ground (CG). An electrode is live and all the others are connected to the ground. The live electrode sweeps the electrode array under the control of an electronic multiplexing. Practically, the current flows from the active (live) electrode to its nearest two neighbors.

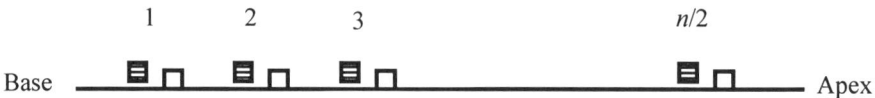

Figure 22. Electrode organization by pairs.

Another possibility (Figure 22) is to pair the electrodes and the pairs are electrically separated. This configuration divides by two the number of possible excitation sites; information is reduced, but independence is increased. The Clarion system uses the repartition indicated in Figure 22.

4.5. Other systems

Several other systems can be seen on the market; it is not possible to list them all, but we can see two of them which have interesting features.

Austrian Combi®
The Austrian system (Combi) [30] is manufactured by Med-El in Innsbruck. The electrical information is distributed to 8 pairs of electrodes in order to get a local stimulation. The stimulation rate is high, and the speed is up to 12,120 pulses per second corresponding to 1,500 per channel. This rate is useful in transmitting transient information; however, it may be doubtful that it is a key factor for the implantees. The rest of the system is rather classical, with an input stage and a radio frequency transmission.

Belgian Laura®
In this system (manufactured by Antwerp Bionic Systems) [31], two ways of processing the signal are used according to the decision of a voice pitch detection function (Figure 23). The electrical information is distributed over 8 pairs of electrodes, corresponding to the repartition indicated in Figure 22.

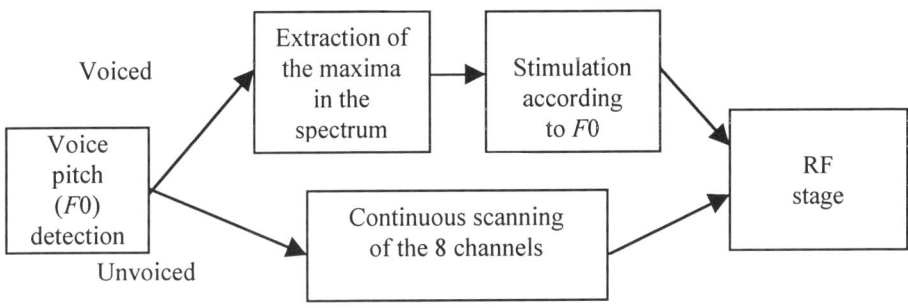

Figure 23. Separation and processing of the voiced
and unvoiced segments in the signal.

On the "voiced way" a "phase-lock" procedure is introduced; the excitation on low frequency channels is delivered synchronously with the maxima of the signal. This property corresponds to the normal response of neurons seen in experimental conditions. However, it is not yet established whether this is a key improvement in coding.

4.6. Surrounding facilities

Back telemetry

The response of the auditory fibbers can be sent back to the speech processor, allowing the clinician to know what is going on in the implanted side (Figure 24). After every stimulation, the response of the electrodes is monitored and transmitted backward. Consequently, the clinician is informed on the efficiency of the stimulation on the target electrodes, and on the response on the side electrodes, showing the dependency. Back telemetry provides some other information:

- impedance of the electrodes;
- current delivered on the electrodes;
- voltage on the electrodes.

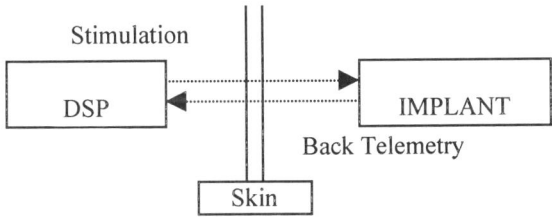

Figure 24. Principle of back telemetry.

Setting of the system

The signal processing performed by the DSP must be adapted to the patient's auditory nerve condition. It is clear that a sophisticated analysis will be useless if it cannot be forwarded to the brain, for instance when it is delivered at the end of dead fibbers. Then, the loudness sensation (comfort level) can be reached more or less quickly, according to the auditory nerve state. This adaptation needs a special skill, and in every clinic there is one (or more) specialist in charge of this task. Also, the number of electrodes which can be used varies from one patient to another, and the grouping of spectrum lines must be done efficiently.

Evoked potential

An efficient stimulation on an electrode triggers a neural response on the auditory pathway's response, which can be recorded in electrophysiology. This information is useful to understand what goes wrong when the results are far from the expectation. In addition, it provides objective data, which are very useful where young children are concerned. Consequently, intelligence in cochlear implantation is to assist and give as much information as possible to use efficiently the reconstruction of the acoustic signal provided by the machine.

4.7. New trends in research

Hearing and cognition

The understanding of speech is a complicated phenomenon. The brain guesses what should come and tries to organize the acoustic cues. We have seen that, usually, the guess concerns several situations, which are sorted out using the acoustic information.

This balance between semantics and pattern recognition is done more or less consciously, and it has led to a lot of representations, such as the Markov models [32] where speech is taken as a chain of symbols and where the tests are performed in a dynamic and probabilistic way.

Many experiments have been conducted to estimate the relative importance of semantics and acoustical cues. In these experiments, words were distorted in continuums going from logical to totally illogical, such as moving from "How to milk a goat" to "How to milk a coat," in a typical study previously mentioned [3]. Meaning strongly influences the phoneme categorization at the acoustic level. Illogical meanings are rejected until the acoustic signal becomes perfectly clear. It is also possible to show subliminal images to the subject to influence him/her before the acoustic wave is played.

Mathematics and psychology are deeply mixed in these experiments, and it is necessary to have a good knowledge of human behavior before making intelligent machines.

Fuzzy discrimination

A way to deal with the acoustic signal complexity is to use fuzzy and probabilistic methods. The basic idea lies in the variability of speech and the polymorphism of the utterance for the same phoneme. In a safe strategy, when the recognition fails, it is possible to come back at uncertain nodes and to restart the logical path with a new idea. This behavior can be seen in everyday life when someone does not understand a problem; he/she can restart where the situation began to become unclear and he/she tries again to follow new ideas.

A typical case when uncertainty should be considered is the influence of the noise. The S/N (signal to noise) ratio plays an important part in the recognition of the acoustical message. In order to understand this influence, techniques that use "intelligent" signal extraction and are relatively immune to noise are worthy to be seen. The method based on artificial neural networks is one of them.

These techniques have been used, for example, in the University College of London (UCL/Phonetics department), to extract cues in the acoustic signal and use them in the SiVo (Sine Voice) hearing aid [33], [34]. The features extracted in the SiVo system are complementary to the visual assistance (lip reading):

- the voice fundamental frequency ($F0$);
- the amplitude of the signal;
- the energy in the lower half of the spectrum;
- the energy in the upper half of the spectrum.

The extracted cues can be transmitted to the auditory system by means of normal hearing aids or by a cochlear implant, and both versions have been developed. The "hunt for cues" is open [35], [36], [37]; we recall that the cues strongly depend on the patient.

Frequency-time representations and wavelets

The acoustic signal is usually represented based on frequency-time methods. The main idea is to attach to the signal, at a given instant t, a vector made of several coefficients, usually associated to the frequency. Each coefficient is denoted $R(t,c)$. For details on these technical aspects, the reader is referred to textbooks in the field and to the Bibliographic Note at the end of this chapter.

Fast Fourier Transform (FFT)

The classical form of frequency-time representation is the Fast Fourier Transform (FFT), where the integration time is limited to the interval [-T, T], and a weighting of the signal is introduced by the function $f(u-t)$:

$$R(t,\omega) = \int_{-T}^{+T} f(u-t).x(u).e^{-i\omega u} du$$

This formula is widely used in the cochlear implant systems, in order to calculate the spectrum lines. With cochlear implants, it was seen that the coefficients are the spectrum lines and they are grouped and distributed to the electrodes. Other transformations are under investigation; they have advantages and drawbacks. Their use in cochlear implants is similar to the Fourier spectrum use.

Cohen formula

Representations based on the Cohen formula use the pulsation ω (ω = 2πf), where f is the frequency, attached to the coefficient c. The Cohen formula is:

$$R(t,\omega) = \iint_D \Phi(u-t,\tau) \cdot x\left(u+\frac{\tau}{2}\right) \cdot x^*\left(u-\frac{\tau}{2}\right) \cdot e^{-j\omega t} du d\tau$$

where $R(t,\omega)$ is the coefficient attached to f, at the time t, $x(t)$ is the signal and $x^*(t)$ its conjugate ($x(t) = x^*(t)$ in the case of real signals), $\Phi(t,\tau)$ is the kernel of the representation, D is the integration domain, $D = \mathbf{R}^2$, with R = (-∞,∞).

Wigner-Ville representation

Another way to decompose the signal and to derive specific coefficients is provided by the Wigner-Ville transform:

$$R(t,\omega) = \int_{-\infty}^{\infty} x(t+\tau/2) \, x^*(t-\tau/2) \, e^{-i\omega\tau} \, d\tau$$

Considering that the integration interval runs from -∞ to ∞, it is not possible to use the above formula in practice. A limitation is introduced in the pseudo Wigner-Ville transform:

$$R(t,\omega) = \int_{-T}^{T} x(t+\tau/2) \, x^*(t-\tau/2) \, \{f(\tau/2)\}^2 \, e^{-i\omega\tau} \, d\tau$$

where $f(\tau/2)$ introduces a weighting of the signal over the analysis interval [-T, T].

Wavelets transform

It is also possible to replace the classical trigonometric functions in the FFT by a function ψ(t) representing oscillations with decreasing amplitude when the signal is moving away from the instant *t*:

$$R(t,a) = \int_{-\infty}^{\infty} f(\tau) \cdot \frac{1}{\sqrt{a}} \Psi\left(\frac{\tau-t}{a}\right) \cdot d\tau$$

where $\frac{1}{\sqrt{a}}$ is introduced for the normalization of the energy. A classical approach is to take the Morlet's wavelet:

$$\Psi(u) = e^{-\alpha u^2/2} e^{i\omega u}, \text{ with } u = \frac{\tau-t}{a}.$$

In these formula, ω characterizes an oscillation, α shapes the descent of the amplitude toward zero, *a* is a time scale factor, and *t* is the point where the wavelets are calculated.

Practically, considering the fast decent of $\Psi(u)$ toward zero, the integral is calculated over a limited interval [-T, T], where T depends on the scale factor; the larger *a*, the smaller T. Considering the spectrum of the Morlet's wavelet, we can see that T is small when ω is large (ω = 2π*f*, T = 1/*f*), and a transient phenomenon, which is rich in high frequencies, can be analyzed more precisely.

The field of applying transforms is opened to compare the efficiency of the existing different methods, in theory and with the patients.

Future implants

The above report shows that intelligence in speech processing needs a close adaptation to the patient and should give to the implantation team as much information as possible on the patient and on the technology [38]. It is also important to assist the patient and the speech therapists. The family and the work colleagues have an important part to play in the communication network.

For a long time, medical skill aimed to keep people alive; nowadays, this goal is insufficient. We are in a world of communication, which should be shared by everybody. But, every human being is different, and technology is powerful enough to be adapted to everybody. It is important that advances in knowledge also benefit people at the lower end of the performance spectrum. A team is not good only for its star patients, but also by the efforts it makes to help the other implantees. Then, implants in adverse conditions need to be studied [39].

Another suggestion is the use of large arrays of electrodes. For each signal, only a small subset should be concerned. Let us recall that a normal cochlea has about 3,500 sensory cells, but it is unclear now if we need to closely mimic the nature, as far as many parameters remain unknown.

Intelligence in cochlear implants is to take the best advantage of the patient's possibilities. Electrophysiology, mainly with back telemetry and evoked potentials, provides key information. Then, a long rehabilitation, under the assistance of specialized speech therapists, helps the patient to make the best use of his machine. Objective tests can provide a biofeedback to motivate the patient and to assess his/her progression. Another form of intelligence is in the price of the machine. It is useless to have a powerful system nobody can use because it is not affordable. Thus, it is not easy to establish what are intelligent techniques in deafness rehabilitation. What is intelligent today may not be so bright tomorrow.

5. Future prospects

Nowadays, numeric evolution allows many possibilities of smearing the signal. This is a powerful tool of investigation.

5.1. Simulation of the pathology

A simple question needs to be raised at this point: what is deafness? Brian Moore, in the Department of Experimental Psychology in Cambridge, tries to bring up answers [5]. He established several tests to know more about hearing impairment. It is not obvious to define the differences between a "normal" and a "deaf" person. Smearing the signal can simulate deficiencies and can help to understand this point even if some controversies come out of this approach. Four steps are identified when this procedure is considered:

- How to smear the signal?
- What is achieved by a patient having a "pure" deficiency?
- What are the performances of control subjects when they are submitted to a smeared signal?
- What are the results obtained with mathematical methods working on the "pathological" (smeared) signal?

The last step is useful for an analytical approach, because it is difficult to assimilate a patient to a mere equation ignoring the high levels in the language. Then, results obtained at all the stages need to be compared.

5.2. Classical simulations

In this subsection, we consider several classical simulations of hearing impairments.

Hearing threshold and dynamic range

The simplest smearing of the signal is the attenuation of the high frequencies, corresponding to presbyacousy (Figure 8). Sentences (or words) are digitized at a given sampling frequency, and a pre-emphasis (action of the middle ear) is done. The speech signal is then submitted to a Fourier analysis, and the spectrum lines are grouped according to a filter organization. Then the energy in the high frequency bands is attenuated, and a new signal is reconstructed from this spectrum. Many parameters can be set in the transformation of the spectrum, according to the effect to be studied.

Influence of temporally coded acoustic patterns

Smearing of the signal can affect the temporal aspects. The following items can be studied:
- transition time (which is supposed to play a key part in several pathologies, such as the comprehension of consonants by dyslexic children);
- presence or absence of laryngeal excitation (voicing);
- temporal rhythm which is more or less perceived by hearing impaired people;
- influence of amplitude envelope variations on speech understanding [40].

The signal can be accelerated or slowed down to show the effect of the time micro-organization. Psychoacoustics are then brought in to evaluate the consequence of the signal modification.

Simulation of the diminution of the frequency discrimination

Once more, the idea is to produce a pattern similar to the excitation expected to occur in an impaired ear receiving an acoustic signal. In the case of reduced frequency discrimination, smearing the signal starts with a filtering of the signal. Broad frequency bands are constructed and noise may be added. The construction of frequency bands results in smoothing the signal. Then, the modified spectrum is reconverted into time samples with an inverse FFT. In the reconstruction, close frequencies are not separated. The addition of noise worsens the performance [41], [42].

Simulation of loudness recruitment

In an impaired ear (deafness), a small increase of amplitude stimulates a large number of new nerve fibbers. In a normal ear, the auditory range is from

0 dB (auditory threshold) to 100 dB (discomfort level). In the case of cophosis, a variation from 60 dB to 100 dB spans from threshold to discomfort. This behavior can be mimicked by splitting the signal into frequency bands. A threshold and a dynamic expansion are introduced before reconstruction. In this situation, a small variation of amplitude is magnified, and it may be similar to what happens in pathology. Simulation with control subjects gives an idea of what can be expected with the best hearing impaired patients. Then, corrections are tested and the results are assessed. This approach helps to understand human behavior. Adapted algorithms are established belonging to the "intelligent procedures" category.

Introduction of new technologies

The power of speech processing techniques needs to be fully investigated. Classically, artificial neural networks perform well (better than classical methods) in noisy conditions. They have been used in the detection of speech cues, such as voicing, in noisy conditions. We have seen, already, that, normally, the spectrum is split into frequency bands according to the filter model of the cochlea. Other frequency-time representations are available in the package of the speech-processing engineer, such as wavelets, Wigner-Ville, or Gabor transforms. Each one is worthwhile to be investigated, and this is done in specialized laboratories.

5.3. Discussion

Models of pathology are attractive means to see hearing impairment. But how relevant are they? Results obtained with control subjects submitted to smeared signals are usually higher than those seen with hearing impaired persons. The reason lies in the accuracy of the model. Several reasons may explain this difference:

- The simulation does not mimic accurately the effect of the pathology.
- Other factors (not coming from the ear) introduce further deficits. Handicaps are, usually, polyhandicaps, and a simple model is not sufficient.
- An impaired ear deteriorates with the time, because an organ insufficiently used worsens.
- Deafness mechanisms vary along the cochlea, and some regions work better than others do. Consequently, a simple model cannot reflect properly the behavior of the organ.

Models are necessary to understand the pathology, but we must not forget their limits, which are high, when mankind and especially the human mind are the objects of the simulation.

6. Conclusions

Sensorial rehabilitation raises the question "of life and communication" and what is "intelligent or not" in the assistance. How to decide that a technique is intelligent and another is not is unclear. It is more or less admitted that a technique is intelligent if it processes human concepts and if it can simulate human behavior. In that sense, the techniques described in this chapter are intelligent.

In our case, the reconstruction of the signal done by cochlear implants is supposed to mimic a "high level" human function. However, to what extent is this simulation valid? Then, when the reconstruction delivers to the patient blocks of data compatible with the linguistic theory, the results can be quite different of the expectation made with the consideration of the spectral representation. In fact, the machine reflects our knowledge on the procedures used by human beings to understand the language. We learn from our failures, and the implantation in the machine of the evolution of the "state of the art" makes the machine "more intelligent."

It is true that computers and integrated circuits have changed our approach on deafness rehabilitation. We moved from amplification and compression of the signal and from the adjustment of onset and offset times to a full reconstruction of the message. In order to handle the new technology, audiologists will have to adapt their practice. Setting up all the parameters of a cochlear implant or a numeric hearing aid must be mastered by skilled specialists. We need a good setting of the machine, in order to use efficiently the patient's possibilities. We cannot put in the machine the knowledge we don't have, but we can make the assistance increasingly accurate, provided we establish what is needed for this assistance (in other words, what is needed to characterize and correct the impairment).

Of course, it is important to keep people alive, and the development of powerful machines to assist the vital functions of our body is necessary. Nevertheless, the communication, in our world of media, is not a luxury, and the assistance to sensory handicaps is worthwhile to be enhanced because it cannot be accepted that some people are let down.

Close cooperation between powerful machines and patients will have fruitful effects. We must not forget the fantastic plasticity of the human brain, and we must introduce in the machine the elements characterizing our sensorial system. This is another challenge, and we are far from knowing the rules.

Acknowledgments. The author thanks Professor Lionel Collet, head of the laboratory, for the strong support given in this field and Professor Horia-Nicolai L. Teodorescu for the correction and assistance in editing the manuscript.

References

[1] Grant, W., Walden, E., and Seitz, F.: Auditory visual speech recognition by hearing impaired subjects: consonant recognition, sentence recognition and auditory-visual integration, *J. Acoust. Soc. Am.*, vol. 103, pp. 2677-2690, 1998.

[2] Ehret, G. and Romand, D.: *The Central Auditory System*, Oxford Press, New York, 1997.

[3] Borsky, S., Tuller, B., and Shapiro, L.P.: How to milk a coat: the effect of semantic and acoustic information on phoneme categorisation, *J. Acoust. Soc. Am.*, vol. 103, pp. 2670-2676, 1998.

[4] Killion, M.C.: Hearing aids: past, present, future: moving toward normal conversation in noise, *Brit. J. Audiology*, vol. 31, pp. 141-148, 1997.

[5] Moore, B.C.J.: *Perceptual Consequences of Cochlear Damage*, Oxford Medical Publication, 1995.

[6] Killion, M.C.: The SIN report: circuits have not solved the hearing in noise problem, *Hearing J.*, vol. 50, pp. 28-32, 1997.

[7] CALLIOPE: *La parole et son traitement automatique*, Coll. Technique & Scientifique of French Telecom., Masson, 1989.

[8] Lombard: Le signe de l'élèvation de la voix, *Annales des maladies de l'oreille et du larynx*, vol. 37, pp. 101-119, 1911.

[9] Hansen, J.H.L. and Bria, O.N.: Lombard effect compensation for robust automatic speech recognition in noise, *Int. Spoken Language Processing* (Kobe, Japan), Proc., pp. 1125-1128, 1990.

[10] Dillion, H.: Compression? Yes but for low or high frequencies, and with what response time?, *Ear & Hearing*, vol. 17, pp. 287-307, 1996.

[11] Berger-Vachon, C., Collet, L., and Morgon, A.: An optimised model of the audiogram, *Annals of Telecom.*, vol. 49, pp. 625-639, 1994.

[12] Allen, J.B., Hall, J.L., and Jeng, P.S.: Loudness growth in 1/2-octave bands (LGOB): a procedure for the assessment of loudness, *J. Acoust. Soc. Am.*, vol. 88, pp. 745-753, 1990.

[13] Chouard, C.H., Les protheses numeriques, *Les Cahiers de l'Audition*, vol. 10, pp. 6-12, 1997.

[14] Byme, D.: Hearing aid selection for the 1990s: where to?, *J. Am. Acad. Audiol.*, vol. 7, pp. 377-395, 1997.

[15] Chouard, C.H.: *Entendre sans oreilles*, Robert Laffont, Paris, 1978.

[16] Djourno, A. and Eyries, C.: Prothese auditive par excitation electrique a distance du nerf sensoriel a l'aide d'un bobinage inclus a demeure, *Presse Med.*, vol. 35, pp. 1417-1423, 1957.

[17] Bogli, H. and Dillier, N.: Digital speech processor for the Nucleus 22 channel cochlear implant, *IEEE Eng. in Med. & Biology Safety*, vol. 13, pp. 1901-1902, 1992.

[18] Blamey, P.J. and Clark, G.M.: Place coding of vowel formants for cochlear implant patients, *J. Acoust. Soc. Am.*, vol. 88, pp. 667-673, 1990.

[19] Perrin, E., Berger-Vachon, C., Kauffmann, I., and Collet, L.: Acoustical recognition of laryngeal pathology using the fundamental frequency and the first

three formants of the voice, *Med. Biolog. Eng. Computing*, vol. 35, pp. 361-368, 1997.
[20] Tyler, R.S., Murray, N.T., Moore, B.C.J., and McCabe, B.F.: Synthetic two formant vowel perception by some of better cochlear implant patients, *Audiology*, vol. 28, pp. 301-315, 1989.
[21] Gantz, B.J., Tyler, R., Kunton, J.F., and Woodworth, G.: Evaluation of 5 different cochlear implants design: audiologic assessment and predictors of performance, *Laryngoscope*, vol. 90, pp. 1100-1106, 1988.
[22] Shiroma, M., Honda, K., Yamanaka, N., Kawano, J., Yakawa, K., Kumakawa, K., and Funasaka, S.: Factors contributing to phoneme recognition ability of users of the 22 channel cochlear implant system, *Ann. Otol. Rhinol. Laryngol.*, vol. 101, pp. 32-37, 1992.
[23] Berger-Vachon, C., Djeddou, B., and Morgon, A.: Model for understanding the influence of some parameters in cochlear implantation, *Annals Otol., Rhinol., Laryngol.*, vol. 101, pp. 42-45, 1992.
[24] Fu, Q., Shannon, V., and Wang, X.: Effect of noise and spectral resolution on vowel and consonant recognition: acoustic and electric hearing, *J. Acoust. Soc. Am.*, vol. 104, pp. 3586-3596, 1998.
[25] Wilson, B.S., Finley, C.C., Farmer, J.C., Lawson, D.T., Walford, R., Eddington, and D.K., Rabinowitz, W.M.: Better speech recognition with cochlear implants, *Nature*, vol. 352, pp. 236-238, 1991.
[26] Berger-Vachon, C. and Morgon, A.: An evaluation of auditory performances in patients with cochlear implants, *Speech Com.*, vol. 7, pp. 87-95, 1988.
[27] Belaieff, M., Dubus, P., Leveau, J.M., Repetto, J.C., and Vincent, P.: Sound processing and simulation coding of Digisonic DX-10, 15-channel cochlear implant, in: *Advances in Cochlear Implants*, I.J. Hochmair-Desoyer and E.S. Hochmaier (Eds.), pp. 198-203, Verlag Vienna, Manz, 1994.
[28] Gallego, S., Luu, B.L., and Berger-Vachon, C.: Modelling of the electrical simulation delivered by the Digisonic cochlear implant, *Advances in Modelling* (Series B), vol. 39, pp. 39-53, 1998.
[29] Kubo, T., Iwaki, T., Ohkusa, M., Doi, K., Uno, A., Yamamoto, K., and Fujii, K.: Auditory plasticity in cochlear implant patients, *Acta Otolaryngol. (Stockh.)*, vol. 116, pp. 224-227, 1996.
[30] Zierhofer, C., Peter, O., Brill, S., Czylok, T., Pohl, P., Hochmair-Desoyer, I., and Hochmair, E.: A multichannel cochlear implant system for high rate pulsatile stimulation strategies, in: *Advances in Cochlear Implants*, I.J. Hochmair-Desoyer and E.S. Hochmaier (Eds.), pp. 204-207, Verlag Vienna, Manz, 1994.
[31] Marquet, J., Van Durme, M., Lammens, J., Collier, R., Peeters, S., and Bosiers, W.: Acoustic stimulation experiments with pre-processed speech for an 8-channel cochlear implant, *Audiology*, vol. 25, pp. 353-362, 1986.
[32] Ramachandrula, N., Sitaram, V., and Sreenivas, T.: Incorporating phonetic properties in hidden Markov models for speech recognition, *J. Acoust. Soc. Am.*, vol. 102, pp. 1149-1158, 1997.
[33] Faulkner, A., Ball, V., Rosen, S., Moore, B. C. J., and Fourcin, A. J.: Speech pattern hearing aids for the profoundly hearing-impaired: Speech perception and auditory abilities, *J. Acoust. Soc. Am.*, vol. 91, pp. 2136-2155, 1992.

[34] Faulkner, A., Walliker, J. R., Howard, I. S., Ball, V., and Fourcin, A. J.: New developments in speech pattern element hearing aids for the profoundly deaf, *Scandinavian Audiology*, Suppl., vol. 38, pp. 124-135, 1993.
[35] Wilson, B.S., Lawson, D.T., Walford, R., and Eddington, D.K.: Coding strategies for multichannel cochlear prostheses, *Am. J. Otol.*, Suppl. 12, pp. 56-61, 1991.
[36] Pfingst, B., Telman, S., and Sutton, D.: Operating ranges for cochlear implants, *Am. Otol. Rhinol Laryngol.*, vol. 89 Suppl. 66, pp. 1-4, 1980.
[37] Berger-Vachon, C., Gallego, S., Morgon, A., and Truy, E.: Analytic importance of the coding features for the discrimination of vowels in the cochlear implant signal, *Annals Otol. Rhinol. Laryngol.*, Suppl. 166, pp. 351-353, 1995.
[38] Wilson, B.S.: The future of cochlear implants, *Brit. J. Audiology*, vol. 31, pp. 205-225, 1997.
[39] Fu, Q., Shannon, R.W., and Wang, X.: Effect of worse and spectral resolution on vowel and consonant recognition: acoustic and electric hearing, *J. Acoust. Soc. Am.*, vol. 104, pp. 3586-3596, 1998.
[40] Shannon, R.V., Zeng, F.G., and Wygonski, J.: Speech recognition of altered spectral distribution of envelope cues, *J. Acoust. Soc. Am.*, vol. 104, pp. 2469-2476, 1998.
[41] Beattie, R., Barr, T., and Roup, C.: Normal and hearing impaired word recognition scores for monosyllabic words in quiet and noise, *Brit. J. Audiology*, vol. 31, pp. 153-164, 1997.
[42] Agnew, J.: Directionality in hearing... revisited, *Hear. Rev.*, vol. 3, pp. 20-26, 1996.

Bibliographic Note. The following references are particularly useful in the field of signal representation methods referred to in this chapter:

Cohen, L.: Time-frequency distribution-a review, *Proceedings IEEE*, vol. 77, pp. 941-981, 1989.
Auger, A. and Doncarelli, C.: Some remarks about recently proposed time-frequency representations, (in French), *Traitement du Signal*, vol. 9, pp. 3-25, 1992.
Claasen, C.M. and Mecklenbauer, W.F.G.: The Wigner distribution in discrete signals, *Philips J. Research*, vol. 35, pp. 276-300, 1980.
D'Alessandro, C.: Time-frequency speech transformation based on an elementary waveform transformation, *Speech Com.*, vol. 9, pp. 419-431, 1990.
Holschteiter, M.: General inversion for wavelets transforms, *J. Math. Phys.*, vol. 34, pp. 4190-4198, 1993.

A commented list of texts on wavelet transforms is:
Teodorescu, H.N.: Further reading on wavelet decomposition, in Teodorescu, H.N. Kandel, A. and Jain, L.C.: *Soft Computing in Human-Related Sciences*, CRC Press, Boca Raton, 1999, pp. 233-234.

A discussion of wavelet transforms and of fuzzy techniques can be found in:
Beksac, S. *et al.*: Intelligent diagnostic systems in maternal and fetal medicine. Chapter 6, Teodorescu, H.N., Kandel, A., and Jain, L.C.: *Soft Computing in Human-Related Sciences*, CRC Press, Boca Raton, 1999, pp. 137-197.

Part 3.

Locomotor prostheses

Chapter 4

Sensory feedback for lower limb prostheses

Daniela Zambarbieri, Micaela Schmid,
and **Gennaro Verni**

In this chapter, we deal with biofeedback techniques for rehabilitation of the lower limb prosthetic subjects. The general theories of motor control are first discussed to explain the role of sensory feedback for the reconstruction of the internal model. Since sensory feedback from lower limbs is lacking in amputee subjects, employing an artificial feedback can improve subject performance in using his or her artificial leg. Auditory, visual and tactile biofeedbacks are described and discussed. A portable device for sensory substitution of the ground pressure information in the prosthetic foot is detailed and the evaluation procedure for assessing system performance is presented.

1. Introduction

An internal model of the human body is used by the central nervous system to decide the adequate motor commands needed to execute movements [5], [6]. The presence of lesions, such as limb amputation, induces a mismatch between the output predicted by the internal model and the movement actually executed by the body. Thus, a reorganization of the motor strategies is needed to readapt and update the internal model. Rehabilitation of the prosthetic subjects can induce the update of the internal model. If the subject is provided with some kind of artificial sensory information, he or she is likely to assume that the process of updating the internal model can be improved. Moreover, the availability of biofeedback can help the prosthetic subject during his everyday life activities.

For lower limb amputees the most important information that is lacking is the pressure exerted by the prosthetic foot on the ground. An artificial substitution of the natural feedback, the latter provided by tactile and proprioceptive input to the central nervous system, must therefore be able to measure the location, and eventually the amount, of foot pressure. In addition, it should transmit this information toward the nervous system, by using both direct connections to the nervous system or sensory substitution.

Few examples are available in the literature concerning sensory feedback for lower limb prostheses [8], [17], [32]. The most part of the effort made in the field of prosthetic limbs has been devoted to upper limb prostheses in which the control of the grasping is of course of great importance for the return of the patient to the normal life [2], [7], [31], [33], [35-39], [42].

Nevertheless, even in the case of lower limb amputee subjects, the functionality that the prosthesis can give is not only that of walking. Even for these subjects a device able to return some sensorial information could play a fundamental role in the perfect reinsertion of the subject in everyday life.

In this chapter, we investigate this topic by first examining some general concepts about the theories on movement control. A brief review will be presented on the physiology of the natural sensory feedback from lower limbs. Then, possible solutions for the realization of an artificial feedback will be discussed together with a description of those studies published in the literature. Finally, the system we have developed in our laboratory is discussed and its application during the rehabilitation process is described.

2. Theories of movement control

When a subject decides to move from one point in space to another, the consequent motor act implies a complex coordination not only of the lower limbs, but also of the upper limb and the trunk. In fact, during displacement, the central nervous system has to control that the movement reaches its goal and that balance is preserved.

In controlling every body movement, the general problems can be summarized as follows: a motor act implies a progressive modification of posture, every posture modification implies a balance problem, therefore during motor act execution the central nervous system has to control, at the same time, movement, posture and balance. Moreover, during movement execution some body segments must be kept stationary since they act as reference for the movement to be achieved. For instance, during walking and running, the head inclination is kept stable to allow clear vision of the external world [30].

2.1. Coordination between posture and movement

A movement can be considered as a series of successive postures and it is due to a progressive modification of the static balance between forces exerted by agonist muscles. This corresponds to the "balance point" theories proposed by Bernstein in 1967 [5]. The continuous shift from one point of equilibrium to another would be produced by a central nervous command that controls the ratio between muscle forces.

Posture control is used not only to produce the movement but also to prepare its execution, a situation that has been named "readiness to move" after Bernstein. Some postural adjustment actually precedes the beginning of movement. This anticipatory characteristics of postural control during movement is the best demonstration that posture is not only the result of some servo-mechanisms able to correct the error between the actual and the desired position, but it is part of the general planning of the motor act. Bernstein proposed the idea of the "action-perception cycle." Fundamental components of this conceptual model are the *programmer* that decides the motor program, the *comparator* that provides the relevant command, and a *regulator* that processes the commands and activates the relevant muscles.

The programmer receives information on the motor act to be executed and sensorial information from peripheral receptors. The output of the programmer is sent to the comparator, which also receives sensorial information. The action of the comparator is threefold: comparison between the actual and the desired movement to produce the correction signals; identification of the movement completeness and activation of the succeeding motor act; modification of the movement trajectory in the case of inadequacy during the execution of the movement.

The coordination of a motor act would require the control of a great number of degrees of freedom. A way to reduce the number of degrees of freedom to be controlled is to make use of *synergies*, which are elementary motor actions, implying the coordination among different body segments. In other words, a synergy is a specific configuration of muscle activation aimed to obtain a specific posture. These concepts have been introduced by Bernstein [5] and later by Nashner [23], Gahery and Massion [14], and Cordo and Nashner [9], by suggesting the existence of a synergy repertoire that can be activated by sensory input induced by external disturbance or by internal commands for voluntary movements. Synergies are not strictly pre-programmed, but they can be adapted and the choice of a specific synergy can depend on the support condition [20], [21], [26], [28].

A fascinating hypothesis suggests that some basic synergies are innate, being part of the genetic resources, and other are acquired from the interaction with the environment. When the situation of interaction with the environment is modified, a learning process would take place, resulting in the substitution of the old synergy with a new one. The use of a specific synergy or a sequence of synergies to perform a motor act represents a *motor strategy*. The choice of the motor strategy that best fits the required action is the higher level function performed by the nervous system in the control of movement.

2.2. The internal model

In order to be able to select the most appropriate motor strategy to perform a motor act, the existence of an internal model of the system must be hypothesized. Among all possible motor strategies and synergies, the internal model selects those better matching the action to be accomplished. Then, based on the knowledge of the geometry, kinematics and dynamics of the body segments of the initial and current state of the system, the internal model decides the motor commands needed to perform those postural variations that produce the desired movement. The internal model represents a synthesis of the experience acquired in programming and executing different motor acts.

In 1988, Droulez and Berthoz [12] suggested that the brain has a dual mode of movement control. The first mode operates in a continuous way following the classical scheme of servosystems; the second mode simulates the movement in order to predict its consequences and therefore to choose the better motor strategy.

During motor acts executed at very high speed, as for instance skiing down the hill, the brain has no time to continuously control the information coming from sensory receptors. It can be assumed therefore that the brain makes use of an internal representation of the movement and checks sensory re-afference, that means information from sensory feedback arising in the periphery, in a sampled way.

The first control mode operates in a closed loop by using sensory re-afference and pre-programmed motor acts. The second control mode makes use of internal maps where the movement can be simulated without execution. A map is a pool of neurons that, in a specific area of the brain, contains a topographical representation of the external world characteristics. Even if sensory re-afferences are checked in a discontinuous way, the control is maintained through simulation.

In both control modes, sensory re-afference plays a fundamental role. In the first mode, it is used to build up and update the internal model and to choose the most appropriate synergies. In the second mode, sensory re-afference provides information on the actual state of movement execution.

When changes occur such as modifications in environmental conditions (i.e., microgravity) or the presence of lesions in the nervous and muscle-skeleton apparatus, the internal model becomes inadequate. It results in a lack of correspondence between the movement predicted by the internal model and the movement actually executed. If the central nervous system is able to detect this mismatching by means of the sensory re-afferences, an adaptation process can take place, which updates the internal model. The lack of a lower limb and its substitution with a prosthesis represent an internal modification of the system which requires a reorganization of the motor strategies and synergies involved to accomplish a movement of the amputee limb.

In lower limb amputations, functional reeducation has the task of making the subject able to walk correctly again. The lack of one, or two, lower limb needs to develop new motor strategies which allow the subject to use his prosthesis in the right way, by distributing the weight on both legs, and to walk with the minimum energy waste. The movements that a prosthetic subject has to learn in order to control his prosthesis correctly during walking may be completely different from those of the natural leg. The rehabilitation program represents the only way for the prosthetic subject to become aware of this new condition, learning how to use his residual functionality and that of the prosthesis in the best way. An update of the internal model is likely to occur during rehabilitation.

3. Natural feedback

Sensory receptors are neural structures that provide information from the external world and from within our body. Sensory systems are divided into three categories: exteroreceptive, proprioceptive, and interoceptive [16]. Exteroceptive systems are sensitive to external stimuli (vision, audition, skin sensation, and chemical senses); proprioceptive systems provide information about body position in space and the relative position of body segments to one another. Interoceptive systems are those concerned with internal events in the body and often the signals they provide do not reach consciousness.

The somatic sensory system can be considered belonging to all the three classes previously described. It comprises different perceptual modalities, in particular tactile sensations, proprioceptive sensations, thermal sensations, and pain sensations. For the purpose of our study, only the first two classes of sensations are relevant: tactile sensations are elicited by mechanical stimulation applied to body surface, and proprioceptive sensations are elicited by mechanical displacements of muscles and joints.

Without going into anatomical details, it is important to note that a somatic stimulus is perceived at the periphery, and processed and relayed to higher level of the nervous system through the spinal cord or the medulla.

3.1. Tactile sensation

Tactile sensation is mediated by a class of receptors that are called mechanoreceptors. There are different types of mechanoreceptors that can be divided into two major groups: the slowly adapting mechanoreceptors, which respond continuously to an enduring stimulus, and the rapidly adapting mechanoreceptors, which respond only at the onset of the stimulus.

Glabrous skin contains two kinds of rapidly adapting mechanoreceptors, the Meissner and the Pacini corpuscles, and two kinds of slowly adapting mechanoreceptors called the Merkel receptors and the Ruffini corpuscle. Tactile corpuscles described by Meissner are located in the papillae of the corium of the hand and foot, the front of the forearm, the skin of the lips and the mucous membrane of the tip of the tongue. Pacini corpuscles are found in the human subject chiefly on the nerves of the palm of the hand and the sole of the foot, lying in the subcutaneous tissue. Merkel has described tactile corpuscles as occurring in the papillae and epithelium of the skin of man and animals, especially in those parts of the skin devoid of hair. Ruffini has described a special variety of nerve endings in the subcutaneous tissue of human finger.

Each different mechanoreceptor is able to mediate different sensations, from light touch to deep pressure. The complex natural stimuli characteristics experienced in everyday life activate different combinations of mechanoreceptor classes.

3.2. Proprioceptive sensation

Proprioception includes the sense of balance, primarily mediated by the vestibular apparatus, the sense of stationary position of the limbs, and the sense of limb movement (kinesthesia). During voluntary limb movements, a corollary discharge of the motor command is also available that could be used for proprioception sensation. Nevertheless, several experimental studies have demonstrated that even during voluntary movements, the senses of the limb position and movement are actually mediated by peripheral receptors.

Three main types of peripheral receptors are able to provide information about the stationary position of the limb and the speed and direction of limb movement. The three classes of peripheral receptors are the mechanoreceptors located in the joint capsules, the cutaneous mechanoreceptors, and the mechanoreceptors located in the muscle and transducing muscle stretch. Muscle spindles are located within the belly of the muscle. Because they are attached in parallel with the other muscle fibers, they are stretched whenever the muscle is stretched. A receptor in each spindle responds to an increase of muscle length and its output is sent to the spinal cord. There is another type of stretch receptor in skeletal muscle, the Golgi tendon organs, which responds to an increase in tension rather than length. Tendon organs are located at the junctions of muscle fibers and their tendons and thus they are in series with the contractile parts of the muscles as opposed to the spindles, which are in parallel. They measure the forces produced by the contracting fibers and send impulses to the spinal cord.

4. Artificial feedback

When a sensory system (visual, auditory, or somatic) is lacking or it is damaged, several approaches can be followed to replace the lost functionality. We can in principle distinguish between *natural* prostheses or *substitutive* prostheses. Natural prostheses are those that replace the peripheral part of the damaged system and are connected to the central nervous part of the system itself. Some examples can be found in the case of blind subjects. A video camera perceives the scene of the external world and converts it in electric pulses that are transmitted to the cerebral cortex. In the cerebral cortex an array of microelectrodes is implanted in the visual area and electric signal transmission can be obtained with a percutaneous cable connection (with a high degree of infections risks) or by induction [24], [37].

Substitutive prostheses are those that use a different sensory system to provide some of the information that the damaged system is no longer able to produce. Still using blind people as an example, there are prostheses that permit the subject to read a text not Braille printed, or that permit the subject to navigate in the environment avoiding obstacles. The auditory and the tactile systems remain available in these patients and the information collected from these substitutive prostheses are converted into auditory or tactile signals for the subject.

The situation of a limb amputee subject can be considered from two different points of view. A leg is needed as a support during walking, and this function is successfully replaced with the prosthesis. But during walking or any other activity, the information provided by the tactile and proprioceptive systems that make part of the closed loop described in the first paragraph is also important.

In an amputee subject, independently from the level of amputation, tactile information from the foot sole is lacking; moreover, proprioceptive information from muscles is no longer reliable since those muscles remaining after amputation are no longer efficient as normal muscles. The only information that can be reasonably measured with sensors is foot pressure. This is used in the examples described in the literature and in the system we have recently developed.

To create an artificial feedback to the central nervous system, we could therefore identify natural and substitutive solutions, comparable to those described for the blind subjects. The natural approach makes a direct connection between the pressure sensors and the nervous pathway toward the central nervous system. The substitutive approach can use the visual system, the auditory system or the tactile system itself but in different regions of the body surface. In the latter case, the kind of information processed by means of the tactile system will of course be different from that normally performed in the intact limb.

5. Center of pressure

The most important need for lower limb amputees, especially at the beginning of rehabilitation, is that of maintaining balance both in static and dynamic conditions. The balance is achieved when the ground projection of the body center of mass (CM) lies inside the support surface. CM position is a quantity not directly detectable. It must be reconstructed through the internal model from the information provided by the muscle-tendon receptors and the cutaneous receptors of the foot sole.

The latter also provide the central nervous system with signals that can be used to obtain the position of the center of pressure (CP). The amputee, deprived of these sensory re-afferences, has some difficulties in controlling his CM position. Reaching the right posture to maintain balance therefore becomes a very difficult task. Usually, rehabilitation trains the patient to execute movements without the help of the lost sensorial re-afferences.

5.1. Instrumentation for center of pressure (CP) evaluation

CP position can be evaluated as the point of application of the vertical component of the resulting force of ground reaction. Instrumentation for CP evaluation must therefore have sensors able to measure the intensity of ground reaction forces on the foot surface and a system – either software or hardware – to compute the resulting force. Different devices are at present available for measuring the force exerted at ground level during walking.

5.1.1. Forceplates

The forceplate is used to measure the forces and the torque moments during the foot contact with the ground in the stance phase. In particular, three components, namely vertical, anterior-posterior, and medial-lateral, can be obtained for the resulting force, but only the component relative to the vertical axis for the moment. In fact, the moment components that lie on the gait plane are equal to zero, due to the impossibility of exercising traction forces during stance. It is also possible to obtain the coordinates of the instantaneous center of pressure.

The various types of forceplate differ in the transducer they use. Transducers can be piezoelectric or resistive sensors, optical systems, or deformable metals. In gait analysis laboratories, the Kistler (Kistler Instruments Corp., Amherst, NY) and the AMTI (Advanced Mechanical Technology Inc., Watertown, MA) forceplates are widely used. In Kistler forceplates, the four piezoelectric cells are placed at the vertices and measure all three components of the applied force. The piezoelectric cells are quartz transducers, which generate an electric charge when stressed. They do not require a power supply to excite the transducers; however, special charge amplifiers and low noise coaxial cables are required to convert the charge to a voltage proportional to the applied load. The transducers are calibrated at the factory and no recalibration is necessary. In general the Kistler platforms are more sensitive and have a greater force range than the stain gauge type. AMTI forceplates instead use strain gauges to measure the stress in specially machined aluminium transducer bodies (load cells) when a load is applied. They do not require the special cabling and charge amplifiers of the piezoelectric type; however, they do require excitation of the strain gauge bridge circuit. Data acquisition can also vary among different forceplates. In all cases, however, the amount of analog signals that can be manipulated is not limited, since the device is fixed on the ground and it is directly connected to the computer.

During gait analysis, the use of the forceplate has some disadvantages. First, only one single step for each foot can be measured; second, it is necessary that the foot entirely fall on the plate surface. This last constraint can significantly influence the normal walking pacing of the examined subject.

5.1.2. Sensorized insoles

Sensorized insoles are normally placed inside the subject's shoes. They can be made of a few sensors placed on specific zone of the foot surface, or they can be arranged as a matrix covering the entire foot surface. In the latter case, a better resolution in CP position evaluation is obtained. The number of sensors in the matrix can vary from about 60 up to 960 as in the F-Scan sensorized insoles (Tekscan Inc., Boston, MA).

The F-Scan system uses the patented Tekscan sensor, a flexible and trimmable sensor with 960 sensing locations distributed evenly across the entire plantar surface. The sensor feeds data into the computer for analysis and display. Each sensing location is continuously sampled up to 165 times per second as the patient walks, runs or jumps. It is possible to view the sampled data in real time, and data can be recorded for detailed review and analysis. Recordings can be viewed in motion or studied a frame at a time. Summary screens can show peak force versus time, pressure versus time, peak pressure versus time and pressure profile [18], [41]. The advantage of these devices is primarily the fact that the subject can walk on every type of surface and successive gait cycles can be analyzed.

In sensorized insoles, data acquisition is realized in different modes. A cable can be used to connect the insoles worn by the subject to the computer. Therefore, there is no limitation in the number of transferred analog signals; however, the presence of the cable limits the length of subject displacement and could sometimes interfere with his movements. Another possibility that some devices have adopted is that of using an A/D converter which is attached to the subject's belt. The subject is therefore completely free to move, but data analysis is performed only at the end of the experiment when the stored data are transferred to the computer [1]. A third solution we have implemented in our system makes use of the telemetric connection between the subject and the computer. No cables are needed. Consequently, no cable interferes with the subject walking, but only a limited number of data can be transferred to the computer.

5.1.3. Telemetric acquisition of CP

We have used in our experiments a device for CP evaluation that allows on-line computing of the CP position during movement execution. On-line availability of CP positions information is of course an essential requirement for realizing sensory feedback. This system is a prototype recently developed at the Istituto Superiore di Sanità in Italy [19]. The insoles are made of a matrix of 64 pressure sensitive sensors. The analog signals provided by each sensor are locally processed by means of a small sized resistive circuit connected to the insole. The circuit provides in real time the X and Y coordinates of the CP position and the vertical component of the resulting forces. The analog output from the insole can be used to directly control biofeedback devices. Alternatively, the insole output is connected to a small lightweight device, which performs A/D conversion at a frequency of 60 HZ. By using telemetry, the digital output of this device is transmitted in 7 byte records to the serial port of the personal computer, and the subject is therefore free to move without any constraints. Both the A/D converter and the transmitter are held by the subject in a small bag, fastened as a belt. We have used this device for examining CP trajectories during walking and for the visual and auditory biofeedback that will be described later.

5.2. Normal trajectory of CP during walking

The *gait cycle* or *stride* is defined as the set of movements and events that take place between two successive initial ground contacts with the same foot [10], [11], [15], [29], [43]. The gait cycle can be divided into two principal phases: the *stance phase*, during which the foot remains in contact with the ground, and the *swing phase* during which the foot is brought forward. In normal subjects, the stride cycle begins with *heel-strike* and terminates with another heel-strike of the same foot.

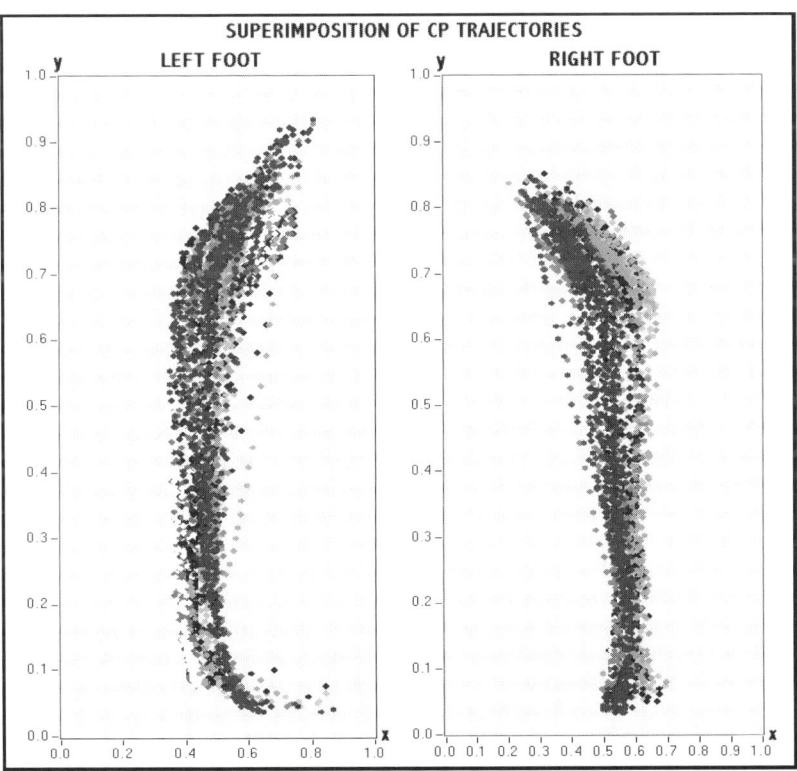

Figure 1. Superposition of CP trajectories obtained during walking in a normal subject. Twenty steps for each foot are presented and shadings indicate different trials.

The stance phase continues with the entire foot in contact with the ground and then the heel rise and terminates with *toe-off*; the swing phase begins with toe-off, continues with the passage through the zenith of the swinging limb and terminates with a new heel-strike.

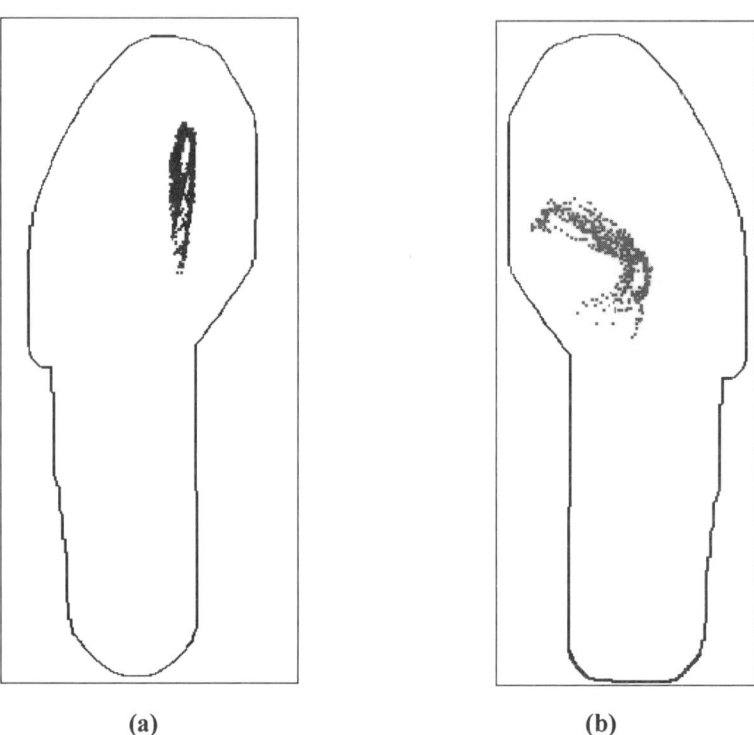

(a) (b)

Figure 2. (a) CP trajectories in a patient with transtibial amputation of the left leg. (b) CP trajectories in a patient with congenital lack of the right leg.

Several studies are available in the literature that examine the plantar pressure distribution in normal subjects during walking and in addition compare barefoot conditions and shod conditions [3], [4], [22], [25], [40]. In Figure 1, we provide examples of CP trajectories in a normal subject during walking. At the beginning of the single stance phase, CP lies on the medial-posterior heel and then it moves through the mid-foot region, and continues towards the forefoot, crossing the metatarsal heads and terminates in the region of the great and second toe. During successive steps, even in the same subject, the trajectories of CP are not always perfectly the same. Superposition of CP trajectories during successive steps results therefore in an "area" on the foot surface. We have decided to quantify this "area" in order to have a reference for the evaluation of walk. By using a polynomial interpolation of this trajectory an analytical expression can be calculated that can be used to test whether the incoming signal provided by the sensorized insole lies inside or outside this area [44].

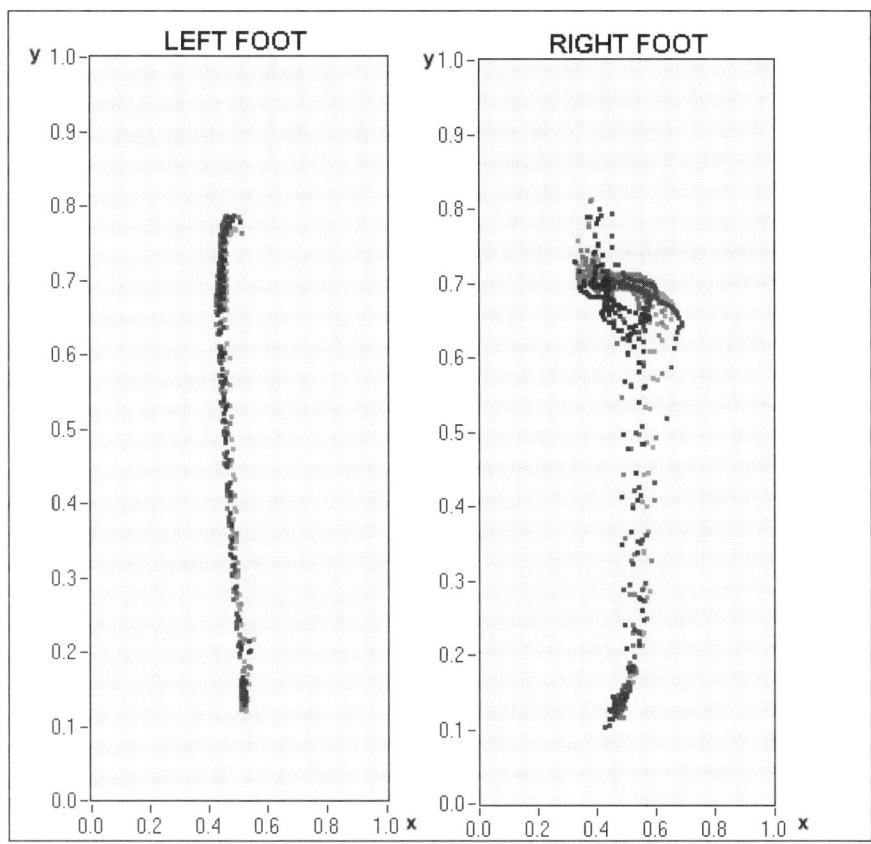

Figure 3. CP trajectories of the prosthetic (on the left) and the natural (on the right) foot in a patient with transfemoral amputation of the left leg. Data have been recorded at the end of the rehabilitation process.

In amputee subjects of course CP trajectories of the prosthetic foot can vary dramatically with respect to normal subjects, mainly during the first period of rehabilitation. Figure 2a shows the example of a patient with a transtibial amputation due to a car accident, recorded after one week of prosthesis fitting. It can be easily appreciated that the patient was not able to strike the heel of the prosthetic foot, but he was not aware of this until the visual feedback was used. In Figure 2b, we provide another example of the wrong strike in a young patient with a congenital lack of the right leg. The heel-strike of this patient was almost absent and he only used the anterior part of the foot by executing a partial rotation of the foot during the stance phase.

Figure 3 shows an example of a subject with left transfemoral amputation wearing a modular prosthesis with an electronic knee and a dynamic foot. Data have been recorded at the end of the rehabilitation process. It can be observed that CP trajectories of the prosthetic foot are almost straight along the foot surface from the heel towards the forefoot and are perfectly suprimposed step after step. In contrast, CP trajectories of the natural foot show the variability already observed in normal subjects (Figure 1).

6. Visual and auditory feedback

6.1. Visual feedback

Visual biofeedback is achieved by showing the CP position on a screen, while the subject is carrying out the movement. In particular, two images are presented which correspond to the left and right foot. For each foot, the area in which CP trajectory should be maintained (reference area) is also presented. According to what has been discussed in the previous section, the reference areas are different for the prosthetic and the natural feet. The points falling outside the reference area are shown in a different color, providing the subject with information on how much he is deviating from the desired performance.

Visual biofeedback is very easy to carry out and provides the patient with information, not only on CP trajectory, but also on its movement. The presentation of the visual image, however, disturbs the normal role that vision plays in the control of posture and locomotion. Therefore, the patient may have difficulty in watching the screen and simultaneously correcting his mistake, mainly during the initial phases of the reeducation.

Thus, the visual representation of CP movement seems to be more useful to the physiotherapist, rather than as biofeedback technique. The physiotherapist, following on-line the trajectory of CP position, can better understand how to instruct the subject for the next trials.

6.2. Acoustic biofeedback

Acoustic biofeedback is realized by using sounds to make the patient aware of the CP distance from the reference area. The deviations towards the inside of the foot are signaled with one sound and those towards the outside are signaled with a second and different sound. Simple tones or recorded sounds, such as two distinct vowels, are used as acoustic biofeedback. The use of more complex acoustic messages to signal not only the direction of the deviation, but its amplitude is not advisable, because complex messages confuse the subject.

To avoid instantaneous correction, with the risk of creating instability, the acoustic signaling is provided only if the subject leaves the area of reference for at least 50 ms. The main advantage of this biofeedback system is that it does not employ the sensory pathways normally used to control movement. In addition, the simplicity of the message, obtained by reducing the amount of information sent to the subject, makes his task easier. Even this system can be used only for experimental purposes, since in everyday life the patient would not accept such a "noisy" device.

7. Tactile and proprioceptive biofeedback

Tactile and proprioceptive feedback substitution for artificial limbs can use direct neural stimulation, transcutaneous stimulation, or mechanical vibrators. Several attempts have been made concerning the application of electric stimulation in upper limb prostheses in order to control prehension force and these systems are described in another chapter of the book.

Few studies, however, are available in the literature related to sensory substitution in lower limb prostheses. In 1981, Kawamura et al. [17] used surface electrocutaneous signals to provide foot sole pressure information. Four independent tape switches located on the sole of the prosthetic foot drive four surface electrodes placed on the thigh in above-knee amputees. The same authors have also implemented a system for the detection of prosthesis knee angle.

Direct peripheral nerve stimulation was used in leg prostheses by Clippinger et al. [8]. Four platinum-iridium electrodes were inserted in the sciatic nerve of patients. The frequency of electrical stimulation was modulated according to the bending moment registered through strain gauges placed on the pylon of the prosthesis.

More recently, Sabolich and Ortega [32] have proposed a non-invasive system to restore a sense of feeling to amputees. Transcutaneous electrical stimulation is provided to the sense organs at the interface between the residual limb and the socket. Two pressure transducers are incorporated in the sole of the artificial foot and respond proportionately to pressure on individual areas of the foot and send tingling signals to the amputee's residual limb. Even if the system is still under testing in a prototype form and is not yet available on the market, the authors indicate some benefits emerging from its use, such as the improvement in weight distribution, step length and stance time.

8. A portable device for tactile stimulation

8.1. The system

We have recently developed a very simple, low cost, totally portable device to provide mechanical tactile stimulation for artificial sensory feedback. The system is made of two sensors, a circuit, and two small eccentric DC motors (Figure 4).

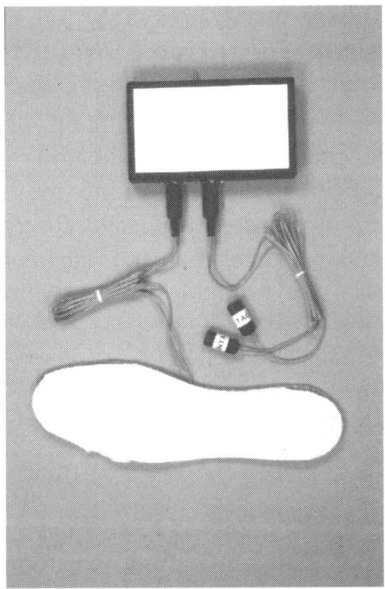

Figure 4. The portable device for tactile stimulation includes a leather sole containing two force-sensing resistors, a box containing the electronic circuit, the power supply, and two mechanical stimulators.

It is a common experience that a vibrating mechanical stimulus applied to the body surface evokes a sensation that human beings identify as quantitatively different from other mechanical stimuli. At a frequency of 2-40 Hz the feeling is one of cutaneous flutter, which passes over into a sense of mechanical hum characterized by the word "vibration." Flutter-vibration is a derived form of mechanoreceptive sensibility, which depends for its unique qualities upon the temporal pattern of the neural inputs evoked.

The sensors used in the system shown in Figure 4 are force-sensitive resistor devices (FSR) that superficially resemble a membrane switch, but unlike the conventional switches, they change resistance inversely with applied force. These sensors are ideal for touch control, are inexpensive, thin (>0.15 mm), durable (10,000,000 actuations), and environmentally resistant. The box containing the electronic circuit and the power supply is lightweight (220 g) and small (160 mm × 95 mm × 35 mm). It can be easily attached to the patient belt by means of the incorporated clip.

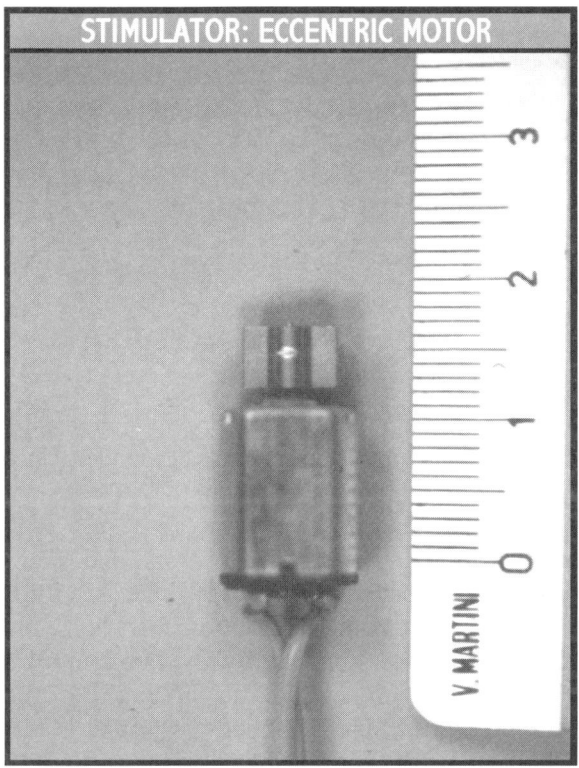

Figure 5. The eccentric motor used to provide the stimulation (Unit: cm).

The sensors are positioned on a leather sole inserted into the patient shoe. Normally the two sensors are placed at the heel and at the toe, but different positioning can be used according to specific needs of the subjects.

The eccentric motors are of the type commonly used in mobile phones (Figure 5). In the below-knee amputee, the two vibrators are placed on the thigh in the anterior and posterior positions in order to maintain spatial correspondence with the sensors. In the above-knee amputee, the vibrators are placed on the trunk. In developing the system, we have decided to make it totally external with respect to the prosthesis for at least two reasons. The first one is that of not increasing the cost of the prosthesis itself, the second one is for leaving the subject to decide when to use it in everyday life activities, after the initial period of rehabilitation.

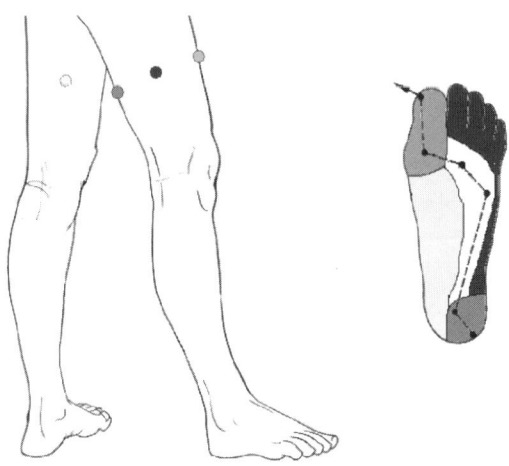

Figure 6. The four stimulation system, with correspondence between sensors and stimulation.

A more complex system with four sensors and four corresponding stimulators is under development (Figure 6). There is no limitation, from a hardware point of view, to the number of sensors that can be placed on the foot sole and the number of tactile stimulators they can control. More likely, an implicit limitation exists which is related to the ability of the subject in the discrimination among a great number of sensors placed in different positions on his residual limb or on his trunk. Not only does a limitation exist in the spatial discrimination ability in tactile stimulation, but also a too complex system would require a constant conscious effort from the subject. This is not acceptable if the system is designed to help not only rehabilitation but also the normal activity in everyday life.

8.2. Rehabilitation protocol

The portable device of Figure 4 has been designed with a twofold purpose. First it is used during the rehabilitation procedure that follows the first fit of the prosthesis to the patient, and second it can be worn by the amputee during his normal activities to improve the prosthesis functionality. Giving the subject sensory feedback on the pressure exerted by artificial foot on any surface could even permit the subject to use automobile clutch, brake, or bicycle pedals.

At present we are still dealing with the first phase of the project. The device has been fitted in a small population of amputee subjects in order to obtain qualitative evaluation of the system performances. The four examined subjects were below-knee amputees and they wore the device during the period spent at the INAIL Centro Protesi in Italy. The subjects have been asked for their personal sensations and they have easily accepted the device without problems. The awareness of prosthetic foot contact to the ground seems to help the patients during the rehabilitation process.

Starting from these positive results, we have developed a protocol for a rigorous quantitative evaluation of subject performances during the rehabilitation process. The rehabilitation protocol, which is normally used at the INAIL Centro Protesi, can be summarized in four successive steps. Step I corresponds to orthostatic exercises to obtain static balance. During step II, the patient begins to walk inside the parallel bars. Step III starts when the subject begins to walk with some auxiliary device, such as crutches, and goes on by reducing successively the number of supports. Step IV corresponds to the subject walking without any auxiliary device.

Starting from the third step of rehabilitation, a quantitative evaluation of the walking performance is done twice a day, untill the end of the rehabilitation. During each test the subject is asked to walk at his natural speed along a 10 m length platform, five times in the same direction. The first daily test is performed in the morning and the second one late in the afternoon in order to evaluate both the improvement produced by rehabilitation and its retention from one day to the following one. Quantitative evaluation of walking is performed by using simultaneously the ELITE system for the analysis of body segments movement, the F-Scan sensorized insole for the measure of ground pressure, and a video recording to observe the general feature of the walking performance.

ELITE (Elaboratore di Immagini Televisive, BTS Inc., Milano, Italy) is a completely automatic system for kinematics and kinetic analysis of movement [13]. It is based on the processing of television images according to criteria of pattern recognition, and it is capable of synchronizing these images with the data deriving from the force platform and from other similar instruments, in our case the F-Scan insoles and the video controller. The system is able to extract, from whatever complex scene, the coordinates of passive markers placed on the anatomical landmarks whose spatial trajectories have to be measured. The passive markers are small spheres or half-spheres (diameter 1.5 cm) covered with retroflective tape.

A population of 20 below-knee amputees will be examined during this quantitative evaluation experimental phase. Ten subjects will follow the standard rehabilitation protocol and the other ten subjects will wear the tactile sensory feedback shown in Figure 4 starting from the beginning of step III of rehabilitation. Subjects are selected according to some criteria in order to obtain a uniform and comparable population. They must have an amputation due to accidents or traumas to avoid other pathological implications and must be in a range of age between 18 and 50 years. Successively, the same experimental protocol will be applied to a population of above-knee amputee subjects.

The main goal of this experimental protocol, which is at present still in progress, will be that of quantifying the advantage of the tactile sensory feedback in reducing the duration of the rehabilitation process needed to obtain a correct gait cycle in the amputee subjects.

9. Conclusions

Lower limb prostheses have reached, at present, a significant level of quality and performances, and amputee subjects are able to walk almost normally, to run and to practice some sports. Nevertheless, even if the mechanical aspects of walking are restored, prostheses still lack the possibility to provide the sensation of ground pressure of the artificial foot. This information would play an important role in the control and coordination of walking, running, and performing other activities.

In fact, according to the general theories on motor control, the central nervous system needs sensory re-afference in order to be able to update and maintain the internal model used to decide the most appropriate motor strategies. If the amputee subject is provided with some kind of artificial sensory information substituting the lacking natural re-afference, it is likely to assume that the process of updating the internal model for motor control can be improved.

In this chapter, we have described first the general theories on motor control and the role of the natural sensory feedback. Then we have described the possible solution for creating an artificial sensory feedback for lower limb amputee subjects. In fact, it is possible to measure the ground pressure by using simple devices and to feed back to the patient this information by using different techniques. The few examples available in the literature make use of electrical stimulation applied directly to the nerve or on the intact skin at the level of the residual limb.

At the University of Pavia and in collaboration with the Istituto Superiore di Sanità and the INAIL Centro Protesi in Italy we have developed some artificial biofeedback systems that make use of different sensory inputs, such as visual, auditory and tactile inputs. One of the systems has been developed to be completely wearable by the subjects and makes use of vibration stimulations. The system is low cost, simple to use, and comfortable to wear.

It provides the subject information on the heel-strike and toe-off of the artificial foot during gait. The system has been fitted in a population of amputee subjects in order to verify the level of acceptance and comfort of the subjects.

Because the examined subjects have been demonstrated to appreciate the system and the kind of information it is able to provide, and the use of the device has not induced any inconvenience, we have started a rigorous clinical testing of the device. The testing includes examining a wide population of amputee subjects during their rehabilitation process. Quantitative analysis of gait performances is performed on two groups of subjects, one wearing the device and the other following the normal rehabilitation protocol. Final results on the effect of the use of sensory feedback during rehabilitation will be available of course only when enough data for a rigorous statistical analysis has been collected from amputee subjects. However, preliminary results seem to indicate that the use of the device makes the subjects aware of the foot contact on the ground and they are therefore able to learn easily the correct pattern of gait of their prosthetic leg.

Acknowledgments. This work has been supported by Centro Protesi INAIL di Vigorso di Budrio (Bologna, Italy) and by the Istituto Superiore di Sanità (Roma, Italy).

References

[1] Abu-Faraj, Z.O., Harris, G.F., Abler, J.H., and Wertsch, J.J.: A Holter-type, microprocessor-based, rehabilitation instrument for acquisition and storage of plantar pressure data. *J. Rehabilit. Res. Dev.*, vol. 34, pp. 187-194, 1997.

[2] Agnew, P.J. and Shannon, G.F.: Training program for a myo-electrically controlled prosthesis with sensory feedback system. *Am. J. Occup. Ther.*, vol. 35, pp. 722-727, 1981.

[3] Alexander, I.J., Chao, E.Y.S., and Johnson, K.A.: The assessment of dynamic foot-to-ground contact forces and plantar pressure distribution: review of the evolution of current techniques and clinical applications. *Foot & Ankle*, vol. 11, pp. 152-167, 1990.

[4] Bennet, P.J. and Duplock, L.R.: Pressure distribution beneath the human foot. *J. Am. Podiatr. Med. Assoc.*, vol. 83, pp. 674-678, 1993.

[5] Bernstein, N.: *The Co-ordination and Regulation of Movements*, Pergamon Press, Oxford, 1967.

[6] Berthoz, A.: *Le sens du movement*, Editions Odile Jacob, Paris, 1997.

[7] Clippinger, F.W., Avery, R., and Titus, B.R.: A sensory feedback system for an upper-limb amputation prosthesis. *Bull. Prosth. Res.*, vol. 247, pp. 10-22, .

[8] Clippinger, F.W., Seaber, A.V., McElhaney, J.H., Harrelson, J.M., and Maxwell, G.M.: Afferent sensory feedback for lower extremity prosthesis. *Clin. Orthop. Relat. Res.*, vol. 169, pp. 202-206, 1982.

[9] Cordo, P.J. and Nashner, L.: Properties of postural adjustment associated with rapid arm movement. *J. Neurophysiology*, vol. 47, pp. 287-302, 1982.

[10] Craik, R.L. and Oatis, C.A.: *Gait Analysis, Theory and Application*, Mosby Year Book Inc., St. Louis, 1995.

[11] DeLisa, J.A. (Ed.): *Gait Analysis in the Science of Rehabilitation*, Monograph 002, Departments of Veterans Affairs, 1998.

[12] Droulez, J. and Berthoz, A.: Servo-controlled (conservative) versus topological (projective) mode of sensory motor control. In: *Disorders of Posture and Gait*, W. Bles and T. Brandt (Eds.), Elsevier, Amsterdam, pp. 83-97, 1988.

[13] Ferrigno, G. and Pedotti, A.: ELITE: a digital dedicated hardware system for movement analysis via real-time signal processing. *IEEE Trans. BME*, vol. 32, pp. 943-950, 1985.

[14] Gahery, Y. and Massion, J.: Coordination between posture and movement. *TINS*, vol. 4, pp. 199-202, 1981.

[15] Giannini, S., Catani, F., Benedetti, M.G., and Leardini, A.: *Gait Analysis: Methodologies and Clinical Applications*. IOS Press, Amsterdam, 1994.

[16] Kandel, E.R. and Schwartz, J.H. (Eds.): *Principles of Neural Science*, Elsevier, Amsterdam, 1985.

[17] Kawamura, J., Sweda, O., Kazutaka, H., Kazuyoshi, N., and Isobe, S.: Sensory feedback systems for the lower-limb prosthesis. *J. Osaka Rosai Hosp.*, vol. 5, pp. 102-109, 1981.

[18] Luo, Z.P., Berglund, L.J., and An, K.N.: Validation of F-Scan pressure sensor system: Technical note. *J. Rehabilit. Res. Dev.*, vol. 35, pp. 186-191, 1998.

[19] Macellari, V. and Fadda, A.: Italian Patent nr. 1289231/1999. Apparecchiatura per la telemetria delle forze di interazione piede-suolo in un soggetto deambulante. Istituto Superiore di Sanità, Roma, Italy, 1999.

[20] Macpherson, J.: How flexible are synergies? In: *Motor Control: Concepts and Issues*, D.R. Humphrey and H. J. Freund (Eds.), John Wiley, Chichester, pp. 33-47, 1991.

[21] Macpherson, J.: The neural organization of postural control. Do muscle synergies exist? In: *Posture and Gait: Development, Adaptation, and Modulation*, B. Amblard, A. Berthoz, and F. Clarac (Eds.), Elsevier, Amsterdam, pp. 381-390, 1988.

[22] McPoil, T.G. and Cornwall, M.W.: Variability of the center of pressure pattern integral during walking. *J. Am. Podiatr. Med. Assoc.*, vol. 88, pp. 259-267, 1998.

[23] Nashner, L.: Fixed patterns of rapid postural responses among leg muscles during stance. *Exp. Brain Res.*, vol. 30, pp. 13-24, 1977.

[24] Normann, R.A.: Visual neuroprosthetics. Functional vision for the blind. *IEEE-EMB Magazine*, vol. 14, pp. 77-83, 1995.

[25] Nyska, M., McCabe, C., Linge, K., and Klenerman, L.: Plantar foot pressures during treadmill walking with high-heel and low-heel shoes. *Foot & Ankle*, vol. 17, pp. 662-666, 1996.

[26] Oddsson, L.: Control of voluntary trunk movements in man. Mechanisms for postural equilibrium during standing. *Acta Physiol. Scand.*, vol. 140 (Suppl. 595) (thesis), 1990.

[27] Patterson, P.E. and Katz, J.A.: Design and evaluation of a sensory feedback system that provides grasping pressure in a myoelectric hand. *J. Rehabil. Res. Dev.*, vol. 29, pp. 1-8, 1992.

[28] Pedotti, A., Crenna, P., Deat, A., Frigo, C., and Massion, J.: Postural synergies in axial movements: short and long term adaptation. *Exp. Brain Res.*, vol. 74, pp. 3-10, 1989.

[29] Perry, J.: *Gait Analysis, Normal and Pathological Function*. Slack Inc., NJ, 1992.

[30] Pozzo, T., Berthoz, A., and Lefort, L.: Head stabilisation during various locomotor tasks in humans. *Exp. Brain Res.*, vol. 82, pp. 97-106, 1990.

[31] Prior, R.E., Lyman, J., and Case, P.A.: Supplemental sensory feedback for the VA/NU myoelectric hand: background and feasibility. *Bull. Prosth. Res.*, vol. 10, pp. 170-191, 1976.

[32] Sabolich, J.A. and Ortega, G.M.: Sense of feel for lower-limb amputees: a phase-one study. *J. Prosth. Orthotics*, vol. 6, pp. 36-41, 1994.

[33] Schmidl, H.: The importance of information feedback in prostheses for upper limbs. *Prosth. Orthot. Int.*, vol. 1, pp. 21-24, 1977.

[34] Schmidt, E.M., Bak, M.J., Hambrecht, F.T., Kufta, C.V., O'Rourke, D.K., and Vallabhanath, P.: Feasibility of a visual prosthesis for the blind based on intracortical microstimulation of the visual cortex. *Brain*, vol. 119, pp. 507-522, 1996.

[35] Scott, R.N.: Feedback in myoelectric prostheses. *Clin. Orthop.*, vol. 256, pp. 58-63, 1990.

[36] Scott, R.N., Brittain, R.H., Caldwell, R.R., Cameron, A.B., and Dunfield, V.A.: Sensory-feedback system compatible with myoelectric control. *Med. Biol. Eng. Comput.*, vol. 18, pp. 65-69, 1980.

[37] Shannon, G.F.: A comparison of alternative means of providing sensory feedback on upper limb prostheses. *Med. Biol. Eng. Comput.*, vol. 14, pp. 289-294, 1976.

[38] Shannon, G.F.: A myoelectrically-controlled prosthesis with sensory feedback. *Med. Biol. Eng. Comput.*, vol. 17, pp. 73-80, 1979.

[39] Shannon, G.F. and Agnew, P.J.: Fitting below-elbow prostheses which convey a sense of touch. *Med. J. Aust.*, vol. 24, pp. 242-244, 1979.

[40] Soames, R.W.: Foot pressure patterns during gait. *J Biomed. Eng.*, vol. 7, pp. 120-126, 1985.

[41] Sumiya, T., Suzuki, Y., Kasahara, T., and Ogata, H.: Sensing stability and dynamic response of the F-Scan in-shoe sensing system: Technical note. *J. Rehabilit. Res. Dev.*, vol. 35, pp. 192-200, 1998.

[42] Tura, A., Lamberti, C., Davalli, A., and Sacchetti, R.: Experimental development of a sensory control system for an upper limb myoelectric prosthesis with cosmetic covering. *J. Rehabil. Res. Dev.*, vol. 35, pp. 14-26, 1998

[43] Winter, D.A.: *A. B. C. of Balance During Standing and Walking*. Waterloo Biomechanics, Ontario, Canada, 1995.

[44] Zambarbieri, D., Schmid, M., Magnaghi, M., Verni, G., Macellari, V., and Fadda, A.: Biofeedback techniques for rehabilitation of the lower limb amputee subjects. *Proc. VIII MEDICON*, CD-ROM Medicon '98, ISBN 9963-607-13-614-17, Lemesos, Cyprus, June 1998.

Chapter 5

Multifunction control of prostheses using the myoelectric signal

Kevin Englehart, Bernard Hudgins, and Philip Parker

Myoelectric control of a multifunction artificial arm has been an elusive goal for researchers over the past 30 years. This chapter provides an historical perspective of multifunction myoelectric control and introduces several current research efforts that are addressing this difficult problem.

1. Introduction

1.1. Externally powered prostheses

During the last three decades, aids for physically challenged individuals have improved considerably, mainly by "piggybacking" progress in modern electronics and mechanical technology. In the first generation, the upper-limb prostheses were simple, passive accessories that served mainly as a cosmetic replacement for the missing limb. Prior to 1960, any active upper-extremity prostheses were controlled and powered almost exclusively by gross body movements, which offered limited functionality to amputees.

In the middle of the 1940's, it was suggested that myoelectric signals detected in the stump muscles of an amputee could probably be used for the control of a mechanical hand [1], but this work ended without clinical implementation. A few clinical investigations and some marginal developments took place in the 1950's [2], [3]. It was in the next decade, however, that an intensive development of prostheses and control systems was initiated; research centers arose in many countries, spurred on by transistor technology, which was then becoming available. It is interesting to note that the emergence of this research in the 1960's was markedly dispersed, apparently disjointed and quite unaware of Reiter's pioneering work. Investigations had begun in the USSR [4], England [5], Sweden [6], Japan [7], the United States [8] and Canada [9].

The Russian electric hand was the first clinically viable myoelectric prostheses; a limited quantity found export to England and Canada. In the 1960's, many powered devices (hooks and hands) were designed, though most of this work was commercial and remains unpublished.

A conference in the former Yugoslavia (initiated in 1963) called "*External Control of Human Extremities*" attracted the international research community; this conference was held there every third year from 1966 to 1984. The proceedings of the "Dubrovnik Conferences" are a singular record of the international developments in powered limb research and development during this period.

Myoelectric control received a major boost in North America as a result of a 1966 symposium in Cleveland, Ohio (at Case Western Reserve University) which was entitled "*Myoelectric Control Systems and Electromyographic Kinesiology.*" Bottomley [10] demonstrated an elegant new myoelectric system at that meeting. The meeting was also attended by Professor Robert N. Scott of the University of New Brunswick. Scott headed a group that pioneered the first myoelectric control mechanism in North America.

From mostly small-scale production emerged a supplier – Otto Bock (Duderstadt, Germany) – which gained a strong market position by offering a versatile range of well-designed hands. It was around 1967 that it became possible to purchase a powered prosthesis commercially in North America (the *Viennatone hand*) manufactured by Otto Bock and Viennatone (Austria) [11].

The Veterans Administration Prosthetics Center (VAPC) improved this design with a controller developed at Northwestern University [12] and contracted Fidelity electronics (Chicago, Illinois) to produce a hand which was marketed for a while. Schmidl [13] was fitting many upper-limb amputees in Italy, establishing clinical significance with powered limbs well before this may be said to have happened in North America. Schmidl's group experienced some success with fittings of multifunctional limbs, but the means of control proved to be cumbersome. Engineers at Temple University [14] had some laboratory success using pattern recognition to actuate multifunction control, but the necessary hardware (and computing power) obviated a clinical solution at the time. The Institute of Biomedical Engineering at the University of New Brunswick (UNB) has played an active role in developing control methods for powered limbs and is well known for three-state control design and development [9]. The institute at UNB has also contributed one of the most clinically viable systems of sensory feedback [15].

In the late 1960's and 1970's, much experimentation and development were engendered in the field of external electric power. A Japanese development specified a highly functional myoelectric hand [16]. Scientists at the Massachusetts Institute of Technology (MIT) designed the Boston arm [17], the first myoelectrically controlled elbow. The Boston Elbow was redesigned to become the Liberty Mutual Powered Elbow [18], available through Liberty Mutual Insurance Company (Hopkinton, Massachusetts). This elbow was most likely a stimulus to Steven Jacobsen, who did his graduate studies at MIT and who later developed the highly functional Utah Arm [19]. The Ontario Crippled Children's Center (OCCC) Elbow was developed in the late 1960s and is still in use today.

It was approximately 1977 that powered upper-limb prostheses might be said to have become clinically significant in North America. Otto Bock remains the preeminent supplier of hand and wrist units today, although some companies – Hugh Steeper (London, England), Systemteknik (Lidingo, Sweden), Fidelity Electronics (Chicago, Illinois) and Hosmer Dorrance (Campbell, California) – are pressing for market share with technical innovations. Major vendors of prosthetic elbow units include Variety Ability Systems Inc. (Toronto, Ontario), Liberty Mutual (Hopkinton, Massachusetts) and Motion Control (Salt Lake City, Utah).

1.2. Clinical impact

The original reports from the USSR in 1960 about myoelectric prostheses were received with some skepticism in North America. The success of the Otto Bock company's fittings attracted media attention and incited research interest, but these systems generally lacked the technology to make them genuine clinical solutions. At the time, prosthetists were unprepared to utilize the potential of this new contribution.

Powered prosthetics and prosthetic control remained active fields of research in the next decade, mostly at centers funded as research rather than service. It was gradual progress in the materials and electronics requirements of the devices and development of expertise in clinical application of the devices that eventually led to their clinical significance.

By the 1970's, myoelectric prostheses were routinely fitted and clinical investigations of the functional benefit of the new prostheses were performed. The myoelectric signal proved to be superior in many ways to the gross body movements in the control of prosthetic devices [20], [21], [22], [23]. Actuation of the prosthesis by gross body movements is accomplished by relevant movements of body musculature, transmitted to the prosthesis by a Bowden cable. The return motion is executed by means of gravity or, in some cases, a spring. This arrangement restricts the number of possible movements of a prosthesis. Furthermore, this type of control requires great concentration and effort by the amputee. In order to obtain a substantial movement in the prosthesis, large muscle forces and displacements are required. The effort of meeting these demands can cause muscle fatigue and loss of interest for the amputee.

Electrically-driven prostheses with myoelectric control have since dominated prosthetic development because they have several advantages over other types of prostheses: the user is freed of straps and harnesses; the myoelectric signal is noninvasively detected on the surface of the skin; the electric battery is possibly the most convenient form of power supply that can be incorporated into a prosthesis; they can be adapted to proportional control with relative ease; the required electronic circuits (whether analog or digital) can be continuously improved and miniaturized; and they appear to have the prospect of better long-term reliability.

The clinical success of myoelectric prostheses is, however, a very difficult thing to measure. Statistics that are used to convey a measure of success usually express the percentage of amputees that wear their prosthesis regularly. There is great discrepancy among various studies reporting the rate of acceptance of myoelectric prostheses. The findings from various follow-up studies depend upon the types of prostheses and the means of control, the degree of training given to the subjects, sociological and cultural influences, and many other parameters. Some indicate rather high rates (80 to 100%) of acceptance of myoelectrically-controlled prostheses [21], [24]; some are rather condemning of the technology [25]. The main point to be taken from these studies is that the greatest deficiency of prosthetic systems is the inadequate controllability of the prosthesis, as perceived by the amputee – specifically, the lack of intuitive actuation and dexterous control. For myoelectric prostheses, the control limitations involve the lack of robustness of the processing of the input (the myoelectric signal) to specify the output (joint-space kinematics) and the disparity of the means of manipulation from natural motor control and learning.

When evaluating the adequacy of prostheses, it is necessary to more deeply examine the specific needs of the population of amputees. An amputee (the term amputee will imply those afflicted by a congenital defect or an acquired amputation) who has one normal arm can usually live an independent lifestyle without a prosthesis of any kind. The most common condition for which a prosthesis is prescribed is a below-elbow amputation, where elbow function is retained. These cases require a replacement for hand function and appearance and the terminal device is usually designed to look as much like a hand as possible. For unilateral amputees, the prosthetic terminal device is used mostly as an assistive device. Tasks requiring fine manipulation or sensory feedback are performed by the normal hand. If the amputation is bilateral, there is a much more urgent need for finer grasp control.

The prosthetic replacement of limbs amputated above the elbow is a much more complex problem. Comfortable and secure fitting of the prosthesis is often difficult to provide. The complexity of function increases rapidly when additional degrees of freedom of movement must be controlled. The capability of the amputee to operate these functions by harnessing body movement (via straps and cables) is severely limited. It is in cases of high-level amputation, especially those with bilateral loss, that a powered prosthesis is most needed. With unfortunate irony, however, most powered prostheses in use today – for reasons of technical feasibility rather than clinical priority – are fitted to unilateral, below-elbow amputees.

Indeed, in the period from 1960 to 1980, myoelectric controls research had two distinct goals. One, based upon immediate clinical solutions, attempted to supply useful devices for below-elbow amputees as soon as possible. The motivation for this work was that these cases represented the considerable majority of upper-extremity amputees. Also, the inherent technical problem was much less severe than above-elbow fittings, meaning that the probability of acceptance was much higher.

The other focus of research was based on the conviction that the most urgent need for externally powered prostheses was in high-level amputation. The efforts put forth to meet the intrinsic technical challenge of this complex control problem have produced anatomical and physiological models and have drawn upon statistical signal processing methods to maximally extract information from the myoelectric signal.

Present systems provide less than satisfactory solutions however, owing to one or more of the following reasons: an encumbering number of electrode sites (and associated hardware), an unacceptable discrimination among classes of movement, an excessive degree of conscious effort required during manipulation, an unnatural means of actuation and nonanthropometric movement. The manner of affecting multijoint control of the prosthesis bears little resemblance to physiological motor learning and control strategies. Conscious (cortical) influence appears only to direct the endpoint of the limb; lower neural processes appear responsible for mapping this movement to "joint space" and coordinating the appropriate scheme of muscle recruitment and innervation [26]. This means of control is very difficult if not impossible to achieve in a prosthesis. In fact, control schemes have evolved very little since their introduction; from a functional point of view, many unilateral above-elbow amputees probably have little more reason to wear arm prostheses today than they did thirty years ago.

The state of upper-limb prosthetics today may be summarized in the context of the needs of amputees.

Unilateral below-elbow amputees are fairly well-served by their prostheses. Technical progress in materials, electric motors and rechargeable batteries has provided reasonable function and durability.

- Bilateral below-elbow amputees lack the dexterous control of prehension and wrist orientation necessary to function well.
- Above-elbow amputees (particularly those afflicted by a bilateral deficiency) are in need of a means of multijoint control that can position and orient the limb without an excessive burden on the central nervous system. This implies that the nature of control should resemble physiological motor control and learning: the actuation should involve normal muscle synergies, joint positioning and orientation should be based upon endpoint manipulation, and the overall movement should be anthropomorphic.

In light of the above discussion, the state of prosthetic technology appears most limited by the means of the control interface. The issue of multifunction myoelectric control shall be the focus of this chapter. The next section describes the work that has been done in myoelectric control research to the present.

2. Myoelectric control

2.1. An overview

The exquisite control that normally-limbed individuals possess depends upon a closed-loop control system. Motor (command) signals from the central nervous system are used in the forward path; sensory signals, such as those from the proprioceptive receptors in muscles and joints, are used in the feedback path. The (ideal) prosthetic replacement of a limb should interface the remaining neuromuscular system in a manner as close to its physiological counterpart as possible. Figure 1 depicts a block representation of a prosthesis interacting with the body's neuromuscular system in a closed-loop fashion. The shaded regions indicate problematic areas that must be perfected to achieve a more symbiotic relationship between an amputee and the prosthesis. Both the forward (motor) and the feedback (sensory) paths of prosthetic systems today are far from the functionality of an intact physiological system.

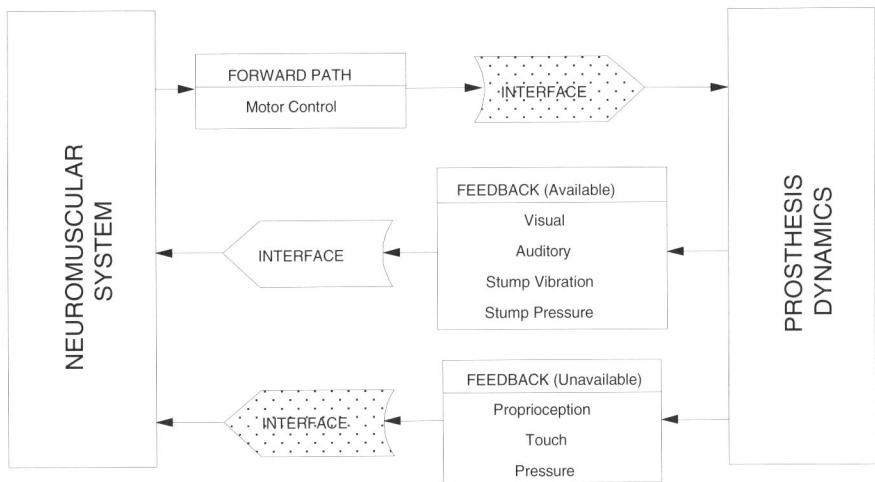

Figure 1. Block diagram illustrating the interface between the neuromuscular system and typical upper-limb prosthesis. The shaded regions indicate problematic areas.

It is generally regarded that an improved quality of feedback to the central nervous system would be desirable. Efforts have been made (using a variety of interfaces) to provide proprioceptive and/or sensory feedback, but none have found clinical acceptance [11], [15], [27], [28]. Undeniably, the sensory and proprioceptive feedback from a human hand is essential to its elegant dexterity. Deficient feedback may not be as consequential for limb positioning tasks, however. Experimental investigations have demonstrated that intact proprioceptive sensory feedback is not essential for controlling limb movements. Primates with inhibited proprioceptive pathways were capable of performing positioning tasks – essentially in open-loop mode (no visual feedback, either) – even if the afferent nerves were severed at birth [29]. In studies of arm movement accuracy in primates, Pollit and Bizzi [30] demonstrated that, following a period of retraining, deafferented monkeys could accurately point to visually presented targets without visual contact with the moving limb. This experiment demonstrated that, within the limits of accuracy imposed by the experimenters, practiced accurate movement could be accomplished in the absence of any sensory feedback. This "open-loop" strategy of movement control would be useful to develop in high-level amputees, where proprioceptive feedback from the limb is minimal or altogether absent, since it would obviate most of the requirement for close visual attention to the moving prosthetic arm. Visual guidance of the arm could be delayed until just before the endpoint of movement, at which time precise, visually-guided corrections could be employed to obtain fine control. This strategy corresponds to that which has been suggested to occur in normal movement, where accurate endpoint control is obtained through a series of approximations [31]. In consideration of these findings, it is conceivable that substantial improvements in prosthetic control lie in the capabilities of the forward path man-machine interface.

The concern for this man-machine interface is as old as the development of the devices themselves. Today, the most widely used devices are the simplest: most systems use myoelectric control to actuate a single device (such as a hand, an elbow, or a wrist). A control signal is derived from the myoelectric signal as a measure of its amplitude [9] or of the rate of change of its amplitude [32]. These systems typically use either one or two myoelectric channels. Single channel control will segment the range of the input signal (amplitude or rate) to effect one of three states (for a prehension device: 1 = off, 2 = open, 3 = close). Two channel systems determine the channel with the higher level of activity, and specify the device state accordingly. Once the state is selected, the joint speed may be constant (ON/OFF control), or it may be determined by the level of myoelectric activity (proportional control).

The approaches using myoelectric control that have been investigated may be roughly classified into two groups: those that use control sites associated with muscles not necessarily related to the desired movement [33], and those that use control sites directly related to the desired movement [34], [35], [36] [37]. The latter approach is obviously more desirable in the context of yielding a more "natural" control interface.

The ability to control a single device depends only upon one (possibly, two) control site. The success of these types of fittings has shown that this control scheme does not place an unreasonable burden upon the human operator. The extension of myoelectric control to multiple degrees of freedom simply cannot originate from multiple control sites that are not related to the desired movement: this requires too much conscious effort. Training the user to isolate the required number of control muscles is impractical if not impossible [38]. The natural way of activating a muscle is within a complex pattern of movement. The best performance of a control system will be obtained when the remaining muscles are used in the same way as they functioned before amputation (for an acquired amputation). Since most individuals with acquired amputations retain a cortical image of the lost limb, they are able to reproduce complicated patterns of muscle contraction in the stump. It is not clear that this is true for a congenitally limb-deficient individual; their remaining musculature is generally unknown in form and function and in who may not have an innate sense of "natural" manipulation in the deficient limb. The most successful results in "natural" multiple degree of freedom control have required the use of several electrodes sites for detecting patterns from functionally distinct muscle groups, and statistical pattern recognition methods to classify muscle activity during natural movements as *intent* in one (or more) degree of freedom.

The use of several recording sites represents two technical problems. First, the impedance of each differential electrode pair must be maintained reasonably stable with respect to each other. This is a significant problem if the user perspires: the electrolyte accumulation on the skin provides an enhanced conductive path between the two electrodes of a differential pair; a severe common-mode to differential voltage conversion may ensue. The second – perhaps more obvious – problem is that all electrode pairs must be consistently placed and maintained in the same location above the muscles each time the prosthesis is replaced on an amputee. Both of these problems will cause variations in the signal patterns, which correspond to distinct degrees of freedom.

2.2. Multifunction control research

The following is an historical perspective on multifunction prosthetic control research: a discourse of the methods, the successes, and the drawbacks of prior work. The intent here is to provide a proper context to discuss the problems that have beset some very good efforts and to highlight the technologies that may hold promise.

2.2.1. Control based on myoelectric statistical pattern recognition techniques: Temple University

Engineers at Temple University and the Moss Rehabilitation Hospital in Philadelphia were probably the first to attempt multifunctional control of elbow, humeral rotation, and wrist rotation. The team was funded by the Veteran's Administration and the Office of Naval Research, and included F. Ray Finley, Donald R. Taylor, and Roy W. Wirta. They realized that a one-muscle-for-one-motion control scheme required excessive mental burden in the control of multiple axes of motion; in normal movement activity, individual muscle groups do not respond in isolation but do so in synergistic groups. A simple motion such as elbow flexion involves a complex combination of both prime movers and joint stabilizers. The shoulder in some ways may be considered the "foundation" of the arm. Motion of the humerus and the forearm generates reaction forces and torques at the shoulder that must be counteracted by shoulder, chest, and back muscles to stabilize the shoulder joint. The goal of this work was to characterize the resultant muscle synergies using pattern recognition.

Their initial work [39] produced "myocoder" instrumentation capable of collecting, amplifying, and quantifying six channels of myoelectric signals. Data were acquired from the anterior and posterior deltoid groups, the long and short heads of the biceps, the lateral head of the triceps, and the pronator teres.

Myoelectric activity was monitored during isometric contractions of forearm pronation-supination and elbow flexion. Multivariate pattern recognition techniques were used [35], [40] on myoelectric signals from multiple muscle sites of the upper arm and shoulder in an attempt to optimally discriminate among the target movement types. Under controlled laboratory conditions, with normally-limbed subjects who had received moderate training producing isometric contractions, the authors reported 92% accuracy for elbow flexion and 97% accuracy for forearm pronation and supination.

Later work [14] considered multiple-axis control for an above-elbow amputee with a short residual limb, such that muscle control sites were limited to those not distal to the deltoids. Eight sites were used: the anterior, middle, and posterior deltoid, the manubrial pectoralis major, the upper and lower-middle trapezius, the rhomboideus major, and the teres major. Five normally-limbed adult males were subjects in tests to determine performance accuracy. The myoelectric data were acquired from isometric contractions at roughly 5% of maximal effort, maintained for 10 seconds. Among four motion types, the performance accuracy was measured to be:

Elbow flexion -   97 %
Elbow extension -   96 %
Humeral rotation (out) - 95 %
Humeral rotation (in) -   43 %
Forearm supination -   70 %
Forearm pronation -   65 %

Not included in these accuracy specifications is the "crosstalk" or simultaneous activation of more than one axis when only one was intended. This was especially prevalent in inadvertent elbow flexion when only supination was desired. These results represent controlled laboratory tests with healthy, normally-limbed, and moderately trained subjects. The control actuation was static (isometric) and not dynamic (phasic); the isometric contractions were very long (10 seconds) _ at least in terms of an acceptable delay in system response. The system was implemented in analog hardware, due to a lack of available microprocessor technology. The inflexibility of a hardware implementation was the reason that the group chose to fix the decision boundaries of the pattern recognition circuit, rather than tailor the classifier to more adequately match the natural muscle synergies of each subject. The authors claimed that the relative variations in myoelectric signals which may be expected as a result of variations in load, day-to-day differences, and isometric versus isotonic muscle usage would not be so great as to markedly deteriorate the patterns of muscle synergy in normal arm movements. These claims were never substantiated by quantitative analysis.

A 1978 paper [14] served as a record of the work done by the team. The project ended as a result of shifting priorities of funding agencies, and a conviction that the control approach needed a sensory feedback system to become truly effective.

2.2.2. Control based on myoelectric statistical pattern recognition techniques: Swedish research

Research at the Chalmers University Hospital in Göteborg, Sweden developed myoelectric statistical pattern recognition techniques for the control of a three degree of freedom below-elbow prosthesis [41]. The classification network was trained to suit individual subjects. The goal was to isolate a sufficient number of hand movement signals without resorting to time multiplexing, level-coded signals, mode switches, *etc.*, all of which increase training time, detract from naturalness, and thus, decrease acceptance of the prosthesis. Simultaneous control of the three degree of freedom Swedish hand [41] was achieved using six electrode pairs placed on the below-elbow stump. The pattern recognition method was easily realized in hardware electronics and brought satisfactory results without excessive training. Later work saw the development of a six degree of freedom hand [42], which showed respectable classification performance and functionality in active daily living tests. Clinical experience with the multifunction hands [42] showed that their movements were cosmetically more appealing than simple prehension hands, but that the reliability and hardware development (weight and compactness) were inferior.

2.2.3. Control based on myoelectric statistical pattern recognition techniques: UCLA research

A research group at the University of California, Los Angeles (UCLA) has also suggested the use of pattern recognition methods [43]. The work originated from studies done by John Lyman while he was with the U.S. Air Force [44], mapping synergistic muscle activity during selected arm movements. At the Biotechnology Laboratory at UCLA, Dr. Lyman and Amos Freedy sought to refine multifunction control of upper-limb prostheses. In their pursuit, they concluded that there is a basic limitation on the ability of a user to supply the control information required for adequate performance [45]. The group approached prosthetic control as an information transfer problem, drawing upon the evolving technologies of pattern recognition, information theory, and adaptive systems.

The research focus of the UCLA group echoed the sentiments of many participating in the Dubrovnik symposia in the early 1970's. The need for trajectory- or endpoint-based control was expressed by those participants with a background in robotics and intelligent control [46], [47], [48], [49]. The contributions at this time were mostly conceptual, with an eye to what might be eventually possible, and what benefits might be gained.

Indeed, the first work by the group described the concept of limb tracking and adaptive aiding [50], incorporating an autonomous control subsystem (ACS) capable of supplementing the operator's own conscious control. The ACS is a sequential algorithm that generates future endpoint positions based upon previous and present states. The learning subsystem may be characterized by

$$\hat{a}_{n+1} = \Phi(X_n, \mathbf{P}_n)$$

where $\hat{a}_{n+1}$ refers to the predicted position of the endpoint of the device at the $(n+1)^{th}$ trial, X_n is the system state vector describing the nth endpoint position, and $\mathbf{P}_n$ is a nonstationary stochastic matrix of conditional probabilities $P(x_j^n | i)$, the probability that the condition represented by x_j^n occurs preceding occupation of position i. Using a maximum likelihood decision rule, the predicted position can be accepted or rejected with respect to some confidence threshold. As the number of trials (n) progresses, the $\mathbf{P}_n$ matrix converges toward an optimal set of probabilities, and the learning subsystem predicts the ensuing motion with greater accuracy, gradually assuming a greater portion of the decision load, reducing the mental decision load of the operator.

Pilot work was done which attempted to demonstrate the feasibility of adaptive aiding: an experimental learning subsystem was applied to trajectory control of artificial arms [51], [52] and remote manipulator control [53]. The scope of the realized system was much simpler than the proposed theoretical model both in terms of degrees of freedom (due to computational burden) and in the size of the $\mathbf{P}_n$ matrix (due to memory limitations). The experimental system was far removed from an actual prosthetic application: the control inputs were either via body movements (one for each degree of freedom to be controlled) or by joystick control (a joystick tends to be rather more predictable and noise-free than myoelectric control sites).

A related research effort of this group was that of resolved motion (or endpoint) control, which is addressed in the next section.

2.2.4. Endpoint control

The object of endpoint control is to relieve the operator of part of the control responsibility, and to provide a more natural control interface: our cognitive task space most often tends to be in Cartesian endpoint coordinates.

There have been a number of research efforts directed at endpoint control problems; these are summarized below.

UCLA Research. The goal of this effort was to produce a control algorithm that would allow the user to specify direction and speed of the endpoint along some natural set of coordinates, producing coordinated endpoint movement without having to simultaneously control several joint motors [54].

Specifically, a three degree of freedom joystick input was mapped to the appropriate three degree of freedom joint angle vector needed to emulate upper-limb positioning: shoulder rotation, shoulder flexion-extension, and elbow flexion-extension. A real-time coordinate transformation algorithm was implemented on an Interdata 70 minicomputer. No attempt was made by the group to use myoelectric sites as the input to an endpoint control scheme.

Manipulation of the intact upper limb involves not only endpoint positioning control, but also orientation control usually in simultaneity. Zadaca *et al.* combined resolved endpoint control with heuristic rules to control orientation in three degrees of freedom [54]; these were humeral rotation, forearm rotation (pronation-supination), and terminal device prehension. The inputs to the heuristic algorithm were direction, position, and speed of the prosthetic joints. The heuristic rules may be summarized as:

- *Prehension.* When reaching out to grasp an object, open the terminal device. If a reaching motion is sensed and the terminal device is not loaded, the terminal device will be opened during positioning. This saves time and emulates normal reaching movements.
- *Humeral rotation.* The idea behind this rule is to use humeral rotation instead of shoulder rotation when the upper limb is nearly vertical. When a shoulder rotation command is issued, the program checks if the current upper-limb position is nearly vertical. If so, shoulder rotation is canceled, and a proper humeral rotation command is issued.
- *Wrist rotation.* The wrist rotation rule attempts to orient the terminal device in the direction of motion.
- *Stop motors to prevent collision damage.* This rule provides protection from possible collision damage to the arm by checking current positions to previous positions when motion was intended.

Although a rule-based approach does reduce the dimensionality of the control problem, movement is constrained to that specified in the heuristic program; this was discovered by the group as they attempted active daily living tasks.

With the advent of microprocessor technology, and under the directed funding of the Veteran's Administration, the UCLA research effort turned to producing a clinical solution. The control system used the same pattern recognition approach as demonstrated by Wirta *et al.*, and attempted to extend it to provide adaptive mapping to optimize the pattern recognition system for individual users' myoelectric patterns. Myoelectric signals from nine sites of the shoulder musculature were chosen to control three degrees of freedom: humeral rotation, elbow flexion-extension, and wrist pronation-supination. The smoothed, rectified myoelectric signal from each electrode was quantized into 5 levels to yield a control input vector $E = (e_1, e_2, e_2, \ldots, e_9)$ capable of 9 sites × 5 levels = 45 discrete states. For each of the three degrees of freedom, there were three possible states: move positive (+1), move negative (-1), or stay still (0). Thus, 3×3 = 27 possible control outputs d_j, were possible. A matrix of the a *priori* probabilities $p(e_i = e_i | d = d_j)$ representing the likelihood of an input (e_i) given an output (d_j) would have 45 inputs × 27 outputs = 945 elements. Two pattern classification rules were used: the Maximum Likelihood Decision (MLD) network and the Nearest Neighbor Classifier (NNC).

The pattern recognition classifier was trained by comparing myoelectric data from an instrumented shoulder/limb to goniometer readings from the contralateral side as both were moved in unison. Amputees were asked to move their "phantom limb" in parallel with their sound limb. Performance was measured by asking the subjects to move to a specified endpoint (each relative directional movement constituted a control decision), and then measuring the time required to reach the proper position. Of the two types of discriminant functions, the NNC proved to be superior to the MLD classifier; subjects were able to train in shorter periods of time, and more directions could be trained.

Performance was judged as a function of both (*i*) the number of trained movements and (*ii*) the number of electrode sites. What the authors characterize as "excellent" performance (proper movement was obtained in less than 0.5 s and during execution, 2-or-less erroneous decisions were made) was achieved with a 9-electrode, 3-direction control system. As the number of trained directions increased from 3 to 5 to 9 performance steadily decreased. Similarly, performance suffered as the number of electrode sites decreased from 9 to 8 to 7 to 6.

Although the researchers suggested that endpoint control and adaptive aiding might eventually be incorporated into a clinical microprocessor-based system, no evidence of this application has been reported.

Swedish Efforts. Lawrence and Lin [55] developed statistical decision procedures to control a modified seven degree of freedom Rancho Arm. The goal was to allow the user to input endpoint position in Cartesian coordinates to allow the user to coordinate the actuators (in seven dimensions) in a space of lower and more natural dimension. The input included a three-dimensional vector $X=(x_1,x_2,x_3)$ which specified the spatial position of the wrist, and $H=(\theta_1,\theta_2,\theta_3)$ (θ_1 = forearm supination, θ_2 = wrist flexion, θ_3 = prehension).

The controller then computed the proper joint space equivalent of {X,H}. Computing the proper shoulder and elbow angles is difficult because (*i*) there are multiple solutions to a given endpoint position in joint space and, (*ii*) once resolved, the problem requires solution of inverse kinematic equations, which can be computationally intensive.

Lawrence and Lin proposed a solution to this problem by using pattern recognition to classify the motion, based on the input {X,H}, into distinct movement tasks derived from a set of exoskeletal goniometer recordings of typical daily tasks. Given the endpoint position, X, and the movement task, the elbow angle was estimated using a regression function, again based upon the kinematic data. Once elbow angle was known, the rest of the joint angles were computed without ambiguity.

The authors suggested that the means of control input should be via body segment position or myoelectric signals from shoulder and/or back muscles. The discrete nature of the required input vectors {X,H} means that inputs from either of these sources will be artificially contrived. The work, as presented, did not address the clinical issues of body or myoelectric control input; X and H were input using a three-dimensional joystick and a keyboard, respectively.

The Feeder Arm. The emphasis of the work by these individuals at Case Western Reserve University was the development of an orthotic device — dubbed the "feeder arm" — that would allow a user to select one of a variety of complex programmed functions [56]. This control scheme was adapted to control the Rancho orthotic arm [57]. The endpoint algorithm provided movement of the hand along rectangular coordinates in four degrees of freedom: shoulder rotation, shoulder flexion-extension, humeral rotation, and elbow flexion-extension. An heuristic rule was used to assure a level hand orientation during motion.

The Use of Heuristic Rules. This work attempted to provide coordinated control by applying heuristic rules to govern multijoint movement [49]. Shoulder movements provided the control input to the coordination algorithm; one of two heuristic rules governed motion:

    i) *Tangential coordination.* "At every point of the wrist trajectory, the hand is colinear to the direction of wrist velocity." This is a useful rule as the hand is ready to grasp an object as soon as the object is reached. The terminal device points toward the object to be grasped, which helps the operator control the endpoint motion.

    ii) *Translational coordination.* The terminal device motion is coordinated with the endpoint motion so as to keep the initial orientation of the hand constant with respect to the shoulder. Such coordination is important in object displacement movements.

Later work by this group [58] established four basic coordinated actions: *Reach, Move, Orient,* and *Grasp-Release*. The tangential coordination rule embodied the *Reach* motions. *Orient* motion starts immediately when the endpoint velocity drops to zero. The *Move* action used the translational coordination rule.

The Berkeley Multi-Mode Arm. Carlson and Radcliffe [59] developed a three degree of freedom pneumatically powered above-elbow prosthesis, termed the Berkeley multi-mode arm. They used *kinematic coupling* to coordinate elbow flexion, wrist flexion, and wrist rotation, using four distinct modes of operation:

    i) *Parallel mode.* The terminal device is kept parallel to its initial position at all times.

    ii) *Coupled mode.* Wrist rotation and wrist flexion are coupled to elbow flexion, providing a very natural motion useful in eating.

    iii) *Wrist flexion mode.* With the elbow locked, the wrist may be flexed over 180°, enabling the amputee to bring the terminal device nearer the body.

    iv) *Wrist rotation mode.* With a locked elbow, 130° of supination-pronation is allowed, useful in eating and rotational activities such as turning a doorknob.

Body-powered microswitches under the arms provided the means for mode selection. Shoulder flexion was used as the control input such that elbow flexion was proportional to the gleno-humeral angle.

Ocular Control. This project provided ocular control of the Rancho Arm. Initially [60] a mechanical conversion was used to supply three-dimensional spherical coordinates (azimuth, elevation, and range) to control four degrees of freedom (shoulder rotation, shoulder flexion-extension, humeral rotation, and elbow extension). Later, ocular signals (with an electronic coordinate converter) provided the control inputs [61], using infrared reflection to monitor eye motion. The coordinate conversion, performed on a minicomputer, eased the conscious effort of positioning tasks by computing the appropriate joint velocities, providing rate-coded endpoint control.

Resolved-Motion Rate Control. At the MIT Draper Laboratory, Whitney [62] developed a resolved-motion rate control technique for the control of six degree of freedom remote manipulators. The objective was to allow the operator to command motion rates of the endpoint along coordinate axes, which are convenient and visible to the operator, by computing the appropriate joint velocities. A direct transformation algorithm was successfully developed.

Binary-Coded Control. A project at Rensselaer Polytechnic Institute sought to provide endpoint control of a two degree of freedom (elbow flexion-extension, wrist flexion-extension) prosthesis using a single myoelectric control interface [63]. From an arbitrary anatomical site, a binary word is generated from the myoelectric signal envelope as a sequence of long (binary 1) and short (binary 0) bursts. A series of n binary digits would yield a repertoire of 2^n different commands. A five-bit binary word allows the user to move the arm in one of two modes. In mode "A", one of seven endpoint directions is chosen, along which the wrist will follow a straight-line trajectory. In mode "B", the user first positions the wrist; subsequent elbow extension-flexion will cause the wrist to follow a path parallel to the pre-selected wrist orientation, thus offering a higher degree of precision than mode "A".

Although this control technique did produce coordinated motion in positioning the endpoint, it offers little functional benefit to the user for normal active daily living tasks. Actuation of *any* motion required that the user produce a five-digit binary word – an obviously inconvenient means of manipulation.

2.2.5. Extended physiological proprioception

At the University of Edinburgh, Simpson and Kenworthy [64] developed a four degree of freedom pneumatically actuated prosthesis. The user controls the arm by clavicular movement relative to the harness supporting the prosthesis. With a position-servo system, it was asserted that proprioception is to some extent extended into the prosthetic arm, providing a position awareness of the arm (prompting the name *extended physiological proprioception*-EPP). Four control movements are possible by moving the shoulder up-down, forward-back, transmitted by Bowden cables to the pneumatic actuators. A proportional force feedback from a return cable transmitted position proprioception. Prehension required a separate body-movement control.

Simpson also provided stabilization of the hand about the horizontal axis, at right angles to the plane of the arm, keeping the terminal device parallel to its initial position at all times. The hand would not rotate in the vertical plane during elbow flexion and arm elevation; this device was justifiably termed "Simpson's Parallelogram Feeder".

Almost a decade after Simpson's published work, the promise of EPP control became the research interest of James Doubler, a Ph.D. candidate at Northwestern University under the supervision of Dudley Childress. This work presented an analysis of EPP as a prosthetic control technique: a communication systems model represented operator error in tracking experiments, yielding an information theoretic measure to describe the rate of information transmission by the subject to the control system. The results of the study showed that, for a hypothetical prosthesis mechanism with nonlimiting dynamic response characteristics, an EPP-controlled prosthesis in which wrist rotation and elbow flexion are controlled by shoulder elevation-depression and protraction-retraction could exhibit extremely functional tracking capabilities. The results also indicated that shoulder-affected position control of prosthesis function has control performance superior to velocity control as defined by information transmission bandwidth from simulation results [65] and from data acquired from an experimental prototype [66].

At the University of Edinburgh, David Gow continues the work proposed by Dr. Simpson. More recent research [67] is directed at implementing an electro-mechanical version of the pneumatic version designed by Simpson.

At the University of Ottawa, David Gibbons, Michael O'Riain and Sebastian Phillippe-Auguste have proposed a control technique loosely based upon the EPP paradigm [68]. Their scheme uses shoulder flexion-extension as a control input to actuate elbow flexion; wrist rotation is functionally related to elbow angle by means of programmed linkages [69], although the "unbeatable-servo" concept introduced by Simpson has been abandoned due to the inherent mechanical complexity. The control scheme is undergoing performance evaluation (assuming ideal prosthesis dynamics), using computer graphics simulation [70].

2.2.6. Modeling of musculo-skeletal dynamics

The Boston arm, designed by MIT scientists, was the first myoelectrically controlled elbow [17]. An ambitious adjunct to this developmental work was investigation into a sophisticated approach to myoelectric control. Robert Mann and Steven Jacobsen (in his doctoral dissertation) proposed an elegant control theory employing statistical techniques coupled with a mathematical formulation of musculo-skeletal dynamics to estimate desired limb motions [36], [71].

The core of what they termed a "postulate-based controller" was the Lagrangian equations describing the dynamics of an intact arm-prosthesis combination. These can be expressed in linear matrix form as

$$\mathbf{M}(\theta, \dot{\theta}) = \mathbf{P}(\theta)\ddot{\theta} + \mathbf{Q}(\theta, \dot{\theta}) + \mathbf{R}(\theta)$$

where:
- θ is an $N = n + p$ vector of joint positions (n = 'natural', p = 'prosthetic' degrees of freedom),
- P   is the generalized inertia matrix of the limbs,
- Q   is the vector incorporating centripetal and Coriolis forces,
- R   is the vector of gravitational forces, and
- M   is the net moment vector containing moments due to muscles and prosthetic actuators.

The postulate states that by detecting the mechanical force output of selected intact muscles (measured indirectly as integrated myoelectric signal activity), and by monitoring the kinematic state of the joints (with appropriately selected constraints on prosthetic degrees of freedom), the amputee's intended limb motion can be interpreted. The torques in the shoulder and clavical joints are determined by means of myoelectric signals from a set of shoulder muscles. The transfer function is found experimentally. By means of the torques and experimentally determined movement equations, the controller applies torques to the prosthetic joints so that the prescribed constraint is satisfied.

In the case of an amputee, the linkage consists of two parts: the remnant natural joints, and the prosthetic joints, thus the linkage moment, position, velocity, and acceleration vectors may be partitioned:

$$\mathbf{M} = \begin{bmatrix} \mathbf{M}_N \\ \mathbf{M}_P \end{bmatrix}, \; \theta = \begin{bmatrix} \theta_N \\ \theta_P \end{bmatrix}, \; \dot{\theta} = \begin{bmatrix} \dot{\theta}_N \\ \dot{\theta}_P \end{bmatrix}, \text{ and } \ddot{\theta} = \begin{bmatrix} \ddot{\theta}_N \\ \ddot{\theta}_P \end{bmatrix}.$$

If the vector of prosthetic moments $\mathbf{M}_P$ were known, the prosthetic control problem is solved. Unfortunately, both $\ddot{\theta}$ and $\mathbf{M}_P$ are unknown, giving an underdetermined set of equations. In this approach, the key to solving the equations lies in the assumption that not all the elements of θ are independent in normal use of the natural limb. The postulate here is that, for most arm tasks, clavicular motion is correlated with arm motion. Thus, θ may be repartitioned as:

$$\theta = \begin{bmatrix} \theta_C \\ \theta_F \end{bmatrix}$$

where θ_C is the vector of constrained angles and θ_F are the free angles, such that:

$$\theta_C = \tilde{\eta} \theta_F.$$

The constraint matrix $\tilde{\eta}$ relates the "free" degrees of freedom (the prosthetic joints and some natural joints) to the constrained degrees of freedom (a number of natural joints, determined by the number of degrees of freedom that must be eliminated to solve the equations). For the case of amputation at mid-humerus, elbow flexion and wrist rotation torques are unknown. To solve the controller equations it is necessary that two degrees of freedom be constrained. For a seven degree of freedom system, clavicular flexion and abduction are constrained, while shoulder flexion and abduction, humeral rotation, elbow flexion, and wrist rotation are free. The optimal choice of $\tilde{\eta}$ would place minimal constraint on natural motion.

The solution of the controller equations for $\mathbf{M}_P$ requires two inputs, $\tilde{\eta}$ and the vector of natural moments, $\mathbf{M}_N$. The constraint matrix (with kinematic data) will specify $\mathbf{P}$, $\mathbf{Q}$, and $\mathbf{R}$. Since, after all, the goal here is myoelectric control, the vector of natural moments must be determined from selected cutaneous electrode sites. An analytical derivation of the EMG-torque relation is confounded by the many factors influencing surface myoelectric recordings. This led to the investigation [72] of an experimental method of relating EMG to torque to fit the model, using a transfer function model which they termed the *vectormyogram*:

$$\mathbf{M}_N = \tilde{\mathbf{G}}(\theta,\dot{\theta})\mathbf{E} + \mathbf{N}(\theta,\dot{\theta}).$$

By recording the multichannel myoelectric activity, $\mathbf{E}$, and actual joint moments throughout normal motion and torque space, the matrix $\tilde{\mathbf{G}}$ and the vector $\mathbf{N}$ were determined using multivariable linear regression.

Drs. Jerard and Jacobsen realized a digital implementation of the postulate-based controller [72] and performed a laboratory evaluation of its performance. The control of a single prosthetic joint (the elbow) was functional, but more difficult than conventional biceps-triceps myoelectric control. The control of multiple degrees of freedom was difficult. Independent control of humeral rotation and elbow flexion was possible with some effort. Wrist rotation was controllable but was inadvertently affected during voluntary shoulder flexion and humeral rotation. Simultaneous control was possible to a limited degree, but was hardly effortless; the control was not "natural" in the sense that it did not respond accurately to subconscious effort.

The key problems and drawbacks of this novel control approach may be attributed to the following factors.

- Knowledge of the model parameters is incomplete: the physiological and anatomical parameters of muscle stiffness, viscosity, inertia and their dependence upon kinematic state and myoelectric activity present a challenging measurement problem. The quantification of shoulder anatomy was undertaken by J.E. Wood et al. [73] to refine force-to-moment conversion in the model. The conclusion of this work was that the determination of dynamical model parameters is very much an exercise in "hitting a moving target". Accurate parameters were determined for one subject, but inter-subject variability is such that generalization is not feasible while maintaining an accurate model.
- Estimation of joint moments via the vectormyogram has too many nonstationary variables, including electrode placement, skin impedance, arm position, and arm velocity. The determination of the $\tilde{\mathbf{G}}$ matrix and the $\mathbf{N}$ vector are dependent on all of these effects. The

experimental data included only that from a single static position. The vectormyogram equation should not be fixed, but dependent upon position and velocity. The problems of electrode placement and skin impedance must be dealt with separately.

- The postulate might not be representative of what actually happens in limb positioning tasks. The inherent assumption in the postulate control theory is that natural control occurs as the central nervous system simultaneously (and subconsciously) issues the appropriate innervation patterns to initiate motion and achieve joint stabilization. In the case of the upper limb, the muscles that cause elbow flexion and the muscles that immobilize the shoulder muscles may be considered to be co-initiators. This *may not* be what actually happens. A plausible argument may be made that the elbow and the shoulder are not co-initiators but rather, that shoulder stabilization is achieved by a postural mechanism that merely *reacts* to any forearm motion in an attempt to immobilize the humerus. This is likely the role of the cerebellum [90]. This may explain why the controller responded poorly to subconscious effort from amputee subjects, requiring instead intentional shoulder contraction (resembling reaction) resulting in considerable genuine effort to affect control.

Dr. Jacobsen continued research in his postulate-based control theory as a faculty member at the University of Utah. The difficulty of completing an appropriate set of anatomical parameters for each subject, and the sensitivity of the algorithm to day-to-day variations in the myoelectric control sites precluded a viable clinical solution. The lure to satisfy clinical and fiscal realities led the research toward development of the Utah Arm [19]. The development of the Utah Arm became the property of a private interest (Motion Control Inc.) under the direction of Howard Sears. Dr. Jacobsen has redirected his research interests to intelligent robotic control. The original research work at MIT undoubtedly influenced Neville Hogan, who embarked upon research with a thesis that elbow compliance is the salient parameter to be controlled via myoelectric signals. The evolution of Dr. Hogan's work will be detailed in a later section.

2.2.7. Statistical features for control

George Saridis built a research background, beginning at Purdue University, in hierarchical, self-organizing control and fuzzy set theory. In the mid-1970s he, and a series of colleagues, endeavored to apply these concepts to robust, distributed control of multiple degree of freedom prosthetic devices [74].

Their first effort produced an hierarchical approach to prosthetic control, the essence of which were three hierarchically-related levels of control. From highest to lowest, they were: (*i*) the *organization level* (description of movement intent), (*ii*) the *coordination level* (generation of the appropriate joint-space kinematics), and (*iii*) the *control level* (actuation to produce desired dynamic response). This approach allowed the decomposition of control (at the lowest level) into seven isolated dynamic control subsystems – one per degree of freedom [75]. This work was mostly analytical; some simulation was carried out demonstrating the feasibility of a reduced version of the control problem. The suggested control input was a binary-coded word from a pulsed myoelectric pattern.

The research efforts of Saridis *et al.* shifted to the problem of the control interface. They were among the first to suggest the use of statistical properties (other than integrated amplitude) as a means of conveying the information content of the myoelectric signal from a given control site [76]. They chose to apply pattern recognition techniques to the synergistic myoelectric signal patterns of the biceps and triceps to control a six degree of freedom prosthesis.

The correlation dimension of the myoelectric feature space from both channels was investigated [77], [78]. The features of the myoelectric signals which formed a sample basis of this space were the mean absolute value (MAV), the variance σ^2, the magnitude of the third moment $|\sigma^2|$, zero crossings (ZC), the autocorrelation function $R(\tau)$, and the power spectral density $S(\omega)$. A statistical analysis of these features during simple motions (one-joint) and combined motions (two- and three-joint) allowed those which contained the maximum information for pattern separation to be identified. Hand grasp/release yielded no measurable myoelectric response. Zero crossings and signal variance were found to provide the best classification of the remaining motions. This conveniently reduced the pattern feature space such that feature extraction and linear discriminant function classification might be performed using a general purpose microprocessor.

Figure 2a shows the grouping of three classes of motions in the feature space of biceps and triceps variance. Clearly, these motions occupy closed regions in this space, and may be classified by linear discriminants. Figure 2b depicts the behavior of the feature set during combined motions and with different contraction strength.

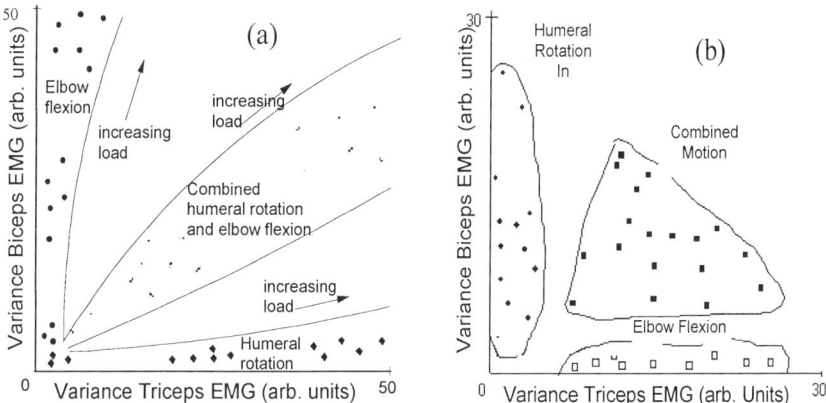

Figure 2. (a) Three motions depicted in biceps-triceps feature space. (b) The effect of loading upon the variance feature set during simple and combined motions (adapted from [76]).

This author stated that the variance subspace of a combined motion was the linear superposition of the variances of simple motions, justified in this case due to the uncorrelated signal data from the biceps and triceps. Saridis went further to include the dependency of muscle activity upon magnitude and rate of contraction by defining a region which contains all instances of the feature set under varying load and velocity conditions. The classification of movement intent is thereby robust under different load and velocity conditions, as evident in Figure 2b.

Still further, the classifier continuously updated the decision boundaries, allowing adaptive Bayesian discrimination. The locus of the feature vector in the feature space determined limb function. The level of myoelectric activity was used to select one of three speeds for the selected function. The past history of the limb motion was used to enhance the performance accuracy of limb function and speed estimation. The average classification rate for all motions was 91% using motion prediction enhancement, 85% without.

The conclusions of this work were presented at a Robotics Forum in Ottawa [79]; the report summarized the signal analysis and classification, the modeling aspects, and the control theory established by his group. The project was at the stage of microprocessor implementation of the control algorithm (using a Texas Instruments TM990 microcomputer); laboratory trials demonstrated fair success in classification of the motion primitives and compensation for loading and velocity effects upon the pattern clusters in feature space.

This work is important because it demonstrates that the control of simultaneous motions of two or three functions is possible using a pattern recognition scheme.

2.2.8. Autoregressive models

Daniel Graupe and colleagues, at the Illinois Institute of Technology, attempted to address the problems imposed by multichannel systems [80], [81], [82], [83]. The hardware and interfacing problems associated with many electrode sites can make multichannel systems unwieldy. A further limitation is that only one or two parameters of the myoelectric signal are being used in the description of the patterns; any other information which the signal may contain at each site is lost.

In light of the desire to have as few myoelectric channels as possible, Graupe and his colleagues proposed that greater information dimension could be extracted from each control site by time-series analysis. At a given electrode site, the myoelectric signal is the temporal and spatial summation of the motor unit action potentials of all active muscle fibers within the detection region of the electrodes. In the cross-section of muscle during a contraction, the active motor units will differ (in general) with respect to their action potential shape and their innervation pattern; the electrical manifestation of this activity at the recording site will also be influenced by the fiber geometry with respect to the electrode and the tissue filtering effect of the conduction medium.

Different limb functions require a different ensemble of muscle activation patterns. This has two effects at a recording site:
1. The composite of active fibers will distinguish the nature of the muscle activity, due to their characteristic action potential shape and recruitment pattern.
2. The spatial location of the active fibers will vary with the type of contraction. The tissue filtering will distinguish remote units from proximal units due to the low-pass filtering effect of dispersive conduction.

A feature set extracted from the myoelectric signal which captures the spectral differences caused by active units of differing action potential shape or proximity to the recording site will necessarily contain more information than simply a measure of amplitude. Unlike multichannel systems – which attempt to isolate the activity of functional groups of muscle, and in which crosstalk is considered noise – a feature set capable of spectral discrimination uses inter-muscular crosstalk as information.

Specifically, Graupe proposed a feature set derived from the coefficients (a_j) of an autoregressive time-series model:

$$y(k) = \sum_{j=1}^{p} a_j y(k-j) + e(k).$$

Two assumptions underlie this model: (*i*) the myoelectric signal from each site must be stationary during the measurement and (*ii*) must be linearly related to muscle force. These assumptions are easily violated in general (for most dynamic movements), requiring specific intent by the subject to maintain a constant level of force.

A model order of $p = 4$ was chosen, which was considered small enough to limit computational time (to keep limb actuation delays small) and large enough to ensure that the residual error in the model, $e(k)$, was sufficiently white. The coefficients a_j, $j = 1,2,3,4$ were computed using both least mean squares (LMS) and recursive least squares (RLS). These coefficients specified a four-dimensional feature space upon which a subspace could be defined for each limb function. During the operation phase any pattern produced was compared in this feature space to determine if it fell within the classification domain of a movement type. If it did, that movement was selected.

If limb function discrimination is to be performed in the feature space of AR parameters, the identification procedure must be done *on-line* for each set of data; a computationally intensive task in 1982. For this reason, Graupe proposed an alternative means of discrimination: AR parameters for each limb function would be performed *off-line*, and only simple filtering would be performed during the operation of the prosthesis. The intent here was to discriminate in the space of the *mean square error* (MSE) associated with each limb function. Computed *off-line*, the MSE associated with limb function i is:

$$E_i = \overline{e(k)} = \frac{1}{(N-p-1)} \sum_{k=P+1}^{N} \left(y(k) - \sum_{j=1}^{p} a_{j,i} y(k-j) \right)$$

where $a_{j,i}$ is the jth AR coefficient of the ith limb function. During *on-line* discrimination, data was fed through each AR model (a simple transversal filter) to compute an MSE estimate $\hat{E}_i$ for each. The minimum of this group was selected and compared to the value of MSE for that function which was computed in the calibration run. Limb function i was selected if the signal level surpassed a threshold and if:

$$\hat{E}_i \leq \gamma_i E_i$$

where γ_i is a weighting coefficient greater than 1.

The performance evaluation of this control system as described by Graupe is somewhat ambiguous. After 12 hours of training, ten above-elbow and shoulder disarticulation amputees achieved successful classification in 99% of four to six limb functions. The muscular activation was not based upon phantom perception (as described by Herberts), but instead by contriving contraction schemes which maximally separated the AR parameters into three ranges in feature space. Discrimination into six classes of movement intent was attained by specifying two ranges of signal variance for each of the three ranges distinguished by AR parameters. The nature of the muscular contraction that an amputee must deliver to effect control may not have any physiological relation to the intended limb function.

The most promising aspect of Graupe's work was that it demonstrated that multifunction control is feasible with a limited number of control sites. The drawbacks were the computational complexity of the algorithm (although this is much less a problem today), and roundoff errors in computation of the AR parameters. The choice of the free parameter γ_i was never explained by Graupe, as well as the means of determining the contraction types to separate AR parameters in feature space. It is likely that Graupe's definition and assessment of signal stationarity were less than robust; nonstationary behavior would likely bias the AR feature set.

Graupe's research shifted to other interests before the problems of computational burden and algorithm stability were fully investigated, although others have applied the techniques introduced in his work.

At MIT, Doershuk et al. [84] adopted Graupe's time-series approach, and extended it to a multiple-site control system. The multichannel autoregressive model of order p is given by:

$$y(k) = \sum_{j=1}^{p} A_{m,j} y(k-j) + e_m(k) \quad m = 1, ..., M$$

where $y(k)$ is the $L \times 1$ vector of the myoelectric signal at L electrode sites at time (sample) k.

Here, m is the limb function being modeled, M is the total number of limb functions, $A_{m,1}, ..., A_{m,p}$ are $L \times L$ coefficient matrices, and $e_m(k)$ is the $L \times 1$ one-step prediction error vector for the AR model when modeling the mth limb function. The crosstalk between signals is included in the model as off-diagonal terms in the $A_{m,j}$ matrices and in the covariance matrix S_m of the prediction error vector e_m; thus, inter-electrode crosstalk becomes part of the model. The model incorporates information of a given myoelectric signal source from the most proximal electrode, as well as the influence of this source upon the remaining electrodes.

Doershuk investigated the classification performance of various AR structures, and the effect of the number of myoelectric channels. A full AR matrix (with cross-correlation terms) proved superior to classification without cross-correlation terms. With a full AR structure, four channels (positioned around the forearm) exhibited a substantial improvement in correct limb function discrimination compared to a single-site system. The test conditions were not specified very well however; it is difficult to conclude that their results indicate better algorithmic performance.

The closely-spaced bipolar electrode pairs used in the four-site arrangement had quite a limited pickup area. Increasing the spacing between the electrodes of a bipolar pair will increase the effective pickup area: Graupe placed a bipolar pair on opposite sides of the upper arm, thereby detecting the global activity within the limb. The aggregate of the data acquired by Doershuk's arrangement contains much of the same information as Graupe's measurement scheme. Doershuk stated that multiple sites are superior to single sites in the case of the failure of one of the channels. Multiple sites, however, mean additional hardware and noisier signals (signal to noise ratio degrades as additional channels must be processed using an amplifier with finite CMMR). Moreover, the probability of electrode failure increases with additional channels; the most common type of failure is loss of electrode contact, which swamps the system with 60 Hz noise.

This work provided some information (on a conceptual basis) of the influence of inter-site correlation as applied to the time-series model discrimination approach. Doershuk's data were acquired from nonamputees, and no details were given concerning computational delay times. This work ended with Doershuk's computer simulation results.

2.2.9. Equilibrium-point control

At MIT, Neville Hogan brought together the work established by Steven Jacobsen (postulate-based multi-axis control) and by Emilio Bizzi (equilibrium-point physiological control theory). Whereas Jacobsen's contribution proposed a biomechanical-mathematical formulation of upper-limb muscular synergies for the purpose of prosthetic control, Bizzi's work proposed an hypothesis explaining the neuromuscular schema of human posture and movement [30], briefly summarized here.

THE EQUILIBRIUM-POINT HYPOTHESIS

The hypothesis states that the central nervous system (CNS) generates movement as a shift of the limb's equilibrium position. The equilibrium position, and the stiffness of a joint at that position are specified as a point on the locus of intersecting muscle length-tension curves (or equivalently, agonist-antagonist torque-angle curves). The CNS input to this model is simply the ensemble of muscle activations to properly set muscle elasticity. Arm trajectories are generated through a series of equilibrium postures. This hypothesis drastically simplifies the requisite limb dynamics computations for multijoint movements and mechanical interactions. Due to the "springlike" dynamics of the musculo-skeletal system, the instantaneous difference between the arm's actual position and the equilibrium position specified by the neural activity can generate the requisite torques, obviating the complex "inverse dynamic" problem of computing the torques at the joints.

The transformations that are thought to occur in a reaching task start with integration of sensory inputs (visual and proprioceptive) to form a neural code representing the location of an object with respect to the body and head [92]. Next, planning of hand trajectory is performed; it has been suggested that this planning stage is carried out in extrinsic, likely Cartesian coordinates that represent the motion of the hand in space [85]. Indeed, recordings from single cells in the motor cortex of the brain have shown a correlation between their firing pattern and the direction of movement [86]. Subsequent representation in body-centered coordinates (e.g. joint angles or muscle lengths) may also occur at some level of motor control [26]. The final step is to transform the desired trajectory into the appropriate ensemble of muscle activations. The equilibrium-point hypothesis is related to this final step and the communication between the processes of movement planning and movement execution.

Hogan proposed that a control system based upon the concepts of equilibrium-point and joint stiffness (joint "impedance" is the term he uses) would constitute a more natural control interface than velocity-controlled systems [87], [88]. An elbow control system was derived from a model in which the forearm is treated as an inertial body, driven by moments due to the muscular forces of the biceps and triceps, and external loads as depicted in Figure 3.

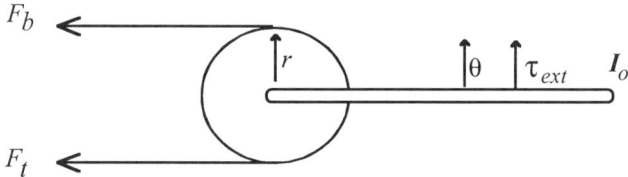

Figure 3. A free-body diagram of the forearm.

The torques generated by the muscles are:

$$\tau_b = rF_b = K_b(\theta_{max} - \theta) - B_b\dot{\theta}$$
$$\tau_t = rF_t = K_t(\theta - \theta_{min}) + B_t\dot{\theta}$$

where the subscripts b and t refer to biceps and triceps. The coefficients K and B are the muscles' contributions to the joint stiffness and damping, respectively; θ_{max} and θ_{min} are angles at which the biceps and the triceps are at rest (zero torque). The muscle stiffness and damping factors are given by:

$$K_i = K_{0i}\alpha_i \quad \text{and} \quad B_i = B_{0i}\alpha_i$$

where i is b for biceps and t for triceps, K_{0i} and B_{0i} are positive constants representing maximum muscle stiffness and damping about the joint, and α_i is the level of activation of the muscles ($\alpha_i = 1$ indicates maximum voluntary contraction). The dynamic behavior of the elbow is given by:

$$I_0 \ddot{\theta} = \tau_b - \tau_t + \tau_{ext}$$

If the net elbow stiffness is defined as $K_0 = K_{0b}\alpha_b + K_{0t}\alpha_t$, the net viscous damping as $B_0 = B_{0b}\alpha_b + B_{0t}\alpha_t$ and the parameter $\tau_{vir} = K_{0b}\theta_{max}\alpha_b + K_{0t}\theta_{min}\alpha_t$, then the equation of motion is:

$$I_0 \ddot{\theta} + B_0 \dot{\theta} + K_0 = \tau_{vir} + \tau_{ext}$$

or equivalently,

$$I_0 \ddot{\theta} + B_0 \dot{\theta} = K_0 (\theta_{vir} - \theta) + \tau_{ext}$$

where $\theta_{vir} = \tau_{vir}/K_0$ is the equilibrium point. The inputs to the controller are the estimates of muscle activity from the biceps (α_b) and triceps (α_t). This specifies the equilibrium point θ_{vir} and thus, the dynamics of the model limb.

Functional evaluation of the control strategy applied to control of a powered elbow has indicated its superiority to conventional velocity control in positioning and dynamic resistance tasks [89], [90], [91], [92], [93].

2.2.10. Pattern recognition-based control using the transient myoelectric signal

The Institute of Biomedical Engineering at the University of New Brunswick in Canada has been developing and fitting myoelectric control systems since the 1960s. The research from this group has been primarily on single function control (UNB 3-state) and sensory feedback, but recently, with collaborative funding from Hugh Steeper Ltd. (UK), they have developed a three degree of freedom myoelectric control system. Their approach uses patterns in the instantaneous myoelectric signal to define a signature for a particular limb function.

The myoelectric signal is very complex as it is influenced by many factors due to the electro-physiology and the recording environment. It is the complexity of the MES that has presented the greatest challenge in its application to the control of powered prosthetic limbs. In most myoelectric control systems, information from the *steady-state* MES (that produced during constant effort) is used as the control input. The steady-state MES however, has very little temporal structure due to the active modification of recruitment and firing patterns needed to sustain a contraction [94]. This is due to the establishment of feedback paths, both intrinsic (the afferent neuromuscular pathways) and extrinsic (the visual system). In a departure from conventional steady-state analysis, Hudgins [95], [96] investigated the information content in the *transient burst* of myoelectric activity accompanying the onset of sudden muscular effort. A substantial degree of structure was observed in these transient waveforms. Data were acquired during small but distinct isometric and anisometric contractions, using a single bipolar electrode pair placed over the biceps and triceps muscle groups. This arrangement was intended to allow a large volume of musculature to influence the measured activity. Figure 4 shows typical patterns corresponding to flexion/extension of the elbow and pronation/supination of the forearm.

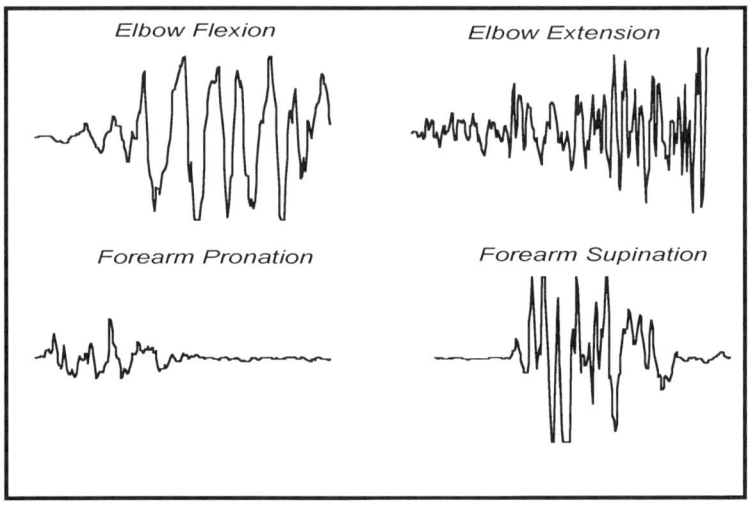

Figure 4. Patterns of transient MES activity recorded using a single bipolar electrode pair, placed over the biceps and triceps.

These patterns exhibit distinct differences in their temporal waveforms. Within a set of patterns derived from the same contraction, the structure that characterizes the patterns is sufficiently consistent to maintain a visual distinction between different types of contraction. Hudgins aligned the patterns using a cross-correlation technique and showed that the ensemble average of patterns within a class preserves this structure.

The question is: why do these structured patterns occur? The amplitude envelopes of these classes of contraction certainly differ, but the degree of structure in the patterns cannot be explained by the gross activity of different muscle groups. This structure suggests that it is likely that a "motor plan" exists for simple, ballistic contractions. In this scenario, an orderly scheme of recruitment and neural discharge is responsible for initiating a contraction. The absence of concrete evidence of this phenomenon is due to the difficulty in identifying motor unit recruitment and firing activity in such a short, dynamic interval. The following observations can be made, however:

1. Weirzbicka *et al.* [97] have identified that the onset of rapid contraction (both isometric and anisometric) produces a transition from tonic to phasic[1] muscle activation, and that a brief interval of silence (inactivity) exists between these states. This suggests the initiation of a new motor program.
2. It has been observed that motor unit recruitment order appears stable for a given task, once the task has been learned [98]. Further, consistent feedforward commands from the motor cortex have been observed during goal-directed movements, such as arm positioning tasks [86].
3. The propagation delays in the neuromuscular system's afferent feedback pathways prohibit modification of motor activity immediately following initiation of a spontaneous contraction. The *stretch reflex* regulates motion as negative-feedback servomechanism, relying on proprioceptors which sense muscle length and tension. The *short-loop* stretch reflex completes its feedback path at the spinal level, resulting in a propagation delay of 30-50 ms. The *long-loop* stretch reflex must consult the cerebellum, resulting in a delay of 50-80 ms [99]. Therefore, the neuromuscular system is operating either partially or fully in an "open-loop" condition for the first 30-80 ms [109]. Indeed, the greatest degree of structure is seen in this early portion of the transient MES patterns.

It is possible that the structure may be due to factors that are not of neuromuscular origin. An obvious mechanism that could impose a deterministic effect is movement artifact (motion of the electrodes relative to the skin). Attempts to reproduce the patterns by passive movement of the limb and rapid electrode lead motion however, have failed [96]. Yamazaki et al. [100] simultaneously recorded patterns of rapid isometric contraction of the biceps using surface bipolar surface electrodes and needle electrodes inserted into the muscle. The needle electrode recordings were highly correlated with the surface recordings, demonstrating fairly conclusively that the activity is not due to movement artifact. Other possible sources of modulation, such as the motion of the active muscle fibers (relative to the electrode), have not been disproved.

Subtle changes in the nature of a contraction however, can introduce variability into the recorded MES. In an ensemble of patterns produced by similar contractions, there are visually perceptible similarities among waveforms, but the local characteristics may vary tremendously. Identifying this loosely defined structure is a challenging pattern recognition task. Hudgins

---

[1] Tonic motor units are those responsible for sustaining force; phasic motor units are those responsible for building force.

used an approach in which he segmented the initial 240 ms of unprocessed MES following a threshold trigger into several time segments as shown in Figure 5.

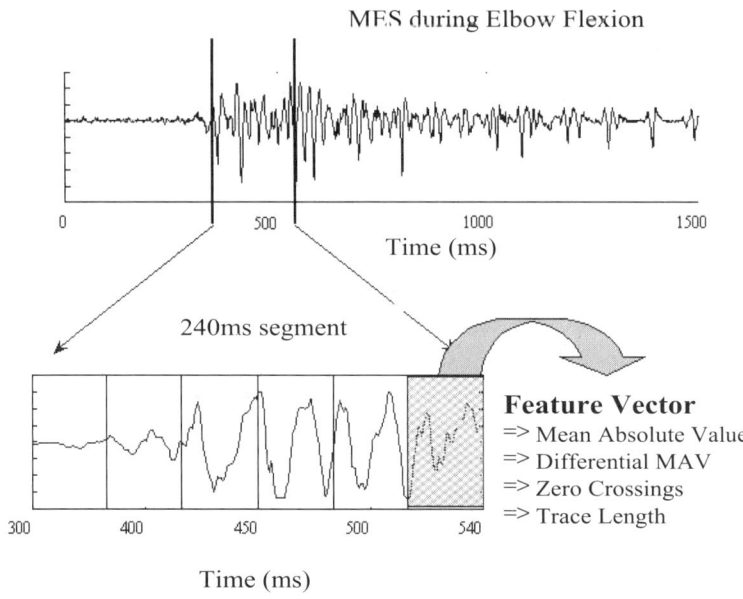

Figure 5. In Hudgins' approach, the features are extracted from several time segments of the unprocessed MES.

A control system based on Hudgins' work was designed at UNB. This system used a simple multilayer perceptron (MLP) artificial neural network as a classifier of the time-domain feature set (zero crossings, mean absolute value, mean absolute value slope and trace length) extracted from the single channel MES. The controller identified four types of muscular contraction using signals measured from the biceps and triceps. A block diagram of the UNB control scheme is shown in Figure 6. A set of time-domain features is extracted from a transient burst of one-channel MES. An MLP classifier is trained upon an ensemble of patterns derived from contractions of (up to) four movement types.

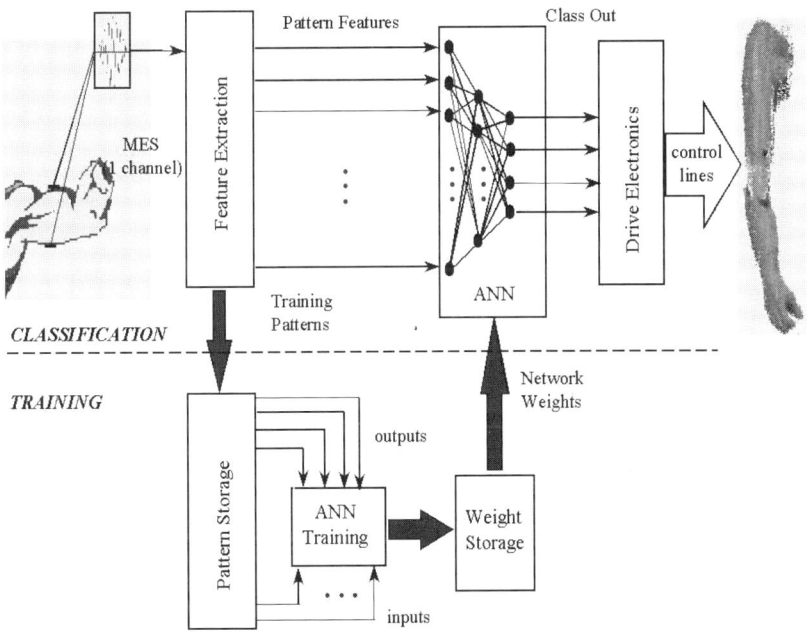

Figure 6. The UNB multifunction control scheme.

Not only does this system provide multifunction control from a single site, but the control signals can be derived from natural contractions, thereby minimizing the conscious effort of the user. The control system was realized in hardware, and improvements to the original design have been suggested to allow it to be used for degree of freedom (DOF) selection [101] and to improve its classification performance [102]. The current system has several modes of operation as shown in Figure 7. Initially, the control system is trained on the distinct MES patterns of the amputee. This information is downloaded into the control system. The control system can then be used to control a 3 DOF prosthetic arm or used to control a virtual arm simulation on a computer screen.

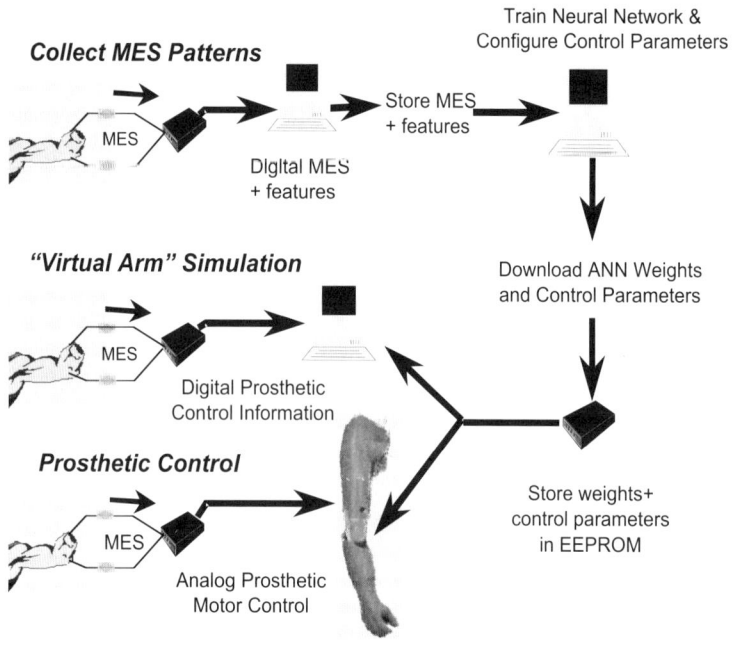

Figure 7. Modes of operation of the UNB multifunction control system.

2.3. Significant contributions of previous work

None of the research efforts described in the previous section could be considered an unqualified success – adequate multifunction control is still an elusive goal. To gain from the efforts of the past, it is imperative to recognize the strengths in ideas introduced in previous work, and identify which technologies may hold promise in an improved control strategy. The following are the significant contributions from previous work, which warrant consideration as elements of a robust multifunction control system.

Muscle Synergy Classification. The attempts to capture and categorize synergistic muscle action represent a direct way to accommodate actuation by natural contraction and to provide a control input of high information dimension. The pattern recognition approaches of Wirta *et al.*, Lyman *et al.* and Herberts *et al.* relied upon multiple electrode sites, from which myoelectric amplitude information was extracted during isometric contraction. The classifier used by Wirta's group had fixed discriminant boundaries; the latter two had adaptable boundaries, which were trained to an individual's own pattern of muscular activity. The concept of adaptive aiding, proposed by Lyman's group, could possibly take synergistic classification a step further by allowing a learning subsystem to assume some degree of control, or to act as an error filter or momentum factor to add robustness during coordinated endpoint movement.

Anatomical Models. The task of transforming body actuated control signals into limb function intent can utilize some *a priori* knowledge if an appropriate anatomical model is assumed. Jacobsen *et al.* envisioned the shoulder and upper-limb dynamics to be characterized by the active torques and the inertial-viscous properties of the upper-limb musculature. In the prosthetic situation, an appropriate estimation of the remaining shoulder muscle torques (via processed myoelectric activity) would allow an analytical solution for the torques of the missing degrees of freedom. Hogan used the equilibrium-point hypothesis to define elbow action with respect to biceps-triceps activity, effectively specifying elbow position and stiffness.

Trajectory Primitives and Kinematic Linkages. The use of predefined trajectories based upon the limb kinematics of useful tasks has been successfully used to reduce the dimension of the control problem. Though fixed trajectories serve a useful dedicated purpose, interactive control of individual degrees of freedom is hindered; tasks that require manipulation that do not match the preassigned functions may be difficult to accomplish. Context-based (adaptive) or interactive trajectory modification may offer a solution to this drawback.

Some solutions to resolved motion (endpoint) control have been offered, insofar as allowing the control input to be specified in endpoint coordinates rather than joint space coordinates. A natural and convenient way for an amputee to transmit endpoint coordinates to the controller has yet to be proposed.

Feature Selection. Graupe, Saridis and Hudgins demonstrated that extraction of meaningful features from the myoelectric signal (in addition to amplitude) can increase the information dimension from each control site, allowing the number of sites to be reduced. Limb function classification can be performed in a decision space defined by multiple features from a few sites, instead of simply amplitude level from many sites. This approach reduces the hardware complexities and fitting problems associated with multichannel systems, although at the expense of added signal processing required for feature extraction.

Some problems associated with using feature vectors to define a decision space (and this includes the multichannel, amplitude-based systems) are the dependence of the features upon the level of contraction and the kinematic state of the limb. The methods used by Graupe and Saridis (and those preceding them) require isometric contractions (velocity is zero).

Temporal Structure in the Myoelectric Signal. Hudgins has proposed the only approach which exploits semi-determinism in the myoelectric signal at the onset of contraction. All other approaches have assumed stationary, isometric signals bearing no instantaneous structure. By extracting a meaningful feature set, retaining the temporal excursion of the feature set, and applying a nonlinear classifier, Hudgins demonstrated that reliable limb function discrimination is possible from only one or two sites.

3. Research directions

As described in the previous section, there has been a considerable history to multifunction control research. Although significant advances have been made, a convenient and robust means of multifunction control has yet to be achieved. Looking toward where research in the field is heading, one must consider that there are two fundamentally different approaches to multifunction control:

1. **Sequential control**. The degrees of freedom to be functionally replaced are actuated one at a time, in a sequence, as one executes a multifunction task.
2. **Simultaneous, coordinated control**. The degrees of freedom are actuated simultaneously, in a coordinated fashion, as one executes a multifunction task.

Clearly, simultaneous, coordinated control is the more desirable of the two, as it promises to replicate the kinematics and dynamics of normal human upper-limb movement. It is also necessarily a longer-term goal, as the problems of sequential control must be solved first. The following sections will describe current research efforts toward these two modalities of control.

3.1. Sequential control

In sequential (or *state-based*) control, each degree of freedom (usually, each prosthetic joint) is independently controlled. This is an obvious, albeit cumbersome approach to replacing the lost axes of manipulation. Nonetheless, an accurate and robust means of sequential multifunction control would greatly enhance the functionality of today's prosthetic devices.

The sequential control task is essentially a pattern recognition problem. If N degrees of freedom are to be controlled, the problem becomes that of N-class discrimination. Once the appropriate class (degree of freedom) is selected, actuation can take a conventional form (e.g., speed proportional to the amplitude of the MES). It is instructive to decompose the pattern recognition problem into its constituent stages: these are signal acquisition, feature extraction, and classification, as illustrated in Figure 8.

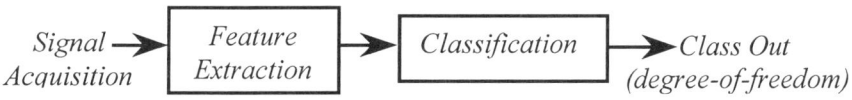

Figure 8. The stages comprising the pattern recognition problem.

The primary goal of sequential control is to maximize the classification accuracy of the MES pattern recognition. There are efforts to improve the classification accuracy at each of these stages, as summarized below.

3.1.1. Signal acquisition

The focus of improving signal acquisition is to maximize the amount of information in the measured MES. Whereas researchers rejected multielectrode configurations as recently as a decade ago, improvements in electronics, fabrication, and packaging have justified their use today.

It has been demonstrated that multiple channels of MES do offer improved classification accuracy over a single-site configuration. Kuruganti *et al.* [101] demonstrated the superiority of a two-channel electrode configuration over a one channel configuration when using Hudgins' neural network based classifier. Leowinata *et al.* [103] used a four channel configuration and demonstrated very good classification accuracy using a very simple classifier. Others are investigating the use of multichannel electrode arrays. With more electrode sites, one obtains a more resolved measure of localized muscle activity, and avoids destructive cancellation of information when muscle activities are superimposed in single channel recording with a large pickup area.

The prospect of using multiple sites for myoelectric control has yet to be fully explored, especially when coupled with powerful feature extraction methods, the subject of the next section.

3.1.2. Feature extraction

It was Saridis *et al.*, Graupe *et al.*, and Doershuck *et al.* who realized the importance of effective feature extraction in the early 1980's. It is realized that this is crucial to the success of a pattern recognition based control system. The most recent work has employed time-frequency analysis to extract features that capture the nonstationary behaviour of the MES. Perhaps the first work of this type was that of Hannaford and Lehman [104]. The STFT was used to track temporal variations of the MES spectrum accompanying rapid movements of the head and wrist. Although no attempt was made to perform pattern recognition, repeatable structure was identified in the MES spectrogram. Gallant [105] and Farry [106] investigated the use of the short-time Fourier transform (STFT) with good success. Englehart *et al.* [102] compared features based on the Hudgins' time-domain features, STFT, the wavelet transform, and the wavelet packet transform. The wavelet packet transform was found to offer the best feature set for classification purposes, followed by the wavelet transform, and the STFT.

Fundamental to the success of the work of Gallant and Englehart was the use of *dimensionality reduction*, a scheme of reducing the number of features in the feature set so as not to overwhelm the classifier. Gallant used an iterative technique called *projection pursuit*, which seeks to map a higher dimensional space (the STFT features) onto a lower dimensional space using a metric which tends to cluster the data. Englehart used a simpler projection method, *principal components analysis*, which projects the higher dimensional space onto a lower dimensional space such that the reconstruction error is minimized. This method has the advantage of having a well-understood, easily computed analytic solution. Both projection pursuit and principal components analysis dramatically improve the classification results when using features based upon the STFT, the wavelet transform, or the wavelet packet transform.

There is much left to be done in the field of feature extraction for classification. Quadratic time-frequency methods hold promise if their computational complexity can be sufficiently reduced so as to be feasible for real-time implementation. Nonlinear projection methods have recently been introduced [107]; these may offer greater class discrimination capabilities than projection pursuit or principal components analysis.

3.1.3. Classifiers

If the feature set extracted from the MES contains complex boundaries, which distinguish the classes of motion, a powerful classifier can improve the accuracy of classification. This was investigated by Hudgins *et al.* [96], who demonstrated that a multiplayer perceptron neural network exhibited superior performance to a linear discriminant classifier, when applied to a simple time-domain feature set. This result suggests that nonlinear boundaries exist between the classes of time-domain features.

Others have investigated MES pattern recognition using more exotic forms of classifiers. Farry *et al.* have reported extremely good discrimination results when using a genetic algorithm [108]. Similarly, Leowinata *et al.* have had very good success using a fuzzy logic classifier [103]. Others have applied hidden Markov models and nonlinear system identification methods with mediocre success.

There is an inherent tradeoff, however, in the degree of sophistication of the classifier and of the feature set. It has been shown by Englehart *et al.* [102] that the choice of classifier matters little if the class discrimination is achieved by the feature extraction. In this work, the use of time-frequency based features, coupled with principal components analysis, produced a feature set with essentially linear class boundaries. In this case, a linear discriminant performed as well as a neural network classifier. It is clear that the feature extraction process may effectively assume the burden of class discrimination.

One approach to classification that may significantly enhance state based control is that which seeks to identify patterns in a continuous stream of MES activity. As opposed to requiring a period of inactivity before eliciting a contraction, continuous classification would allow a user to dynamically switch between degrees of freedom. Preliminary work in continuous classification has been done using dynamic feedforward neural networks [109], [110].

3.2. Simultaneous, coordinated control

Most active daily living tasks require simultaneous and coordinated control of multiple joints. We are capable of this type of control at a subconscious level. There is evidence to suggest that humans plan upper-limb activities in three-dimensional Cartesian coordinates [111], and that this target activity is transformed into the joint space forces (muscle activity) required to produce the desired limb dynamics [112]. Therefore, the conscious command input consists of little more than an *endpoint*, and the neuromuscular and skeletal system take care of the kinematics and dynamics of the joints.

This physiological analog suggests a desirable strategy for multifunction control of prostheses. It is unreasonable to expect that sufficient information could be extracted from the MES to control many degrees of freedom in a coordinated manner; the dimensionality of the problem is simply too high, given the limited amount of information in the MES. If we reduce the problem to that of specifying an endpoint however, the dimensionality of the problem is significantly reduced. In this case, an intelligent subsystem must augment the endpoint command to infer the kinematic and dynamic behavior of the prosthetic limb.

Recent approaches to robotic manipulator control have followed the model of biological systems, attempting to transform task space targets into joint space actuator forces. This is a very difficult and computationally intensive problem, and requires precise knowledge of the kinematic and dynamic parameters of the limb. An understanding of how learning in motion and control occurs in biological systems has motivated model-free connectionist approaches to robot control.

Manipulator control involves three fundamental problems: task planning, trajectory generation and motion control. *Task planning* is the high-level, goal-oriented coordination of movement. *Trajectory generation* is the assignment of finding the sequence of points through which the manipulator endpoint must pass, given initial and goal coordinates, possibly with some intermediate (via) points and motion constraints. The *motion control* problem consists of finding the joint torques that will cause the arm to follow a specified trajectory while satisfying some measure of accuracy. Artificial neural networks have found application in each of these three problems, but it has been in trajectory generation and motion control that the most useful work has been done; these will be discussed here.

3.2.1. Trajectory generation

The fundamental problem in trajectory generation is determining joint space coordinates from Cartesian space coordinates, the *inverse kinematic* solution [113]. The joint coordinates _ are related to the Cartesian coordinates **x** by the forward kinematic equation

$$\mathbf{x} = \mathbf{f}(\theta).$$

Consider the simple two-link case depicted in Figure 9, where $\mathbf{x} = \begin{bmatrix} x \\ y \end{bmatrix}$ and $\theta = \begin{bmatrix} \theta_1 \\ \theta_2 \end{bmatrix}$.

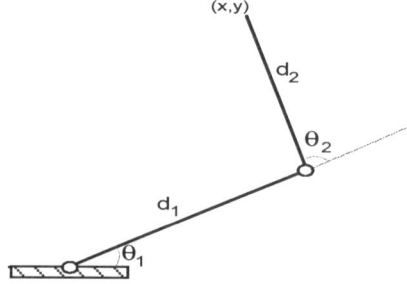

Figure 9. A two degree of freedom arm.

The corresponding kinematic equations are

$$\begin{bmatrix} x \\ y \end{bmatrix} = \begin{bmatrix} d_1 \cos\theta_1 + d_2 \cos(\theta_1 + \theta_2) \\ d_1 \sin\theta_1 + d_2 \sin(\theta_1 + \theta_2) \end{bmatrix}.$$

For three-dimensional manipulation, x is specified by three positional degrees of freedom and three orientational degrees of freedom. The joint space dimension depends on the number of linkages and the nature of the joints. To plan the trajectory in joint space, the kinematic equations must be inverted. This problem, termed *position-based inverse kinematic control*, is not always well-behaved and, without constraints, may contain multiple solutions. Often, the trajectory contains velocity specifications; by differentiation, the representative forward kinematic equation is

$$\dot{x} = J(\theta)\dot{\theta}$$

where the elements of the Jacobian matrix **J** are the partial derivatives

$$\frac{\partial x_i}{\partial y_i} \quad \forall\, i, j.$$

The inverse solution is

$$\dot{\theta} = J^{-1}(\theta)\dot{x} .$$

Thus, at any position _, a given Cartesian velocity specification of the endpoint ($\dot{x}$) can be converted into the appropriate joint velocities ($\dot{\theta}$). This type of trajectory planning is referred to as *velocity-based kinematic control* (or *inverse Jacobian control*). A typical neural network-based inverse Jacobian control system is shown in Figure 10.

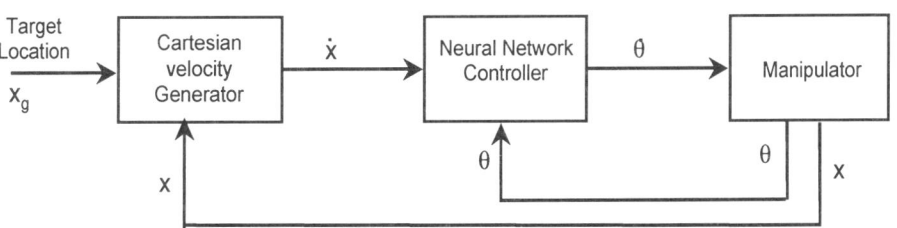

Figure 10. An inverse Jacobian controller.

Successful application of inverse kinematic methods require efficient and stable matrix inversion and accurate knowledge of manipulator kinematic parameters. Neural network approaches are model free (they do not need *a priori* knowledge of parameters) and estimate the inverse solution in a look-up table fashion rather than by solving the control equations. For these reasons they are attractive alternatives to analytical inverse methods.

One of the first neural network approaches to manipulator control was the *Cerebellar Model Articulation Controller* (CMAC), a three-layer network which used random weights in the first layer (making table look-up distributed in nature), and adjustable weights in the second [114]. With no prior knowledge of the structure of the system being controlled, the network can be trained to perform the manipulator control task, provided that there are sufficient adjustable and random connections. Others have investigated inverse kinematic control using the backpropagation algorithm for learning [115], [116]. Attempts to apply backpropagation to systems with more than two or three degrees of freedom have not been very successful, due to the high-order nonlinearities inherent in the problem and hence, slow learning rates. One strategy to improve convergence time in learning involves decomposing the systems into smaller subsystems, which are more linear.

A *context-sensitive network* is one in which the set of input variables is partitioned into two groups. As shown in Figure 11, one set is used as the input to the network which approximates the basic mathematical operation being modeled (the function network), and the second set defines the context within which the function is determined. In the case of manipulator control, the context is the spatial location of the manipulator.

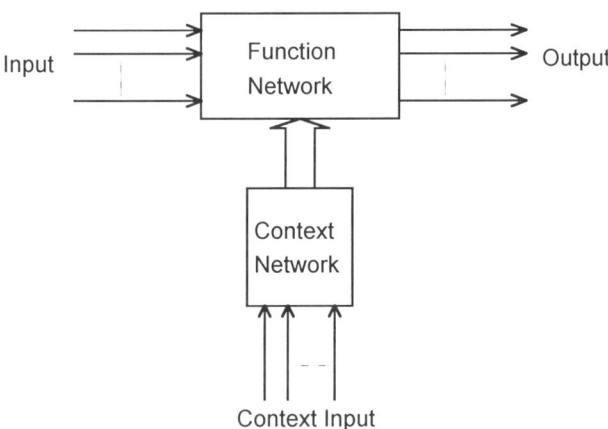

Figure 11. The structure of a context-dependent network.

An n degree of freedom arm requires a function network with n inputs and n output units. The output units have no bias terms and their activation function is simply the identity function $f(x)=x$; thus, the n^2 weights correspond to entries in the inverse Jacobian matrix $\mathbf{J}^{-1}(\theta)$ evaluated at θ. The context network consists of n^2 decoupled subnetworks each of which is responsible for learning a single scalar function (in θ) corresponding to one entry in the inverse Jacobian. Decoupling an n-to-n^2 mapping into n^2 n-to-1 functions simplifies the learning problem, since the role of each subnetwork is clearly defined. The learning rate of this architecture has been shown to be superior to a single "naive" network with both $\dot{\mathbf{x}}$ and θ as inputs [117].

3.2.2. Motion control

The final stage of control is to compute the necessary joint torques to drive the arm, leg or mechanical manipulator through a desired trajectory. The dynamic motion will generally be subject to constraints or performance criteria such as maximum overshoot, minimum energy or minimum time. Two competing models which propose constraints on the physiological upper limb are minimum torque change [118] and minimum jerk [119].

The computation of the necessary torques requires consideration of dynamical properties such as inertia and damping of the members. There are added complications: arm segments are coupled, which means that the inertia matrix is not diagonal and the dynamical equations are highly nonlinear. Gravitational and, to a lesser extent, Coriolis forces influence the dynamics as well. A simplified form of the dynamics equations can be expressed as [120]:

$$\tau = \mathbf{M}(\theta)\ddot{\theta} + \tau_v(\theta,\dot{\theta}) + \tau_g(\theta) + \tau_f(\theta,\dot{\theta})$$

where τ is the torque vector, $\mathbf{M}(\theta)$ is the mass matrix, $\tau_v(\theta,\dot{\theta})$ is a vector of centrifugal and Coriolis forces, $\tau_g(\theta)$ is a vector of gravity terms, and $\tau_f(\theta,\dot{\theta})$ is a vector of friction terms. To obtain the inverse dynamic solution, recall first the forward kinematic relationship:

$$\mathbf{x} = \mathbf{f}(\theta).$$

Differentiating twice yields:

$$\ddot{\mathbf{x}} = \mathbf{J}(\theta)\ddot{\theta} + \mathbf{H}(\theta)\dot{\theta}$$

where the matrix of the second derivative, $\mathbf{H}(\theta)$, is known as the Hessian. Solving this equation for $\ddot{\theta}$, and substituting into the torque equation above, yields:

$$\tau = \mathbf{M}(\theta)\mathbf{J}^{-1}(\theta)\ddot{\mathbf{x}} - \mathbf{M}(\theta)\mathbf{J}^{-1}(\theta)\mathbf{H}(\theta)\dot{\theta} + \tau_v(\theta,\dot{\theta}) + \tau_g(\theta) + \tau_f(\theta,\dot{\theta})$$

which, for small values of angular velocity $\dot{\theta}$ and neglecting the effects of gravity, can be approximated as:

$$\tau' = \mathbf{M}(\theta)\mathbf{J}^{-1}(\theta)\ddot{\mathbf{x}}$$

which looks suspiciously similar to the inverse kinematic relation:

$$\dot{\theta} = \mathbf{J}^{-1}(\theta)\dot{\mathbf{x}}.$$

Indeed, there is a linear relation between the torques τ' and the Cartesian acceleration $\ddot{\mathbf{x}}$ for a given angle θ. Hence, it follows that a context-sensitive neural network controller applies to this simplified version of the inverse dynamics problem.

Considerably less work has been done on the application of neural networks to dynamic control than to kinematic control. Although similar in form, as shown above, the dynamics problem is much more nonlinear and more susceptible to coupling between variables and variation in manipulator parameters [121]. Hence, techniques based on learning without accurate knowledge of the system are appealing.

Virtually all proposed neural network dynamic control schemes rely on feedback from the controlled system. This immediately prompts the question of control architecture, since most popular learning algorithms (such as backpropagation) are useful only with feedforward networks. Perhaps the most complete solution to this problem has been proposed by Kawato *et al.* [122], [123]. Their work is based on studies of movement control in the neuromuscular system. Basically, they assume that within the central nervous system an internal model of the inverse dynamics of the musculoskeletal system is acquired while monitoring a desired trajectory and the associated motor commands.

The general form of their feedback-error learning scheme is shown in Figure 12. Here, a conventional feedback controller (CFC) guarantees stability of the system while serving as an inverse reference model of the response of the controlled object. This CFC processes the differential trajectory to yield the control torque, τ_c. The CFC chosen was a linear controller equivalent to Hogan's impedance controller [87]. An adaptive nonlinear neural network feedback controller (NNFC) is used to model the inverse dynamics of the controlled object. The sum of the output of the CFC τ_c and the external input τ_{ext} for a controlled object is fed to the NNFC as the error signal τ_i. As the neural network acquires the inverse dynamics model of the controlled object, the output responses of the controlled object are governed by the inverse reference model implemented as the CFC. In the absence of external inputs after learning, the actual responses coincide with the reference responses.

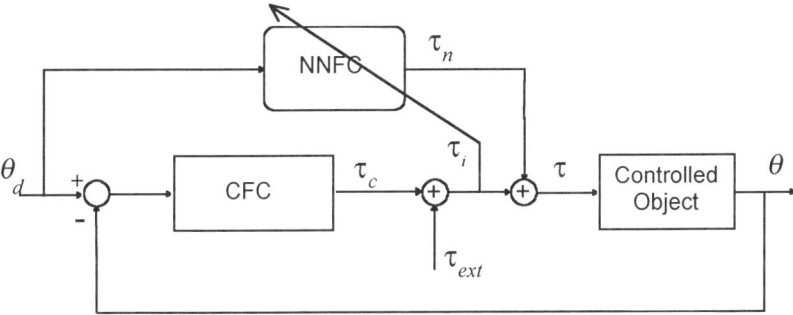

Figure 12. The Feedback Error Learning Model of Kawato *et al.*

The physiological analog to learning control for voluntary movement is demonstrated in Figure 13. Represented here is the control and learning of a novel, consciously-controlled motion emanating from the pre-motor cortex.

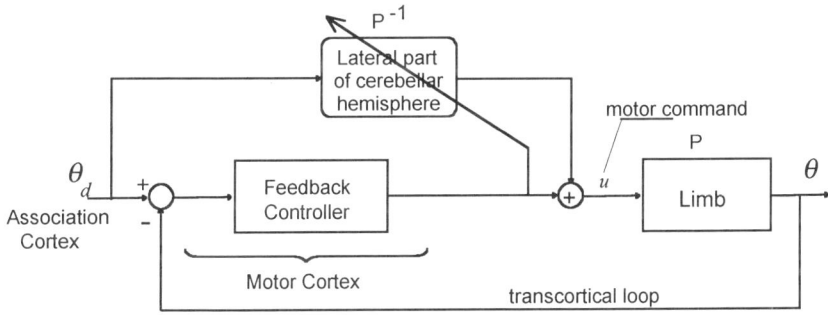

Figure 13. Learning control for voluntary movement.

The endpoint trace is formed in the pre-motor association cortex, defining a desired trajectory. Motion intent is actuated by the motor cortex in the context of motor activity (u) actuating limb motion (θ). The motor cortex contains a fixed, general inverse model of the limb dynamics, and thus initial movements executed by the motor cortex will have relatively high error. Any discrepancy between desired and actual limb position is accommodated via the proprioceptive feedback provided by muscle spindles and the Golgi tendon organs. The cerebellum monitors the motor activity (via the inferior olivary nucleus) associated with this novel pattern of limb motion, and begins to contribute corrective influence as it learns, refining the movement and reducing the feedback error. As the cerebellum continues to learn, it assumes a greater share of the forward processing of the movement. If the motion pattern has been fully learned by the cerebellum (an inverse filter of the limb dynamics has been fully trained), the feedback error approaches zero, no cortical motor activity occurs, and the motion is then a subconscious, learned movement.

The performance of Kawato's system is impressive. With adequate training, the final system was able to generalize movements quite unlike those used for training.

3.3. Discussion

This chapter has provided an historical account of the progress made in multifunction control since the 1940s. Clearly, a great deal of research effort has been devoted to providing a solution, with the motivation of improving the quality of life of those with upper-limb deficiencies. It is obvious however, that an acceptable solution has yet to be found.

Why haven't we solved the problem yet?
The rationale for using the surface myoelectric signal for control purposes is that it provides an autonomous means of eliciting control from the remaining musculature, it is relatively easy to acquire, and its acquisition is noninvasive. For this reason, a substantial amount of research has focused upon maximizing the information content that may be extracted from the surface MES.

It is an unavoidable reality however, that the surface MES conveys the control information elicited by the neuromuscular system as a second-order effect. It is a by-product of the complex temporal and spatial pattern of motor unit innervation that constitutes a specific voluntary contraction. What we measure as the surface MES is the superposition of this exquisitely complex activity, and inevitably, spatial and temporal information is lost.

As a consequence, the amount of information that may be conveyed by the surface MES is a subset of that delivered to the muscles by the motor neurons. We have done our best to maximize the capacity of this information, but it is nonetheless limited. The ability to control an upper limb with the dexterity of a normally-limbed individual however, requires all of the information delivered by the nervous system. Therefore, the prospect of simultaneous, coordinated control is beyond the capability of the surface MES alone.

This is not to say that an acceptable compromise cannot be found. Although the dimensionality of the control problem is beyond that of the information that may be derived from the surface MES, the controllability may be augmented by the presence of an intelligent control subsystem. The purpose of this subsystem should be to assume the responsibility of certain aspects of control, such as defining pre-programmed linkages, planning trajectories,

providing inverse-kinematic solutions, and resolving anthropometric dynamic behavior. This is the domain of robotics research, which has refined these techniques to the point of a matured discipline. There are a couple of issues, however, that must be considered when considering the prospect of a subsystem of intelligent control:
1. There is a tradeoff between the degree to which the subsystem assumes control, and the degree to which the system is under the intentional control of the user. An extreme example of a subsystem taking control is the Case Western Reserve Feeder Arm [56]. Some compromise as to the degree of intervening control must be determined.
2. The prosthetic control problem bears similarity to the robotic control problem, but there are many differences. A prosthesis is worn by an individual, and consequently there are issues such as fitting, spatial translation of the mounting point, and limitations on the prosthesis dynamics. These factors may limit the applicability of robotics techniques to the prosthetics problem, which possesses some unique constraints.

A possible avenue that appears to be very promising is the prospect of providing a direct interface to the motor neurons that innervate the upper limb. There was a period of very encouraging research and development at Stanford University directed toward providing a sustainable direct neural contact by means of regenerating nerve fibers through a conducting sieve constructed of biocompatible materials [124]. This project has been suspended due to lack of funding.

A general commentary may be appropriate at this point. Although significant progress has been made over the decades toward providing a solution to the multifunction control problem, efforts have been hampered due to the lack of economic justification; the percentage of those afflicted by limb deficiencies is relatively small, and of those, only about 15% have above-elbow deficiencies. The efforts of most teams mentioned in this chapter ended because of insufficient financial support. This, coupled with a resistance to an invasive approach (as is required of a direct neural interface, or a skeletal attachment of the prosthesis), has precluded the formation of a large, sustained effort by a team of engineering, surgical, and clinical specialists.

The future may hold promise however, for such a team has been brought together for a current effort funded by the European Commission. Entitled "A Total Modular Prosthetic Arm with High Workability" (TOMPAW), it is a collaborative effort between research labs, clinical centers, and industry in England, Scotland, and Sweden. This multi-degree-of-freedom arm will combine various aspects of the modular arm developed by the Edinburgh group [125] with the hierarchically controlled Southampton hand [126]. Osseo-integrated (direct skeletal) attachment of the arm will also be considered using techniques developed by Brånemark in Sweden [127]. Although this effort will lead to a more functional prosthetic limb, its success will again depend upon the control system.

References

[1] Reiter, R.: "Eine neu elecktrokunstand," *Grenzgebiete der Medicin*, 1, 4, pp. 133-135, 1948.

[2] Berger, N. and C.R. Huppert: "The use of electrical and mechanical forces for control of an electric prosthesis," *American Journal of Occupational Therapy*, 6, 110, 1952.

[3] Battye, C.K., Nightengale, A. and J. Whillis: "The use of myoelectric current in the operation of prostheses," *J. Bone Joint Surgery*, 37-B, 506, 1955.

[4] Kobrinski, A. E. *et al.*: "Problems of bioelectric control," in Automatic and Remote Control, *Proc. 1st IFAC Int. Cong.*, Vol. 2, Coles, J.F. (Ed.), Butterworths, p. 619, 1960.

[5] Bottomley, A.H.: "Working model of a myoelectric control system," *Proceedings of the International Symposium of Applications in Automatic Control in Prosthetics Design*, Belgrade, 1962, 37, 1962.

[6] Herberts, P.: "Myoelectric signals in control of prostheses," *Acta Orthop. Scandinavica,* Suppl. 124, 1969.

[7] Kato, I., Okazaki, E. and H. Nakamura: "The electrically controlled hand prosthesis using command disc or EMG," *J. Soc. Inst. and Control Eng.*, 6, 236, 1967.

[8] Weltman, G., Groth, H. and J. Lyman: "An analysis of bioelectric prosthesis control," *Biotechnology Laboratory Rep. No. 1*, University of California, Los Angeles, 1959.

[9] Dorcas, D.S. and R.N. Scott: "A three-state myoelectric control," *Med. Biol. Eng.*, 4, 367, 1966.

[10] Bottomley, A.H.: "Design considerations for a prosthetic prehension device," Proceedings of the International Symposium on External Control of Human Extremities, Dubrovnik, Yugoslavia, pp. 82-84, 1966.

[11] Childress, D.S.: "Closed-loop control in prosthetic systems: Historical perspective," *Annals of Biomed. Eng.*, 9, 293-303, 1980.

[12] Childress, D.S. and J.N. Billock: "Self-containment and self-suspension of externally powered prostheses for the forearm," *Bull. Prosth. Res.*, BPR 10-14, 4-21, 1970.

[13] Schmidl, H.: "The I.N.A.I.L. experience fitting upper-limb dysmelia patients with myoelectric control," *Bull. Prosth. Res.*, BPR 10-27, 17-42, Spring, 1977.

[14] Wirta, R.W., Taylor, D.R. and F.R. Finley: "Pattern recognition arm prosthesis: A historical perspective - Final Report," *Bull. Prosth. Res.*, BPR 10-30, 8-35, Fall, 1978.

[15] Scott, R.N., Brittain, R.H., Caldwell, R.R., Cameron, A.B. and V.A. Dunfield: "Sensory feedback system compatible with myoelectric control," *Med. and Biol. Eng. & Comp.*, Vol. 18, No. 1, pp. 65-69, 1980.

[16] Kato, I. et al.: "Multifunctional myoelectric hand prosthesis with pressure sensory feedback system - WASEDA Hand - 4P," *Proceedings of the 3rd International Symposium on External Control of Human Extremities*, Dubrovnik, Yugoslavia, pp. 155-170, 1969.

[17] Mann, R.W.: "Cybernetic limb prosthesis: The ALZA distinguished lecture," *Annals of Biomed. Eng.*, Vol. 9, pp. 1-43, 1981.

[18] Williams, T.W.: "Clinical applications of the improved Boston Arm," *Proc. Conf. on Energy Devices in Rehab.*, Boston (Tufts), 1976.

[19] Jacobsen, S., Knutti, D., Johnson, R. and H. Sears: "Development of the Utah arm," *IEEE Transactions on Biomedical Engineering*, BME-29, No. 4, pp. 249-269, 1982.

[20] Feeny, R.J. and I. Hagaeus: "Evaluation of the EMG-controlled hand prosthesis," *Proc. 3rd Int. Symp. on External Control of Human Extremities, ETAN*, Dubrovnik, Yugoslavia, 1970.

[21] Soerjanto, R.: "*On the application of the myoelectric hand-prosthesis in the Netherlands*". Thesis. Report 1.1, 59-3, Institute of Medical Physics, TNO, Utrect, 1971.

[22] Schmidl, H.: "Funktionelle möglichkeiten bei einseitig und beidseitig amputierten, mit mioelektrischen prosthesen ausgestattet. Sensible informationsrückmeldung bei blinden doppelamputierten," *Proc. 1st Int. Congr. on Prosthetics Techniques and Functional and Functional Rehabilitation*, 2, Wien, 1973.

[23] Kondraschin, N.I., Yakoson, Ya.S. and L.M. Voskobojnikova: "Stand und perspektiven der entwicklung des bioelektrischen steuerungssystems bei der prothesenversorgung der oberen extremitäten in der UdSSR," *Orthopädie-Technik*, 26, 4, 1975.

[24] Northmore-Ball, M.D., Heger, H. and G.A. Hunter: "The below-elbow prosthesis," *J. Bone Joint Surgery*, 62B, 363, 1980.

[25] Atkins, D., Donovan, W.H. and A. Muilenberg: "Retrospective analysis of 87 children and adults fitted with electric prosthetic componentry," *Proc. Assoc. Children's Prosthetic-Orthotic Clinics Conf.*, St. Petersburg, Fla., p. 4, 1993.

[26] Bernstein, N.: *The Co-ordination and Regulation of Movements*, Pergamon Press, Oxford, 1967.

[27] Mann, R.W.: "Force and position proprioception for prostheses." In: *The Control of Upper Extremity Prostheses and Orthoses*, Edited by P. Herberts, P. Kadefors, R. Magnusson and I. Petersen, Thomas, Springfield, Ill., pp. 201-209, 1974.

[28] Solomonow, M., Lyman, J. and A. Freedy: "Electrotactile two-point discrimination as a function of frequency, body site, laterality and stimulation codes," *Annals of Biomed. Eng.*, 5, 47-60, 1977.

[29] Taub, E., Perella, P. and G. Barro: "Behavioral development after forelimb deafferentiation on day of birth in monkeys with and without blinding," *Science*, 181, 959-960, 1973.

[30] Pollit, A. and E. Bizzi: "Characteristics of motor programs underlying arm movements in monkeys," *J. Neurophysiol.*, 39, 435-444, 1976.

[31] Greene, P.H.: "Problems of organization of motor systems," In: Rosen, R. and F. Snell (Eds.). *Progress in Theoretical Biology*, Vol. 2, Academic Press, New York pp. 303-338, 1972.

[32] Childress, D.S.: "A myoelectric three-state controller using rate sensitivity," in *Proc. 8th ICMBE*, Chicago, IL, S4-5, 1969.

[33] Schmidl, H.: "Funktionelle möglichkeiten bei einseitig und beidseitig amputierten, mit mioelektrischen prosthesen ausgestattet. Sensible informationsrückmeldung bei blinden doppelamputierten," *Proc. 1st Int. Congr. on Prosthetics Techniques and Functional and Functional Rehabilitation*, 2, Wien, 1973.

[34] Herberts, P., Almstrom, C., Kadefors, R. and P. Lawrence: "Prosthesis control via myoelectric patterns," *Acta Orthop. Scandinavica*, 44, pp. 389-409, 1973.

[35] Wirta, R.W., Taylor, D.R. and F.R. Finley: "Engineering principles in the control of external power by myoelectric signals," *Archives of Physical Medicine and Rehabilitation*, May, pp. 294-296, 1969.

[36] Jacobsen, S.C. and R.W. Mann: "Control systems for artificial arms," *IEEE Conference on Systems, Man and Cybernetics*, 5-7, November, Boston, 1973.

[37] Freedy, A., Lyman, J. and M. Solomonow: "A microcomputer aided prosthesis control," *Proc. Second International Conference on the Theory and Practice of Robots and Manipulators*, Warsaw, Poland, September, pp. 110-122, 1976.

[38] Cordo, P.J.: "Controlling multiple degree of freedom powered prostheses," in *Proc. of the IEEE Frontiers of Engineering and Computing in Health Care*, Columbus, OH, pp. 1.5.1-1.5.5, 1983.

[39] Finley, R.R. and R.W. Wirta: "Myocoder studies of multiple myocoder response," *Archives of Physical Medicine and Rehabilitation*, 48, 598, 1967.

[40] Wirta, R.W. and D.R. Taylor: "Development of a multi-axis myoelectrically controlled prosthetic arm," *Proc. of the Third International Symposium on External Control of Human Extremities*, Dubrovnik, Yugoslavia, 1969.

[41] Lawrence, P., Herberts, P. and R. Kadefors: "Experiences with a multifunctional hand prosthesis controlled by myoelectric patterns," in *Advances in External Control of Human Extremities*, Gavrilovic and Wilson, Eds., Etan, Belgrade, pp. 47-65, 1973.

[42] Almstrom, C., Herberts, P. and L. Korner: "Experience with Swedish multifunction prosthetic hands controlled by pattern recognition of multiple myoelectric signals," *Int. Orthopaed.*, vol. 5 pp. 15-21, 1981.

[43] Lyman, J.H., Freedy, A. and R. Prior: "Fundamental and applied research related to the design and development of upper-limb externally powered prostheses," *Bull. of Prosth. Res.*, Spring, pp. 184-195, 1976.

[44] Sullivan, G.H., Mitchell, M.B., Lyman, J. and F.C. DeDiasto: "*Myoelectric servo control*," Technical Documentary Report No. ASD-TDR-63-70, Bionics Branch, Electronics Technology Division, Air Force Systems Command, Aeronautical Systems Division, Wright-Patterson Air Force Base, Ohio, 1963.

[45] Freedy, A. and J. Lyman: "*An information theory approach to control of externally powered artificial arms*," University of California, Los Angeles, School of Engineering and Applied Science; Biotechnology Laboratory Technical Report, 1967.

[46] Tomovic, R.: "Control theory and signal processing in prosthetic systems," *Proc. of the First International Symposium on External Control of Human Extremities*, Washington, D.C., pp. 221-226, 1966.

[47] Tomovic, R.: "Multilevel control of mechanical multivariable systems as applied to prosthetic," *IEEE Transactions on Automatic Control*, February, pp. 72-74, 1968.

[48] Vukobratovic, M. and D. Juricic: "Note on a way of moving the artificial upper extremity," *IEEE Transactions on Biomedical Engineering*, Vol. BME-16, No. 2, April, pp. 113-115, 1969.

[49] Gavrilovic, M.M. and M.R. Maric: "An approach to the organization of artificial arm control," *Proc. of the Third International Symposium on External Control of Human Extremities*, Dubrovnik, Yugoslavia, pp. 307-322, 1969.

[50] Freedy, A. and J. Lyman: "Adaptive aiding for powered prosthetic control," *Proc. of the 3rd International Symposium on External Control of Human Extremities*, pp. 155-170, Dubrovnik, 1969.

[51] Freedy, A., Hull, F.C., Lucaccini, L.F. and J. Lyman: "A computer-based learning system for remote manipulator control," *IEEE Transactions on Systems, Man and Cybernetics*, SMC-1, No. 4, October, pp. 356-363, 1971.

[52] Freedy, A., Hull, F. and J. Lyman: "A learning system for trajectory control in artificial arms," *Proc. of the Fourth International Symposium on External Control of Human Extremities*, Dubrovnik, Yugoslavia, pp. 303-317, 1972.

[53] Freedy, A., Hull, F. and J. Lyman: "Adaptive aiding for artificial limb control," *Bull. of Prosth. Res.*, Fall, pp. 3-15, 1971.

[54] Zadaca, H., Lyman, J. and A. Freedy: "*Studies and development of Heuristic endpoint control for artificial upper limbs*," University of California, Los Angeles, School of Engineering and Applied Science Report UCLA-ENG-74-79; Biotechnology Laboratory Technical Report No. 54, 1974.

[55] Lawrence, P.D. and W.C. Lin: "Statistical decision making in the real-time control of an arm aid for the disabled," *IEEE Transactions on Man, Systems and Cybernetics*, Vol. SMC-2 No. 1, pp. 35-42, 1972.

[56] Reswick, J.B., Merler, H.W., Do, W.H., Taft, C.K., Brunell, J.H., Corell, R.W., Thomas, D.H., Griggs, K.M. and D.J.Gawlowicz: "*Conscious control of programmed motions in orthotics and prosthetics*," Report EDC4-62-2, Case Institute of Technology, Cleveland, OH, 1962.

[57] Apple, H.P. and J.B. Reswick: "A multi-level approach to orthotic/prosthetic control system design," *Proc. of the Third International Symposium on External Control of Human Extremities*, Dubrovnik, Yugoslavia, pp. 323-338, 1969.

[58] Maric, M.R. and M.M. Gavrilovic: "An evaluation of synergistic control for the rehabilitation manipulator," *Proc. of the 4th International Symposium on External Control of Human Extremities*, Dubrovnik, Yugoslavia, pp. 277-287, 1972.

[59] Carlson, L.E. and C.W. Radcliffe: "A multi-mode approach to coordinated prosthesis control," *Proc. of the 4th International Symposium on External Control of Human Extremities*, Dubrovnik, Yugoslavia, pp. 185-196, 1972.

[60] Moe, M.L. and J.T. Scwartz: "A coordinated, proportional motion controller for an upper-extremity orthotic device," *Proc. of the 3rd International Symposium on External Control of Human Extremities*, Dubrovnik, Yugoslavia, pp. 295-305, 1969.

[61] Moe, M.L. and J.T. Scwartz: "Occular control of the Rancho Electric Arm," *Proc. of the 4th International Symposium on External Control of Human Extremities*, Dubrovnik, Yugoslavia, pp. 288-302, 1972.

[62] Whitney, D.E.: "The mathematics of coordinated control of prostheses and manipulators," *Proc. of the 3rd Annual Conference on Manual Control*, University of Michigan, May, pp. 207-220, 1972.

[63] Ailon, A.: "End-point control via binary coded EMG signal," *Proc. of the 5th Annual IEEE EMBS Conference*, Sept. Columbus, OH, pp. 1-4, 1983.

[64] Simpson, D.C. and G. Kenworthy: "The design of a complete arm prosthesis," *Biomedical Engineering*, pp. 56-59, February 1973.

[65] Doubler, J.A. and D.S. Childress: "An analysis of extended physiological proprioception as a prosthesis-control technique," *Journal of Rehabilitation Research and Development*, Vol. 21, No. 1, BPR 10-39, pp. 5-18, 1984.

[66] Doubler, J.A. and D.S. Childress: "Design and evaluation of a prosthesis control system based on the concept of extended physiological proprioception," *Journal of Rehabilitation Research and Development*, Vol. 21, No. 1, BPR 10-39, pp. 19-31, 1984.

[67] Gow, D.: "Physiologically appropriate control of a multi-degree of freedom upper limb prosthesis - or Where prosthetics meets robotics," *Proc. JCF IARP Workshop*, Ottawa, pp. 18.1-18.3, 1988.

[68] Gibbons, D.T., O'Riain, M.D. and S. Philippe-Auguste: "An above-elbow prosthesis employing programmed linkages," *IEEE Transactions on Biomedical Engineering*, Vol. BME-34, No. 7, July, pp. 493-498, 1987.

[69] Gibbons, D.T., Phillippe-August, J.S. and M.D. O'Riain: "An above-elbow prosthesis employing extended physiological proprioception and programmed linkages," *Proc. JCF IARP Workshop*, Ottawa, pp. 16.1-16.5, 1988.

[70] Gibbons, D.T., Philippe-Auguste, S. and M.D. O'Riain: "Performance evaluation of an artificial arm based on a virtual reality simulation," *Proc. of the 19th Conference of the Canadian Medical and Biological Engineering Society*, Ottawa, pp. 132-133, 1993.

[71] Jacobsen, S.C.: *"Control Systems for Artificial Arms,"* Doctoral Dissertation, M.I.T, 1973.
[72] Jerard, R.B. and S.C. Jacobsen: "Laboratory evaluation of a unified theory for simultaneous multiple axis artificial arm control," *J. Biomechanical Engineering*, Vol. 102, pp. 199-207, 1980.
[73] Wood, J.E., Meek, S.G. and S.C. Jacobsen: "Quantitation of human shoulder anatomy for prosthetic arm control - I. Surface modelling," *J. Biomechanics*, Vol. 22, No. 1, pp. 273-292, 1989.
[74] Saridis, G.N. and H.E. Stephanou: "Fuzzy decision-making in prosthetic devices," in M.M. Gupta and G.N. Saridis (Eds.), *Fuzzy Decision Making in Prosthetic Devices*, Elsevier, New York, pp. 387-402, 1977.
[75] Saridis, G.N.: *Self-Organizing Control of Stochastic Systems*, Marcel Dekker, New York, 1977.
[76] Saridis, G.N. and T. Gootee: "EMG pattern analysis and classification for a prosthetic arm," *IEEE Transactions on Biomedical Engineering*, BME-20, June, pp. 403-409, 1982.
[77] Lee, S.: *"Intelligent Control of a Prosthetic Arm by EMG Pattern Recognition,"* Ph.D. Thesis, Dept. of Electrical Engineering, Purdue University, West Lafayette, IN, 1982.
[78] Lee, S. and G.N. Saridis: "The control of a prosthetic arm by EMG pattern recognition," *IEEE Transactions on Automatic Control*, AC-29, No. 4, April, pp. 290-302, 1984.
[79] Saridis, G.N.: "EMG trained, prosthetic control," *Joint Coordinating Forum for the International Advanced Robotics Programme*, Ottawa, Canada, pp. 15.1-15.9, 1988.
[80] Graupe, D. and W.K. Cline:, "Functional separation of EMG signal via ARMA identification methods for prosthetic control purposes," *IEEE Transactions Systems, Man and Cybernetics*, SMC-5, No. 2, pp. 252-259, 1975.
[81] Graupe, D., Magnussen, J. and A.A. Beex: "A microprocessor system for multifunctional control of upper-limb prostheses via myoelectric signal identification," *IEEE Transactions on Automatic Control*, Vol. AC-23, No. 4, pp. 538-544, 1978.
[82] Graupe, D., Salahi, J. and K.H. Kohn: "Multifunction prosthesis and orthosis control via microcomputer identification of temporal pattern differences in single-site myoelectric signals," *J. Biomed. Eng.*, Vol. 4, pp. 17-22, 1982.
[83] Graupe, D., Salahi, J. and D. Zhang: "Stochastic analysis of myoelectric signal temporal signatures for multifunctional single-site activation of prostheses and orthoses," *J. Biomed. Eng.*, Vol. 7, January, pp. 18-29, 1985.
[84] Doershuk, P.C., Gustafson, D.E. and A.S. Willsky: "Upper extremity limb function discrimination using EMG signal analysis," *IEEE Transactions on Biomedical Engineering*, Vol. BME-30, No. 1, pp. 18-28, 1983.
[85] Morasso, P.: "Spatial control of arm movements," *Experimental Brain Research*, Vol. 42, pp. 223-22, 1981.

[86] Georgopoulos, A.P., Caminiti, R., Kalaska, J.F. and J.T. Massey: "Spatial coding of movement: A hypothesis concerning the coding of movement direction by motor cortical populations," *Experimental Brain Research* (Supp.), Vol. 7, pp. 327-336, 1993.

[87] Hogan, N.: "Impedance control: An approach to manipulation," *Journal of Dynamic Systems, Measurement and Control*, Vol. 107, pp. 1-24, 1985.

[88] Abul-Haj, C.J. and N. Hogan: "An emulator system for developing improved elbow-prosthesis designs," *IEEE Transactions on Biomedical Engineering*, Vol. 34, No. 9, September, pp. 724-736, 1987.

[89] Hogan, N.: "Quantification of the functional capability of upper extremity amputees," *Rehabilitation Research and Development Progress Reports*, pp. 16-17, 1989.

[90] Abul-Haj, C.J. and N. Hogan: "Functional assessment of control systems for cybernetic elbow prostheses - Part I: Description of the technique," *IEEE Transactions on Biomedical Engineering*, Vol. 37, No. 11, November, pp. 1025-1036, 1990.

[91] Abul-Haj, C.J. and N. Hogan: "Functional assessment of control systems for cybernetic elbow prostheses - Part II: Application of the technique," *IEEE Transactions on Biomedical Engineering*, Vol. 37, No. 11, November, pp. 1037-1047, 1990.

[92] Mansfield, J.M. and N. Hogan: "Paradoxes in control: Prostheses versus myoelectric signals," *Proc. Myoelectric Controls Conference (MEC'93)*, August, Fredericton, pp. 105-110, 1993.

[93] Russell, D.L.: "Energy expenditure in upper limb prostheses performing constrained movements," *Proc. Myoelectric Controls Conference (MEC'93)*, August, Fredericton, pp 98-104, 1993.

[94] DeLuca, C.J.: "Control of upper-limb prostheses: a case for neuroelectric control," *J. Med. Eng. Technol.*, vol. 2, No. 2, 1978.

[95] Hudgins, B.S.: "*A Novel Approach to Multifunction Myoelectric Control of Prostheses*," Ph.D. Thesis, Dept. Electrical Engineering, University of New Brunswick, Fredericton, New Brunswick, Canada, 1991.

[96] Hudgins, B.S., Parker, P.A. and R.N. Scott: "A new strategy for multifunction myoelectric control," *IEEE Transactions on Biomedical Engineering*, Vol. 40, No. 1, pp. 82-94, 1993.

[97] Weirzbicka, M., Wolf, W., Staude, G., Konstanzer, A. and R. Dengler: "Inhibition of EMG activity in isomerically loaded agonist muscle preceding a rapid contraction," *Electromyography and Clinical Neurophysiology*, 33, pp. 271-278, 1993.

[98] Basmajian, J. and C.J. DeLuca: *Muscles Alive*, Baltimore: Williams and Wilkins, 5th Ed, 1985.

[99] Schwartz, A., Kettner, R.E. and A.P. Georopoulos: "Primate motor cortex and free arm movements to visual targets in three-dimensional space. I. Relations between single cell discharge and direction of movement," *The Journal of Neuroscience*, Vol. 8, No. 8, pp. 2913-2927, 1988.

[100] Yamazaki, Y., Suzuki, M., and T. Mano: "An electromyographic volley at initiation of rapid contractions of the elbow," *Brain Research Bulletin*, Vol. 30, pp. 181-187, 1993.

[101] Kuruganti, U., Hudgins, B. and R.N. Scott: "Two-channel enhancement of a multifunction control scheme," *IEEE Transactions on Biomedical Engineering*, Vol. 42, No. 1, 1995.

[102] Englehart, K., Hudgins, B., Parker, P.A., and M. Stevenson: "Classification of the myoelectric signal using time-frequency based representations," *Medical Engineering and Physics,* (Special issue: Intelligent Data Analysis in Electromyography and Electroneurography, Fall 1999).

[103] Leowinata, S., Hudgins, B., and P.A. Parker: "A multifunction myoelctric control strategy using an array of electrodes," *Proc. 16th Annual Congress of the International Society Electrophysiology and Kinesiology*, Montreal, P.Q., Canada, 1998.

[104] Hannaford, B. and S. Lehman: "Short-Time Fourier analysis of the electromyogram: Fast movements and constant contraction," *IEEE Transactions on Biomedical Engineering*, Vol. BME-33, No. 12, pp. 1173-1181, 1986.

[105] Gallant, P.J.: "*An Approach to Myoelectric Control Using a Self-Organizing Neural Network for Feature Extraction*," Master's Thesis, Queens University, Kingston, Ontario, 1993.

[106] Farry, K., Walker, I.D. and R.G. Baraniuk: "Myoelectric teleoperation of a complex robotic hand," *IEEE Transactions on Robotics and Automation*, 12 (5), pp. 775-788, 1996.

[107] Kramer, M.A.: "Nonlinear principal component analysis using autoassociative neural networks," *AIChe Journal*, 37 (2), pp. 233-243, 1991.

[108] Farry, K., Fernandez, J., Abramczyk, R., Novy, M. and D. Atkins: "Applying genetic programming to control of an artificial arm," *Proc. Myoelectric Controls Conference*, Fredericton, N.B., Canada, pp. 50-55, 1997.

[109] Atsma, W.J., Hudgins, B. and D.F. Lovely: "Classification of raw myoelectric signals using finite impulse response neural networks," *Proc. 18th Annual International Conference of the IEEE EMBS*, Amsterdam, The Netherlands, paper 916, 1996.

[110] Ward, M.: "*Detection and classification of transient underwater sounds by a finite impulse response neural network*", M.Sc. Thesis, University of New Brunswick, Fredericton, N.B., Canada, 1998.

[111] Bizzi, E., Hogan, N., Mussa-Ivaldi, F.A. and S. Giszter: "Does the nervous system use equilibrium-point control to guide single and multiple joint movements?," *Behavioral and Brain Sciences*, Vol. 15, pp. 603-613, 1992.

[112] Srinivasan, S.: "*A Rhythmic Movement Control Scheme Using Artificial Neural Networks*," Ph.D. Dissertation, University of Saskatchewan, Sasketoon, Saskatchewan, 1992.

[113] McKerrow, P.J.: *Introduction to Robotics*, Addison-Wesley, Sydney, 1991.

[114] Albus, J.: "A new approach to manipulator control: The cerebellar model articulation controller," *J. Dynamic Systems, Measurement and Control*, Vol. 97, pp. 270-277, 1975.
[115] Josin, G., Charney, D. and D. White: "Robot control using neural networks," *Proc. Intern. Conf. on Neural Networks*, pp. 625-631, 1988.
[116] Elsley, R.K.: "A learning architecture for control based on back-propagation neural networks," *Proc. IEEE Conf. on Neural Networks*, pp. 587-594, 1988.
[117] Yeung, D.-T. and G.A. Bekey: "Using a context-sensitive learning network for robot arm control," *Proc. IEEE Intern. Conf. on Robotics and Automation*, pp. 1441-1447, 1989,
[118] Wada, Y. and M. Kawato: "A neural network model for arm trajectory formation using forward and inverse dynamics models," *Neural Networks*, Vol. 6, pp. 919-932, 1993.
[119] Flash, T. and N. Hogan: "The coordination of arm movements: An experimentally confirmed mathematical model," *The Journal of Neuroscience*, Vol. 5, No. 7, pp. 1688-1703, 1985.
[120] Craig, J.J.: *Introduction to Robotics*, Addison-Wesley, Reading, MA, 1986.
[121] Psaltis, D., Sideris, A. and A. Yamamura: "Neural controllers," *Proc. IEEE Conf. on Neural Networks*, pp. 551-558, 1987.
[122] Miyamoto, H., Kawato, M., Setoyana, T. and R. Suzuki: "Feedback-error-learning neural network for trajectory control of a robotic manipulator," *Neural Networks*, Vol. 1, pp. 251-265, 1988.
[123] Gomi, H. and M. Kawato: "Neural network for a closed-loop system using feedback-error learning," *Neural Networks*, Vol. 6, pp. 993-946, 1993.
[124] Wan, E.A., Kovacs, G.T., Rosen, J. and B. Widrow: "Development of neural network interfaces for direct control of neuroprostheses," in *Proc. International Neural Networks Conference*, pp. II.3-II.21, Washington, D.C., 1990.
[125] Gow, D.: "Development of the Edinburgh Modular Arm System," *Proc. MEC'99 Conf.*, University of New Brunswick, Canada, pp. 64-66, 1999.
[126] Kyberd, P., Evans, M. and te Winkel, S: "An intelligent anthropomorphic hand, with automatic grasp", *Robotica*, Vol. 16, pp. 531-536, 1998.
[127] Brånemark, R.: "Osseointegration in prosthetic orthopaedics," *Proc. 8th World Congress of ISPO*, pp. 163, 1995.

Chapter 6

Selective activation of the nervous system for motor system neural prostheses

Warren M. Grill

Electrical activation of the nervous system is a technique to restore function to individuals with neurological disorders. In this chapter, approaches to selective stimulation of the nervous system are reviewed. Neural prostheses need an interface that enables selective activation of specific groups of neurons. The requirements and performance of muscle-based electrodes, nerve-based electrodes, and centrally-based electrodes are presented. Centrally-based electrodes provide an opportunity for a new approach to motor system neural prostheses. Rather than activating the last-order neuron, as with muscle- and nerve-based electrodes, central stimulation targets higher-order neurons. This may enable exploitation of the biological neural networks for control and thereby simplify control of complex functions.

1. Introduction

Neural prostheses are an emerging technology that uses electrical stimulation of the nervous system to restore function to individuals with disability due to damage of the nervous system [48]. Clinical applications of neural prostheses are in both sensory and motor systems, with perhaps the cochlear implant being in the most widespread use. In this chapter, the focus is on electrical activation for restoration of motor function. Further, the focus is on fundamental research and development rather than clinical applications, which have been reviewed elsewhere [48], [136].

Electrical activation of intact lower motor neurons is used to restore functional movements to individuals paralyzed by spinal cord injury, stroke, or head injury. Clinical applications to date include restoration of bladder, bowel, and sexual function [25], electrophrenic respiration [21], restoration of hand grasp and release [108], and standing and stepping [70], [74]. These systems have demonstrated the potential of motor prostheses for restoration of useful function in individuals with paralysis.

Motor prosthesis research is aimed at restoring movement to individuals with neurological impairment who maintain healthy lower motor neurons. According to the Office of Technology Assessment [106], this population consists of more than 180,000 spinal cord injured patients and 2,800,000 stroke patients in the United States. The medical expenses and lost income of this population exceeds $2,000,000,000 each year. Thousands of new patients are added to this group each year. Spinal cord injuries occur mostly in younger people with the most common age at injury being 19 years and the mean age at injury being 29 years [156]. In the paraplegic individual, the very basic movements required to walk or simply stand from a chair are restricted or lost. Quadriplegic individuals will have lost, in addition, some or all of the ability to manipulate and control their environment. Motor function can be provided by electrically activating paralyzed muscles, and thereby contribute significantly to rehabilitation of these individuals. In addition to the decreased financial drain on the resources of their families and our society, rehabilitation increases these individuals' independence and their quality of life.

A fundamental requirement of neural prostheses is an interface that enables selective, and often graded, activation of specific groups of neurons (nerve fibers). Fully implantable electrodes, leads, and stimulators are required in these systems to provide adequate function and long-term reliability. These devices must remain stable and functional for periods of decades and must not damage the tissue they are intended to stimulate. In this chapter, the approaches to interfacing with the nervous system will be reviewed. Below, the specifications for safe and efficacious implanted neural prostheses electrodes are presented, the current approaches to meeting these specifications are reviewed, and some directions for future research are considered.

2. Fundamental considerations for neural prosthesis electrodes

Neural prosthesis electrodes require a conductor for current delivery, an insulating carrier for the stimulating element, a conductive lead, and lead insulation. Electrodes must provide selective, graded, and maximal activation of the targeted tissue in a stable and repeatable fashion with minimal activation of neighboring tissue. Implantable electrodes must be both passively and actively biocompatible. Passive biocompatibility refers to the tissue reaction to the composition, shape, and mechanical properties of the electrode materials. Active biocompatibility refers to the performance of the device under stimulation and has several components. First, passage of current through the electrode must not cause electrochemical reactions that lead to formation of toxic chemical species around the electrode [117] or activate the tissue at a level to cause neuronal damage [2]. Second, the level of activation and the position of the electrode must be maintained under dynamic conditions where movement could induce tissue injury and a chronic foreign body response.

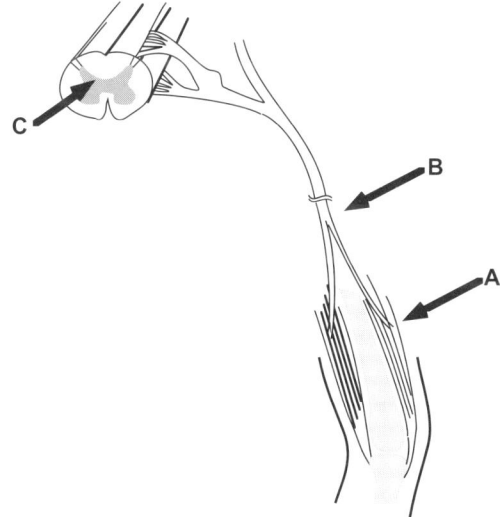

Figure 1. Approaches to electrical activation of the motor system. Lower motor neurons can be activated using either muscle-based (A) or nerve-based electrodes. Activation of higher-order neurons is accomplished by electrodes placed within the spinal cord (C).

3. Approaches to the nervous system

There are several levels at which the motor system can be approached. These are outlined in Figure 1 and include electrodes placed in or on individual muscles; in, on, or around individual nerve branches; electrodes placed in, on, or around multiple component nerve trunks; electrodes placed at the level of the spinal root; and electrodes placed in the spinal cord. In all cases but the latter, the electrodes are all activating muscles by stimulation of motor nerve fibers (i.e., the axons of alpha-motoneurons). Current flow of the appropriate polarity depolarizes the nerve membrane, creating an action potential that travels to the end of the nerve to effect control of the end organ, which in the case of motor prostheses is a muscle. Membrane depolarization, at the terminal end of the motor nerve, leads to release of the neurotransmitter acetylcholine at the neuromuscular junction. Acetylcholine binds to ligand gated sodium channels on the post-synaptic membrane causing an increase in sodium conductance of the muscle membrane. Sodium influx causes initiation of a muscle action potential and subsequent contraction of the muscle. Note that, from the perspective of the end organ, the artificial generation of the action potential is transparent.

3.1. Muscle-based electrodes

Electrodes placed in or on skeletal muscle are used to excite the terminal endings of motor nerve fibers as they enter the muscle. Muscle-based electrodes (MBEs), including intramuscular wires and epimysial disks, have well established records of safety and efficacy. MBEs are physically removed from the nerve fibers and have little possibility of mechanically damaging the tissue they are intended to stimulate. However, MBEs can damage the muscle fibers which surround them due to mechanical stress or electrochemical products formed if the reversible charge injection limits of the chosen metal are exceeded. Furthermore, relative movement between the electrode and the tissue can induce a chronic foreign body reaction or lead to mechanical failure of the electrode.

Excitation of a motor nerve fiber is achieved by creating an electric field that causes currents to flow within the neural tissue. Skeletal muscle fibers can also be excited by an extracellular electric field. Thus, passage of current with electrodes placed in or on a muscle will cause depolarization of both nerve and muscle fibers. In innervated muscle, the terminal motor nerve fibers are excited at lower stimulus intensities than required for direct activation of muscle fibers [23]. Therefore, muscle-based electrodes stimulate nerves which, in turn, leads to subsequent contraction of skeletal muscle.

Coiled wire intramuscular electrodes that can be placed percutaneously or fully implanted [17], [94], [95], [98], [125], and implanted epimysial electrodes [3], [39] are two of the better electrode designs available. Both designs possess the advantage of good selectivity (recruit force in one muscle, but not others), and have little risk of inducing nerve damage since the electrodes are physically removed from the motor axons.

Muscle-based electrodes also have complex recruitment characteristics (i.e., the relationship between the evoked force and the stimulus amplitude or pulsewidth) [24], [111]. These are caused by the non-uniform distribution of terminal motor nerve fibers in the muscle that lie at different distances from the electrode, and create regions of variable recruitment slope or gain. In regions of low gain, large changes in the stimulus amplitude or pulsewidth generate only small changes in force, while in regions of high gain small changes in stimulus amplitude or pulsewidth generate large changes in force. In cases where the user voluntarily grades the stimulus parameters, the changes in gain produce poor control characterized by deadbands, overshoot, and hunting behavior [56].

An additional problem with muscle-based electrodes is electrode displacement, relative to the motor nerves that are to be activated, that occurs during limb motion, giving rise to position-dependent variations in muscle recruitment [24], [39]. This makes recruitment a non-unique function of the stimulus parameters.

Intramuscular electrodes are susceptible to fracture and displacement of their stimulating tip due to the large stresses they experience within a contracting muscle or when crossing tissue planes. In the upper extremity, 20% of percutaneous intramuscular electrodes fail within the first year and there is less than a 50% probability that the seven electrodes required for functional grasp will last just two years [94]. In the upper extremity of an adolescent population, 45% of percutaneous intramuscular electrodes failed within the first year [131]. Most failures were the result of altered response indicative of electrode migration, although the failure mode varied with time post-implant [131]. In the lower extremity, only 25% of all electrodes survive more than two years [85]. More recently, modified electrode designs with more robust lead and barb configurations have improved dramatically the stability and lifetime of intramuscular electrodes. The double helix percutaneous intramuscular electrode has reduced first year failures to less than 30% [125], and all surgically implanted tandem-wound intramuscular electrodes were still functional after 10-33 months implantation in dogs [95].

The primary method of enhancing the function of motor prostheses is to activate additional muscles. In systems employing muscle-based electrodes, the necessity to implant at least one electrode per muscle has required that only a subset of muscles be chosen for stimulation, thereby limiting the function of these prostheses. Unfortunately, each additional channel requires an additional electrode; thus increasing device complexity, making implant surgery more difficult and lengthy, and increasing the probability of device failure. In addition, the anatomical location of the motor point of certain muscles, for example the hamstrings, make repeatable and accurate placement of muscle electrodes difficult [85]. It is increasingly clear that alternative methods of stimulation are required to further advance the function of motor prostheses for paralyzed muscles.

3.2. Nerve-based electrodes

Nerve-based electrodes overcome many of the disadvantages of muscle-based electrodes; however, they also introduce a host of new challenges [101]. The electrodes may be placed in areas of relatively low stress, minimizing the chances of mechanical failure of the electrodes or leads. Nerve-based electrodes are also unlikely to be subject to length-dependent recruitment properties, as the electrodes do not move relative to the motor nerve fibers. Durfee and Palmer [31] implanted cuff electrodes on the tibial and common peroneal nerves of cats and measured recruitment curves at different lengths of the medial *gastrocnemius* and *tibialis anterior* muscles. There were no differences between the recruitment properties at different muscle lengths when the curves were normalized to maximum force at each muscle length, indicating that the recruitment properties were independent of muscle length. In acute experiments we have found that the recruitment properties of multiple-contact nerve cuff electrodes implanted on the sciatic nerve did change, as the ankle joint angle was changed [42]. However, in contrast to the results obtained during acute experiments, chronically implanted cuff electrodes exhibited stable recruitment properties with changes in the ankle position [45]. These results indicate that tissue encapsulation acted to stabilize the cuff electrode and prevent relative movement between the cuff and the nerve trunk during changes in limb position.

Nerve-based electrodes have excitation thresholds that are one order of magnitude lower than those of intramuscular and epimysial electrodes. The use of lower excitation currents permits the use of smaller electrode surfaces to increase selectivity without the risk of corrosion. The lower power requirements of nerve-based electrodes also make them an ideal component of a fully implanted neural prostheses system.

Nerve-based electrodes also offer the opportunity for more controlled activation of nerve fibers and thus more refined control of muscle contraction. Physiological recruitment order (i.e., activation of small diameter nerve fibers before large diameter nerve fibers) can be achieved using cuff electrodes and specialized stimulus waveforms. Large amplitude (several times threshold), long duration (≥ 350 μsec) quasi-trapezoidal stimulus pulses block propagation of action potentials in the largest nerve fibers via anodal hyperpolarization [32], [144]. Thus, action potentials are propagated to the muscle only in the larger diameter nerve fibers, and physiological recruitment order is achieved [32]. Similarly, nerve cuff electrodes employing quasi-trapezoidal stimuli can generate unidirectionally propagating action potentials and thus block neural transmission via collision block [144]. Long duration ($\geq$ 500 μsec) sub-threshold depolarizing pulses applied immediately before the stimulus pulse elevate the threshold of large diameter nerve fibers and also allow selective stimulation of small nerve fibers [43]. Very large amplitude depolarizing stimuli (5-7 times threshold) can create an anodal block of propagation in large nerve fibers at the virtual anodes formed around the central cathode or at the virtual anodes at ends of a monopolar cuff electrode [116], [140], [143]. Finally, small electrodes placed very close to the targeted nerve fibers (i.e., intraneural electrodes placed less than 1 internodal length from the fibers) activate smaller nerve fibers at lower currents than larger nerve fibers (i.e., physiological recruitment order) [119], [147].

In addition to stimulation, nerve-based electrodes can record afferent activity in peripheral nerves that can be used as a prosthesis command signal or for closed-loop control. Lichtenberg and De Luca [79] demonstrated the feasibility of spatially selective neural recordings using a rigid multiple contact cuff-type electrode. The electrode allowed the intraneural location of stimulus evoked antidromic activity to be determined by potential measurements on the surface of the nerve trunk. Intrafascicular electrodes can record signals from single afferent nerve fibers, and thus may provide large numbers of feedback or command control signals [76]. Cuff electrodes have been used to record the activity of cutaneous afferent fibers in a nerve trunk [52], and this information has been used as a feedback signal in closed-loop control of intramuscular stimulation of the cat hindlimb [53].

Nerve-based electrodes also present additional challenges that are not such a concern with muscle-based electrodes. First, since they are in direct contact with neural tissue, nerve-based electrodes are more likely to cause neural damage than muscle-based electrodes [101]. There is typically a large mismatch between the mechanical properties of the electrode and the mechanical properties of the underlying nervous tissue. Second, muscle-based electrodes can be placed in a relatively straightforward implant procedure, either through on open incision or percutaneously. Nerve-based electrodes require open surgical exposure of the targeted nerve trunk, mobilization of the nerve trunk over some distance, and in some cases identification of individual nerve components. Selective activation of individual muscles is also more challenging with nerve-based electrodes.

Muscle-based electrodes are placed directly in or on the muscles targeted for activation. While nerve-based electrodes could potentially be placed directly in or on particular nerve branches innervating individual muscles, such an approach makes for a very difficult implant procedure and requires that a separate electrode be placed to activate each targeted muscle.

3.3. Anatomy of peripheral nerves

The intraneural topography of peripheral nerves provides an opportunity to activate selectively many muscles with a single nerve-based electrode. The anatomical studies of Sunderland [138] showed that, in the more distal sections of a nerve trunk, motor axons are arranged into discrete fascicles that eventually branch from the main trunk to innervate single muscles or small groups of muscles. This conclusion has been corroborated by other anatomical studies [60] and studies employing electrical stimulation applied to the surface of exposed nerve trunks [75].

Sunderland [138] implied that at locations proximal to the branching point, the topographic organization of the nerve trunk is lost and nerve fibers intermingle and cross between fascicles. However, recent data support the retention of topography at more proximal levels. Intraneural microstimulation has revealed that sensory fibers remain grouped even in the more proximal regions of peripheral nerve trunks [50], [124], and HRP staining has demonstrated that the digital axons within the median nerve of the monkey remain as discrete geometrical groups from the carpal tunnel to the proximal arm [13]. These data are consistent with the view that the nervous system repeatedly employs and maintains topographic organization of nerve fibers over long distances. Based on these findings, it is likely that motor fibers, like sensory fibers, also retain a topographic organization over distances that extend more proximal than implied by Sunderland [138].

Detailed studies of human peripheral neuroanatomy reviewed by Sunderland [138] make it clear that peripheral nerve implant sites exist where nerve fascicles are not intermixed. Selective activation of individual muscles using nerve-based electrodes can be achieved by localizing the region of excitation to specific fascicles or regions of fascicles within a nerve trunk. Thus, an electrode with sufficient spatial selectivity should allow selective activation of an individual muscle without activation of other muscles served by different regions of the same nerve trunk.

A successful nerve-based electrode must allow selective and independent control of multiple muscles innervated by a common nerve trunk, it must minimize the potential for damage to the neural tissue, and it must be able to be simple to implant. The various electrode designs that could be considered for spatially selective activation of peripheral nerve trunks are reviewed below.

3.4. Intraneural electrodes

Intraneural or intrafascicular electrodes, designed to reside within a nerve fascicle, have been proposed for selective activation of peripheral nerve trunks. Modeling studies have suggested that the intrafascicular approach would allow more selective activation of regions of the nerve trunk than the extraneural approach [146]. However, this prediction has not yet been demonstrated in experimental studies. The theoretical and experimental studies of Rutten et al. [119] indicate that intrafascicular electrodes have to be spaced at least 250 μm apart to excite discrete regions of a fascicle. Thus, only 3 or 4 electrodes would be available for activation of a typical fascicle.

Veltink et al. [148] measured the forces evoked in tibialis anterior and extensor *digitorum longus* muscles of rat when electrical stimuli were applied via intraneural and extraneural electrodes placed on the common peroneal nerve. With intrafascicular stimulation, the two muscles were recruited simultaneously, indicating that there was limited selectivity available with the intraneural electrodes. However, some separation of recruitment was reported for extraneural electrodes. Furthermore, much larger forces were developed with the extraneural electrodes than with the intraneural electrodes, and less current was required to obtain maximum force.

Koole et al. [72] implanted 25 μm intrafascicular wire electrodes in the tibial and common peroneal fascicles of the rat sciatic nerve. Forces were recorded from extensor digitorum longus (EDL, innervated by the common peroneal division) and soleus (SOL, innervated by the tibial division), and EMGs were recorded from EDL, SOL, tibialis anterior (innervated by the common peroneal division), and medial gastrocnemius (innervated by the tibial division). Their data demonstrate a very limited degree of selectivity between the fascicles. Significant overlap of recruitment was found, even at low stimulus amplitudes.

Yoshida and Horch [155] implanted pairs of Pt-Ir wire electrodes in the medial gastrocnemius nerve and lateral gastrocnemius/soleus nerve of cats in acute experiments to assess the selectivity between fascicles and within fascicles. The degree of overlap between the two fascicles ranged from 0.8 to 15.6% (5.5±2.2%, mean ± s.e.) of the maximum force, and the degree of overlap within a fascicle ranged from -11.2 to 66.5% (26.6±8.4%). The maximum forces reported (12.9±2.9N) indicate that two electrodes, even when maximally activated, were only stimulating a portion of the nerve fascicle.

Implantation of intrafascicular electrodes compromises the perineurium and the blood/nerve barrier, which serve to maintain the chemical and mechanical micro-environment necessary for the continued function of nerve fibers [123]. Although the perineurium retains many of its barrier properties after physical insults such as ischemia and stretching [81], compression [121], and neurolysis [122], the blood/nerve barrier is damaged more easily [82].

Damage to the perineurium or blood/nerve barrier leads to endoneurial edema, an increase in endoneurial pressure, nerve fiber compression, and loss of nerve fibers with the larger nerve fibers being the most vulnerable [123]. This sequence of events has been observed with chronically implanted intraneural electrodes [9], demonstrating that the electrodes carry a significant risk of nerve trauma [2].

Chronic studies using intrafascicular electrodes have shown endoneurial fibrosis and edema [120], loss of nerve fibers [76] with the large myelinated fibers being the most susceptible [9], and variable shifts in threshold [9]. A bulbous enlargement forms at the point of electrode penetration, which is associated with nerve fiber compression, demyelination, edema, and proliferating fibroblasts [9], [88].

Implantation and stabilization are other potential problems with intraneural electrodes. Implantation of a large number of electrodes into multiple fascicles, as required for control of multiple muscles, will require mobilization and identification of the nerve branches. Secondly, introducing an electrode into the fascicle requires some means to pierce the perineurium, which is an extremely tough membrane. Finally, once an electrode is implanted, some method is required to anchor it and ensure first that it stays within the fascicle and second that it does not move within the fascicle.

3.5. Epineural electrodes

The epineurium is a loose connective tissue matrix that is located between individual fascicle, surrounds the entire nerve trunk, and is believed to have a role in protecting the nerve against compression and mechanical injury [83]. The amount of epineurium varies among different nerve trunks and along the lengths of individual nerves, and the thickness of the epineurium has been observed to be greater where nerves cross joints or bony structures [138].

Electrodes sutured to the epineurium have been used by one research group to activate the phrenic nerve in a diaphragm pacing application [141], and for activation of the femoral nerve for ambulation [58]. Another group has used epineural electrodes placed on the median and radial nerves to activate the muscles of the hand [67], [68], [107]. Few data have been published to demonstrate the degree of selectivity available with this approach [51], but several factors suggest that it will be limited. Epineural electrodes are not surrounded by a layer of insulation, and therefore precise control of the excitatory field within the nerve trunk is not possible. Current can spread to excite neighboring nerve branches and may result in activation of unwanted muscles. In their present implementation, epineural electrodes are used in a bipolar configuration to pass current in a transverse direction. Significantly more current is required to excite nerve fibers when a transverse field is applied than when a longitudinal field is applied [139], although recent results suggest that this is a means to achieve selectivity [29]. Neural damage including endoneurial edema, loss of axons, and thinning myelin has already been reported as a result of application of epineural electrodes [34], [71].

Clippinger et al. [22] employed 2 mm × 1 mm Pt-Ir electrodes with a Dacron skirt sutured to the epineurium of the human sciatic nerve to provide sensory feedback to 13 amputees using below knee prostheses. Patients reportedly benefited from a frequency coded feedback signal of the phase of gait, and there were no reported complications for use as long as six years. Although this was a four-electrode system, there was no information in the report about selectivity between the four electrodes.

Koole et al. [73] conducted modeling studies and acute experimental testing of a novel multiple groove electrode designed to accept individual branches of a multifascicular nerve trunk after surgical separation. The model results suggested that the electrode would allow selective stimulation of fascicles placed within grooves when the inter groove partitions were at least as high as the fascicle diameter. The results also indicated that smaller electrode contacts produced a recruitment curve with a lower slope, and that multiple small contacts would allow selective stimulation of regions of a fascicle within a single groove. Potential problems with this approach are the mechanical impedance mismatch between the electrode array and the nerve fascicles and the surgical skill required for implantation. Additionally, since no provision was made for swelling of the fascicles within the grooves, post-surgical edema may lead to compression induced neural damage [123]. Finally, surgical separation of the nerve fascicles provides the possibility of epineural fibrosis which could lead to compression induced injury [122].

Rather than requiring surgical separation, Tyler and Durand [142] introduced a penetrating interfascicular electrode that was designed to use mechanical energy stored by elastic deformation of the electrode structure to place electrode contacts between fascicles within the nerve trunk. Results from acute experiments on the cat sciatic nerve demonstrated that the electrode penetrated into the nerve within 24 h, and that contacts at different locations on the penetrating element generated different torque vectors at the cat ankle joint.

3.6. Cuff electrodes

Cuff-type electrodes are another electrode design for selective activation of peripheral nerve trunks. Cuff electrodes provide a more stable interface between the electrode and the nerve fibers than intrafascicular electrodes, and should therefore provide more stable recruitment patterns over time. Bowman and Erickson [9] reported large shifts in stimulation thresholds and Lefurge et al. [76] reported changes in the population of nerve fibers that were recorded from chronically implanted intraneural wire electrodes. The impedance and stimulation thresholds of cuff electrodes have been reported to be remarkably stable over time [88], [89] and chronically implanted cuff electrodes provide stable long-term recordings [28], [135]. We have found that there is some variability of the recruitment properties of chronically implanted multiple-contact nerve cuff electrodes even after tissue encapsulation [45]. Cuffs also afford the opportunity for retrieval and replacement in the event of a failure, whereas such a procedure would be difficult with intrafascicular electrodes.

Implantation of cuff electrodes should place minimal demand on both the patient and the surgeon, as large nerve trunks are relatively easy to access throughout the body. Furthermore, previous clinical success with nerve cuff electrodes suggests that they may be more readily accepted by the surgical community than intrafascicular designs. Clinical applications have included correction of footdrop [88], [151], [152], with some implants still functioning after longer than twelve years, pain suppression [109], phrenic nerve pacing for respiratory assist [36], and stimulation of the spinal roots for micturition assist [11], [12], [126], [127]. Cuff electrodes have also been used to record chronically [28], [57], [135] from peripheral nerve trunks in efforts to obtain prosthesis control signals and to study the role of afferent feedback in normal motor control.

Generally, cuff electrodes produce a sigmoidal recruitment curve with a high gain [37] because of the sharply peaked axon diameter distribution in motor nerves [10]. Short pulsewidths increase the threshold difference between different diameter nerve fibers [37] and nerve fibers lying at different distances from the electrode [41]; thus recruitment curves with lower gain [37], [41], [91], [111].

Selective activation of peripheral nerve trunks using cuff electrodes has been demonstrated in acute and chronic animal studies. Starbuck et al. pioneered the idea of a multiple-contact extraneural electrode array for selective activation of peripheral nerve trunk regions [133], [134]. A four-contact monopolar cuff electrode was used to alternately excite different portions of the medial gastrocnemius nerve in cats in an effort to reduce muscle fatigue. Caldwell [16] reported electromyographic studies indicating selective activation of the *gastrocnemius* and *tibialis anterior* muscles of the rabbit using eight wire electrodes positioned around the sciatic nerve. McNeal used a rigid cuff-type electrode, placed on the sciatic nerve of the dog, to demonstrate selective activation of the ankle flexor and extensor muscles [87]. It was concluded that the selectivity was highly dependent on the electrode orientation and required that the electrode fit snugly around the nerve trunk [90]. Foster [33] proposed a bipolar cuff electrode employing four field steering elements that were intended to modify the region of activation generated by the bipolar band electrodes. The field steering elements, however, were not located in the region of excitation and thus would have had little if any effect on selectivity. Sweeney et al. [139] conducted computer modeling and acute animal studies to examine the efficacy of a tripolar (cathode between two anodes) electrode configuration with an additional anode located across the nerve trunk from the tripole to steer the electric field. It was concluded that, with careful positioning of the electrodes, it was possible to activate selectively and maximally the fascicle innervating the medial gastrocnemius muscle. Addition of the transverse field steering current significantly improved the selectivity.

More recently, we have demonstrated that multiple-contact spiral nerve cuff electrodes can be used to effect selective activation of peripheral nerve trunk fascicles. The key developments in this technology were a cuff that can expand and contract to provide a snug yet non-compressing fit to the nerve [100], and a distributed array of contacts which made the performance of the electrode independent of the positioning of the cuff around the nerve [42], [149]. The results of these studies demonstrated that a multiple-contact cuff could activate selectively and maximally individual fascicles of a nerve trunk. Further, these results have been replicated in long-term chronically implanted electrodes, which demonstrate that selectivity is maintained over time [45].

Centrally-based electrodes

Interfacing with the nervous system at the level of the motor neuron, as with muscle- and nerve-based electrodes, presents fundamental problems for control of complex behaviors involving the interaction of multiple muscles. It requires implantation and maintenance of a large number of electrodes and associated stimulation hardware. Furthermore, methods must be developed to coordinate artificially the timing and levels of muscle contractions to produce functional movements. Activation of the motor system at the lowest level may also lead to unnatural patterns of activation that compromise the function of the prosthesis. For example, preferential recruitment of large force-producing rapidly fatiguing motor units by extracellular stimulation leads to difficulty in force regulation and fatigue.

Potential of exploiting biological control circuits

To restore complex motor functions, it may be advantageous to access the nervous system at a higher level and use the intact neural circuitry to control the individual elements of the motor system. There is abundant evidence in animals, and increasing evidence in humans, that the interneuronal circuitry of the spinal cord is capable of generating complex movements with coordinated muscle activity. Behaviors that can be mediated by isolated spinal cords include reaching-like limb movements [35], standing [129], locomotion [4], [38], [80], [129], scratching [7], micturition [26], [112], [128], and defecation [27]. In most cases generation of these behaviors has been by systemic administration of pharmacological agents, but recently these circuits have been activated by epidural [59] and intraspinal electrical stimulation [35], [44], [47],

[77], [78]. Further, evidence supports that spinal locomotor control circuits are present in humans, and are maintained after spinal cord injury [15], [30], as are those for defecation [84].

Thus, as recognized by Burke [14], "One of the major challenges facing clinical neurobiologists is how to exploit the untapped reserves of coordinated movement contained in the spinal cord circuits of patients with a functionally isolated spinal cord." Intraspinal microstimulation is one method to activate intact neural circuits. Again, as stated by Burke, "The complexity of the spinal circuitry implies that if a supraspinal trigger could generate movement it would need to be a highly focused drive onto a select populations of interneurons" [14]. Thus a neural prosthesis using microstimulation of the spinal cord will require selective and controlled activation of specific populations of interneurons.

In this section, work on microstimulation of the spinal cord is reviewed. Specifically, three fundamental questions related to neural prostheses based on intraspinal microstimulation will be addressed. First, where in the spinal cord are the neurons that regulate behaviors of interests? Second, what are the physiological effects evoked by intraspinal microstimulation? Third, how can targeted groups of neuronal elements be stimulated selectively?

Identification of spinal neurons

Conventional retrograde tracers, such as horseradish peroxidase (HRP), can be used to identify the location of motor neuron cell bodies and afferent terminals in the spinal cord, e.g., [145]. Higher-order neurons can be identified using transynaptic viral tracers [137] or injections of retrograde tracers in target regions [40]. These methods can be used to identify connectivity of neuronal networks, but do not yield information on which neurons participate in control of specific behaviors. For this purpose, activity-dependent neuronal tracers are necessary.

There are several methods of activity-dependent neuronal tracing. There is evidence that HRP conjugated to wheat germ agglutinin can move retrogradely across synapses in an activity-dependent manner [61]. Sulforhodamine can be used to identify active neurons through pinocytosis [69]. The most widespread activity-dependent neuronal marker has been immediate early gene expression.

The immediate early gene c-fos is rapidly and transiently expressed in neurons whose level of electrical activity has been increased [97]. The c-fos gene encodes mRNA that leads to production of the c-Fos protein, which can be detected using immunochemistry [20]. Expression of c-Fos like immunoreactivity has been used previously to map the location of neurons involved in reflex control of scratching [6], locomotion [18], [62], reflex control of vomiting [96], reflex erection [113], and reflex micturition (Figure 2A) [46]. These results serve to identify regions of the spinal cord that contain neurons that are active during specific behaviors of interest and thus are regions to target with microstimulation to replicate those behaviors.

Physiological effects of intraspinal stimulation

As described above, the spinal cord contains at lest some portion of the neuronal neural networks that regulate motor behaviors. Thus, it might be possible to electrically activate these neurons to restore function following neurological injury or disease. Below, we review results on the physiological responses evoked in the genitourinary (bladder and urethra) and motor systems by intraspinal microstimulation.

Genitourinary system

A significant component of the neural control of the genitourinary system resides within the sacral spinal cord, and control of micturition by spinal stimulation has been an active area of research. Nashold *et al.* pioneered this approach and implanted penetrating electrodes into the spinal cords of individuals with paraplegia [103]. Ten of 14 individuals were able to void large volumes of urine using the device [102]. Importantly, the early human studies demonstrated the feasibility of chronic intraspinal microstimulation. However, further investigations employing fixed electrodes at only a few locations have failed to identify a micturition center in the sacral spinal cord [8], [19], [64].

We recently completed a series of experiments employing multiple penetrations to identify regions of the sacral spinal cord where microstimulation generated selective contraction of the bladder (i.e., without co-contraction of the urethral sphincter) and regions where microstimulation generated reductions in urethral pressure [47]. The results demonstrated that regions are present in the sacral spinal cord of the spinal intact anesthetized cat where microstimulation generated either selective contraction of the bladder without increases in urethral pressure or small reductions in urethral pressure. Importantly, these data also indicated that microstimulation around the central canal produced micturition-like responses in anesthetized spinal intact animals (Figure 2B). Note that this was an area that was identified to contain many active neurons during reflex micturition (Figure 2A). These data suggest that microstimulation can be used to achieve micturition and demonstrate the utility of combining activity-dependent neuronal tracing and microstimulation mapping to replicate reflex behaviors.

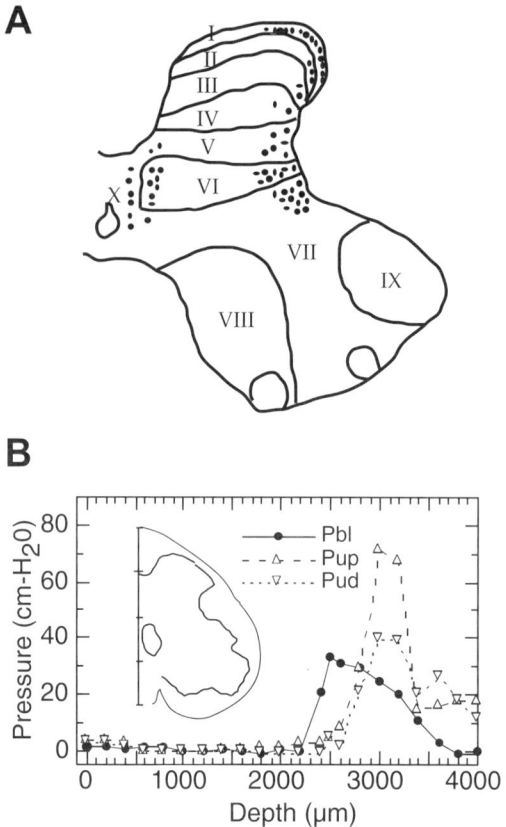

Figure 2. Identification and effects of stimulation of spinal neurons regulating reflex micturition. (A) Distribution of neurons in the S2 spinal cord of a male cat expressing c-Fos protein after 2 hours of isometric reflex micturition. The increase in c-Fos protein was activity dependent and indicates neurons that were active during reflex micturition. (B) Bladder and urethral pressures evoked by intraspinal microstimulation along a penetration passing the central canal in the S2 spinal cord of a male cat. Stimulation near the central canal generated selective increases in bladder pressure and voiding of small amounts of fluid from the bladder.

Motor system

Intraspinal microstimulation has been proposed as a method to achieve selective stimulation of motor neurons via electrodes placed in the ventral horn [99]. However, the potential benefit of stimulating the spinal cord does not lie in stimulation of motoneurons. As reviewed above, this can be accomplished with muscle- and nerve-based electrodes. Rather, the potential of intraspinal microstimulation lies in the ability to activate higher-order neurons [5]. Microstimulation of spinal interneurons around the central canal generates micturition-like responses [47], and recent data suggest that microstimulation of spinal interneurons may also simplify control of complex motor functions [35], [77], [78].

We have recently begun to map systematically the motor responses evoked by microstimulation of the lumbar spinal cord in the cat [44]. Maps of the isometric knee torque evoked by intraspinal microstimulation revealed a rostrocaudal, mediolateral, and dorsoventral organization of regions of the spinal cord that evoked motor responses about the knee joint. At L6 and L7, stimulation in the ipsilateral dorsal aspect of the cord produced strong flexion torques. Weaker flexion torques were also produced by microstimulation at the lateral aspect of the intermediate region. In the ipsilateral ventral horn, extension torques were produced at locations that were lateral to locations producing flexion torques, and stronger flexion torques were produced by microstimulation over a larger area in L7 than in L6. EMG recordings indicated that microstimulation in the ipsilateral dorsal, intermediate, and medial ventral locations activated knee flexors selectively, while microstimulation in lateral ventral locations activated knee extensors selectively. The results of these studies identify regions of the lumbar spinal cord that when stimulated electrically generate hindlimb motor responses. Maps demonstrated segregation of responses in the ventral horn that correlate with previous anatomical tracing studies. Stimulation in the dorsal aspect of the cord generated ipsilateral flexion and contralateral extension, which suggests that microstimulation can generate electrically two classical spinal reflexes: flexion withdrawal and crossed extension.

Recently, we have been extending these studies to further characterize the hindlimb motor response evoked by intraspinal microstimulation of the cat lumbar spinal cord [77], [78]. Endpoint forces at the paw were measured in the sagittal plane at 9-12 locations covering the hindlimb's workspace. The forces evoked at the limb endpoint were represented as a force field constructed by dividing the workspace into triangles and estimating the force vectors within a triangle by a linear interpolation. The magnitude and direction of the endpoint forces evoked at superficial and intermediate depths varied with limb configuration, and at some stimulation sites exhibited a point of convergence where the net endpoint force was zero (Figure 3A). Active force fields at more ventral depths did not show convergence (Figure 3B) and were likely the result of direct motor neuron activation; similar fields were evoked by intramuscular stimulation of single muscles. These results suggest that microstimulation of the mammalian spinal cord can be used to activate groups of muscles to produce organized force patterns at the limb's endpoint, paralleling results reported for the frog [35].

Taken together the results obtained in the genitourinary system and motor system by intraspinal microstimulation support the notion that electrical activation of higher-order neurons can be used to simplify generation of complex behaviors by electrical stimulation.

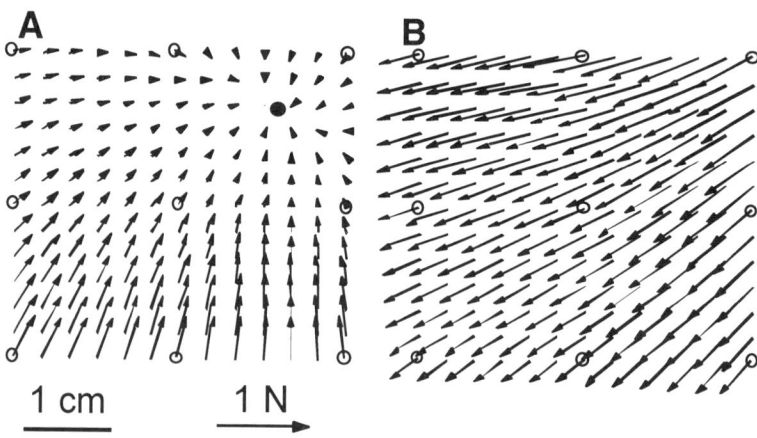

Figure 3. Endpoint forces evoked by microstimulation of the lumbar spinal cord at the L6/L7 border. Each arrow shows the force vector measured at the paw. The length of the vector is proportional to the magnitude of the force, its direction indicates the direction of the force, and its location indicates the location of the hindlimb in the workspace where that force was measured. The open circles are the locations where evoked forces were measured. (A) Forces evoked by microstimulation in the intermediate region (depth = 3400 μm) using a 0.5 s, 40 Hz train of 100 μA, 100 μs pulses. (B) Forces evoked by microstimulation in the ventral region (depth = 5200 μm) using a 0.5 s, 40 Hz train of 15 μA, 100 μs pulses.

Extracellular stimulation of central neurons

Our knowledge of what neuronal elements are activated by microstimulation is lacking and has advanced little since the seminal review of Ranck [114]. Furthermore, techniques to activate selectively targeted neurons are inadequate [154]. While the technology for fabrication of high-density arrays of microelectrodes for insertion in the CNS has advanced greatly, our knowledge of neuronal activation patterns has not.

The spinal cord is a geometrically and electrically complex volume conductor containing cell bodies, dendrites, and axons in close proximity. When a stimulus is applied within the spinal cord, cells and fibers over an unknown volume of tissue are activated, and there can be direct excitation as well as trans-synaptic excitation/inhibition from stimulation of pre-synaptic axons and cell bodies.

We have recently undertaken a computer-based modeling study of extracellular stimulation of CNS neurons [92]. We first sought to address the question of what neuronal elements are activated by microstimulation. A cable model of a neuron including an axon, initial segment, axon hillock, soma, and simplified dendritic tree was used to study excitation with an extracellular point source electrode. The site of action potential initiation was a function of the electrode position, stimulus duration, and stimulus polarity. The axon or initial segment was always the site of action potential initiation at threshold. This finding is in accord with experimental work both in vivo [49] and in vitro [104], [105], which found action potentials initiated in the initial segment or axon even for electrode positioned over the cell body. In contrast to results in uniform axons [150] and predictions based on the gradient of the extracellular electric field [115], the site of maximum depolarization in the central neuron model was not always an accurate predictor of the site of action potential initiation. Rather, the temporal evolution of the changes in membrane potential played a strong role in determining the site of excitation. Although the model used scaled Hodgkin-Huxley membrane dynamics, it was able to reproduce a wide range of experimentally documented extracellular excitation patterns, and the results were insensitive to changes in the maximum conductances in the different segments of the model.

Applications using microstimulation of the CNS will require selective and controlled activation of populations of neurons. However, experimental measurements indicate that fibers and cells have similar thresholds for excitation [49], [118]. Also, the thresholds for generating direct and synaptic excitation of motoneurons are quite similar [49], and the thresholds of differently sized motoneurons are not significantly different [132]. Thus, with conventional stimulation techniques, the thresholds for activation of different neuronal elements are quite similar, and it is difficult to isolate stimulation of particular neurons.

Using our computer model, we examined selectivity between stimulation of a neuron with the cell body positioned under the electrode and stimulation a neuron with the axon positioned under the electrode [92]. With the electrode in close proximity to the neuron (<100 µm), short duration cathodic pulses produced lower thresholds with the electrode positioned over the axon than over the cell body, and long duration stimuli produced the opposite relative thresholds. These results suggested that selective stimulation of neuronal elements could be achieved by modulation of the stimulus duration.

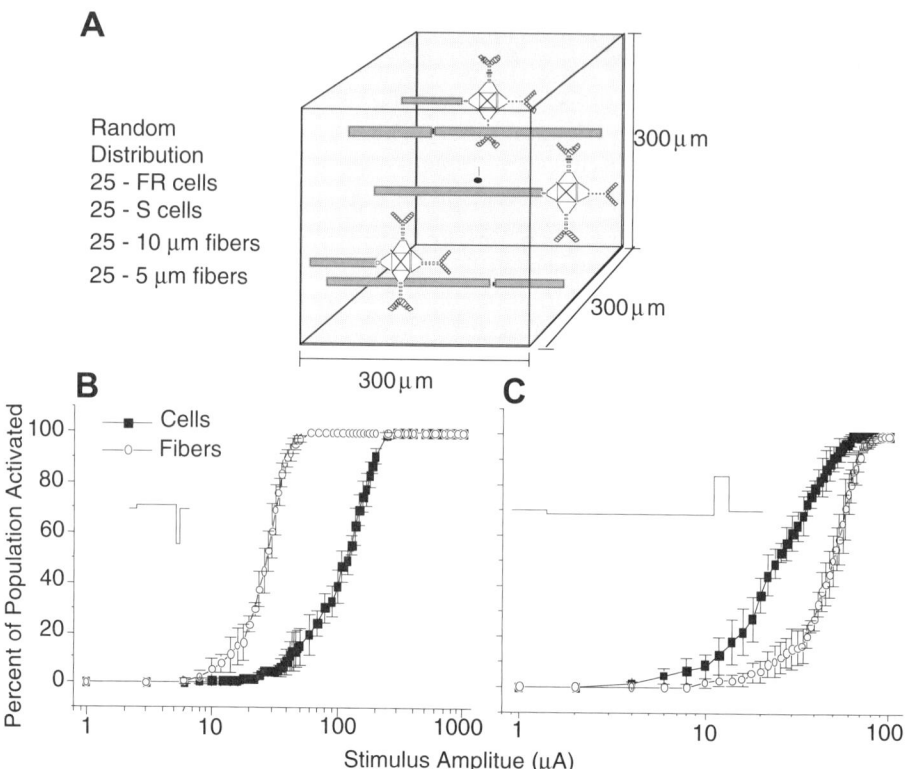

Figure 4. Design of stimulus waveforms for selective stimulation in the central nervous system. (A) Excitation of cable models of spinal motoneurons was studied by randomly distributing a population of 50 cells (25 type-S and 25 type-FR motoneurons) and 50 fibers (25 5-μm and 25-10 μm diameter fibers) about a point source electrode in the center of a 300 μm × 300 μm × 300 μm box. (B, C) Input-output relations for populations of neurons with charge-balanced biphasic stimuli. Anodic first, cathodic second stimuli (B) enabled selective stimulation of cells, while cathodic first, anodic second stimuli (C) enabled selective stimulation of fibers.

Using a second-generation computer-based model of a spinal motor neuron, we have continued to develop techniques that enable selective stimulation of different neuronal populations [93]. In these studies, rather than comparing the threshold of single neurons, we compared activation of populations of cells and fibers, positioned at random locations around an electrode (Figure 4A). This population-based approach has yielded important insights that were not apparent when comparing activation of single cells. In contrast to our prediction using single cells, conventional rectangular pulses produced limited selectivity between neural elements. For example, monophasic cathodic stimuli (duration = 0.20 ms) that activated 70% of the fibers also activated 20% of the cells. Therefore, we designed new waveforms designed to take advantage of the non-linear properties of the ionic conductances in the neurons. Asymmetric charge-balanced biphasic stimulus pulses substantially improved selectivity between neural elements (Figure 4B, C). Anodic first cathodic second charge-balanced stimuli that activated 70% of the fibers activated only 5% of the cells. Similarly, cathodic first anodic second stimuli that activated 70% of the cells activated only 15% of the fibers. These results demonstrate that these novel biphasic stimulus waveforms substantially improved selectivity between activation of fibers and cells in the CNS. Further, these waveforms are charge balanced, which will reduce the possibility of electrode corrosion or stimulus induced tissue damage.

Interfacing with the CNS: technical challenges

Electrodes placed in the central nervous system (CNS) enable access to the sensory and motor systems at a higher level. Microstimulation in the CNS can activate populations of neurons with greater specificity than is possible with larger electrodes implanted on the surface of the spinal cord or the brain. The potential thus arises for electrical activation of intact neuronal circuitry, and in turn, generation of distributed and controlled sensory inputs or motor outputs for application in neural prostheses [5]. In the case of motor system neural prostheses, this approach may simplify control by enabling exploitation of intact neuronal control circuits, and in the case of sensory prostheses allow restoration of function when the peripheral structures are damaged. The CNS, however, poses a challenging environment in which to make long-lasting stable neural interfaces. Electrodes used in the CNS include discrete wires (stainless steel, platinum-iridium, tungsten, iridium/iridium oxide), bundles of these wires, and multiple site silicon microelectrodes. These materials are well tolerated in the CNS, leading to formation of a thin capsule of glial cells. The strength and stiffness of these materials is adequate to penetrate the pie matter surrounding the brain and spinal cord. However, the mechanical properties of these electrodes are markedly different from those of CNS neural tissue and relative motion leads to destruction of the neural tissue around the electrode [153]. Clearly, alternative approaches are required to make long-term stable interfaces with the CNS.

In addition to a stable mechanical interface, chronic electrical activation of spinal neurons will require knowledge of what stimulation levels can be tolerated by spinal cord tissue. Although non-damaging levels of stimulation have been identified under certain conditions for the cerebral cortex [1], recent studies indicate that non-damaging levels of stimulation in other brain regions (cochlear nucleus) are different than those in the cortex [86]. Thus, differences may also exist between the non-damaging levels for stimulation of the spinal cord and other CNS tissues, and previous data demonstrate that the non-damaging levels of stimulation also depend on the electrode material, electrode geometry, and the temporal pattern of the applied stimuli. Thus, an important question is how much stimulation can be tolerated on a chronic basis by spinal cord tissue [153].

4. Conclusions and future prospects in motor system neural prostheses

Current state of the art neural prostheses include fully implanted electrodes, leads, and stimulators that are powered and controlled via a transcutaneous radio frequency link [66]. These devices are in clinical use restoring significant function to individuals with neurological impairment. For example, cochlear prostheses for restoration of hearing have been implanted in more than 30,000 individuals, motor system neural prostheses for restoration of micturition have been implanted in over 1000 individuals, and motor system neural prostheses for restoration of hand grasp and release have been implanted in over 130 individuals. Recent clinically deployed innovations include a fully implanted joint angle transducer that is used to generate command signals for hand opening and closing [63], and a implantable stimulator-telemeter that can recover biopotential signals for use in command and control [130]. These developments eliminate the daily task of mounting a control transducer and provide more repeatable sources of command signals. Other innovations include using implanted cuff electrodes to record form intact afferent nerve fibers to recover sensory information. Such devices have been used to obtain trigger signals in foot drop correction [54] and slip signals for adjustment of grasp force [55]. The use of implanted sensors, both artificial physical sensors and sensors designed to recover information from biological sensors, will lead to improvements in control of motor system neural prostheses.

The development of new stimulation technologies, as described in this chapter, will lead to wider application of motor prostheses and enhanced function. For example, multiple-contact cuff electrodes that allow controlled activation of multiple muscles using a single implanted device should simplify implantation and allow more function than muscle-based systems. Further work on intrafascicular and interfascicular electrodes will increase the density of implanted electrodes, leading to improvements in actuation and sensing and subsequent improvements in function. Further use of reflexes and biological neural networks will lead to improved control of complex motor functions. The presence of neural control circuitry in the spinal cord below the level of the lesion provides the opportunity for reflex-based control of motor function. For example, the flexion withdrawal reflex, elicited by electrical stimulation of the common peroneal nerve, has been used as a component of neural prosthetic stepping. Challenges to using these reflex functions include accommodation of the response, as well as state-dependence: in many cases, the output generated by the same input depends on the state of the system. However, these biological control systems provide a wealth of opportunity for simplifying neural prosthetic control of complex functions.

Rapid advances in knowledge and application of neuronal regeneration, tissue engineering, and cell transplantation will be combined with advances in microelectronics to develop hybrid neural prosthesis implants. Examples of hybrid devices include the cone electrode which is seeded with peripheral nervous tissue to promote integration following implantation in the cortex [65], and the cultured neuron probe which contains cultured neurons places within electrode wells on a silicon substrate [110]. The concept is that following implantation the cultured neurons will extend processes and establish synaptic contacts with surrounding neurons, thereby establishing electrical contact.

Thus, future neural prostheses will take better advantage of what biology has to offer, including recovering biological control signals, utilizing biological control systems, and maximizing the recovery of function and intimacy of the interface through biological growth and regeneration.

Acknowledgements. Preparation of this chapter and the work reported herein was supported by the NIH Neural Prosthesis Program (NO1-NS-8-2300), the National Science Foundation (NSF BES 9709488), and the Department of Veterans Affairs, Rehabilitation Research and Development Service, Center of Excellence in Functional Electrical Stimulation. Thanks to Dr. Michel Lemay for assistance in preparation of Figure 3, and Mr. Cameron McIntyre for assistance in preparation of Figure 4.

References

[1] Agnew, W.F., D.B. McCreeey, *Neural Prostheses: Fundamental Studies.* Prentice Hall, Englewood Cliffs, NJ, 1990.

[2] Agnew, W.F., D.B. McCreery, L.A. Bullara, T.G.H. Yuen, Effects of prolonged electrical stimulation of peripheral nerve. *Neural Prostheses: Fundamental Studies*, W.F. Agnew and D.B. McCreery, (Eds.), Prentice Hall, Englewood Cliffs, NJ, 1990.

[3] Akers, J.M., P.H. Peckham, M.W. Kieth, K. Merritt, Tissue response to chronically stimulated implanted epimysial and intramuscular electrodes. *IEEE Trans. Rehab. Eng.* Vol. 5, pp. 207-220, 1997.

[4] Barbeau, H., S. Rossignol, Recovery of locomotion after chronic spinalization in the adult cat. *Brain Res.* Vol. 412, pp. 84-95, 1987.

[5] Barbeau, H., D.A. McCrea, M.J. O'Donovan, S. Rossignol, W.M. Grill, M.A. Lemay, Tapping into spinal circuits to restore motor function. *Brain Res. Reviews* Vol. 30, pp. 27-51, 1999.

[6] Barajon, I., J.-P. Gossard, H. Hultborn, Induction of fos expression by activity in the spinal rhythm generator for scratching, *Brain Res.* Vol. 588, pp. 168-172, 1992.

[7] Berkinblit, M.B., T.G. Deliagina, A.G. Feldman, I.M. Gelfand, G.N. Orlovsky, Generation of scratching I. Activity of spinal interneurons during scratching. *J. Neurophysiol.* Vol. 41, pp. 1040-1057, 1978.

[8] Blok, B.F.M., J.T. van Maarseveen, G. Holstege, Electrical stimulation of the sacral dorsal gray commissure evokes relaxation of the external urethral sphincter in the cat. *Neurosci. Lett.* Vol. 249, pp. 68-70, 1998.

[9] Bowman, B.R., R.C. Erickson, Acute and chronic implantation of coiled wire intraneural electrodes during cyclical electrical stimulation. *Ann. Biomed. Eng.* Vol. 13, pp. 75-93, 1985.

[10] Boyd, I.A., M.R. Davey, *Composition of Peripheral Nerve*, E&S Livinstone Ltd., London, 1968.

[11] Brindley, G.S., C.E. Polkey, D.N. Rushton, Sacral anterior root stimulators for bladder control in paraplegia. *Paraplegia* Vol. 20, pp. 365-381, 1982.

[12] Brindley, G.S., C.E. Polkey, D.N. Rushton, L. Cardozo, Sacral anterior root stimulators for bladder control in paraplegia: the first 50 cases. *J. Neurol. Neurosurg. Psychiat.* Vol. 49, pp. 1104-1114, 1986.

[13] Brushart, T.M.E., Central course of digital axons within the median nerve of macaca mulatta. *J. Comp. Neurol.* Vol. 311, pp. 197-209, 1991.

[14] Burke, D., Movement programs in the spinal cord (Commentary). *Behav. Brain Sci.* Vol. 15, p. 722, 1992.

[15] Calancie, B., B. Needham-Shropshire, P. Jacobs, K. Willer, G. Zych, B.A. Green, Involuntary stepping after chronic spinal injury. *Brain* Vol. 117, pp. 1143-1159, 1994.

[16] Caldwell, C., Multielectrode Electrical Stimulation of Nerve. in *Development of Orthotic Systems using Functional Electrical Stimulation and Myoelectric Control*, Final Report Project #19-P-58391-F-01, University of Lubljana, Faculty of Electrical Engineering, Lubljana, Yugoslavia, 1971.

[17] Caldwell, C.W., J.B. Reswick, A percutaneous wire electrode for chronic research use. *IEEE Trans. Biomed. Eng.* Vol. 22, pp. 429-432, 1975.

[18] Carr, P.A., A. Huang, B.R. Noga, L.M. Jordan, Cytochemical characteristics of neurons activated during fictive locomotion. *Brain Research Bull.* Vol. 37, pp. 213-218, 1995.

[19] Carter, R.R., D.B. McCreery, B.J. Woodford, L.A. Bullara, W.F. Agnew, Micturition control by microstimulation of the sacral spinal cord of the cat: acute studies. *IEEE Trans. Rehab. Eng.* Vol. 3, pp. 206-214, 1995.

[20] Chaudhuri, A., Neural activity mapping with inducible transcription factors. *NeuroReport* Vol. 8, pp. iii-vii, 1997.

[21] Chervin, R.D., C. Guilleminault, Diaphragm pacing: Review and Reassessment. *Sleep* Vol. 17, pp. 176-187, 1994.

[22] Clippinger, F.W., A.V. Seaber, J.H. McElhaney, J.M. Harrelson, G.M. Maxwell, Afferent sensory feedback for lower extremity prosthesis. *Clin. Orthop. Rel. Res.* Vol. 169, pp. 202-206, 1982.

[23] Crago, P.E, P.H. Peckham, J.T. Mortimer, J.P. Van der Meulen, The choice of pulse duration for chronic electrical stimulation via surface, nerve, and intramuscular electrodes. *Ann. Biomed. Eng.* Vol. 2, pp. 252-264, 1974.

[24] Crago, P.E., P.H. Peckham, G.B. Thrope, Modulation of muscle force by recruitment during intramuscular stimulation. *IEEE Trans. Biomed. Eng.* Vol. 27, pp. 679-684, 1980.

[25] Creasey, G.H., Electrical stimulation of the sacral roots for micturition after spinal cord injury. *Urol. Clinics North America* Vol. 20, pp. 505-515, 1993.

[26] de Groat, W.C., I. Nadelhaft, R.J. Milne, A.M. Booth, C. Morgan, K. Thor, Organization of the sacral parasympathetic reflex pathways to the urinary bladder and large intestine. *J. Autonomic Nervous System* Vol. 3, pp. 135-160, 1981.

[27] de Groat, W.C., J. Krier, The sacral parasympathetic pathway regulating colonic motility and defecation in the cat. *J. Physiol.* Vol. 276, pp. 481-500, 1978.

[28] De Luca, C.J., L.D. Gilmore, L.J. Bloom, S.J. Thompson, A.L. Cudworth, M.J. Glimcher, Long-term neuroelectric signal recording from severed nerves. *IEEE Trans. Biomed. Eng.* Vol. 29, pp. 393-402, 1982.

[29] Deurloo, K.E., J. Holsheimer, H.B.K. Boom, Transverse tripolar stimulation of peripheral nerve: a modelling study of spatial selectivity. *Med. Biol. Eng. Comput.* Vol. 36, pp. 66-74, 1998.

[30] Dimitrijevic, M.R., Y. Gerasimenko, M.M. Pinter, Evidence for a spinal central pattern generator in humans. *Annals N.Y. Acad. Sciences* Vol. 860, pp. 360-376, 1998.

[31] Durfee, W.K., K.I. Palmer, Estimation of force-activation, force-length, and force-velocity properties in isolated electrically stimulated muscle. *IEEE Trans. Biomed. Eng.* Vol. 41, pp. 205-216, 1994.

[32] Fang, Z.-P., J.T. Mortimer, Selective activation of small motor axons by quasitrapezoidal current pulses. *IEEE Trans. Biomed. Eng.* Vol. 38, pp. 168-174, 1991.

[33] Foster, J.A., Functional neuromuscular stimulation of limbs: a feasibility study. *Bull. Prosthetic Res.* Vol. 16, pp. 409-414, 1979.

[34] Girsch, W., R. Koller, H. Gruber, J. Holle, C. Liegl, U. Losert, W. Mayr, H. Thoma, Histological assessment of nerve lesions caused by epineurial electrode application in the rat sciatic nerve. *J. Neurosurg.* Vol. 74, pp. 636-642, 1991.

[35] Giszter, S.F., F.A. Mussa-Ivaldi, E. Bizzi, Convergent force fields organized in the frog's spinal cord. *J. Neuroscience* Vol. 13, pp. 467-491, 1993.

[36] Glenn, W.W.L., M.L. Phelps, Diaphragm pacing by electrical stimulation of the phrenic nerve. *Neurosurgery* Vol. 17, pp. 974-984, 1985.

[37] Gorman, P.H., J.T. Mortimer, The effect of stimulus parameters of the recruitment characteristics of direct nerve stimulation. *IEEE Trans. Biomed. Eng.* Vol. 30, pp. 407-414, 1983.

[38] Gossard, J.-P., H. Hultborn, The organization of the spinal rhythm generator in locomotion. in *Plasticity of Motoneuronal Connections*, A. Wernig, Ed., Elsevier Science Publishers, pp. 385-404, 1991.

[39] Grandjean, P.A., J.T. Mortimer, Recruitment properties of monopolar and bipolar epimysial electrodes. *Ann. Biomed. Eng.* Vol. 14, pp. 53-66, 1986.

[40] Grant, G., M. Illert, R. Tanaka, Integration in descending motor pathways controlling the forelimb in the cat. *Exp. Brain Res.* Vol. 38, pp. 87-93, 1980.

[41] Grill, W.M., J.T. Mortimer, The effect of stimulus pulse duration on selectivity of neural stimulation. *IEEE Trans. Biomed. Eng.* Vol. 43, pp. 161-166, 1996.

[42] Grill, W.M., J.T. Mortimer, Quantification of recruitment properties of multiple contact cuff electrodes. *IEEE Trans. Rehab. Eng.* Vol. 4, pp. 49-62, 1996.

[43] Grill, W.M., J.T. Mortimer, Inversion of the current distance relationship by transient depolarization. *IEEE Trans. Biomed. Eng.* Vol. 44, pp. 1-9, 1997.

[44] Grill, W.M., B. Wang, Mapping knee torques evoked by intraspinal microstimulation. *Proc. 19th Ann. Int. Conf. IEEE-EMBS*, Vol. 19, 1997.

[45] Grill, W.M., J.T. Mortimer, Stability of the input-output properties of chronically implanted multiple contact nerve cuff stimulating electrodes. *IEEE Trans. Rehab. Eng.* Vol. 6, pp. 364-373, 1998.

[46] Grill, W.M., B. Wang, S. Hadziefendic, M.A. Haxhiu, Identification of the spinal neural network involved in coordination of micturition in the male cat. *Brain Res.* Vol. 796, pp. 150-160, 1998.

[47] Grill, W.M., N. Bhadra, B. Wang, Bladder and urethral pressures evoked by microstimulation of the sacral spinal cord in cats. *Brain Res.* Vol. 836, pp. 19-30, 1999.

[48] Grill, W.M., R.F. Kirsch, Neural prostheses, in *Wiley Encyclopedia of Electrical and Electronics Engineering*, J.G. Webster (Ed.), John Wiley & Sons, Inc., New York, pp. 339-350, 1999.

[49] Gustafsson B., E. Jankowska, Direct and indirect activation of nerve cells by electrical pulses applied extracellularly. *J. Physiol.(London)* Vol. 258, pp. 33-61, 1976.

[50] Hallin, R.G., Microneurography in relation to intraneural topography: somatotopic organisation of median nerve fascicles in humans. *J. Neurol. Neurosurg. Psychiat.* Vol. 53, pp. 736-744, 1990.

[51] Happak, W., H. Gruber, J. Holle, W. Mayr, Ch. Schmutterer, U. Windborg, H. Thoma, Multi-channel indirect stimulation reduces muscle fatigue. *Proc. 11th Ann. Int. Conf. IEEE EMBS* Vol. 11, pp. 240-241, 1989.

[52] Haugland, M., J.A. Hoffer, T. Sinkjær, Skin contact force information in sensory nerve signals recorded by implanted cuff electrodes. *IEEE Trans. Rehab. Eng.* Vol. 2, pp. 18-28, 1994.

[53] Haugland, M., J.A. Hoffer, Slip information provided by nerve cuff signals: application in closed-loop control of functional electrical stimulation. *IEEE Trans. Rehab. Eng.* Vol. 2, pp. 29-36, 1994.

[54] Haugland, M., T. Sinkjær, Cutaneous whole nerve recordings used for correction of footdrop in hemiplegic man. *IEEE Trans. Rehab. Eng.* Vol. 3, pp. 307-317, 1995.

[55] Haugland, M.K., A. Lickel, R.R. Riso, M.M. Adamczyk, M. Keith, I.L. Jensen, J. Haase, T. Sinkjær, Restoration of lateral hand grasp using natural sensors. *Journal of Artificial Organs* Vol. 21, pp. 250-253, 1997.

[56] Hines, A.E., N.E. Owens, P.E. Crago, Assessment of input-output properties and control of neuroprosthetic hand grasp. *IEEE Trans. Biomed. Eng.* Vol. 39, pp. 610-623, 1992.

[57] Hoffer, J.A., Techniques to study spinal-cord, peripheral nerve, and muscle activity in freely moving animals. in *Neuromethods, Vol. 15: Neurophysiological Techniques: Applications to Neural Systems.* A.A. Boulton, G.B. Baker, and C.H. Vanderwolf (Eds.), The Humana Press Inc., Clifton, NJ, pp. 65-145, 1990.

[58] Holle, J., H. Thoma, M. Frey, H. Gruber, H. Kern, C. Schwanda, Walking with an implantable stimulation system for paraplegics. *Proc. Int. Conf. Rehab. Eng.,* Ottawa, Canada, 1984.

[59] Iwahara, T., Y. Atsuta, E. Garcia-Rill, R.D. Skinner, Spinal cord stimulation-induced locomotion in the adult cat. *Brain Research Bull.* Vol. 28, pp. 99-105, 1991.

[60] Jabaley, M.E., W.H. Wallace, F.R. Heckler, Intraneural topography of major nerves of the forearm and hand: a current view. *J. Hand Surg.* Vol. 5, pp. 1-18, 1980.

[61] Jankowska, E., B. Skoog, Labelling of midlumbar neurones projecting to cat hindlimb motoneurons by transneuronal transport of a horseradish peroxidase conjugate. *Neurosci. Lett.* Vol. 71, pp. 163-168, 1986.

[62] Jasmin, L., K.R. Gogas, C. Ahlgren, J.D. Levine, A.I. Basbaum, Walking evokes a distinctive pattern of Fos-like immunoreactivity in the caudal brainstem and spinal cord of the rat. *Neuroscience* Vol. 58, pp. 275-286, 1994.

[63] Johnson, M.W., P.H. Peckham, N. Bhadara, K.L. Kilgore, M.M. Gazdik, M.W. Kieth, P. Strojnik, Implantable transducer for two-degree of freedom joint angle sensing. *IEEE Trans. Rehab. Eng.* Vol. 7, pp. 349-359, 1999.

[64] Jonas, U., J.P. Heine, E.A. Tanago, Studies on the feasibility of urinary bladder evacuation by direct spinal cord stimulation I. Parameters of most effective stimulation. *Invest. Urol.* Vol. 13, pp. 142-150, 1975.

[65] Kennedy, P.R., The cone electrode: a long-term electrode that records from neurites grown onto its recording surface. *J. Neuroscience Methods* Vol. 20, pp. 181-193, 1989.

[66] Kilgore, K.L., P.H. Peckham, M.W. Kieth, G.B. Thrope, K.S. Wuolle, A.S. Bryden, R.L. Hart, An implanted upper extremity neuroprostheses: a five patient review. *J. Bone Joint Surg.* Vol. 79A, pp. 533-541, 1997.

[67] Kiwerski, J., M. Weiss, R. Pasniczek, Electrostimulation of the median nerve in tetraplegics by means of implanted stimulators. *Paraplegia* Vol. 21, pp. 322-326, 1983.

[68] Kiwerski, J., R. Pasniczek, An apparatus making possible restoration of simple functions of the tetraplegic hand. *Paraplegia* Vol. 22, pp. 316-319, 1984.

[69] Kjaerulff, O., I. Barajon, O. Kiehn, Sulphorhodamine-labelled cells in the neonatal rat spinal cord following chemically induced locomotor activity in vitro. *J. Physiol.* Vol. 478, pp. 265-273, 1994.

[70] Kobetic, R., E.B. Marsolais, Synthesis of paraplegic gait with multichannel functional neuromuscular stimulation. *IEEE Trans. Rehab. Eng.* Vol. 2, pp. 66-79, 1994.

[71] Koller, R., W. Girsch, C. Liegl, H. Gruber, J. Holle, U. Losert, W. Mayr, H. Thoma, Long-term results of nervous tissue alteration caused by epineurial electrode application: An experimental study in rat sciatic nerve. *Pacing and Clinical Electrophysiology* Vol. 15, pp. 108-115, 1992.

[72] Koole, P., J.H.M. Put, P.H. Veltink, J. Holsheimer, Muscle selective nerve stimulation. *Proc. 10th Int. Symp. on Ext. Control of Human Extremities*, Dubrovnik, Yugoslavia, 1989.

[73] Koole, P., J. Holsheimer, J.J. Struijk, A.J. Verloop, Recruitment characteristics of nerve fascicles stimulated by a multigroove electrode. *IEEE Trans. Rehabil. Eng.* Vol. 5, pp. 40-50, 1997.

[74] Kralj, A., T. Bajd, R. Turk, J. Krajnik, H. Benko, Gait restoration in paraplegic patients: a feasibility demonstration using multichannel surface electrode FES. *J. Rehab. Res. and Dev.* Vol. 20, pp. 3-20, 1983.

[75] Kraus, W.M., S.D. Ingham, Peripheral nerve topography: 77 observations of electrical stimulation of normal and diseased peripheral nerves. *Arch. Neurol. Psychiat.* Vol. 4, pp. 259-296, 1920.

[76] Lefurge, T., E. Goodall, K. Horch, L. Stensaas, A. Schoenberg, Chronically implanted intrafascicular recording electrodes. *Ann. Biomed. Eng.* Vol. 19, pp. 197-207, 1991.

[77] Lemay, M.A., W.M. Grill, Endpoint Forces Evoked by Microstimulation of the Cat Spinal Cord. 1999.

[78] Lemay, M.A., W.M. Grill, Spinal force fields in the cat spinal cord. *Society for Neuroscience Abstracts* Vol. 25, p. 1396, 1999.

[79] Lichtenberg, B.K., C.J. De Luca, Distribushability of functionally distinct evoked neuroelectric signals on the surface of a nerve. *IEEE Trans. Biomed. Eng.* Vol. 26, pp. 228-237, 1979.

[80] Lovely, R.G., R.J. Gregor, R.R. Roy, Weight-bearing hindlimb stepping in treadmill exercised adult chronic spinal cats. *Brain Res.* Vol. 514, pp. 206-218, 1990.

[81] Lundborg, G., C. Nordborg, B. Rydevik, Y. Olsson, The effect of ischemia on the permeability of the perineurium to protein traces in rabbit tibial nerve. *Acta Neurol. Scand.* Vol. 49, pp. 287-294, 1973.

[82] Lundborg, G., Structure and function of the intraneural microvessels as related to trauma, edema formation, and nerve function. *J. Bone Joint Surg.* Vol. 57A, pp. 938-948, 1975.

[83] Lundborg, G., *Nerve Injury and Repair*. Churchill-Livingstone, London-Edinburgh, 1988.

[84] Mac Donagh, R.P., W. Sun, D. Thomas, R. Smallwodd, N. Read, Anorectal function in patients with complete supraconal spinal cord lesions. *Gut* Vol. 33, pp. 1532-1538, 1992.

[85] Marsolais, E.B., R. Kobetic, Implantation techniques and experience with percutaneous intramuscular electrodes in the lower extremities. *J. Rehab. Res. and Dev.* Vol. 23, pp. 1-8, 1986.

[86] McCreery, D.B., T.G.H. Yuen, W.F. Agnew, L.A. Bullara, Stimulus parameters affecting tissue injury during microstimulation in the cochlear nucleus of the cat. *Hearing Research* Vol. 77, pp. 105-115, 1994.

[87] McNeal, D.R., Selective stimulation. in Annual Reports of Progress, Rehabilitation Engineering Center, Rancho Los Amigos Hospital, Downey, CA, pp. 24-25, 1974.

[88] McNeal, D.R., R. Waters, J. Reswick, Experience with implanted electrodes. *Neurosurgery* Vol. 1, pp. 228-229, 1977.

[89] McNeal, D.R., Experience with implanted electrodes at Rancho Los Amigos Hospital. *Appl. Neurophysiol.* Vol. 40, pp. 235-239, 1978.

[90] McNeal, D.R., B.R. Bowman, Selective activation of muscles using peripheral nerve electrodes. *Med. Biol. Eng. Comput.* Vol. 23, pp. 249-253, 1985.

[91] McNeal, D.R., L.L. Baker, J.T. Symons, Recruitment data for nerve cuff electrodes: implications for design of implantable stimulators. *IEEE Trans. Biomed. Eng.* Vol. 36, pp. 301-308, 1989.

[92] McIntyre, C.C., W.M. Grill, Excitation of central nervous system neurons by non-uniform electric fields. *Biophysical Journal* Vol. 76, pp. 878-888, 1999.

[93] McIntyre, C.C., W.M. Grill, Model-based design of stimulus waveforms for selective microstimulation in the central nervous system. *Proc. 21st Ann. Int. Conf. IEEE-EMBS*, Vol. 21, 1999.

[94] Memberg, W.D., P.H. Peckham, G.B. Thrope, M.W. Keith, T. Kicher, An analysis of the reliability of percutaneous intramuscular electrodes in upper extremity FNS applications. *IEEE Trans. Rehab. Eng.* Vol. 1, pp. 126-132, 1993.

[95] Memberg, W.D., P.H. Peckham, M.W. Keith, A surgically implanted intramuscular electrode for an implantable neuromuscular stimulation system. *IEEE Trans. Rehab. Eng.* Vol. 2, pp. 80-91, 1994.

[96] Miller, A.D., D.A. Ruggiero, Emetic reflex arc revealed by expression of the immediate-early gene *c-fos* in the cat. *J. Neuroscience* Vol. 14, pp. 871-888, 1994.

[97] Morgan, J.I., T. Curran, Stimulus-transcription coupling in the nervous system: involvement of the inducible proto-oncogenes *fos* and *jun*. *Ann. Rev. Neurosci.* Vol. 14, pp. 421-451, 1991.

[98] Mortimer, J.T., Motor Prostheses. in *Handbook of Physiology: The Nervous System II*, V.B. Brooks (Ed.), American Physiological Society, Bethesda, MD, pp. 155-187, 1981.

[99] Mushahwar, V.K., K.W. Horch, Proposed specifications for a lumbar spinal cord electrode array for control of lower extremities in paraplegia. *IEEE Trans. Rehab. Eng.* Vol. 5, pp. 237-43, 1997.

[100] Naples, G.G., J.T. Mortimer, A. Scheiner, J.D. Sweeney, A spiral nerve cuff electrode for peripheral nerve stimulation. *IEEE Trans. Biomed. Eng.* Vol. 35, pp. 905-916, 1988.

[101] Naples, G.G., J.T. Mortimer, T.G.H. Yuen, Overview of peripheral nerve electrode design and implantation. in *Neural Prostheses: Fundamental Studies*, W.F. Agnew and D.B. McCreery (Eds.), Prentice Hall, Englewood Cliffs, NJ, 1990.

[102] Nashold, B.S., H. Friedman, J. Grimes, Electrical stimulation of the conus medullaris to control the bladder in the paraplegic patient. *Appl. Neurophysiol.* Vol. 44, pp. 225-232, 1981.

[103] Nashold, B.S., H. Friedman, J.F. Glenn, Electromicturtion in paraplegia-implantation of a spinal prosthesis. *Arch. Surg.* Vol. 104, pp. 195-202, 1972.

[104] Nowak, L.G., and J. Bullier, Axons but not cell bodies are activated by electrical stimulation in cortical gray matter. I. Evidence from chronaxie measurements. *Exp. Brain Res.* Vol. 118, pp. 477-488, 1998.

[105] Nowak, L.G., and J. Bullier, Axons but not cell bodies are activated by electrical stimulation in cortical gray matter. II. Evidence from selective inactivation of cell bodies and axon initial segments. *Exp. Brain Res.* Vol. 118, pp. 489-500, 1998.

[106] Office of Technology Assessment, Neural Grafting: Repairing the Brain and Spinal Cord, U.S. Government Printing Office Stock #052-003-01212-0, Washington, D.C., September, 1990.

[107] Pasniczek, R., J. Kiwersji, J. Wirski, H. Borowski, Some problems of implant stimulation applied to grasp movements. in *Advances in External Control of Human Extremities*, M.M. Gavibovic and A.B. Wilson (Eds.), Yugoslav Committee for Electronics and Automation, Belgrade, pp. 584-602, 1973.

[108] Peckham, P.H., M.W. Keith, A.A. Freehafer, Restoration of functional control by electrical stimulation in the upper extremity of the quadriplegic patient. *J. Bone Joint Surg.* Vol. 70A, pp. 144-148, 1987.

[109] Picaza, J.A., S.E. Hunter, B.W. Cannon, Pain suppression by peripheral nerve stimulation. *Appl. Neurophysiol.* Vol. 40, p. 223, 1977.

[110] Pine, J., M. Maher, S. Potter, Y.-C. Tai, S. Tacic-Lucic, J. Wright, G. Buzsaki, A. Barin, A cultured neuron probe. *Proc. 18th Ann. Int. Conf. IEEE-EMBS* Vol. 18, 1996.

[111] Popovic, D., T. Gordon, V.F. Rafuse, A. Prochazka, Properties of implanted electrodes for functional neuromuscular stimulation. *Ann. Biomed. Eng.* Vol. 19, pp. 303-316, 1991.

[112] Rampal, G., P. Mignard, Behavior of the uretral striated sphincter and of the bladder in the chronic spinal cat. *Pflügers Arch.* Vol. 353, pp. 33-42, 1975.

[113] Rampin, O., S. Gougis, F. Giuliano, J.P. Rousseau, Spinal Fos labeling and penile erection elicited by stimulation of dorsal nerve of the rat penis, *Am. J. Physiol.* Vol. 272, pp. R1425-R1431, 1997.

[114] Ranck, J.B., Jr., Which elements are excited in electrical stimulation of mammalian central nervous system: a review. *Brain Res.* Vol. 98, pp. 417-440, 1975.

[115] Rattay, F., Analysis of the electrical excitation of CNS neurons. *IEEE Trans. Biomed. Eng.* Vol. 45, pp. 766-772, 1998.

[116] Rattay, F., Analysis of models for extracellular fiber stimulation. *IEEE Trans. Biomed. Eng.* Vol. 36, pp. 676-682, 1989.
[117] Robblee, L.S., T.L. Rose, Electrochemical guidelines for selection of protocols and electrode materials for neural stimulation. in *Neural Prostheses: Fundamental Studies*, W.F. Agnew, D.B. McCreery (Eds.), Prentice-Hall, Englewood Cliffs, NJ, pp. 25-66, 1990.
[118] Roberts, W., D. Smith, Analysis of threshold currents during microstimulation of fibers in the spinal cord. *Acta Physiol. Scand.* Vol. 89, pp. 384-394, 1973.
[119] Rutten, W.L.C., H.J. van Wier, J.H.M. Put, Sensitivity and selectivity of intraneural stimulation using a silicon electrode array. *IEEE Trans. Biomed. Eng.* Vol. 38, pp. 192-198, 1991.
[120] Rutten, W.L.C., H.J. van Wier, J.H.M. Put, R. Rutgers, R.A.I. De Vos, Sensitivity, selectivity and bioacceptance of an intraneural multi electrode stimulation device in silicon technology. in *Electrophysiological Kinesiology*, W. Wallinga, H.B.K. Boom, and J. de Vries (Eds.), Elsevier, Amsterdam, pp. 135-139, 1988.
[121] Rydevik, B., G. Lundborg, Permeability of intraneural microvessels and perineurium following acute, graded experimental nerve compression. *Scand. J. Plast. Reconstr. Surg.* Vol. 11, pp. 179-187, 1977.
[122] Rydevik, B., G. Lundborg, C. Nordborg, Intraneural tissue reactions induced by internal neurolysis: an experimental study on the blood-nerve barrier, connective tissues and nerve fibers of rabbit tibial nerve. *Scand. J. Plast. Reconstr. Surg.* Vol. 10, pp. 3-8, 1976.
[123] Rydevik, B.L., N. Danielsen, L.B. Dahlin, G. Lundborg, Pathophysiology of peripheral nerve injury with special reference to electrode implantation. in *Neural Prostheses: Fundamental Studies*, W.F. Agnew and D.B. McCreery (Eds.), Prentice Hall, Englewood Cliffs, NJ, 1990.
[124] Schady, W., J.L. Ochoa, H.E. Torebjork, L.S. Chen, Peripheral projections of fascicles in the human median nerve. *Brain* Vol. 106, pp. 745-760, 1983.
[125] Scheiner, A.G. Polando, E.B. Marsolais, Design and clinical application of a double helix electrode for functional electrical stimulation. *IEEE Trans. Biomed. Eng.* Vol. 41, pp. 425-431, 1994.
[126] Schmidt, R.A., H. Bruschini, E.A. Tanagho, Sacral root stimulation in controlled micturition: peripheral somatic neurotomy and stimulated voiding. *Invest. Urol.* Vol. 17, pp. 130-135, 1979.
[127] Schmidt, R.A., H. Bruschini, J. Van Gool, E.A. Tanagho, Micturition and the male genitourinary response to sacral root stimulation. *Invest. Urol.* Vol. 17, pp. 125-129, 1979.
[128] Shefchyk, S.J., R.R. Buss, Urethral puidendal afferent-evoked bladder and sphincter reflexes in decerebrate and acute spinal cats. *Neurosci. Lett.* Vol. 244, pp. 137-140, 1998.
[129] Sherrington, C.S., Flexion-reflex of the limb, crossed extension-reflex, and reflex stepping and standing. *J. Physiol.* Vol. 40, pp. 28-121, 1910.
[130] Smith, B., Z. Tang, M.W. Johnson, S. Pourmehdi, M.M. Gazdik, J.R. Buckett, P.H. Peckham, An externally powered, multichannel, implantable stimulator-

telemeter for control of paralyzed muscle. *IEEE Trans. Biomed. Eng.* Vol. 45, pp. 463-75, 1998.

[131] Smith, B.T., R.R. Betz, M.J. Mulcahey, J.J. Triolo, Reliability of percutaneous intramuscular electrodes for upper extremity functional neuromuscular stimulation in adolescents with C5 tetraplegia. *Arch. Phys. Med. Rehab.* Vol. 75, pp. 939-945, 1994.

[132] Spielmann, J.M., Y. Laouris, M.A. Nordstrom, G.A. Robinson, R.M. Reinking, D.G. Stuart, Adaptation of cat motoneurons to sustained and intermittent extracellular activation. *J. Physiol.* Vol. 464, pp. 75-120, 1993.

[133] Starbuck, D.L., Myo-electric control of paralyzed muscles. Report No. EDC 4-67-15. Cybernetic Systems Group, Engineering Design Center, Case Institute of Technology, Cleveland, Ohio, USA, 1967.

[134] Starbuck, D.L., J.T. Mortimer, C.N. Sheally, J.B. Reswick, An implantable electrode system for nerve stimulation. *Proc. 19th Ann. Conf. on Eng. in Med. and Biol.* Vol. 8, pp. 38, 1966.

[135] Stein, R.B., T.R. Nichols, J. Jhamandas, L. Davis, D. Charles, Stable long-term recordings from cat peripheral nerves. *Brain Res.* Vol. 128, pp. 21-34, 1977.

[136] Stein, R.B., P.H. Peckham, D.P. Popovic, *Neural Prostheses: Replacing Motor Function After Disease or Disability*. Oxford University Press, New York, 1992.

[137] Strack, A.M., A.D. Loewy, Pseudorabies virus: a highly specific transneuronal cell body marker in the sympathetic nervous system. *J. Neurosci.* Vol. 10, pp. 2139-2147, 1990.

[138] Sunderland, S., *Nerves and Nerve Injuries, 2nd ed.*, Churchill-Livingstone, NY, 1978.

[139] Sweeney, J.D., D.A. Ksienski, J.T. Mortimer, A nerve cuff technique for selective excitation of peripheral nerve trunk regions. *IEEE Trans. Biomed. Eng.* Vol. 37, pp. 706-715, 1990.

[140] Tai, C., D. Jiang, Selective stimulation of smaller fibers in a compound nerve trunk with single cathode by rectangular current pulses. *IEEE Trans. Biomed. Eng.* Vol. 41, pp. 286-291, 1994.

[141] Thoma, H., W. Girsch, J. Holle, W. Mayr, The phrenic pacemaker: Substitution of paralyzed functions in tetraplegia. *ASAIO* Vol. 10, pp. 472-479, 1987.

[142] Tyler, D.J., D.M. Durand, A slowly penetrating interfascicular nerve electrode for selective activation of peripheral nerves. *IEEE Trans. Rehab. Eng.* Vol. 5, pp. 51-61, 1997.

[143] Ungar, I.J., J.T. Mortimer, J.D. Sweeney, Generation of unidirectionally propagating action potentials using a monopolar cuff electrode. *Ann. Biomed. Eng.* Vol. 14, pp. 437-450, 1986.

[144] van den Honert, C.H., J.T. Mortimer, A technique for collision block of peripheral nerve: single stimulus analysis. *IEEE Trans. Biomed. Eng.* Vol. 28, pp. 373-382, 1981.

[145] Vanderhorst, V.G.J.M., G. Holstege, Organization of lumbosacral motoneuronal cell groups innervating hindlimb, pelvic floor, and axial muscles in the cat. *J. Comp. Neurol.* Vol. 382, pp. 46-76, 1997.

[146] Veltink, P.H., B.K. Van Veen, J.J. Struijk, J. Holsheimer, H.B.K. Boom, A modeling study of nerve fascilce stimulation. *IEEE Trans. Biomed. Eng.* Vol. 36, pp. 683-691, 1989.

[147] Veltink, P.H., J.A. van Alste, H.B.K. Boom, Influences of stimulation conditions on recruitment of myelinated nerve fibers: a model study. *IEEE Trans. Biomed. Eng.* Vol. 35, pp. 917-924, 1988.

[148] Veltink, P.H., J.A. van Alste, H.B.K. Boom, Multielectrode intrafascicular and extraneural stimulation. *Med. Biol. Eng. Comput.* Vol. 27, pp. 19-24, 1989.

[149] Veraart, C., W.M. Grill, J.T. Mortimer, Selective control of muscle activation with a multipolar nerve cuff electrode. *IEEE Trans. Biomed. Eng.* Vol. 40, pp. 640-653, 1993.

[150] Warman, E.N., W.M. Grill, D. Durand, Modeling the effects of electric fields on nerve fibers: determining excitation thresholds. *IEEE Trans. Biomed. Eng.* Vol. 39, pp. 1244-1254, 1992.

[151] Waters, R.L., D.R. McNeal, J. Perry, Experimental correction of footdrop by electrical stimulation of the peroneal nerve. *J. Bone Joint Surg.* Vol. 57A, pp. 1047-1054, 1975.

[152] Waters, R.L., D.R. McNeal, W. Faloon, B. Clifford, Functional electrical stimulation of the peroneal nerve for hemiplegia. *J. Bone Joint Surg.* Vol. 67A, pp. 792-803, 1985.

[153] Woodford, B.J., R.R. Carter, D. McCreery, L.A. Bullara, W.F. Agnew, Histopathologic and physiologic effects of chronic implantation of microelectrodes in sacral spinal cord of the cat. *J. Neuropathol. Exp. Neurol.* Vol. 55, pp. 982-991, 1996.

[154] Yeomans, J.S., *Principles of Brain Stimulation.* Oxford University Press, New York, 1990.

[155] Yoshida, K., K. Horch, Selective stimulation of peripheral nerve fibers using dual intrafascicular electrodes. *IEEE Trans. Biomed. Eng.* Vol. 40, pp. 492-494, 1993.

[156] Young, J.S., P.E. Burns, A.M. Bowen, R. McCutchen, *Spinal Cord Injury Statistics: Experience of the Regional Spinal Cord Injury Systems.* Good Samaritan Medical Center, Phoenix, Arizona, 1982.

Chapter 7

Upper limb myoelectric prostheses: sensory control system and automatic tuning of parameters

Andrea Tura, Angelo Davalli, Rinaldo Sacchetti, Claudio Lamberti, and Claudio Bonivento

A sensory control system for an upper limb myoelectric prosthesis has been designed. Force Sensing Resistor (FSR) sensors have been used to control the strength of the grip on objects. The problem of the object possibly slipping from the grip has been considered also. To this aim a system based on an optical motion sensor has been used. Tests have been carried out on different everyday objects. Moreover, a software package that uses a Fuzzy Logic Expert System to calculate prosthesis parameters has been developed. The system determines the parameter set corresponding to the desired macroscopic behavior of the prosthesis.

1. The sensory control in upper limb prostheses

The hand is a fundamental organ for the demonstrations of creativity that are typical of man. Its loss, either from birth or owing to an accident, is therefore a highly dramatic event, for both the practical and the psychological consequences it entails. In such circumstances, it is advisable to provide a suitable prosthetic device.

The preliminary studies about the possibility of using residual muscles of a residual limb to move prosthesis date from the beginning of this century, but only in the late 1940s, was the importance of myoelectricity completely understood [1-4]. The first myoelectric hand was realized by Reiter in Germany, while significant improvements were made in England and in Moscow [5]. In the last few years, advanced robotic hands have been developed for which it is possible to imagine use in the prosthetic field. For example, the Stanford/JPL hand consists of three fingers, each one with three degrees of freedom, controlled by twelve actuators. The Utah/MIT hand has four fingers, each with four degrees of freedom, and 32 actuators. The Belgrade/USC hand consists of five fingers and four motors; the UBH (University of Bologna Hand) consists of three fingers and eleven actuators [6, 7]. From a prosthetic point of view, there is the difficult problem of the control of these sophisticated devices by the patient, although studies on the subject can already be found in literature [8-10]. However, the versatility and the functionality of an artificial hand are not determined only by the number of degrees of freedom available. An important issue is the presence of a sensorial system that can enable the grip to be optimized and tasks to be carried out efficiently and rapidly.

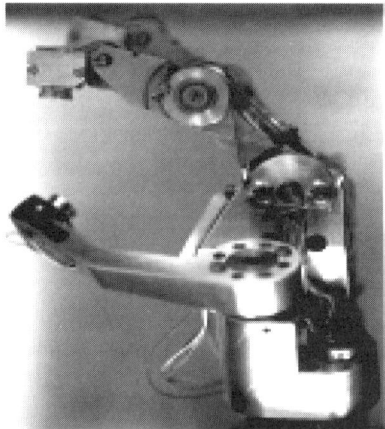

Figure 1. The MARCUS hand.

The central role of the sensorial system in a prosthetic hand has been understood since the 1960s. In those years, the Army Medical Biomechanical Research Laboratory developed the AMBRL hand, which had a slip sensor on the thumb to increase prehension when slip occurred [11]. More recently, pressure sensors along the surface of the fingers and encoders that determine the degree of rotation of the fingers with respect to the palm have been mounted on the above-mentioned Belgrade/USC hand. Significant studies in the field of sensorial systems for prostheses have also been carried out by Chappel and Kyberd at the University of Southampton. They have realized the sensorial system of the MARCUS hand. This is also an example of an advanced prosthesis, which resulted from an EEC project in which the INAIL R&D Department took part [12, 13] (see Figure 1).

The MARCUS hand consists of three fingers: a thumb, an index finger and a middle finger; the last two are connected at the base of the phalanxes. Both the fingers and the palm of the hand have sensors; this enables, in suitable phases of the hand's functioning cycle, the recognition of contact with an object and any possible slipping of the same. Therefore, the motors operate in such a way as to ensure an optimal contact and an increase in the strength of grip sufficient to avoid slipping.

As far as the INAIL R&D Department is concerned, the prosthesis that is generally fitted on patients is the Otto Bock myoelectrically controlled cosmetic hand (Figure 2). This prosthetic hand does not have the same versatility as those mentioned above, since it is characterized by a pincer-like movement (that is, with only one degree of freedom); it is, however, well known for its high reliability, which has contributed to making it a standard [14]. Another issue of importance is the satisfactory cosmetic covering. The Otto Bock hand consists of the mechanical part, an underglove covering it and the actual cosmetic glove, which is available in 18 color shades; consequently, it can be well adapted to the natural skin color of the patient.

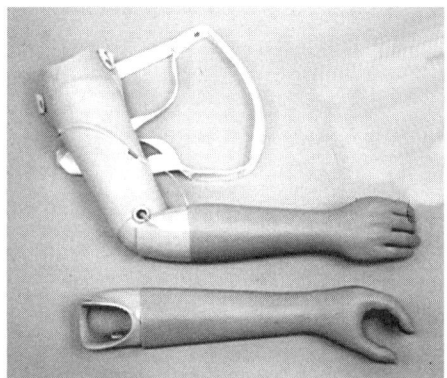

Figure 2. The INAIL myoelectric upper limb prosthesis with Otto Bock components.

To increase the functionality of the Otto Bock hand our aim was to fit it with a sensorial system, bearing in mind that this should not compromise the appearance. This constraint leads to many difficulties. For example, the sensorial system of the MARCUS hand, although advanced, is not capable of functioning if there is a cosmetic glove; the controller continues to receive information from the sensors, but since this is incorrect, it can result in totally inadequate actions.

2. A sensory control system for the Otto Bock prosthesis

2.1. Involuntary feedback in a sensory control system

To allow for the understanding of the sensorial system it is necessary to describe the functioning of a prosthesis without it. The Otto Bock prostheses previously used at the INAIL R&D Department were of the "all or nothing" type. The EMG signal caused by the contraction of two remaining muscles in the stump (typically the flexor and the extensor muscles), detected by means of electrodes, produces the opening or closing of the prosthetic hand at the fastest speed possible for it, for the whole contraction time. The speed depends on the voltage of the power supply. Metering of the movements is thus obtained by means of a sequence of microcontractions. The use of the prosthesis is consequently rather difficult or at least awkward, especially in the manipulation of objects with little mechanical resistance. Recently, the fitting of proportional control prostheses began: the speed of movement and the strength applied to an object in the grip phase are proportional to the intensity of the muscular signal. It is thus possible to better meter these elements, in order to obtain a finer control of the prosthesis.

However, the control system of the above-described prostheses lacks feedback, except the visual feedback of the patient. Visual control does, however, require considerable attention by the patient, which must continually keep his eyes on the actions of the prosthesis, which can be tiring. An important aim is to obtain a subconscious control, similar to the control of natural limbs. In other words, one would like to realize a control system that really depends on feedback that is of an involuntary kind. This means that no explicit patient's act of will is required (Figure 3).

This objective can be achieved by providing the prosthesis with two types of sensors, namely strength sensors and slipping sensors.

The information coming from the strength sensors and the slipping sensors can be sent jointly to the control system, which is in this way informed if the prosthetic hand is grasping an object and if this is done with enough strength to avoid it slipping. In case slipping occurs, the control system can control the actuator of the prosthesis to automatically obtain an increase in the grip strength.

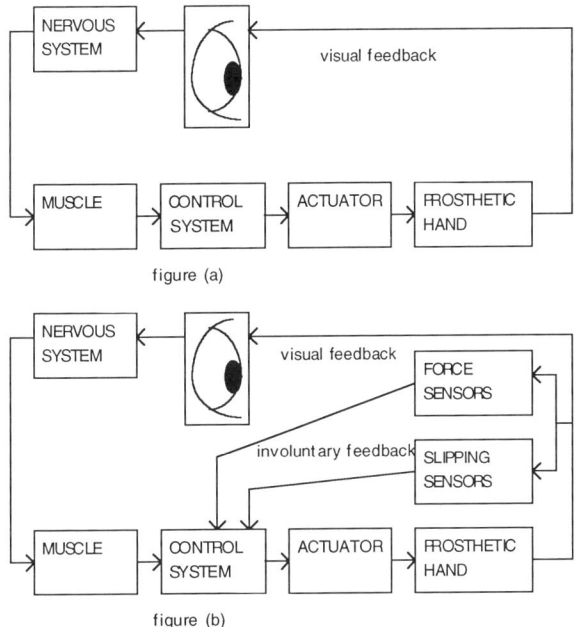

Figure 3. Control system with visual feedback (a) and control system with involuntary feedback (b).

2.2. The microcontroller card for the sensory control system

In practice, to carry out the sensory control system for the Otto Bock hand, a microcontroller card was developed, that processes the EMG signals picked up from the stump and the signals of the sensors to suitably control the actuator of the hand (Figure 4).

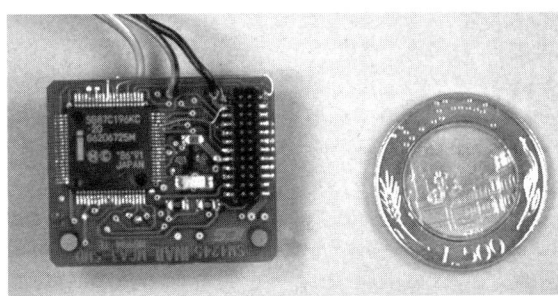

Figure 4. The microcontroller card in SMD technology (33×26 mm).

The EMG signals are picked up by means of surface electrodes and processed, then they are sampled at a frequency of 100 Hz. The value of 100 Hz was found suitable by experimental tests. Finally, the EMG signals undergo a mobile average filtering, with a number <D> of samples. The value of <D>, as the value of other parameters described below, can be set by means of software by linking a terminal to the microcontroller of the card (Figure 5). In this way, the global action of filtering can be modulated based on the EMG signal characteristics of each patient, which may be more or less irregular. Clearly, it is best not to oversize the value of parameter <D>, because that would make the patient's control of the hand unnecessarily less prompt.

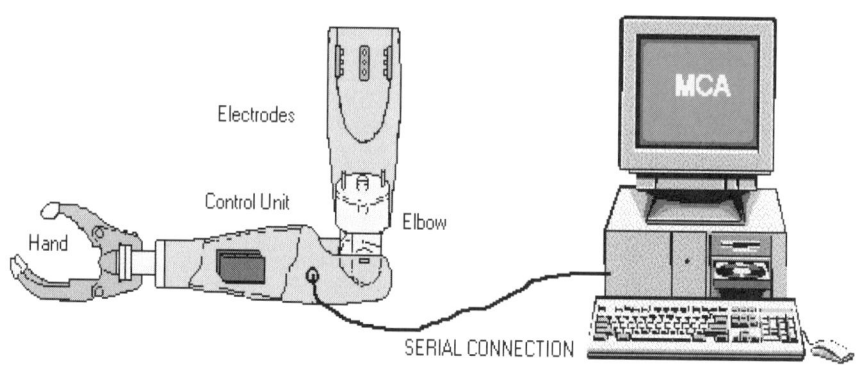

Figure 5. Prosthesis connected with a terminal.

The microcontroller used is a 87C196KC Intel, which is a CMOS technology microcontroller, with various peripheral units incorporated: a PWM signal generator, two timers, a serial port, and an A/D converter with 8 input channels. The other main blocks of the card are the following:

1. Power stage: it is a high performance DC/DC downhill converter that provides the motor of the hand with a voltage that varies between 0 and 7.2 V. The switching network of the converter consists of an H bridge made of four power MOSFETs (two *n*-channel and two *p*-channel).

2. EEPROM memory: this memorizes the optimal value of the parameters of the prosthesis, which can be set by means of software. To enable the prosthesis to work as well as possible, the values of the parameters must be suitably chosen for each patient. Besides, even for the same patient, the optimal values can vary in time, or simply according to the task that he intends carrying out with the prosthesis. Therefore, it was not possible to memorize the

parameters in the EPROM of the microcontroller, where the executable operation code of the hand, the same for all patients, is memorized.

3. Comparator for revival from Power-down: Power-down is a functioning mode of the microcontroller aimed at guaranteeing energy saving. This state is assumed if EMG signals are not picked up for a certain time. The comparator for revival from Power-down is an adder whose output goes high if the sum of the two EMG signals goes beyond a threshold (that can be set with a potentiometer).

4. Voltage regulator: it is a DC/DC converter that, supplied with 7.2 V, provides a nominal output voltage of 5 V, used to supply the microcontroller.

5. LED: two LEDs have the functions of signaling, respectively, the Power-down state and the low battery state. When the card is applied to the prosthesis, the LEDs are placed in two small holes in the cradle, so the patient can see them.

The structure of the software is made up of a set of starting procedures and a set of procedures that are carried out cyclically. This cyclical part of the program carries out the following tasks:

1. Management of the communication with a terminal (or with a PC): this is a serial communication in an 8-bit asynchronous mode, activated by means of an interrupt every 100 ms. This communication enables the operator to set the values of the parameters of the prosthesis, moreover to see on the display how the EMG signals, the sensor signals and the control signals (for example the battery charge level signal) vary in real time.

2. Management of the Power-down state: if a "muscular inactivity counter" reaches a certain value, the system goes into the Power-down state. All the interrupts are switched off, except the one that makes the system come out of this state.

3. Power supply control: it is necessary to make sure that the power voltage remains above a safety threshold (5.6 V), to prevent the microcontroller from carrying out unexpected actions. Actually, the battery is considered insufficient only if the voltage signal is found to be under the threshold for a certain consecutive number of samplings. This is to avoid the system being blocked by a temporary voltage drop due to an absorption peak of the motor. If the battery is found insufficient, the automatic opening of the hand is ordered and the microcontroller is blocked.

4. Management of the EMG signals and the sensor signals: this task, which is the heart of the program, is effected by means of a routine activated by an interrupt every 10 ms. Based on the value of the EMG signals, the sensor signals and some parameters, this routine activates the actuator according to a certain control law.

2.3. The FSR sensors

An important function of the sensory control system is based on the use of sensors called FSR (Force Sensing Resistor) produced by Interlink. An FSR sensor is made up of two thin leaves of polymer (0.2 mm in all), one of which is covered with a network of interlaced electrodes, while the other is covered with a semiconductor material. When no force is applied, the resistance between the electrodes is high; when a force is applied, the semiconductive material comes into contact with the electrodes, creating a short circuit area that determines a drop in resistance. The dynamic range is high (from 2 K_ to 1 M_) and this enables the use of a simple and economic electronic interface, unlike other force sensors. (Extensometers, for example, characterized by a low dR/R require bridge circuits, which are not necessary for FSRs.) The interface used is a simple operational amplifier in non-reversing configuration, with the gain that can be set with a potentiometer. Moreover, the force-resistance characteristic is very regular, and almost perfectly logarithmic. We have tested this on a circular force sensor of 2.54 cm diameter. Increasing loads were applied to this sensor by means of a cylindrical metal probe of 1.27 cm diameter. The characteristic obtained by interpolating the experimental points is shown in Figure 6. Clearly, the regularity of the characteristic is valid in a certain range of applied forces: for high values of force the curve tends to a saturation value, while for very low values of force it tends to rapidly increase. The sensitivity is expressed by the manufacturer in terms of pressure: 0.007 kg/cm^2. This value is even better than the requirements imposed by our application. The repeatability was also found satisfactory: we measured variations of _5% after 10 million activations.

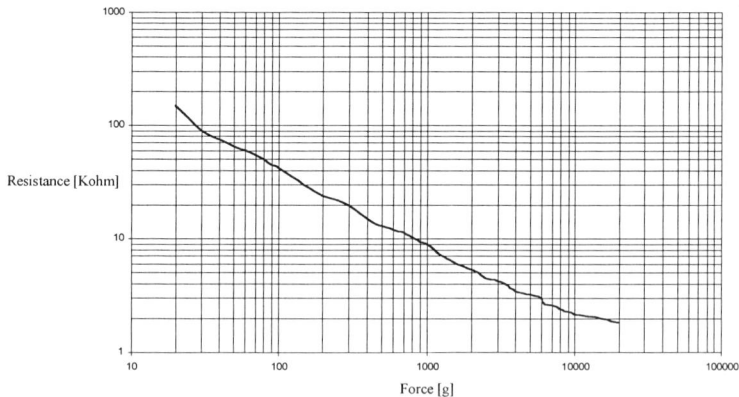

Figure 6. Force-resistance characteristic for a circular FSR.

The FSR sensors are available in various shapes and sizes; for the application on the prosthetic hand, we used the mm strip FSRs and the 5×5 mm^2 FSRs. The former has the advantage that only one element determines a uniform region of sensitivity along the whole finger where it is applied. The latter has been found slightly more sensitive, but at least three connected in parallel are necessary to obtain a sufficiently uniform sensitivity along the finger. This makes installation more difficult and gives the system a lesser degree of reliability. Indeed, the presence of three or more sensors requires a higher number of electrical connections, which are subject to wear and tear owing to the position in which they are situated. Notice that it is important to have the largest possible region of sensitivity along the fingers and not only at the fingertips (as is the case of the MARCUS hand). Since the Otto Bock hand has only one degree of freedom, grasping an object does not necessarily entail contact with the fingertips.

The FSR sensors have been placed on the thumb and index finger of the underglove. To obtain a good fastening of the sensors, we filed the underglove in some points of the fingers, so as to make flat contact areas. Then the sensors were glued with cyano-acrylate glue, moreover fixed with adhesive tape. Moreover, again with the aim of ensuring good fastening, the strip sensors were shortened to 7 cm (this does not cause functional problems) and the edges were cut, to obtain a width of 8 mm (except at the end where the contacts are, that was left to its original width). It is possible to do this since the width of the sensitive part if only 6.5 mm. Finally, the sensors were covered by the cosmetic glove, which makes them invisible on the outside and preserves the natural appearance.

2.4. The "intelligent" hand: automatic touch

An innovation introduced with respect to the proportional control prostheses at the INAIL R&D Department consists in the automatic research for contact with the objects. An EMG signal impulse generated by the contraction of a remaining muscle of the stump is sufficient to obtain the automatic grip with certain strength. On receiving this impulse, the prosthetic hand begins a closing action and goes on closing until the FSR sensors produce a signal that is greater or equal to a certain value called "contact threshold." Then it stops, since the object has been grasped with the required strength of grip. In brief, the patient only gives the "start" order of the grip action, after which the latter occurs automatically without calling further on the patient's will. By the connection between the PC and the microcontroller, the parameters on which the function of automatic grip depends can be set in order to optimize the behavior of the prosthesis, according to the patient's requirements.

The most important parameters concerning this function are:

1. <d>: number of samples for mobile average filtering on the FSR signals.
2. <n1>, <n2>: offset to subtract from the FSR signals of the thumb and the index finger, respectively.
3. <T>: contact threshold; this is the force value theoretically reached in the action of automatic touch.
4. <a>: duration of the opening impulse in the final phase of the action searching for touch. The inertia of the prosthetic hand causes the movement and does not stop immediately at the instant the power supplied to the motor is set to zero. Thus, the contact threshold set for the automatic touch is regularly exceeded. To limit this inconvenience it was found to be useful to provide the hand with a "braking impulse": as soon as the FSR signals reach the contact threshold, instead of zeroing the power, a short opening impulse is supplied, and the power is only subsequently zeroed. Quantitative information about the value of these parameters is given in a subsequent section.

Clearly, once contact with an object has been reached automatically, the patient can further increase the strength of the grip by activating the flexor muscle again. The prosthetic hand goes into the "squeeze" state and starts to work again according to the proportional mode. It should be emphasized that a parameter enables the patient to choose between linear type proportionality and square type proportionality. This is due to different opinions concerning the type of law that best correlates the effort associated with a muscular contraction to the EMG picked up.

2.5. The slipping problem: an optical sensor for motion detection

The grasping of delicate objects is what patients find to be most problematical. Consequently, the automatic grip mechanism becomes particularly useful in this circumstance. To avoid damage to these objects, it is necessary to set a low grip strength value (that is, a low value for the contact threshold). This can determine the slipping of objects weighing more than a certain value that depends on the intensity of the grip strength.

The problem can be solved if the patient orders a further closing of the hand, once the automatic grip has been reached; however, the realization of a feedback control that is really involuntary entails the necessity to automate also any possible increase in grip strength. The objective can be reached by making use of the information coming from one or more slipping sensors.

Bearing in mind the constraint of respect for appearance, besides the small size of the prosthesis, the detection of slipping is not an easy task to solve. An optical sensor with analogic memory for motion detection was thought capable of providing reasonably good results.

The device, whose code name is DIDI, is a 64×64 pixel image sensor with an analogic memory for detecting movement, developed at the Institute for

Scientific and Technological Research (IRST) in Trento (Italy). It is an integrated circuit based on standard CMOS technology, in which the sensitive element consists of a matrix of photosensors fitted with an analogic memory that records the signal of the previous frame. It doesn't need any specific light source, since it works with the light in the environment.

The cells of the sensitive matrix, each of which has a photodiode and a memory capacitance, are directed by means of a line and a column decoder; the selection of the various cells occurs line by line. A series of switches connects the selected cell to the input of a motion processor, which includes a charge amplifier and an analogic subtractor. This processor calculates for every cell the difference between the charge value provided by the photodiode (current frame) and the value memorized in the memory capacitance (previous frame), after which it memorizes the former in the memory capacitance. Finally, there is an output buffer that generates the actual output signal, that is an analogic signal giving the information of the difference pixel by pixel between the current frame and the previous one (Figure 7).

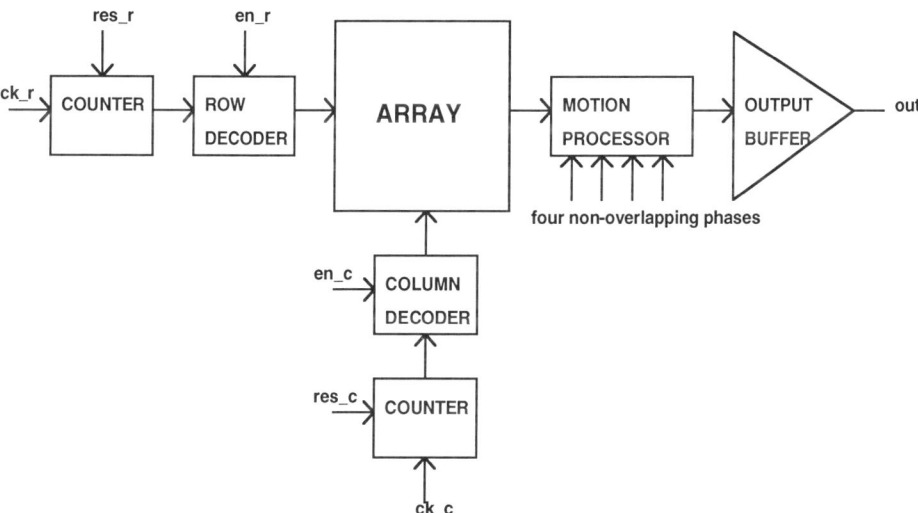

Figure 7. Block diagram of the optical sensor DIDI.

To work correctly, the sensor needs to receive a certain number of signals. These signals are the clocks for the counters, the enable and reset signals for the decoder, four non-overlapping phases for the motion processor and a set of reference voltages for both the processor and the output buffer. The voltages are provided by means of resistive dividers, while the above-mentioned signals are generated by a programmable logic circuit (the Xilinx XC3042 PC84C) that, when the system is switched on, is programmed by means of an EPROM in which the configuration program is situated [15, 16].

The output signal has a theoretical constant value equal to 2.5 V in case of a still image, while it has peaks in case of a moving image. Each peak refers to a pixel of the sensitive matrix and the amplitude is proportional to the degree of light variation in time. Consequently, positive peaks are obtained if the light increases and negative ones in the opposite case.

If it would be possible to position the sensor on the prosthetic hand such that to frame the object during the grip phase, it would be possible to detect any movement, evidence of the beginning of slipping. Indeed, the sensor, on framing a moving image, would produce peaks of the output signal.

To actually obtain useful information, it is necessary to suitably manage the output signal. Two stages of signal processing are located after the sensor, consisting of a precision rectifier and a time integrator. The first stage is required for obtaining peaks of the same sign; to avoid this peaks of different signs compensate each other. Indeed, both positive and negative peaks are evidence of a moving image. Consequently, they must both contribute to the increase of the integrator output. The integration time is equal to the duration of a frame: at the beginning of a new frame the output is reset to ground, and immediately afterwards a new cycle of integration begins. The integrator output referring to the generic i-th frame provides global information about any possible variation between the frame itself and the previous one. At this point, information that can easily be used is available; the microcontroller samples this signal and compares it with a threshold: if the former is found higher, which is evidence of slipping, the order is given to increase the intensity of grip on the object. The power assigned to the motor is maximum, because it is necessary to intervene in time by increasing the strength of the grip, to stop the object from slipping. Clearly, the prosthetic hand must already be in the grip phase (both the FSR signals greater than zero). Moreover, the EMG signals must not be picked up: if they are present, it is correct that they determine the behavior of the prosthesis, since this is the expression of the patient's explicit wish to carry out a certain action, whether a slipping situation is present or not.

The sensor DIDI is not capable of effecting the perfect subtraction between the image at time i and that at i-1; even when there is no movement, its output does not maintain a value that is perfectly constant at 2.5 V (2.5 _ 0.2 V). This influences the later stages and in particular causes the integrator output not to remain constant at 2.5 V: it does increase up to a certain value that depends on the time constant RC of the integrator itself.

It is therefore necessary to choose a compromise. To avoid rapidly saturating the output even when there is no movement, it would be better to choose a high RC value; on the other hand, this choice leads to a reduction in sensitivity in the presence of a meaningful signal. Experimental tests carried out with varying RC values have not led to acceptable results. Consequently, it was decided that an Rr resistance should be placed in parallel with the capacitor. In this way, even with a small RC value, in rest condition, the output has a limited increase, since while the capacitor is charged it is able to partially discharge through the Rr. However, since it is possible to choose a sufficiently small RC value, in at least a few instants of the integration cycle the variation of the output in the presence of a moving image remains satisfactory. Clearly, the behavior of the output is no longer ramp-like; in rest situations, the output appears as in Figure 8 (top).

The value of the plateau reached by the output depends not only on RC and Rr values, but on the level of environmental light as well. We therefore found it convenient to carry out a procedure for self-learning the "slipping threshold" (that is, the value of the plateau), to avoid searching for it manually through interaction with the microcontroller by means of a PC. The procedure samples the signal 20,000 times in about 3 seconds, and then calculates the mean value (that is found reliable with this number of samples). This mean value is then multiplied by a corrective value greater than one; the resulting value is the slipping threshold. At present, this routine is carried out when the system is switched on or reset.

In the presence of movement, the signal is deformed in a somewhat unforeseeable way, so that it is not certain that the maximum is reached at the end of the integration cycle (Figure 8, bottom). As a result, it is not sufficient to sample immediately before the reset instant: it is necessary to have sufficiently dense sampling during the whole integration cycle.

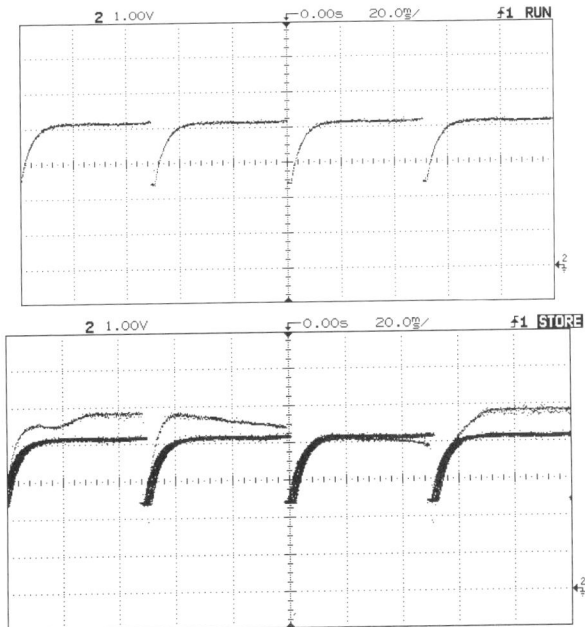

Figure 8. Integrator output in absence of movement (a) and in presence of movement (b).

2.6. Tests on the sensory control system

The experimental tests described below were carried out using a man's hand fixed on a metallic support. A hand that consisted of all new components (mechanical part, underglove, and cosmetic glove) was chosen. The aim that was initially defined was to search for a set of parameters that enabled the most delicate grip possible to be carried out. One of the first problems that occurred in searching for the optimal set of parameters was the variability of the offset of the FSR signals with respect to how open the hand was. The FSRs, even in the absence of grip, give rise to a signal that is greater than zero because of the pressure exercised by the adhesive tape used to fix them, as welll as because of the pressure applied by the cosmetic glove. In addition, the fact that the sensors are slightly curved (to follow the line of the fingers) entails a component of offset. If the offset were constant, it would easily be compensated for by means of the parameters of offset subtraction, <n1> and <n2>. The problem is the variability of the offset with respect to the position of the fingers, owing to the fact that the degree of curving of the sensors (in the part of the sensor corresponding to the base of the fingers) depends on this factor. This forces the selection of high values of <n1> and <n2>, chosen on the basis of the worst case, but this entails a decrease in the sensitivity of the sensors corresponding to the positions of the hand characterized by lower offset. Clearly, the offset is greater the more closed the hand is, because the sensors are more curved in the area around the base of the fingers. This spatial variability of the offset is about 30%. There is also a temporary variability of offset, although it is less pronounced. With the hand closed in a certain position the offset oscillates continuously, about ±5% around the mean value. The variability of the offset also depends on the gain of the FSR signals. (The gain can be set by means of a potentiometer.) This forces limit of the amplification. The variability can, on the other hand, be limited by selecting a high value of the parameter <d> (number of samples of the mobile average filter on the FSR signals); however, this determines less "rapidity" of the microcontroller in recognizing that contact with the object has been reached. It has been found experimentally that an increase in <d> leads to two effects, which compensate for each other, leaving the situation practically unchanged. Since any action on <d> is not a useful strategy, it is left at the default value (<d> = 1) or at the highest value <d> = 2.

In practice, the problem of the offset variability only concerns one of the two FSR sensors. We realized that it is possible to make reaching contact with an object depend on only one FSR signal. This could create problems when the thumb and the opposing fingers do not reach an object at the same time: the hand could stop before it has actually touched the object. However, it has been found that this case is purely theoretical, because the sensitivity of the sensor, once the offset of the worst case has been subtracted, is not sufficient to cause activation in the absence of a suitable resistance coming from the object. This only happens if the opposing fingers contact the object. In particular, it was decided to make the touch depend on the FSR on the thumb, because the thumb must be involved in gripping an object. On the other hand, since there are four opposing fingers, grip could occur without the index finger being involved. However, the sensor on the index finger has not been eliminated, since it has taken on a different function: checking the maximum strength applied to an object during the state of proportional squeeze. The threshold value of maximum strength is a parameter that can be set by means of the software. The FSR signal of the index finger is amplified much less than that of the thumb, because for the function it carries out, great sensitivity is not important; on the contrary, it should not go into saturation for low strength values.

When the strip sensors (7 cm length) are used, the set of values that determines the most delicate grip possible is the following:

$<d> = 2$
$<T> = 1$
$<n1> = 248$
$<n2> = 0$
$<a> = 2$

All these parameters have a range from 0 to 255. Their setting was obtained by trial and error, measuring the strength of the automatic touch with a dynamometer. The minimum value of strength obtained was 2 kg.

For the reasons given above, no offset was subtracted from the FSR signal of the index finger ($<n2> = 0$). The value $<n1>$ is high because the FSR signal of the thumb was highly amplified, to have the greatest sensitivity as possible.

The contact threshold $<T>$ is set to the minimum value. The braking impulse is equal to $2*\Delta t$, with Δt of 130 ms. Braking cannot be too long to prevent the hand from actually carrying out an opening movement, with the object falling from the grip as a result. We have therefore tried to affect the automatic research for contact with everyday objects of various shapes and sizes, also with the characteristic of low mechanical resistance (plastic bottles, pieces of fruit, glasses, etc.). The grip is of such a kind that these objects are not damaged. However, more delicate objects were broken (for example, eggs and paper cups). Thus, in order to obtain a more delicate touch, it was decided to shorten the sensor on the thumb, reducing it from 7 cm to 5.5 cm. This lessens the problem of the degree of curving of the sensor that varies with respect to the position of the fingers, and so reduces the variability of the offset of the signal, enabling the sensor itself to have greater sensitivity.

The shortening of the sensor involves the disadvantage of reducing the sensitive surface. However, the length remains sufficient to cover the thumb from the tip to the base. The whole palm of the hand is not covered, but it is rather unlikely that the grip of an object involves only this part of the hand. In this new arrangement of the sensor, $<n1>$ can be reduced to 150, while the other parameters keep the same values. The minimum strength obtained was 0.6 kg. Therefore, new touch trials were carried out, varying the area of contact of the hand with the object, as happens in reality. In all the trials, the hand started from an opening of 5 cm (distance between the tips of the thumb and the index finger). In this case, even delicate objects such as raw eggs were never broken or cracked. The limit is still found to be paper cups: these regularly undergo significant deformation [17].

The set of trials described was repeated using square 5×5 mm sensors, three in parallel on the thumb. The results were slightly better, but we do not think this justifies the greater constructional complexity and the lower reliability owing to the critical element in the linking between the three sensors.

From these trials, it can be deduced that the choice of the minimum contact threshold enables even delicate objects to be gripped without damaging them. Of course, the heavier the object is, the more it tends to slip. However, weight is not the only factor that determines the tendency of the object to slip, as became clear in other trials on heavier and larger objects (in this case the hand started from the maximum degree of opening, but with the same parameter values). The most significant case in these trials was the grip of an orange with a very porous surface; although weighing 300 g it never slipped from the grip, nor even began slipping, unlike the case of objects that were only about 100 g, but with smoother surfaces. The extension of the area of contact between the hand and the object also has an important role: when the other factors are the same, a larger extension is an obstacle to slipping.

Therefore, in the absence of a slipping sensor, the choice of the value of the contact threshold for the automatic touch is a compromise between two requirements:

1. gripping delicate objects without damaging them (low contact threshold);
2. preventing heavy objects from slipping (high contact threshold).

When a slipping sensor is included it is possible to set the contact threshold to the minimum value (without considering the type of objects to be manipulated), since the slipping sensor automatically increases the grip if necessary. As far as the experimental tests on the slipping sensor DIDI are concerned, it should be pointed out that until now it has not been possible to carry out tests with the sensor actually installed on the prosthesis. We have only carried out a demonstration system based on a master card whose size is not suitable for installation on the prosthesis. However, the dimensions could be drastically reduced, especially because the test card was designed with the aim of constructing a demonstrator, with no attention paid to problems of size; moreover, it was not created *ad hoc* for DIDI, since it was also used for other devices. By designing a card in SMD technology, the whole system could be placed inside the cradle of the prosthesis. The sensor should then be connected to a coherent optic fiber capable of transporting images, one end of which would be placed facing the area of interest - the area of hand-object contact. To do this, it would be necessary to open a small hole in the cosmetic glove, to enable the fiber to "see" the object in the hand's grip. This is undoubtedly a disadvantage, but it is not however something that would seriously damage the appearance.

The experimental tests consisted of moving objects of various shapes, sizes and colors (the above-mentioned objects) within the visual field of the sensor, to simulate manually the movement condition of an object owing to an insufficient grip strength. We checked if the hand automatically carried out a closing movement in such a situation. The best results were obtained by assigning the parameters concerning the management of slipping the following values:

1. parameters of the integrator: $RC = 190$ μs, $Rr = 22$ KΩ;
2. corrective factor for the self-learning procedure of the slipping threshold: $CF = 1.07$.

With this set of parameters, it was observed that the slipping signal (the output of the integrator) in the condition of lack of movement is characterized by a plateau with oscillations lower than 4% with respect to the mean value. On the other hand, when there is movement, the signal increases with respect to the mean value of the signal at rest up to values that are 20% higher. This enables us to detect even slight movements (between 1 and 5 mm) of any object tested; both movements in the orthogonal direction and in the tangent direction to the plane of the sensor are detected. However, it was found that the sensor showed greater sensitivity in recognizing objects of a dark color. With this setting of the parameters, false positives did not occur (that is, erroneous recognition of a slipping condition).

As far as the clinical tests are concerned, it has not yet been possible to carry them out on a large scale; moreover, the tests have only concerned the automatic touch function, since it is not yet possible to install the slipping sensor on the prosthesis.

The first volunteer was a third-mean right forearm amputee (male aged 45). Before trying the automatic touch function, it was necessary to spend a long time on training the patient (it was the first time a myoelectric prosthesis was applied) and on setting the parameters that influence the management of the EMG signals. In fact, he was initially not able to activate the two muscles (flexor and extensor) independently; or rather, in the attempt to activate the flexor, an extensor signal higher than that of the flexor was obtained for the same amplification. Once these problems were solved, the patient only had time to carry out a few automatic touch trials: sitting down, he managed to grip some of the previously mentioned objects arranged on a flat surface.

Fewer problems were encountered with the second patient (male aged 35), disarticulated at the right elbow. The muscles used in this case are the biceps (closing) and the triceps (opening). This patient was able to try out the prosthesis for a whole day, carrying out various activities (also including lunch).

Both patients showed that they immediately understood the functioning philosophy of the "intelligent" hand, particularly appreciating the lower degree of attention necessary for using the prosthesis. Clearly, they both expressed the desire for an automatic increase in grip when an object slips.

2.7. Development of new sensors

Currently, we are working in two different directions. The first one is to improve the above-presented sensorial system, the second one is to develop new force sensors, to be used instead of FSRs. In fact, FSRs have many advantages, but the sensitivity is limited. For example, with FSRs it is not possible to automatically grasp very soft objects (e.g., paper cups). Thus, an important point is the research of new sensor solutions, maintaining compatibility with cosmetics; we are hence working on two possible solutions, which are presented below.

1. *Hall effect sensors.* The main idea consists of the integration of a magnet in the underglove structure, and in modifying the thumb to able the fitting of the Hall sensor (Figure 9).

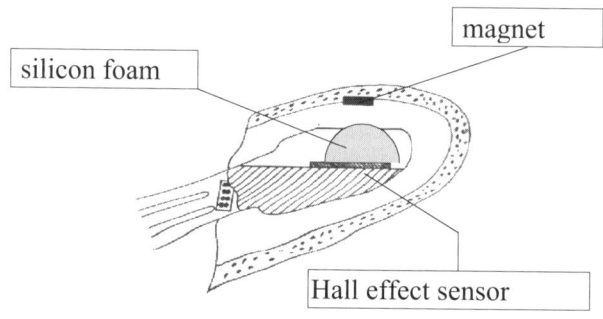

Figure 9. Longitudinal section of the mechanical structure of the thumb with the Hall sensor and the magnet.

In this way, when the prosthetic hand grasps an object, the distance between the magnet and the sensor is reduced, and correspondingly the magnetic field increases. This variation is detected by the sensor, which provides a voltage proportional to the magnetic field. The advantages of this solution are:

a) the output signal doesn't need any additional electronic components, and it can be read directly by an A/D converter;

b) easy to install: the sensor is glued directly on the little hole made on the structure of the thumb; the magnet is fixed with silicon glue on the internal surface of the underglove;

c) low cost: the price of the sensor (also considering the time necessary to install it) is not relevant with respect to the total cost of the prosthesis;

d) the installation phase is not critical during the fitting of the hand into the underglove.

One problem of this solution may be the high power consumption of the sensor. For this reason, the sensors are powered only during the acquisition time, while in the other periods the sensors are switched off.

2. *Thin layer with Strain Gauge sensors.* In this case, the sensor consists of a thin layer applied on the thumb which is provided with Strain Gauges (Figure 10). Its particular shape allows the sensor contact with the underglove also without load (i.e., when the hand doesn't grasp any objects). During the grip, the Strain Gauges provide a signal related to the layer deformation.

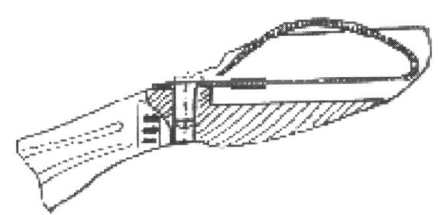

Figure 10. Longitudinal section of the mechanical structure of the thumb with the strain gauge thin layer sensor (dimension: about 7 mm × 15 mm).

The advantages of this solution are:
a) it is not necessary to work on the underglove;
b) good repeatability of the sensor behavior.

The disadvantages are:
a) it needs an electronic circuit to adapt the sensor output signal to the A/D converter input specifications; the Strain Gauge output is very low;
b) the total price (including sensor building and installation) is high.

At this stage of the work, it is not possible to define the best solution between these sensors for the following reasons:
- the interaction between sensors and underglove is still to be investigated, especially when the underglove becomes old;
- we are investigating how the patients use or expect to use the sensorized hand; this information can help us to understand the possible sensor problems.

3. Automatic tuning of prosthesis parameters

3.1. A fuzzy expert system for tuning parameters

As stated above, the upper limbs prostheses developed at the INAIL R&D Department are controlled by a microprocessor system that acquires the EMG signals and, with a particular control law, drives the hand motor. This law is suitable of changes to set the best value of its parameters, in order to allow optimal control of the hand by the patient.

A software package (MCA Auto Tuning System) was developed to realize automatic tuning of myoelectric prostheses by using a Fuzzy Logic Based Expert System [18-21]. Such a system first acquires information regarding the actual artificial arm activity and the desired behavior, then applies a specific set of rules representing expert operator know-how to define the parameter set satisfying the patient requirements. A general scheme of a Fuzzy Logic Based Expert System is shown in Figure 11.

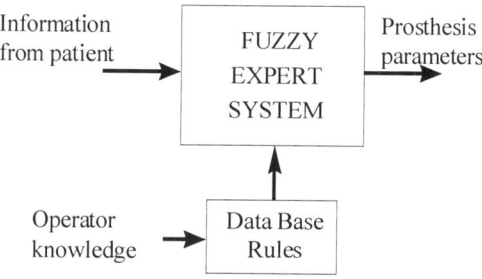

Figure 11. General scheme of a fuzzy logic-based expert system.

This software is an important step of the global INAIL prosthesis project as it allows emulation of a human skilled operator, giving more freedom to prosthesis users and making the work of technicians easier. So far, the tuning process was realized manually by an expert operator able to understand the intrinsic nature of the prosthesis and specialized in using a fairly difficult procedure. From now, thanks to a user-friendly graphical interface and to the inclusion of expert-operator-knowledge, also a low-level user can adjust the parameter values of his/her own prosthesis. In particular, this can help whenever a new setting of the prosthesis is required because of the macroscopic behavior modification due to climatic changes or mechanical and electrical consumption. Moreover, the initial setting, which is generally accomplished by an expert operator and critically depends on EMG signal entity and amputation level, can be easily done by using a solution like the MCA Auto Tuning System.

3.2. Parameters involved in the automatic tuning procedure

The system has been initially applied to the proportional control law of the prosthesis. The control law is customized on each patient using a set of parameters: when the optimal parameters are found, they are stored in a permanent memory and the prosthesis will work with maximum performances. The MCA Auto Tuning purpose is the automatic setting of some of these parameters.

1. Noise <n0>: this value is a measurement of electromagnetic noise that is coupled to the electrodes. The value is subtracted to the A/D converter value so that the disturbance is eliminated. To find the right noise value the expert operator manually sets <n0> equal to zero and reads the EMG signals values while the patient keeps still. The expected signal is null, but if the read value is different from zero then <n0> has to be increased. The same operation is realized by the program: first of all the patient is informed to keep still; then the software acquires the EMG signals values and sets <n0> equal to a proper value based on maximum EMG signal which is as a matter of fact the electromagnetic noise.

2. Inactivity threshold <I>: the <I> parameter allows the selection of opening and closing thresholds under which the acquired signals are not processed. In practice, it is necessary that at least one of the two signals is greater than the <I> value to move the prosthesis. The parameter has been introduced to filter out spurious signals that are generated when the patient moves the body without intention of opening or closing the prosthetic hand. Without this threshold, the spurious signals would move the artificial arm. If the parameter value is too low then also the "physiology noise" produces an imperceptible movement that augments the power consumption overheating the electrical motor. So, the software package increases the <I> value depending on spurious signals entity.

3. Maximum threshold <M>: the <M> value assigns the upper power limit over which the motor gives the maximum power value. The threshold allows the patient to reach the maximum velocity of the prosthesis even if the signal is weak. In order to calculate this value, the software acquires first the patient EMG signals generated in maximum effort conditions and then eliminates spikes.

4. Extensor gain <E> and Flexor gain <F>: these parameters assign the gain connected to extensor and flexor signals, respectively. These values are used to level by software possible differences between the two signals. First the software acquires the EMG signals and then a fuzzy algorithm to increase the gain corresponding to the lower signal is activated.

3.3. Examples of rules of the fuzzy expert system

The more innovative part of the project for the development of the automatic tuning system is the one relating to a fuzzy logic structure which implements the expert system. This expert system is called by two controllers, dedicated to calculate the Inactivity threshold and the Extensor and Flexor gains, respectively.

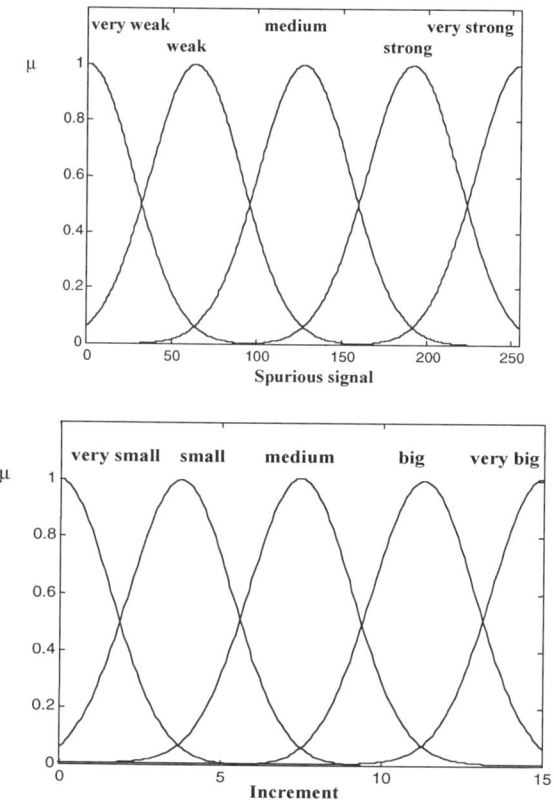

Figure 12. Gaussian-shaped membership function degree to represent spurious signal (input variable) (top) and Inactivity increment (output variable) (bottom).

The Inactivity threshold Fuzzy Logic Controller is a single-input–single-output controller: its input is a value resulting from spurious signal acquisition and filtering processes, while output is the increment to be assigned to the parameter value. The input space has been represented by five Gaussian fuzzy sets uniformly distributed on the whole range and called "very weak", "weak", "medium", "strong" and "very strong", respectively (Figure 12, top).

Similarly, the output variable is represented by five Gaussian fuzzy sets which are labeled as "very small", "small", "medium", "big", and "very big" respectively (Figure 12, bottom).

The implemented rule set is represented as follows:

If spurious signal is very weak then increment is very small.
If spurious signal is weak then increment is small.
If spurious signal is medium then increment is medium.
If spurious signal is strong then increment is big.
If spurious signal is very strong then increment is very big.

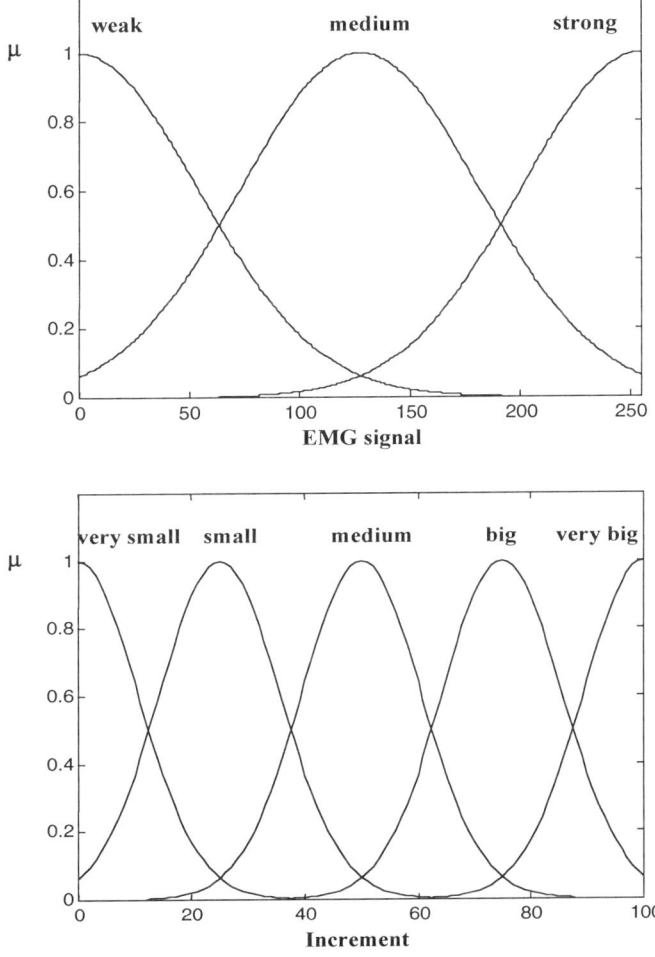

Figure 13. Gaussian-shaped membership function degree to represent EMG signals (input variables) (top) and gain increment (output variable) (bottom).

Regarding the Fuzzy Logic Controller implemented to tune Extensor and Flexor gains, input variables are represented by the EMG signals, called <e> and <f>, respectively. The output variable is the increment to be assigned to the gain corresponding to lower signal so that the final gain values are similar to each other. Every input variable has been described by three fuzzy sets, as in Figure 13, top.

Output variable is represented by five Gaussian fuzzy sets which are labeled as "very small", "small", "medium", "big" and "very big", respectively (Figure 13, bottom). The rules set that resulted from expert operator knowledge is represented as follows:

If <e> signal is weak and <f> signal is weak then increment is very small.
If <e> signal is weak and <f> signal is medium then increment is small.
If <e> signal is weak and <f> signal is strong then increment is very big.
If <e> signal is medium and <f> signal is weak then increment is small.
If <e> signal is medium and <f> signal is medium then increment is very small.
If <e> signal is medium and <f> signal is strong then increment is big.
If <e> signal is strong and <f> signal is weak then increment is very big.
If <e> signal is strong and <f> signal is medium then increment is big.
If <e> signal is strong and <f> signal is strong then increment is very small.

The above-described Fuzzy Logic Controllers allow us to modify the input and output variables range depending on patient signals entity. This is the very important feature since it allows us to overcome the problem of managing people with considerable different EMG signals.

Of course, the parameters determining the macroscopic behavior of the prosthesis are related each other. In order to simplify the project we decided to calculate one parameter at a time, but following a well-defined order not to neglect the mentioned interdependence. Thus, the first parameter which has to be modified is <n0> because it does not depend on other parameters, while all the other parameters depend on it: their regulation is based on EMG signals acquisition which is correct only if the noise has been eliminated by <n0>. After finding the proper value of <I> it is possible to calculate the <E> and <F> gains to make extensor and flexor signals similar; only after "leveling" the two signals it is possible to acquire signals corresponding to sustained forceful contractions to calculate the optimal Maximum threshold <M>.

An experimental test of the system on a limited number of subjects was realized. The testing results show the comparison between manual tuning and automatic tuning. Differences are negligible: this means that the implemented fuzzy rules accurately reproduce the manual tuning procedure adopted by the expert operator (Table 1) [22].

Table 1. Comparison between manual and automatic tuning on a subject.

Parameters	n0	I	E	F	M
Manual Tuning	001	030	255	128	150
Automatic Tuning	003	031	255	129	180

3.4. The tele-assistance project

The MCA Auto Tuning software provides a user-friendly interface for the automatic set-up of the prosthesis parameters. However, this skill can be beyond the possibility of many users, in particular elder people, therefore particular care has been given to provide the MCA software with tele-assistance functionality.

In this operative mode the MCA software runs on two personal computers connected by a fast communication link (i.e., ISDN telephonic line). The first PC hosts the physical link to the patient prosthesis, while the second runs the fuzzy expert system under the supervision of a technician (Figure 14). The patient and the technician communicate through the videoconference utility running on both the PCs. In this way the technician may guide and help the patient during the tuning session, asking him/her to use the prosthesis and then supervising the control parameter calculation performed by the MCA package.

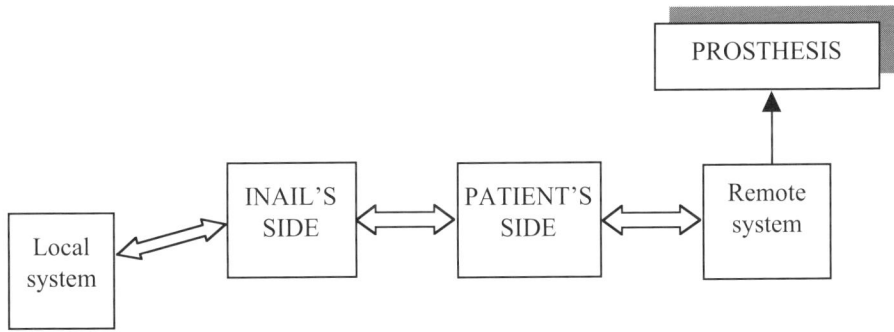

Figure 14. General scheme for the tele-assistance target.

Two tele-assistance approaches have been considered in our project. The first method, called *Application Sharing*, consists of distributing the MCA Auto Tuning and the teleconference software packages to the decentralized assistance points. In this way, the technician can supervise the tuning process using a proper software package, which permits the sharing of applications running on remote personal computers.

However, this solution presents two main disadvantages. The first is that the MCA software should be distributed to the decentralized assistance points, with the risk that unskilled software manipulation could make unusable the system, the second is that a high communication rate is requested to transfer the video map between the two PCs to realize the application sharing.

The second approach, called *Virtual Serial Port*, was to map the local serial signals between the patient's side PC and the prosthesis through the ISDN connection to the technician-side PC. In this way the patient-side PC acts only as front-end for teleconference services and prosthesis hardware interface, while all the MCA software runs only on the technician-side PC. The advantages of this solution are twofold: first a lower data rate is required with respect to the former solution, second the MCA software is centralized at supervisory center, avoiding any risk of software tempering. The tele-assistance project has been tested on real patients to verify the performance in local connection and in remote connection with satisfactory results.

4. Conclusions

A system of sensory control has been developed for an Otto Bock hand prosthesis. The sensory control system consists of two main functions:
1. the automatic search for contact with the object;
2. the detection of the object possibly slipping from the grip.

The first function, based on the use of FSR sensors, has already reached a satisfactory level of development. However, an important improvement is still possible: manufacturing a cosmetic glove in silicone, which has the FSR already incorporated in it. In this way, it will presumably be possible to obtain a more delicate automatic touch than that which can be obtained at present (it is not yet possible to hold a paper cup without damaging it). Different force sensors are also under consideration.

The advantages of the automatic touch can be summarized as:

1. it frees the patient from the need for visual control during the grip action;

2. it lessens the risk of damaging delicate objects (especially in patients new to prostheses, this risk exists even if the action of the prosthesis is followed visually);

3. it increases the speed of the grip: since grip is automatic, the actuator can be given maximum power, thus maximum speed (actually, this advantage also is clear to patients new to prostheses, less for those who already have some experience in using prostheses).

The development of a device managing slipping still requires a great deal of work to miniaturize the system, so that it is effectively suitable for installation on the prosthesis. On the other hand, only the integration of the two functions can give rise to a really efficient sensory control: in this way, not only the contact with the object, but also the increase in the grip when the object starts to slip become automatic.

We also developed a software package, called MCA Auto Tuning system, which is a useful tool, both for expert operator and for the amputees. The amputated user has more freedom, since he/she can automatically tune his/her prosthesis, possibly without going every time to the Prosthesis Center.

The adoption of this program on a large scale may yield considerable economic benefits and improve the service quality supplied to the prosthesis user. The time required to set the prosthesis parameters is remarkably reduced and, consequently, working time of technicians is reduced too, decreasing costs of prostheses producers and providers. Moreover, the software can be distributed to all users using tele-assistance service and network service, decreasing mobility and assistance costs, and providing a better service.

The tele-assistance project, now limited at myoelectric prostheses control, can also be easily used in the area of disabled wheelchairs, where serial communication to set and control parameters is also needed.

References

[1] Hogan, N.: A review of the methods of processing EMG for use as proportional control signal, *Biomed Eng*, March, pp. 81-86, 1976.
[2] Kreifeldt, J.: Signal versus noise characteristics of filtered EMG used as a control source, *IEEE Trans Biomed Eng*, vol. BME-18 (Jan.), pp. 16-22, 1971.
[3] Hogan, N. and Mann, R.: Myoelectric signal processing: optimal estimation applied to electromyography, *IEEE Trans Biomed Eng*, vol. BME-27 (July), pp. 382-410, 1980.
[4] DeLuca, C.: Physiology and mathematics of myoelectric signals, *IEEE Trans Biomed Eng*, vol. BME-26 (June), pp. 313-325, 1979.
[5] Nader, M.: The substitution of missing hands with myoelectric prostheses, *Clin Orthop Related Res*, Sept., pp. 9-17, 1990.
[6] Crowder, R.M.: Local actuation of multijointed robotic fingers. In: *IEE Conference Publication*, pp. 48-52, 1991.
[7] Gruver, W.A.: Intelligent robotics in manufacturing, service and rehabilitation: an overview, *IEEE Trans. on Industrial Electronics*, vol. 41, no. 1, pp. 4-11, 1994.
[8] DeGennaro, R.A. II, Beattie, D., Iberall, T. and Bekey, G.A.: A control philosophy for prosthetic hand. In: *Proceedings, Fifth Annual IEEE Symposium on Computer-Based Medical Systems*, pp. 429-437, 1992.
[9] Farry, K.A. and Walker, I.D.: Myoelectric teleoperation of a complex robotic hand. In: *Proceedings, IEEE International Conference on Robotics and Automation*, pp. 502-509, 1993.

[10] Iberall, T., Sukhatme, G.S., Beattie, D. and Bekey, G.A.: On the development of EMG control for a prosthesis using a robotic hand. In: *Proceedings, IEEE International Conference on Robotics and Automation*, pp. 1753-1758, 1994.

[11] Reswick, J.B. and Vodovnik, L.: External power in prosthetics and orthotics, an overview, *Artificial Limbs,* vol. 11, no. 2, pp. 5-21, 1967.

[12] Kyberd, P.J., Holland, O.E., Chappel, P.H., Smith, S., Tregidgo, R., Bagwell, P.J. and Snaith, M.: MARCUS: a two degree of freedom hand prosthesis with hierarchical grip control, *IEEE Trans. Rehabilitation Engineering,* vol. 3, no. 1, pp. 70-76, 1995.

[13] Kyberd, P.J., Chappel, P.H., Tregidgo, R. and Bagwell, P.J.: *MARCUS. Hand Software Documentation.* Oxford Orthopaedic Engineering Centre, Electrical Eng. Dept., University of Southampton, 1992.

[14] Michael, J.W.: Upper limb powered components and controls: current concepts, *Clinical Prosthetics and Orthotics,* vol. 10, no. 2, pp. 66-77, 1986.

[15] Sartori, A., Simoni, A., Maloberti, F. and Torelli, G.: A 2-D photosensor array with integrated charge amplifier, *Sensors and Actuators,* vol. 46, pp. 247-250, 1995.

[16] Gottardi, M. and Yang, W.A.: CCD/CMOS image motion sensor. In: *ISSCC Digest of Technical Papers,* pp. 194-195, 1993.

[17] Tura, A., Lamberti, C., Davalli, A. and Sacchetti, R.: Experimental development of a sensory control system for an upper limb myoelectric prosthesis with cosmetic covering, *Journal of Rehabilitation Research and Development*, vol. 35, no. 1, pp. 14-26, 1998.

[18] Driankov, D., Hellendoorn, H. and Reinfrank, M. (Eds.): *An Introduction to Fuzzy Control.* Springer-Verlag, Berlin-Heidelberg, 1993.

[19] Legg, G.: Fuzzy-logic design tools help build embedded systems. EDN, Feb. 1995.

[20] Klir, G.J. and Yuan, B. (Eds.): *Fuzzy Sets and Fuzzy Logic: Theory and Applications.* Prentice-Hall, Englewood Cliffs, NJ, 1995.

[21] Fathi, M. and Lambrecht, M.: Ebflatsy: a fuzzy logic system to calculate and optimize parameters for an electron beam welding machine, *Fuzzy Sets Syst*, vol. 69, pp. 3-13, 1995.

[22] Bonivento, C., Davalli, A., Fantuzzi, C., Sacchetti, R. and Terenzi, S.: Automatic tuning of myoelectric prostheses, *Journal of Rehabilitation Research and Development,* vol. 35, no. 3, pp. 294-304, 1998.

Parts of this material originally appeared in the *Journal of Rehabilitation Research and Development*, 1998; 35(1) and 1998; 35(3); reprinted courtesy of the U.S. Department of Veterans Affairs, Rehabilitation Research and Development Service.

Part 4.

Pacemakers and life-sustaining devices

Chapter 8

Computer-aided support technologies for artificial heart control. Diagnosis and hemodynamic measurements

Tadashi Kitamura and **Ken'ichi Asami**

In this chapter, we demonstrate an approach to making an intelligent support system for long-term control and diagnosis of a circulatory system that includes an artificial heart. The proposed intelligent system is designed on the basis of two types of advanced computation techniques. The first is for understanding the artificial heart recipient circulatory system based on a large dynamic circulatory model by ISM (Interpretative Structural Modeling). The second type of an advanced technique is an indirect measurement technique of blood pressure and flow using the linear estimation technique. The use of this technique is necessary for long time measurements for conducting the first technique, because the second technique makes it possible to minimize invasion to a recipient of an artificial heart. The ISM enables visualization of a hierarchy graph of cause and effect relations of the large circulatory model, suggests control and diagnostic information to the model by tracing back a path in the hierarchy, and allows the user to modify the circulatory model. The indirect measurement technique allows for pressure and flow calculations for on-line control, a noninvasive location for the transducers, and easy applicability to other centrifugal blood pump. The efficiency and performance of the proposed intelligent system demonstrates the technical feasibility of the on-line help of the system.

1. Introduction

We describe in this chapter an approach to making an intelligent support system for control and diagnosis of circulatory system state, with specific application to circulatory systems that include an artificial heart. The system is based on a large circulatory model. In long-term monitoring of artificial heart recipients, the advantages of this system could be (i) to provide on-line qualitative diagnostic and control information, and (ii) to offer indirect measurements of blood pressure and volume flow for on-line control of artificial hearts, with a non-invasive location for the transducers. It is important to link these two functions into a unified system because the use of the feature (ii) makes it possible to make long time measurements for conducting feature (i).

A large circulatory system model cannot give precise quantitative information because it is impossible to identify all the system parameters. Nominal estimates are usually given to most of the unknown parameters based on laboratory experiments and standard textbooks of physiology. Despite the parameter uncertainties, a large circulatory system model should be qualitatively reliable, as long as the model equations are verified based on knowledge of circulatory physiology. For a user to understand and modify a circulatory model, its equations and the knowledge supporting them should be transparent. A large circulatory model, therefore, would be more useful if it were able to provide on-line a user with qualitative knowledge linked to quantitative information.

However, most existing codes for large physiological models, such as Coleman's Human model [1], are made only for simulating time course dynamic performances of the system. Their human interfaces are usually not designed so that a user can access the structure of the model, such as cause and effect relations among model variables. Therefore, it is difficult for users to understand and modify structural insufficiencies of the model. Access to the inside of the code requires reading of the manual, if there is one. Even when the user makes up his or her mind to modify the original model, it is difficult to gain systematic access to the structure of the model using the manual. To facilitate understanding and for efficient modification of a dynamic model, therefore, quantitative simulation should be on-line linked to structural information or qualitative concepts of the model.

Several researchers have investigated linkage of a large dynamic model of a physiological system to qualitative data, in an attempt to make an intelligent support system. A rule-based inference system incorporating a circulatory model was designed for diagnosis and decision support [2]. Qualitative reasoning was combined with multi-scale dynamic models of the heart's electrical activity, based on cellular automata [3]. Some design features for diagnosis were discussed in applying fuzzy logic inference to results of dynamic simulation of an artificial heart's assisted circulation [4], [5]. Little attention, however, has been so far paid to the use of structural analysis of the dynamic model for developing core systems.

Techniques of structural analysis were developed in the 1970's for analyzing large scale systems, such as social, biological, and decision making systems. The ISM, i.e., Interpretive Structural Modeling, [10] is one such typical technique. The purpose of these techniques is to output an essential feature of a given system by applying appropriate algebraic operations to graphical expressions of the system, using a large fast computer. The author has been developing a computer-aided support system for understanding and modifying Coleman's *Human* model, based on structural analysis techniques, with the aim of obtaining qualitative information about the model and linking such information to dynamic simulation [6], [7], [8], [9]. The proposed technique for qualitative aids for diagnosis and control attempts to simplify the *Human* model to a reasonable degree and modify it based on the simplified model.

The proposed intelligent support system needs two types of measurements. The first one is data routinely off-line obtained for artificial heart recipients: blood contents and urine contents. The second type of measurements is on-line hemodynamic data of blood pressures and flow. Reliable long-term measurements of these data facilitate responsive control of the circulatory systems using a centrifugal blood pump. Measurements of the pump flow and the pressure differential (the difference in pressure) between the inlet and outlet are helpful in maintaining these parameters within physiological limits to meet the demand of the circulatory system. Due to difficulties mentioned below, however, continuous direct measurements of blood flow and pressures are not attempted in clinical long-term use of artificial hearts.

Use of an extracorporeal pressure transducer connected to a fluid-filled catheter may have the advantage of accuracy for nonpulsatile blood pressures and the ability to compensate for the baseline drift. However, it has three major disadvantages: 1) artifacts are superimposed on pulsatile pressure measurements due to mechanical resonance in the catheter and to changes in the body posture, 2) the catheter can become blocked with thrombus, and 3) the catheter can easily induce septicemia in the recipient. Pressure measurements by an implantable transducer are free from artifacts, but these transducers can also cause blood clot problems. Most importantly, an implantable transducer cannot be recalibrated. Long-term reliable measurements of blood flow are also difficult using an electromagnetic flowmeter *in vivo* with an artificial heart due to thrombus formation and difficulties in recalibration.

Several techniques of indirect measurements of blood flow and pressure for pneumatic pulsatile blood pumps have been studied and proven successful to a certain extent *in vivo* [19], [20], [21], [22], [26]. They use a variety of modeling techniques, from empirical to physical ones. However, it is almost impossible to apply these techniques to centrifugal pumps because their techniques use the models of the drive and artificial heart pump systems in which blood flow and pressures are physically reflected. The development of indirect measurement techniques of blood flow and differential pressure for centrifugal blood pumps is yet under way in the area of artificial heart research, although the necessity of such development was emphasized in several occasions, especially during the 7th International Society of Rotary Blood Pumps, 1999. Some techniques presented there, such as [30], are successful *in vitro* and/or simulation tests. Most of them, however, are not easily applied due to their empirical modeling of the pump systems.

Akamatsu and his group developed an indirect measurement technique of the pressure differential and flow for a centrifugal pump [28]. This technique solves a set of nonlinear algebraic equations for the pressure differential and flow using the motor current and rotation available extracorporeally. Their technique was shown successful in *in vivo* tests, but estimates of the pressure and flow are unreliable in the case when blood viscosity changes. Such a case frequently occurs in clinical circumstances, such as transfusion of water and blood, and misleads the solution of the equations because the equations used have viscosity-dependent coefficients. We have been trying to solve this problem, under the same circumstances, but using a physical model-based approach [27]. Although not completed, the proposed intelligent system is oriented toward the goal of integrating system diagnosis, control, modeling, CAI, and indirect measurements of hemodynamic parameters. In the subsequent sections, we first explain the *Human* model and show the method used for structural analysis, model reduction, and ISM. We then demonstrate a viscosity-independent indirect measurement technique of pressure differential and flow for a centrifugal pump showing fundamental model equations for estimation and the linear estimation technique used. We show some diagnosis results and modeling aids, as well as results of indirect measurements, based on our previous work [27].

2. Method

2.1. Model reduction

A dynamic model can be reduced by eliminating an input-output relationship, whose gain is less than a given value, called threshold ε in this study. A gain is defined as percent change of an output's response to a given input's percent step change. Percent change of a variable is defined as percent deviation from the normal value of the variable. Then, a gain is computed by conducting a simulation of a module of *Human* for a given response time at which the simulation is stopped. The model reduction for a module is completed by making its reduced correlation matrix between inputs and outputs. We take an example of model reduction of the following 3-dimensional simultaneous differential equations:

$$dx_1/dt = -(2x_1 - x_2)^2 + 3u_1 + 0.5x_2 \quad (1)$$

$$dx_2/dt = -u_2 x_1 + 0.08 x_3 \quad (2)$$

$$dx_3/dt = -x_2^2 + 0.1 x_3 u_2 \quad (3)$$

where x_i is output, and u_j is input ($i = 1, 2, 3; j = 1, 2$). A gain, g_{ij} ($i = 1, ..., 5; j = 1, 2, 3$), i.e., x_j's ($j = 1, 2, 3$) response for a given response time, is computed to, for instance, 10% step change of each of x_h ($h = 1, 2, 3; h \neq j$) and u_i ($i = 1, 2$), with other outputs and inputs fixed at their normal values. Given a threshold $\varepsilon_{ij} > 0$, the i-j entry of a correlation matrix is 1 if $g_{ij} > \varepsilon_{ij}$, and otherwise, its entry is 0.

The original correlation matrix, i.e., the correlation matrix for $\varepsilon_{ij} = 0$ ($i = 1, ..., 5; j = 1, 2, 3$), is given in Figure 1(a), where the i-j entry of the matrix is 1 if the variable in the i-th row influences the one in the j-th column, and otherwise, the entry is 0. All the diagonal elements are defined as 0 in a correlation matrix since the identical relation of each variable is trivial, and all the elements of input to input are also 0. An example of a reduced correlation matrix, shown in Figure 1(b), for the system (1), (2) and (3), can be made if x_3 is removed away by assuming $g_{ij} > \varepsilon_{ij}$ ($i = 1, j = 2; i = 2, j = 1$) and $g_{ij} < \varepsilon_{ij}$ ($i = 2, j = 3; i = 3, j = 2; i = 5, j = 3$). Then, the reduced differential equations are given by:

$$dx_1/dt = -(2x_1 - x_2)^2 + 3u_1 + 0.5x_2 \quad (4)$$

$$dx_2/dt = -u_2 x_1 \quad (5)$$

	x_1	x_2	x_3	u_1	u_2
x_1	0	1	0	0	0
x_2	1	0	1	0	0
x_3	0	1	0	0	0
u_1	1	0	0	0	0
u_2	0	1	1	0	0

Figure 1 (a). Original correlation matrix of equations (1), (2) and (3).

	x_1	x_2	u_1	u_2
x_1	0	1	0	0
x_2	1	0	0	0
u_1	1	0	0	0
u_2	0	1	0	0

Figure 1 (b). Reduced correlation matrix of equations (1), (2) and (3).

If an input variable u_i in (4) and (5) is a fixed parameter, its existence in a module is important for diagnosis because the parameter can be a pathological cause of a change in the variable x_i, depending on the parameter as mentioned in Section 4.1. The above process of reduction is first applied to a set of first order differential equations of each module of *Human* to obtain its reduced correlation matrix for a given set of thresholds. Then, the reduced correlation matrix for the full model of *Human* is obtained by combining all the correlation matrices of *Human*'s modules for sets of thresholds given to the modules.

2. 2. Interpretive structural modeling (ISM) [10], [18]

The ISM, Interpretive Structural Modeling, is an algebraic technique for analyzing a directed graph, as illustrated in Figure 2. It reduces a correlation matrix of a system to a hierarchical directed graph [10]. The correlation matrix A in Figure 2(a) equivalently corresponds to the directed graph in Figure 2(b). The matrix A in Boolean sense is said to make a reachability matrix R if a Boolean n-multiple product of $A+I$ uniquely converges to R for all integers $n > n_0$, where n_0 is an appropriate positive integer, I is a Boolean unity matrix, and $+$ is addition in Boolean sense. The reachability matrix or its equivalent graph in Figure 2(c) represents all direct and indirect linkages among S_i ($i = 1, ...,6$), i.e., all directed paths from one node to another. Then, the reachability matrix is reduced to the hierarchy graph in Figure 2(d). This hierarchy is obtained through appropriate algebraic manipulations. The manipulation includes finding a set of nodes that cannot reach other nodes outside the set itself, removing the set out of the original graph and repeating this process to remaining graphs until a unique set of nodes no other nodes can reach is obtained. Eliminating all the redundant links, S_6 to S_5, S_6 to S_1, S_6 to S_3, S_6 to S_4, and S_2 to S_4, out of the graph in Figure 2(d), produces the skeleton graph in Figure 2(e). Here, the redundant link, directed from node S_6 to S_5, is removed out of the graph in figure 2(d), because S_6 can reach S_5 through S_2 and S_1. All these manipulations are on-line performed by the system.

Kitamura and Asami: Artificial heart control support system

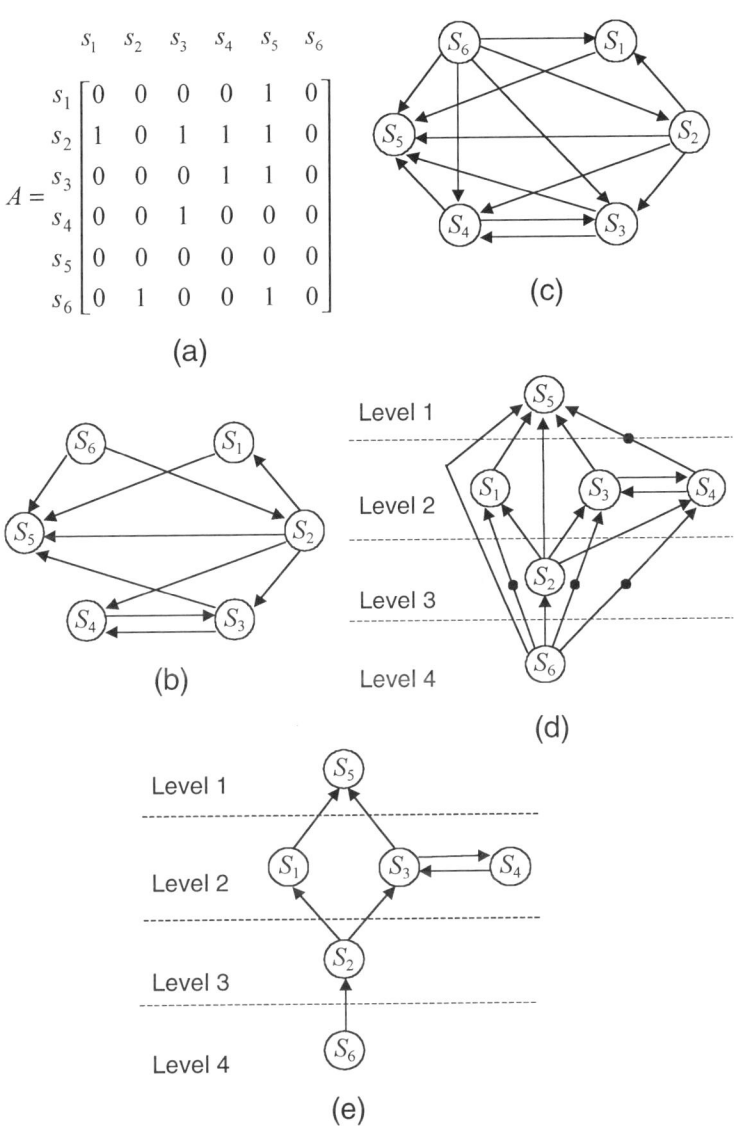

Figure 2. Summary of interpretive structural analysis.

A hierarchical graph of the reachability matrix has all possible relationships among all variables including all existing real links. As Figure 2(d) illustrates, the links with dots (•) do not exist in the original graph in Figure 2(b); they show for example a virtual link produced by the two real links from S_4 to S_3 and from S_3 to S_5. Such a virtual link facilitates knowing if there is an eventual relation among variables. Although a skeleton graph shows a minimized representation of all the direct relations among variables, it may be misleading. Assume that dosing a drug blocks the output of S_2 to S_5 and at the same time, activates the output of S_6 to S_5 in the original graph in Figure 2(b). This can occur in an artificial heart patient post-operatively, when a drug with several side effects is administered. Then, the skeleton under the above assumption is exactly the same one as in Figure 2(e), i.e., it hides the realities of blockage and activation of the links. Taking Boolean OR of Figure 2(b) and (e) and differentiating them on the OR graph can help to avoid the misleading paths.

3. System description

3.1. Structure of the system

The system consists of four major parts, Main Window, Structural Analysis, Simulation, and Data Base, as shown in Figure 3.

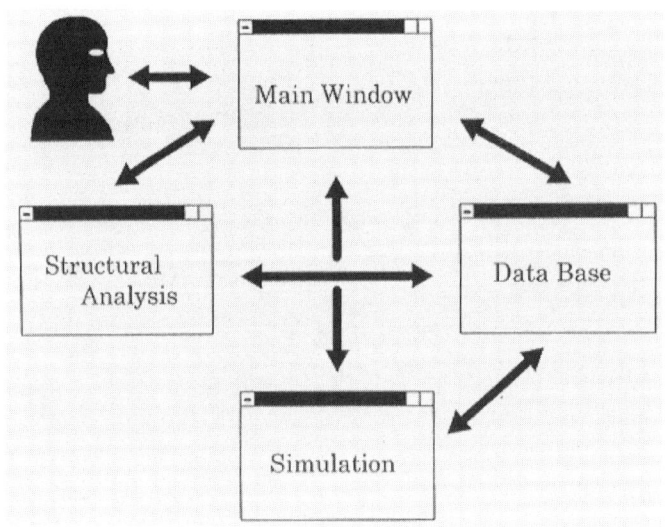

Figure 3. System configuration.

This system, written in C++ on Windows95®, on an Epson™-PC Pentium™ machine, is designed based on object-oriented concepts so that each part of the system can be written independently of and is easily accessible to other parts. The Main Window provides human interface to the other parts, each of which being selectable in the menu. It also provides information on what this system can do for users. The major function of the "Analysis" part, which is linked to the "Simulation" module, is to conduct model reduction and to allow the user to perform the "ISM". The last task means to compute any kind of hierarchy graphs, as illustrated in Figure 2(b) to (e), of a given module of *Human*, based on a specified set of thresholds for a given computation time. Moreover, the ISM indicates the maximum total gain on the path from a given input to a given output of a graph. The *Simulation* computes a time course of a chosen output of a given module with all its inputs given, as well as time courses of the outputs of the full *Human* model. The results of *Simulation* can be stored in the Data Base.

The Data Base, linked to all the other parts of the system, contains the following information about the *Human* model:

(1) a dictionary of all model variables and parameters, giving their meanings, attributes and information, for example, in which module they are initialized and computed;
(2) original correlation matrix of the full model of *Human* and original matrices of all *Human*'s modules;
(3) typical results of Analysis, i.e., reduced correlation matrices for typical 10 sets of thresholds between 0 and 0.3, and their corresponding directed graphs and skeleton graphs;
(4) temporary results of *Analysis* for a given set of thresholds; and
(5) temporary results of *Simulation*, for a given set of thresholds.

Information given in (1) helps to remodel a module by visualizing a structure of its equations, variables, and parameters.

3.2. *Human* model

The *Human* model was developed by Coleman [1] and it is a digital version of Guyton's large circulatory analog model. The model consists of over 25 physiological modules of major circulatory organs and other related functional units with over 200 variables and 60 parameters. The major 25 modules of the *Human* model are: *Control of Exercise, Pharmacology, Reflexes* – Part 1 and 2, *Cardiac Function, Heart-Reflex Interaction, General Circulation, Oxygen Balance, Carbon Dioxide Balance, Control of Ventilation, Gas Exchange, Basic Renal Hormones, Status of Kidney, Renal Excretion, Fluid Infusion and Loss, Water Balance, Sodium Balance, Acid/Base Balance, Urea Balance, Potassium Balance, Protein Balance, Volume Distribution, Blood Volume and Red Cell Mass*, and *Temperature Regulation*. An on-off switch for the artificial heart is included in the module of Heart-Reflex Interaction. In Figure 4 is shown the *Human* block diagram, consisting of 25 modules. The modules are interconnected by a directed link if at least one output variable of the one module is an input to the other.

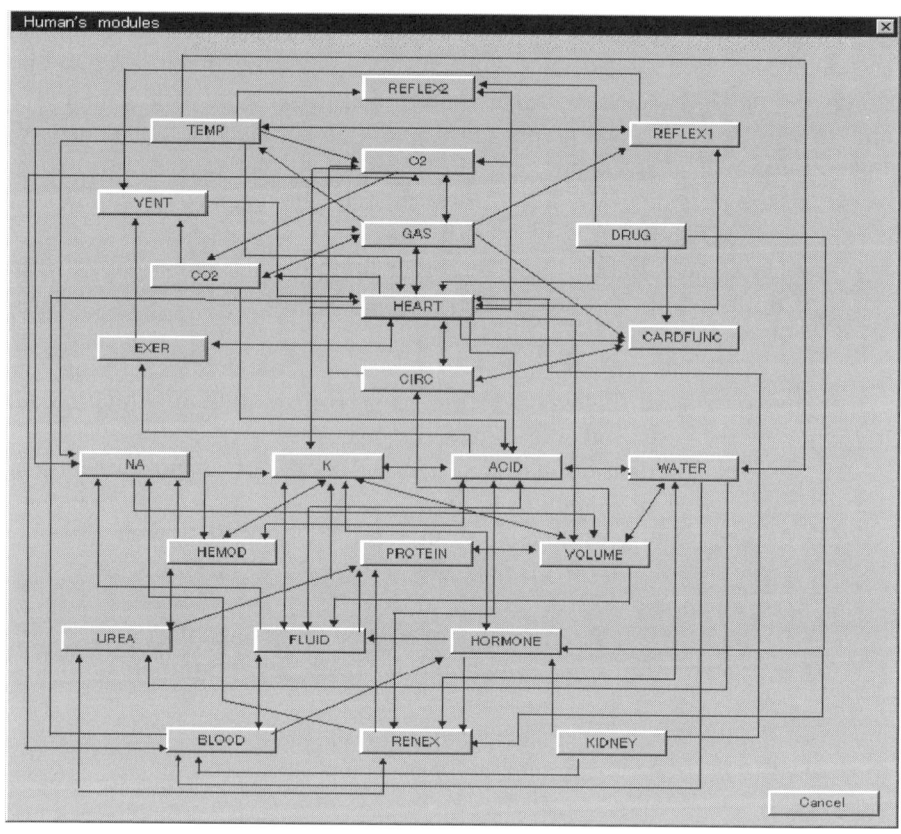

Figure 4. Block diagram of the *Human* model.

We changed the QuickBasic version by Randall [11] into a C-language version to install in the Data Base of the system. The C version takes about five seconds to simulate the processes taking place in a one-month time-period in the natural system modeled by *Human*; the simulation corresponds to a one minute sampling of the physiological processes. It was shown that *Human*'s quantitative accuracy is limited for both short [12] and long-term simulations [13], [15]. Transient tendencies in minutes of *Human*'s hemodynamic variables with the artificial hearts' switch turned on agree with animal data, according to [14]. However, heuristic adjustments of the parameters, as shown in the next section, are necessary to minimize the qualitative discrepancy between *Human* and the animal data in a long time course of over two months.

We organized a dictionary of variables and parameters of *Human* in the database, with the help of the correlation matrices of *Human* and of the modules, for easy accessibility from one variable to another. The dictionary outputs all the variables linked within a module to a specified variable, and is aimed to help consulting, besides demonstrating the definition of the variable. The original IBM-PC version of *Human* in Quick/Basic has no human interface function and consequently the user can neither know the structure of *Human*, or access definitions of variables and parameters. Definitions of variables/parameters are only listed at the beginning of the source code, in the manual [1], and in a textbook for the original *Human* [11].

4. Indirect measurement technique

4.1. Model identification

The proposed technique first estimates blood viscosity by the linear estimation technique, and then solve a set of three equations of the pump system, illustrated in Figure 5 for the mock circulation for total left atrium bypass set-up, to obtain pressure differential and flow. The three equations used for estimation of viscosity are the ones for a simple Windkessel model of a systemic circulation, a centrifugal pump, and rotating parts including the rotor of a DC-motor. They are given as follows. If the difference between left and right atrial pressures is negligible compared to ΔP, the Windkessel model is:

$$\Delta \dot{P} = -\frac{1}{RC}\Delta P + \frac{1}{C}Q \qquad (6)$$

where ΔP is the pressure differential from the intra-aorta through the pump to left atrium, Q is the output flow of the centrifugal pump, R denotes the total systemic resistance, and C is the compliance of the aorta. The equation of the centrifugal pump is:

$$\Delta P + \phi\dot{Q} + c_1 Q\omega + c_2 Q^2 = K_2 \omega^2 \qquad (7)$$

where ω is the rotation speed of the impeller, ϕ is the total inertance of the inlet and outlet cannulas, and c_1, c_2 and K_2 are viscosity-dependent parameters. This equation was obtained by the second order approximation, based on non-dimensional analysis of the relationship between pressure differential and volume flow [28]. The actuator equation is given by:

$$J\dot{\omega} + c_3\omega + c_4 Q\omega + T_R = K_1 i \qquad (8)$$

where i is the DC-motor current, J is the inertia of the whole rotating parts, c_3 and c_4 are the viscosity-dependent parameters, T_R is the dynamic friction coefficient of the rotating axis, and K_1 is the torque constant of the DC-motor. This equation is the equation of motion of the rotating parts of the pump system. The last two equations are the same as those justified for a centrifugal pump in [28].

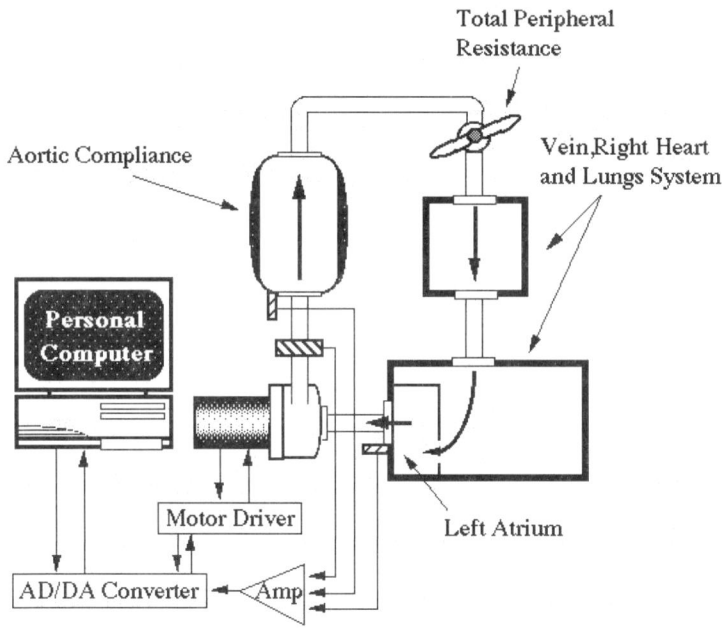

Figure 5. Schematic drawing of the mock circulation.

We carefully off-line identified the coefficients of the equations (6) and (7), dropping the derivative terms for the centrifugal pump [27]. Figure 6 shows *in vitro* data for the static ΔP-Q relationship and that of the i-Q relation using a mock circulatory loop. The *in vitro* experiments for parameter identification showed that c_1 and c_3 are viscosity-dependent, as shown in Figure 7 and Figure 8, while the other parameters can be seen as almost independent of viscosity. In these experiments, the glycerol water temperature was carefully controlled to keep the viscosity constant in the mock circulatory loop. It was verified that c_1 and c_3 were identified as linear functions of 1/8th power of viscosity ν as: $c_1 = ac_1 \nu^{1/8} + bc_1$, $c_3 = ac_3 \nu^{1/8} + bc_3$, respectively, where ac_1, bc_1, ac_3 and bc_3 can be off-line identified.

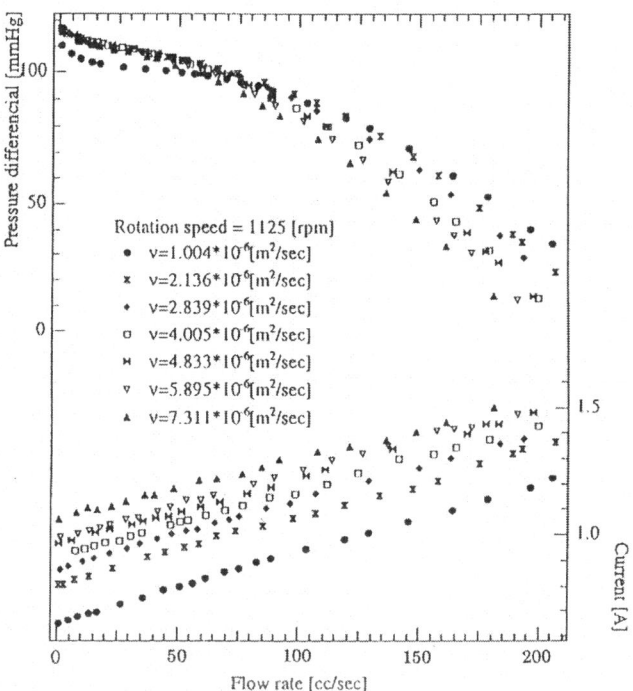

Figure 6. Static relationship of pressure differential to flow rate and that of motor current to flow rate.

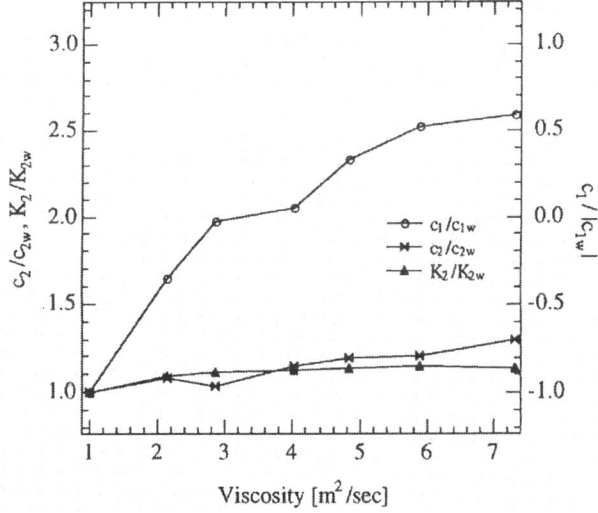

Figure 7. Relationships between the coefficients c_1, c_2 and K_2, and the viscosity; the suffix w denotes water at 20°C.

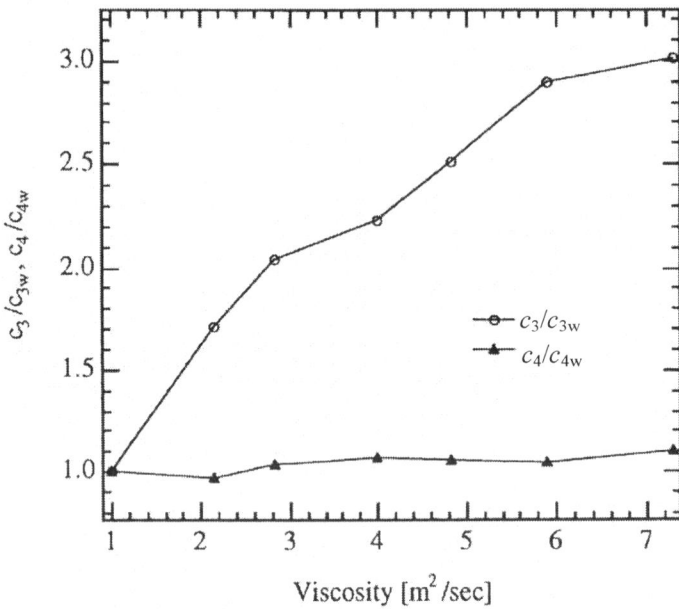

Figure 8. Relationships between the coefficients c_3 and c_4, and viscosity; the suffix w denotes water at 20°C.

4.2. Estimation technique

Estimation of ΔP and Q is made under the driving condition that the motor current i randomly forced for a specified interval of 10 seconds. Such an interval of random drive of the motor is specified about once every 2 minutes, and the blood pump is basically driven at a constant speed for other intervals. The algorithm for pressure and flow estimation is given as follows.

Step 1: Measure the motor current i and rotating speed ω, with forced random current for 10 seconds.

Step 2: Identify viscosity v, R and C in the equations (6), (7) and (8) by the on-line least square method [29] using the data of $i(t)$ and $\omega(t)$ obtained in Step 1.

Step 3: Solve the following two algebraic equations:

$$\Delta P + c_1 Q \omega + c_2 Q^2 = K_2 \omega^2 \tag{9}$$

$$c_3 \omega + c_4 Q \omega + T_R = K_1 i \tag{10}$$

with the substitution of identified ν into the equations, to obtain ΔP and Q. These two equations are obtained from (7) and (8) by equating the derivatives, dQ/dt and $d\omega/dt$, to zero.

The straightforward application of the on-line least square method provides recursive forms of the unknown parameters, ν, $1/R$ and $1/RC$. These parameters are estimated as linear estimates because the nonlinear equations (6), (7) and (8) are linear with respect to the three parameters. However, a set of standard formulas for the on-line linear estimation algorithm using an output error has to be slightly modified into the ones using an equation error for this study, because no measurement of any variables in (6) is available under long-term clinical circumstances

5. Results and Discussion

5.1. Diagnostic aids

A diagnostic problem is defined as follows: Given an output variable y, whose value is out of its normal range, find the causative parameter which reaches y with the maximum sum total gain. The sum total gain is given by summing up all gains from y to the causative parameter. Causative parameters are physiological ones included in the right side of an equation used in *Human*. They are supposed to be diagnosed as causes of an abnormal variation of an output measurement under medical examination. The sum total gain helps decide major causative parameters because the maximum gain says that they can be the most noteworthy variables related to the change of the output. *Reducing* and *Hierarchizing* features, when applied to *Human* by ISM, make it possible for the proposed support system to efficiently detect causative variables or parameters for qualitative diagnosis, as shown in this section. All the gains of each module are necessary to be computed and compared with a given set of thresholds to reduce *Human*. A common threshold to all input-output relationships of *Human* is used in this study to illustrate how the present technique works.

For carrying out diagnosis, the user specifies an output y from the pop-up menu, and then the system searches for all causative parameters which reach y. Consequently, all paths between all such causative parameters, i.e., inputs to *Human*, are shown to the user. The procedure of searching paths is given as follows:

(1) An input variable is stacked up to the list.
(2) A traceable node from the head element of the list is stacked up to the list. When the head isn't able to be traced to any other nodes, it is taken away from the list.

(3) When the head is the output variable *y*, the content of the list is recorded as a path from the input to the output.

The above procedure is continued until the list becomes empty, and the search for all possible paths is finished. The path search, however, cannot be finished if there is a loop connecting variables within a level of the hierarchy. In order to avoid this problem, any path is removed that goes through a node more than two times.

Figure 9(a) shows an example of diagnosis, in which the user needs to know causal parameters for the output variable CO2A (arterial CO2 content) in threshold $\varepsilon = 0.05$. Figure 9(b) shows a result for output AP (arterial pressure). All combinations of paths from all possible input variables are searched for in the model of the hierarchical graph structure. From the screens shown in Figure 9, the user is able to find that abnormal perturbations of both of CO2A and AP are mainly related to the positive change of BODH2O (body water) and NAMASS (extracellular sodium mass). The negative change in KCMASS (cellular protein mass) has the largest influence on both CO2A and AP. Furthermore, as shown in Figure 10, the diagnostic system can also inform about intermediate causal relations between the input and output, where an arrow indicates a causal relation included in the equations.

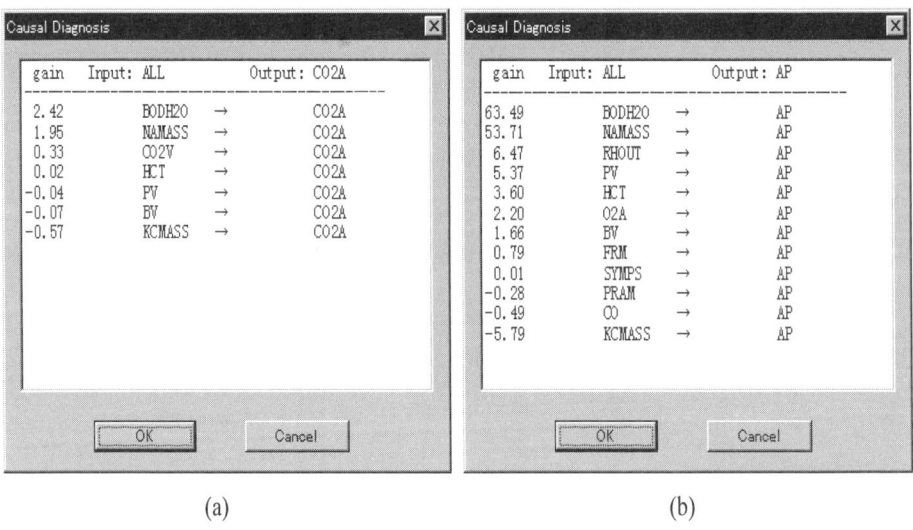

(a)   (b)

Figure 9. Results of influence diagnosis for the output variables CO2A and AP.

When the *Human* model is reduced for a large threshold over $\varepsilon = 0.1$, the total number of paths not only decreases for the same output variable, but also the computation time reduces. On the other hand, computation time of searching paths can become explosive for the reduced model with a small threshold value, because it can include more loop relations among variables. In fact, the use of a small threshold such as $0.01 < \varepsilon < 0.05$ can make diagnosis impossible, unless the model is hierarchized by ISM. Hierarchizing the model reduces the search space by determining the search direction from the bottom level to the top. Hierarchizing removes unnecessary computation for paths from each level to lower levels. Although the total number of loop relations does not change after hierarchizing, dividing the original loop relations into smaller ones within each level also helps reduce computation time. *Hierarchizing*, furthermore, helps the user to visualize the structure of relations among variables.

We compared the computational search time for all paths on the hierarchical graphs and that for their corresponding original models. In these simulations, 120 cases of appropriate input and output variables for threshold ε = 0.03, 0.04 and 0.05 are tested on Windows PC with 166 MHz Pentium Processor and 96 MB RAM. For original models, 31 cases required over 5 minutes for tracing all paths in the model. On the other hand, almost all cases required only one second for the hierarchies. For $0.01 > \varepsilon$, the computation was not finished with any present algorithm, within 24 hours, because the number of loops was explosive.

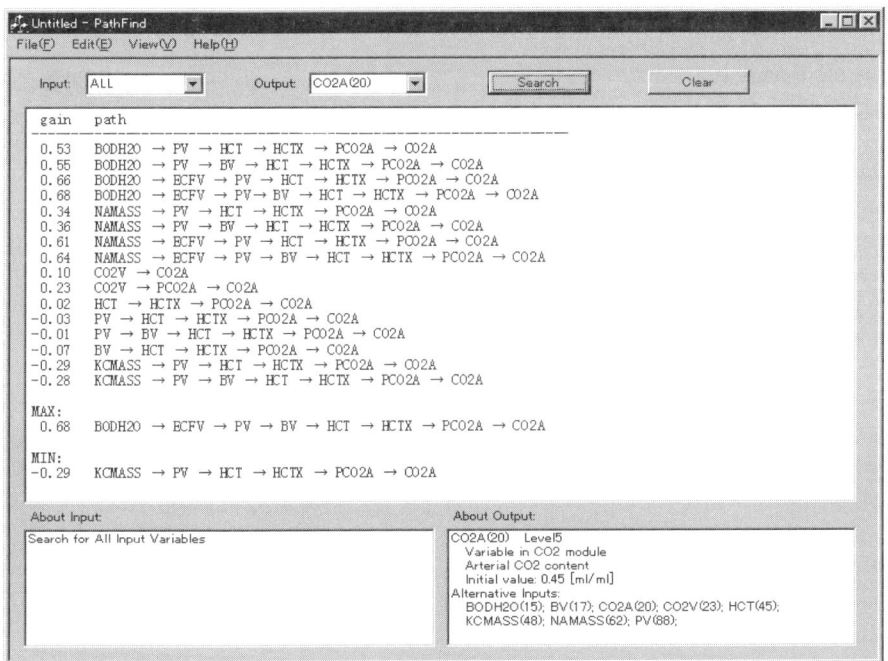

Figure 10. Sample of interface display for detecting causal relations in the *Human* model.

5.2. Analytical and modeling aids

The proposed system also provides users with analytical aids and modeling aids. Details of these aids are shown in [17]. This section briefly introduces these functions. The full *Human* model needs reduction to obtain a hierarchy because the ISM shows that all the elements of the reachability matrix made from the original correlation matrix of *Human* are one, and this means that it cannot be changed into a hierarchy. Applying the ISM to the original correlation matrix of *Human* produces Figure 11 showing a hierarchical graph for the threshold $\varepsilon = 0.07$. In this figure, accessible fixed parameters are differentiated from variables, and a module name is indicated on all the output variables belonging to the module, for better physiological understanding.

Tracing back all paths starting from MUSFLO, muscle blood flow (ml/min), at level 2 in Figure 11 tells the most influential variable to a change in MUSFLO is TEMP at level 5, body temperature, reaching MUSFLO through MMBS at level 3 and BMR at level 4 with total gain 0.3. In this search, TEMP was found out of 11 variables/parameters at the ends of 49 paths comparing total gains, where a total gain is defined as the product of all gains from MUSFLO to a variable/parameter at the end of a path. This search can tell that it is most possible that over 10% change in TEMP is a cause of over 30% change in MUSFLO.

Another computation by the Analysis showed that a path from CO to O2V, mixed venous O_2 content (ml/ml), has a high total gain of 0.25. This justifies the investigation of O2V as a promising index representing blood demand for artificial heart control. Thus, it seems useful to search for measurable variables to which CO is more influential, and to evaluate if they are better-suited indices for artificial heart control. This search should be made for as a small threshold as possible, because the number of variables kept in a reduced model increases with the threshold decrease.

The proposed system also facilitates to modify the circulatory model. A good example of this is the modification for compensation of the discrepancy between long-term experimental data for animals with total artificial hearts and results of the computer simulation by *Human*. Animal experiments with total artificial hearts of fixed cardiac outputs show that the aortic pressure gradually increases for three months [15]. However, under the same conditions as for the animal experiments, the aortic pressure doesn't change in original *Human* [13]. In the *Analysis* mode of the proposed system, clicking AP in the graph of the hierarchy for $\varepsilon = 0.07$ in Figure 11 displays a subset hierarchy including AP at a top, as shown in Figure 12. This figure shows that AP, SYMPS, and SYT are primarily connected with each other, and APAD, an instrumental variable for stable computation, is physiologically equivalent to AP in the program. In this case, because the cardiac output is constant, the

Kitamura and Asami: Artificial heart control support system

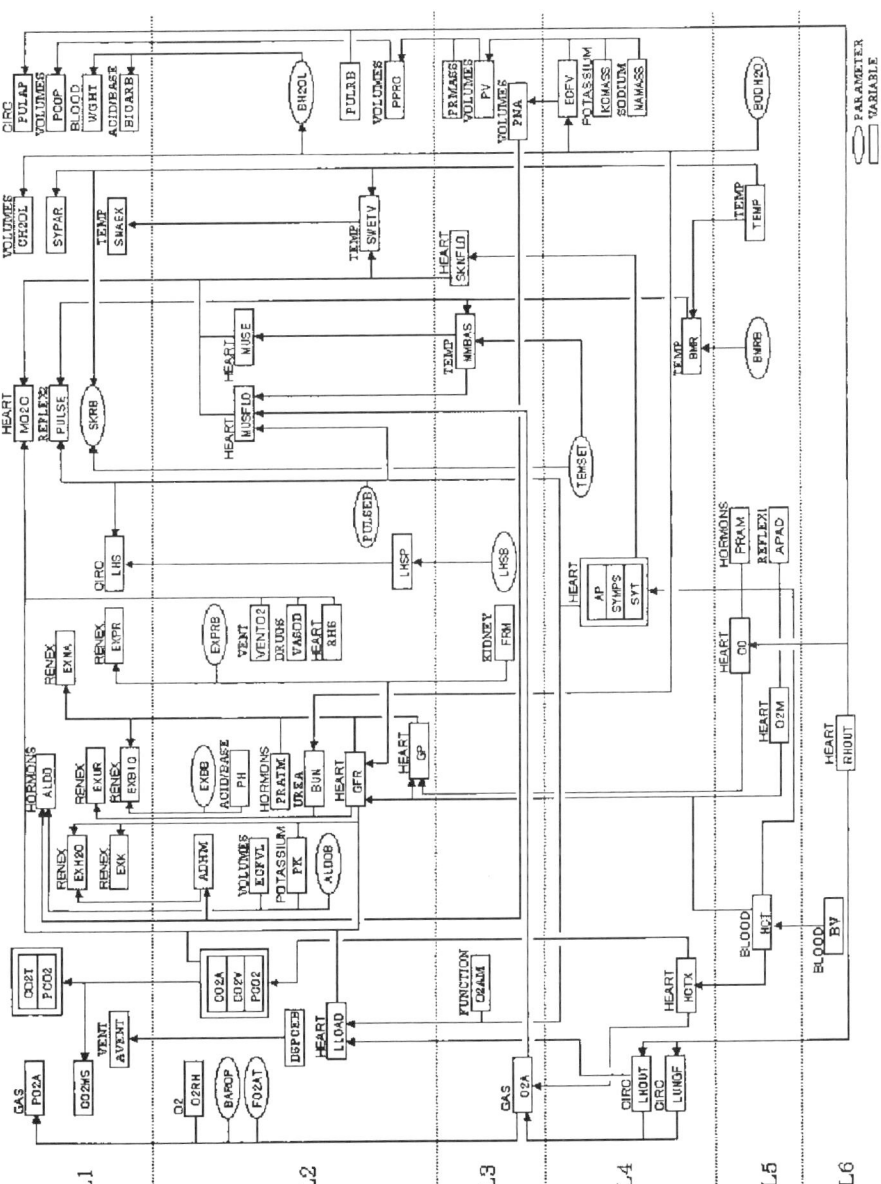

Figure 11. Hierarchy of the whole *Human*; $\varepsilon = 0.07$.

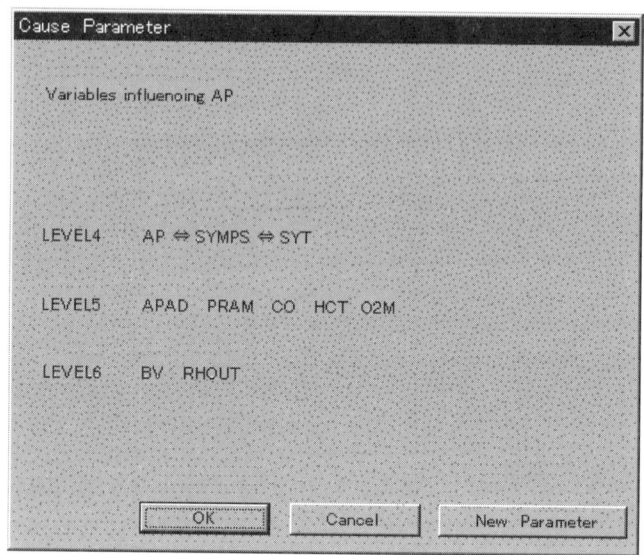

Figure 12. Hierarchy of variables influencing AP.

influences of CO at Level 5 and RHOUT at Level 6 are ignored. All the other variables at levels lower than 4 can be considered almost constant in the experiments. Consequently, we added a term RSYMPS to the equation:

$$SYMPS = PHOXYN*(SYT-0.6+PHEO)+0.6+RSYMPS \qquad (11)$$

where SYMPS is a multiplier for sympathetic nervous activity, PHOXYN is an alpha-blocker multiplier, SYT is a sympathetic total neuro-component, PHEO is a pheochromocytomia, and RSYMPS is the relative strength of sympathetic activity. The addition of RSYMPS is based on the interpretation that the sympathetic nerve activity is relatively dominant after the artificial heart operation [15].

We compared this modified full *Human* model with the results obtained in animal experiments with total artificial hearts. The comparison showed good agreement in the tendency of gradual decrease in GFR – the glomerular filtration rate (ml/min) – of the renal function, for three months [9], [16]. We used a common threshold to all input-output relationships of *Human* for simplicities in model reduction in this study. For more clinical-oriented applications, however, a set of thresholds for model reduction needs to be given depending on each input-output relationship of the module, considering results of gain computation and specific physiology of the module. Such specific physiological knowledge about each module is needed for this purpose. The present technique for model reduction will be useful for collecting information about gain analysis itself, such as information as to which input-output relationship should be removed, since this technique can easily display results of gain analysis to an expert.

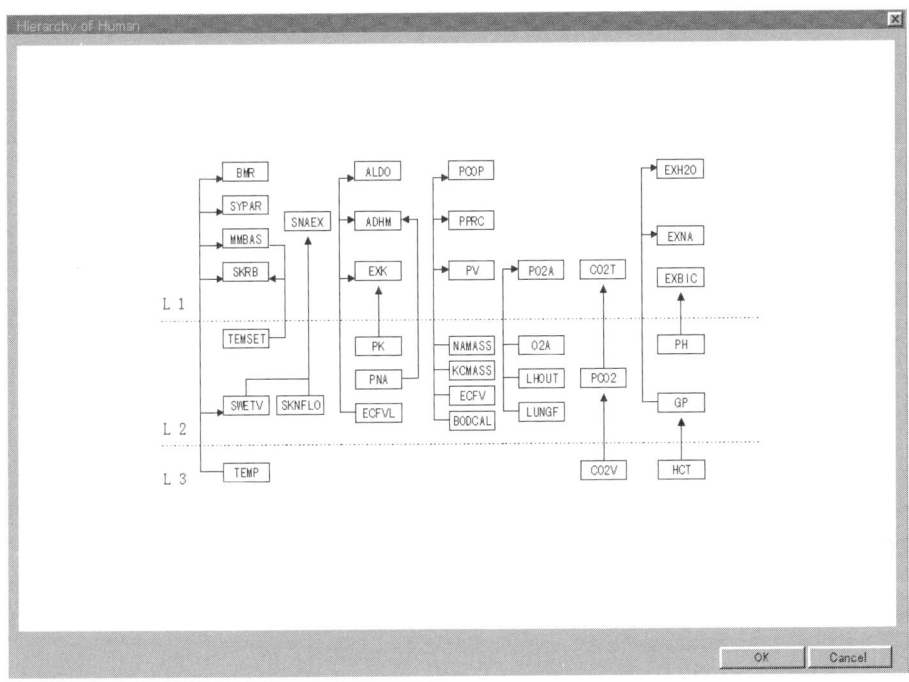

Figure 13. Hierarchy of *Human*; $\varepsilon = 0.2$.

It should be useful that comparison of a reduced model response with a full model response is made in order to find a reduced model valid and simple enough for efficient qualitative simulation. Two additional features would facilitate the Analysis to compare some models. The first function is needed to solve a search problem for an appropriate set of thresholds to which an output variable to be compared can be left in a reduced model. For instance, Figure 13 showing a hierarchy of *Human* for a uniform threshold $\varepsilon = 0.2$ misses AP, one key output in the circulatory control in the module HEART, while AP is kept in Figure 12 for $\varepsilon = 0.07$. To keep AP in a reduced model, it is necessary to find a threshold such that at least one gain in the input and AP relationship of the module HEART is not eliminated for the threshold. The present process of model reduction doesn't have this function. The second function is needed to secure an output of a reduced model. For this, we need to check the mathematical stability of the reduced model, which is a set of nonlinear differential equations. In practice, it should be based on checking the run-time of a reduced model, because a theoretical checking of stability of nonlinear differential equations is in general impossible.

5.3. Indirect measurement

In vitro tests of the estimation algorithm for control of the centrifugal blood pump were carried out using the set-up in Figure 5, with changing the systemic resistance R and viscosity. Figure 14 and Figure 15 show the correlations between actual and estimated values of the pressures differential and the pump flow, respectively. Each correlation is satisfactorily linear although the correlation becomes poor for low differential pressure. Figure 16 shows the comparisons of actual and simulated time course data to a given current. Figure 16(a) shows that viscosity converges within one second after the random current is applied. Figures 14 to 16, however, show that reliability of the proposed technique is good enough to justify the proposed indirect measurement technique. The high accuracy of the estimation in these experimental results validates the use of the mathematical models, from the DC-motor to the pump. The Windkessel model parameters are instrumental, because the derivative of ΔP is formally necessary to run the estimation technique: ΔP would be left unknown if this model were not used. In fact, identified values of R and C are deviated from their real values in most cases; at the cost of their inaccuracy, viscosity converges to its accurate value, and an accurate value of R can be computed by $\Delta P/Q$.

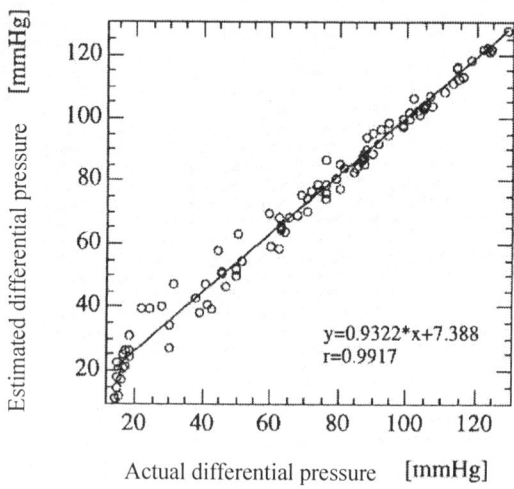

Figure 14. Correlation of actual and estimated differential pressure.

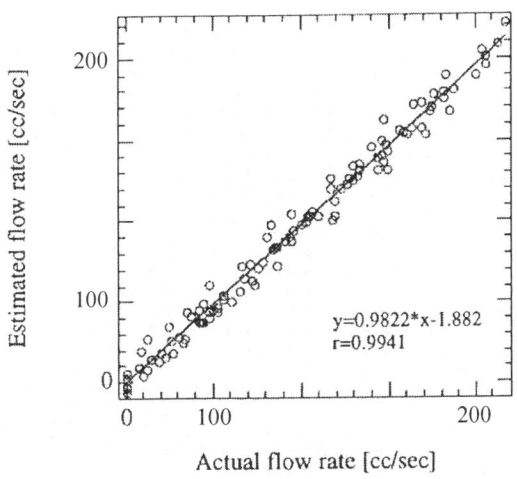

Figure 15. Correlation of actual and estimated flow rate.

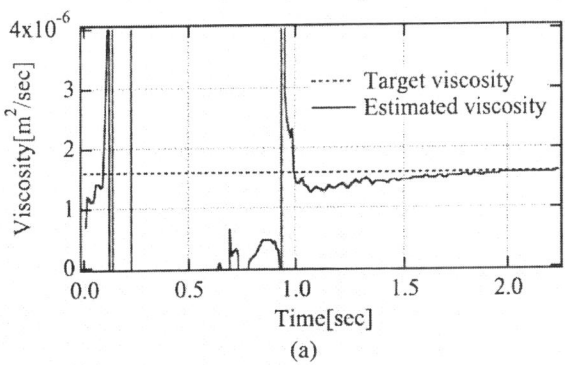

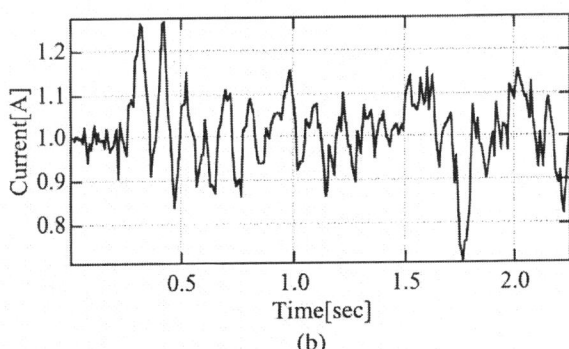

Figure 16 (continued next page).

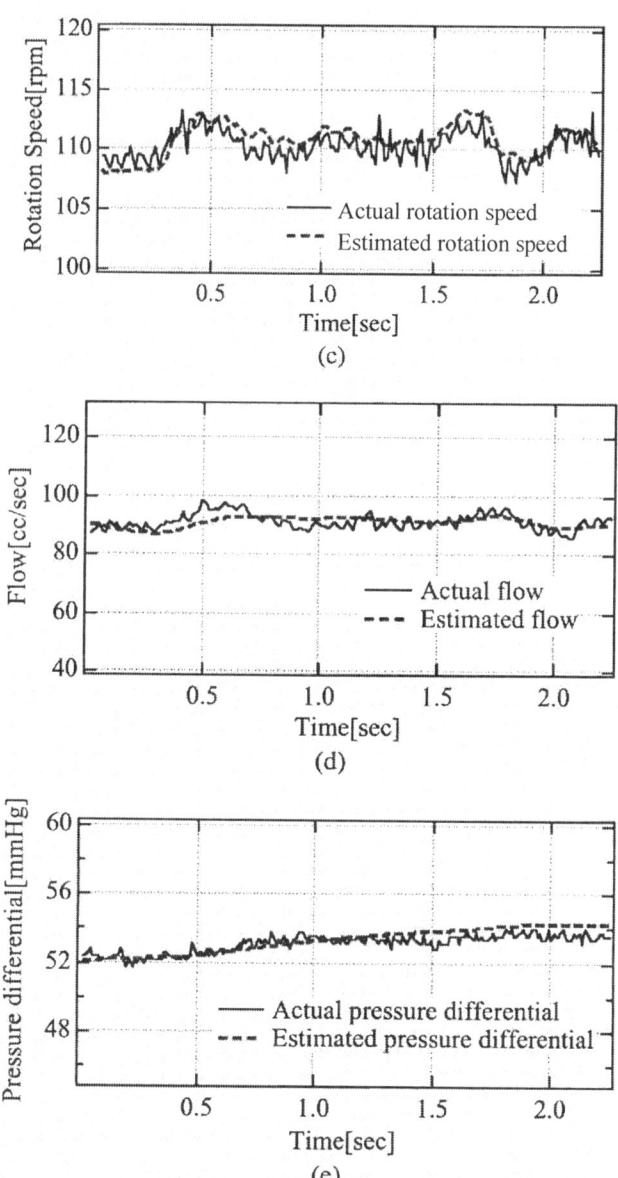

Figure 16. Comparison between actual and simulated time course data forced by random current for linear estimation *in vitro*, (a) viscosity, (b) applied random current, (c) rotation speed, (d) pump Flow, (e) differential pressure.

The Q^2-dependent pressure loss term that includes c_2 in (7) has widely been accepted to describe a pressure-flow relationship along a cannula [24], [25]. Compliance of the cannulas is ignored in the pump equation, but we suppose that this produces no significant errors in estimation [22]. All the parameters except the coefficient c_2 and inertance ϕ can be determined beforehand for an *in vivo* experiment. But these two coefficients are determined on the spot after open surgery, because they depend on their length determined to fit surgical conditions. Because cannula diameters are usually fixed independent of animals, a new technique is necessary to on-line determine these surgery-dependent parameters for the future work.

6. Conclusions

In this study, we described an intelligent diagnostic support system for use in relation to artificial hearts and based on indirect measurements of blood flow and differential pressure of a centrifugal pump. The diagnostic system uses a systems approach based on Coleman's *Human* circulatory model. The system employs two techniques, namely model reduction and ISM, and provides hierarchical graphs of input-output relations whose gains larger than a specified threshold. The indirect measurement technique makes long-term use of the diagnostic function possible.

The proposed system:

(1) enables visualization of a hierarchy graph of cause and effect relations of the large circulatory model,
(2) suggests control and diagnostic information to the model via tracing back through the hierarchy,
(3) allows a user to modify the circulatory model, and
(4) offers blood viscosity-independent indirect measurements of pump pressure differential and blood flow at a noninvasive location for the transducers.

The efficiency and performance of the proposed system demonstrates technical feasibility of on-line long-term diagnosis for circulatory control. Further work is needed to determine specific thresholds using physiological data with the on-line help of the proposed system for diagnostic support. The indirect measurement technique also needs to be tested *in vivo*.

References

[1] Coleman, T. G.: *Human Physiological Basis of a Comprehensive Model for Body Function*. (Manual.) University of Mississippi Medical Center, Mississippi, 1981.

[2] Cramp, D. G., Carson, E. R. and Leaning, M. S.: Some design features for a user-friendly computer-aided decision support system incorporating mathematical models, in *Artificial Intelligence in Medicine*, Eds. Delotto, I. and Stefanelli, M., Elsevier Science Publisher B.V., Amsterdam, pp. 11-20, 1985.

[3] Siregar, P., Sinteff, J-P., Julen, N. and Lebeux, P.: Spatio-temporal reasoning for multi-scale modeling, *Artificial Intelligence in Medicine*, Vol. 10, pp. 41-57, 1997.

[4] Kitamura, T. and Iwaya, F.: Design of a Fuzzy Logic-Based Support System for Artificial Heart Control, *Proc. 7th World Congress of International Society for Artificial Organs*, Sapporo, Japan, pp. 288-290, 1989.

[5] Kitamura, T.: Design of intelligent support system for artificial heart control, *Japanese Journal of Fuzzy Theory and Systems*, Vol. 3, No. 3, pp. 231-240, 1991.

[6] Kitamura, T.: Development of a tool for theoretical analysis in total artificial heart control. Design of a fuzzy logic-based on-line support system coupled to dynamic circulatory models, Abstracts of *Medical & Biological Engineering & Computing*, Vol. 29, Suppl. Part 2, p. 668, 1991.

[7] Kitamura, T.: Diagnostic Support System Design for Artificial Heart Control, *Proc. 14th Int. Conf. IEEE EMBS*, Paris, France, pp. 371-372, 1992.

[8] Kitamura, T.: Graph Analysis of the Coleman's Large Circulatory System Model Human for Diagnosis, *Abstracts of the World Congress on Medical Physics and Biomedical Engineering*, August, Rio de Janeiro, p. 456, 1994.

[9] Kitamura, T.: Structural analysis of a circulatory system for artificial heart control, based on the Coleman's model HUMAN, *Proc. Waseda Intl. Cong. Modeling and Simulation Technology for Artificial Organs*, Tokyo, pp. 107-108, 1996.

[10] Warfield, J. N.: *Societal Systems-Planning and Complexity*, John Wiley & Sons, 1976.

[11] Randall, J. E.: *Microcomputers and Physiological Simulation*, Raven Press, 1987.

[12] Affeld, K., et al.: *Simulierung von Regelungsproblemen beim Totalherzersatz mit Hilfe des Coleman-Kreislauf- Modells*, Springer Verlag, Berlin, pp. 308-328, 1982.

[13] Kitamura, T.: How should we use the Coleman's circulatory model "Human" for artificial heart control. In Sezai, Y. (Ed.), *Artificial Heart*, Harwood Academic Publishers, pp. 129-132, 1993.

[14] Abe, Y.: *Physiological Control of the Total Artificial Hearts -1/R Control*. Ph. D Thesis at University of Tokyo, 1994, (in Japanese).

[15] Nozawa, H., Mabuchi, K., Imachi, K., Chinzei, T., Abe, H., Yonezawa, T., Suzukawa, M., Imanishi, K. and Fujimasa, I.: The influence of total artificial heart on renal functions, *Japanese Journal of Artificial Organs (Jinko-zouki)*, Vol. 20, No. 4, pp. 1347-1356, 1991.

[16] Nagahama, Y.: *Structural Analysis Tool of a Circulatory System-Based on HUMAN*. Master Thesis, Graduate School of Computer Science, Kyushu Institute of Technology, 1997, (in Japanese).
[17] Kitamura, T.: A Computer-aided Approach to the Structural Analysis and Modification of a Large Circulatory System Model, *IEEE Trans. Biomed. Eng.*, Vol. BME 46, No. 5, pp. 485-493, 1999.
[18] Sawaragi, G. and Kawata, K. (Eds.): *Participatory Systems Approach*, Nikkan Kougyo Shinbun-Sha, Tokyo, 1981, (in Japanese).
[19] Affeld, K.: A New Method for the Intermittent Measurement of Atrial Pressure in a Pneumatic Total Artificial Heart, *Tech. Developments. Artificial Heart-A Contribution to Second World Symposium Artificial Heart*, Berlin, pp. 78-84, 1984.
[20] Rosenberg, G., Landis, D. L., Phillips, W. M., Stallsmith, J. and Pierce, W. S.: Determining Atrial Pressure, Left atrial Pressure, and Cardiac Output from the Pneumatic Driveline of the Total Artificial Heart, *Trans. ASAIO*, Vol. 24, pp. 341-344, 1978.
[21] Kitamura, T. and Gross, D. R.: On-line Pressure Estimation for a Left Heart Assist Device, *IEEE Trans. Biomed. Eng.*, Vol. 37, No. 10, pp. 968-974, 1990.
[22] Kitamura, T. and Muramasu, H.: Physical Model-Based Indirect Measurement of Blood flow and Pressures for Pulsatile Circulatory Assist-In Vitro Study, *JSME International Journal*, Series C, Vol. 42, No. 3, pp. 605-611, 1999.
[23] Eykhoff, P.: *System Identification*, John Wiley & Sons, 1974.
[24] Kitamura, T., Kijima, T. and Akashi, H.: Modeling Technique of Prosthetic Heart Valves, *ASME, Trans. Biomech. Eng.*, Vol. 106, pp. 83-88, 1984.
[25] Peskin, C. S.: The Fluid Dynamics of Heart Valves: Experimental, Theoretical, and Computational Methods, *Ann. Rev. Fluid Mechanics*, Vol. 14, pp. 235-259, 1982.
[26] Heimes, P. and Klasen, K.: Completely Integrated Wearable TAH-drive Unit, *Int. J. Artificial Organs*, Vol. 5, No. 3, pp. 157-159, 1982.
[27] Kitamura, T., Matsushima, Y., Tokuyama, T., Kono, S., Nishimura, K., Komeda, M., Kijima, T. and Nojiri, C.: Physical Model-Based Indirect Measurements of Blood Flow and Pressure Differential for Left Heart Assist Using a Centrifugal Pump, *Proc. 7th. Congress of the Int. Soc. Rotary Blood Pumps*, Tokyo, 1999, (to appear).
[28] Tsukiya, T., Akamatsu, T. and Nishimura, K.: Indirect Measurement of Flow Rate and Pressure Difference and Operation Mode of the Centrifugal Blood Pump with Magnetically Suspended Impeller, *Japanese Journal of Artificial Organs*, pp. 249-254, 1996.
[29] Young, P. C., Shellswell, S. H. and Neethling, C. G.: *A Recursive Approach to Time Series Analysis*, University of Cambridge Press, 1971.
[30] Ayre, P. J., Watterson, P. A., Lowell, N. H. and Woodard, J. C.: Sensorless flow and Head Estimation for the Ventrassist Rotary Blood Pump, *Abstracts of 7th ISRP Conference*, p. 52, 1999.

Chapter 9

Diaphragm pacing for chronic respiratory insufficiency

Harish Aiyar and **J. Thomas Mortimer**

Chronic respiratory insufficiency or the inability to independently breathe has a profound impact on the affected individual, his/her family and the health care community as a whole. The treatment of chronic respiratory insufficiency has been traditionally performed with intermittent positive pressure mechanical ventilation. Electrical activation of the diaphragm muscle, by way of the phrenic nerves, offers an alternative to mechanical ventilation, providing an opportunity for improved speech and mobility and reducing many of the problems associated with mechanical ventilation. In this chapter we present the etiology and issues involving chronic respiratory insufficiency and its treatment. In the first section we describe chronic respiratory insufficiency with specific reference to spinal cord injury and central hypoventilation syndromes. Section 2 provides some background into respiration, including its neural control and the muscles involved. In the third section we present diaphragmatic pacing, its history, present status, advantages and disadvantages. The fourth section deals with alternative treatments for chronic respiratory insufficiency. The chapter ends with some conclusions with regards to the treatment of respiratory insufficiency and points to future directions.

1. Respiratory insufficiency

Respiration is generally an involuntary act to efficiently supply the body with oxygen while relieving it of carbon dioxide. This mechanism aims to maintain arterial P_{O_2}, P_{CO_2}, and pH levels within a small range even as the body's respiratory requirements fluctuate through sleep, wakefulness, rest and exercise. Voluntary and involuntary activities of daily living such as talking, eating and coughing also require complex neural control of respiration. In chronic respiratory insufficiency (CRI), this control mechanism is disrupted, resulting in profound, long-term, systemic changes.

The etiology of CRI, or the inability to independently breathe, may be congenital, idiopathic, traumatic, iatrogenic or secondary to disease. In many cases, this condition is temporary, and the individual regains respiratory function. In others, it is permanent and the resulting load, physical, emotional as well as social, that is placed on the individual, his/her family and the health care system in general is enormous. At present, there are a number of different approaches used to supplement or maintain adequate ventilation including pharmacologic, rehabilitative, surgical, mechanical, and prosthetic. Of these, either invasive or non-invasive intermittent positive pressure mechanical ventilation is the most widely used and recognized treatment modality. Prosthetic systems that aim to restore or augment function (e.g., phrenic or diaphragm pacers) have also been used for both part-time and full-time ventilatory support. These phrenic nerve pacing systems, so termed because they electrically activate the phrenic nerves to elicit diaphragmatic contraction for respiration, have been used over the past 25 years in over 1,000 patients worldwide [1-7].

The two main clinical indications for phrenic nerve pacing have been cervical spinal cord injuries and central hypoventilation syndromes. Although both of these conditions manifest in the individual's inability to independently breathe, spinal cord injury involves the disruption of the signal pathway from the respiratory center in the brain to the respiratory nerves (primarily the phrenic nerves) whereas central hypoventilation syndromes generally involve a decreased respiratory drive. In the latter case, the signal from the respiratory center to the phrenic nerves is not generated or sent although the conduction pathway to deliver the signal is intact.

1.1. Spinal cord injury

A major cause of CRI is high cervical spinal cord injury (SCI). Spinal cord injuries are usually secondary to motor vehicle accidents, falls, recreational sporting activities (e.g., diving) or the result of acts of violence [8, 9]. A traumatic injury to the spinal cord results in a loss of function below the level of injury. The "neural drive" to generate the control signal still exists, but the conduction pathways to deliver this signal from the brain to the target muscle(s) have been disrupted. An injury to the spinal cord at the level of C1 to C5 (cervical spinal levels 1 to 5) impacts on the ability of an individual to independently maintain both involuntary and spontaneous respiration. The degree of this impact is highly dependent on the exact level of the trauma. The lower motor neurons of the phrenic nerves originate in the spinal cord at the level of C3, C4 and C5 [10]. If the injury is above C3 or above the origin of the phrenic nerve roots, the lower motor neurons and the phrenic nerves are usually left intact. But, in these cases, the pathway from the medullary respiratory center in the brain to the phrenic nerves has been disrupted. Because function is lost below the level of the injury, this individual no longer has control of the diaphragm and the accessory respiratory muscles (e.g., internal and external intercostals, abdominal muscles). This individual is likely to be CRI, requiring some sort of artificial, full-time ventilatory support. An injury to the cord at the C3-C5 level may disrupt respiration, depending on the extent and severity of the injury. Although functional use of the accessory respiratory muscles is lost, depending on the extent to which the lower motor neurons of the phrenic nerves are damaged, control of the diaphragm muscle may still be intact. These individuals may retain some respiratory function and only need part-time ventilatory support, if any. Damage to the cord below C5 usually does not result in damage to the phrenic nerves, but still affects "normal" respiration. In this case, the phrenic nerves activate the diaphragm, but many of the accessory muscles involved in inspiration and expiration are not activated because the nerves that control these muscles originate below the level of injury, e.g., from the thoracic vertebrae for activation of the intercostal muscles [10].

The number of SCI individuals living in the United States is estimated to be between 183,000 to 230,000 with an annual estimated incidence of 40 cases per million population (or approximately 10,000 new cases per year). This does not include those who do not survive the acute post-injury phase [9, 11]. This number is expected to increase due to advances in acute emergency medical treatment and widespread knowledge of cardiopulmonary resuscitation techniques. Because of its poor mechanical stability, injuries to the cervical spinal cord (C1-C8) resulting in tetraplegia [12, 13] are more prevalent, with complete and incomplete tetraplegia accounting for 18.6% and 29.6% of this population, respectively. With the average age of injury being 31.7 years, the average life expectancy for high tetraplegia (C1-C4) is approximately 56 to 60 years (for those surviving at least one year post-injury). The average life expectancy of ventilator dependent individuals (any level of injury) is approximately 46 to 54 years [9, 11] (see Table 1). Initial costs (health care and living expenses) that are directly attributable to SCI for a high tetraplegic average $529,675 for year one with an average $94,878 for each subsequent year (in 1998 dollars). Based on a life expectancy of 30 years post-injury, the total cost that is directly related to the SCI is approximately $3,376,015 [9, 11]. Not only is there a large variation between levels of SCI (e.g., tetraplegia and paraplegia), there is variation within the levels as well. In estimating the "cost" of respiratory dependence, Whiteneck approximated the cost of care for two groups: high tetraplegics who were ventilator dependent ($n = 24$) and those who could sustain voluntary ventilatory control ($n = 76$). Although there were large variations in cost between individuals, the expenses of the ventilator dependent group averaged approximately three times those of the ventilator independent group for both initial and follow-up care (in 1989 dollars, Initial Costs: $426,592 vs. $150,698; Follow-up Costs: $141,238 vs. $38,512) [14]. These figures do not include any indirect costs including losses in wages, fringe benefits and productivity that vary substantially based on education and pre-injury employment history. Berkowitz et al. estimated that only 35% of the total aggregate costs of SCI to society were direct costs, while 65% were indirect costs [15].

The survival and re-integration of these patients is a great challenge. This is illustrated by the fact that by post-injury year 10, only 23.1% of patients with tetraplegia are employed (including both CRI individuals and those able to breathe on their own) [9]. Where individuals live post-injury is also an indicator of re-integration. As of April, 1999, 91.7% of all persons with SCI (including paraplegia and tetraplegia) who were discharged from a Model SCI Care System were sent to a private residence (primarily their place of residence prior to the injury) [11]. In a study involving 19 SCI patients requiring full-time mechanical ventilation, Carter et al. reported that 6 months post-discharge from their first rehabilitation admission, 10 patients or 52.6% lived at home [16].

Based on data compiled from the National Spinal Cord Injury Data Base, Carter estimated that 4.2% of spinal cord injuries result in long-term to permanent CRI [17]. High tetraplegics outside of this apneic group (C3-C5) may or may not retain respiratory function. These individuals fall into one of two categories: 1) post-injury, the level of injury descends or 2) there is no change post-injury. In the first case, as the level of injury descends, the level of function increases. Those who were originally CRI immediately post-injury may regain control of the phrenic nerves and thus the diaphragm muscle. Early motor recovery may occur with the resolution of spinal cord edema [18] or recovery from neurapraxia [19]. This could take anywhere from days to months. In the latter case, if there is no change in the level of injury, the individual will remain CRI and require some sort of artificial ventilatory support. In one 16 year study involving 107 high level spinal cord injured patients (level of injury was C1 to C4), 31% (or 33 cases) presented diaphragmatic paralysis at the time of injury [20]. Recovery of diaphragm function was seen in seven of these patients between 40 and 393 days (mean 143 days) post-injury. These patients were weaned from ventilatory support. Diaphragmatic recovery was seen at a later stage (between 84 and 569 days post-injury; mean 290 days) in five additional patients. However, these patients remained at least partially dependent on mechanical ventilation [20].

Assuming there are 400 (approximately 4.2% of 10,000 cases per year) high cervical spinal cord injuries (C1-C3) each year in the United States who would suffer from CRI, the direct costs of care of these "new" injuries would total nearly $212 million annually. This figure does not include the annual costs of care for the nearly 8,000 individuals with high tetraplegia and CRI, nor any indirect costs associated with either group.

Table 1. Life Expectancy Following Traumatic High Cervical Spinal Cord Injury

Age at injury	For those who survive the first 24 hours			For those surviving at least 1 year post-injury		
	NO SCI	High Tetra (C1-C4)	Ventilator dependent at any level	NO SCI	High Tetra (C1-C4)	Ventilator dependent at any level
20 years	56.8	32.7	15.3	56.8	36.2	26.5
40 years	38.2	18	6.9	38.2	20.7	13.7
60 years	21.1	6.5	1.1	21.1	8.1	4.1

Data from National Spinal Cord Injury Statistical Center (NSCISC).

1.2. Central hypoventilation syndrome

Central hypoventilation syndrome (CHS) is characterized by the absence or failure of the involuntary central respiratory drive and hypoventilation resulting from inadequate response to hypoxia and/or hypercapnia in the absence of any chest wall and lung parenchymal deformities or respiratory muscle weakness [21-24]. The extent and severity of CHS varies significantly between individuals. Some may be able to supplement breathing during the day with voluntary ventilation. However, during quiet sleep, when involuntary control of breathing is predominant, the effects of CHS may be more pronounced. Thus, CHS is also known as central sleep apnea or Ondine's curse, after the German mythological figure. This term, however, has fallen into disfavor in recent years [22].

The etiology of CHS is unknown, but may be congenital, idiopathic, iatrogenic or traumatic. It may be secondary to injury to the medullary respiratory center resulting from central nervous system infection, tumor, infarction, lesion or stroke. The condition may be observed in association with central nervous system malformations (e.g., Chiari II malformation) or metabolic disease (e.g., Leigh disease). This condition is relatively uncommon as patients with central sleep apnea constitute less than 10% of the patients in most sleep laboratories [23].

Depending on the severity of the condition, patients may require part- or full-time ventilatory support. If only part-time support is needed, a non-invasive approach (e.g., nasal BiPAP) may be employed. A more severe condition that mandates full-time ventilatory support may necessitate a more invasive, "permanent" treatment such as intermittent positive pressure ventilation requiring a tracheostomy. In one study concerning congenital CHS in children, the incidence of mechanical ventilatory support during sleep was 83% and the frequency of tracheostomy was 80% [25].

2. Respiration

To help in understanding the concept and operation of diaphragm pacing systems and their limits, we present in this section an introduction to respiration, its neural control and the involved muscles. The reader familiar with respiratory physiology may skip this section.

Respiration, both involuntary and voluntary, is the end result of a coordinated action of a number of muscles including the diaphragm, internal, parasternal and external intercostals, scalenes, sternocleidomastoids, abdominal muscles and the muscles of the upper airway. The coordinated contraction of these muscles causes pressure changes in the thoracic and abdominal cavities that result in the movement of air into and out of the lungs. These pressure changes must be sufficient to overcome two intrinsic opposing forces: the elastic recoil of the chest and the airflow resistance. The elastic recoil arises from the elastic properties of the lung parenchyma and the surface tension at the alveolar gas-liquid interface. The airflow resistance accounts for the pressure needed to overcome the frictional and viscous forces in the airways [26].

The neural pathways that control this mechanism are illustrated in Figure 1. Involuntary or metabolic respiration primarily depends on the brain stem and on peripheral and central chemoreceptors whereas voluntary or behavioral respiration is mainly under cortical control [24]. In both spinal cord injury and central hypoventilation syndromes, some point of the neural pathway from the brain to the target muscle(s) has been disrupted or is malfunctioning.

Involuntary respiration is controlled by the respiratory control center in the medulla. This control center consists of two groups of neurons known as the dorsal and ventral respiratory groups (DRG and VRG). Afferent signals from the brain, the peripheral and central chemoreceptors and receptors within the lungs and upper airway are integrated in the DRG and VRG with the output relayed to the target muscles and organs (e.g., the lungs) via the spinal cord. The DRG elicits a response from the diaphragm muscle and the VRG from the accessory respiratory muscles [24]. The central rhythm generator, contained within the DRG, initiates the signal that triggers breathing. The rate of this stimulus is influenced by the chemoreceptors and the receptors of the lungs. The peripheral chemoreceptors, consisting of the carotid and aortic bodies, respond primarily to changes in arterial P_{O_2} and pH. These receptors are responsible for the increase rate of ventilation seen as a result of hypoxia. The central chemoreceptors located in the medulla respond primarily to changes in P_{CO_2} and, to a lesser degree, pH. An increase in P_{CO_2} results in an increase in the rate and depth of breathing. The receptors within the lungs and upper airways are influenced by lung inflation, airway tone and mechanical and chemical stimulation of the airways. These receptors, via the vagus nerve, deliver information to the DRG, where it is interpreted along with the signals from the peripheral and central chemoreceptors to maintain homeostasis [24, 27].

Voluntary or spontaneous respiration is controlled by the cerebral cortex and uses neural pathways that are separate from involuntary respiration. The voluntary stimuli bypass the medullary respiratory control center and interact directly with neurons in the spinal cord. This interaction overrides the involuntary respiratory signal to a point. For instance, one is able to hold his/her breath for prolonged periods of time — even though the P_{CO_2} levels have increased beyond the threshold to trigger the DRG to instigate a breath [27].

Normal respiration depends on the coordinated effort of both the involuntary and voluntary neural pathways. The motor neurons within the brainstem and upper cervical spinal cord receive the signals from the cerebral cortex, the DRG and VRG, interpret the information and elicit the appropriate response from the respiratory muscles.

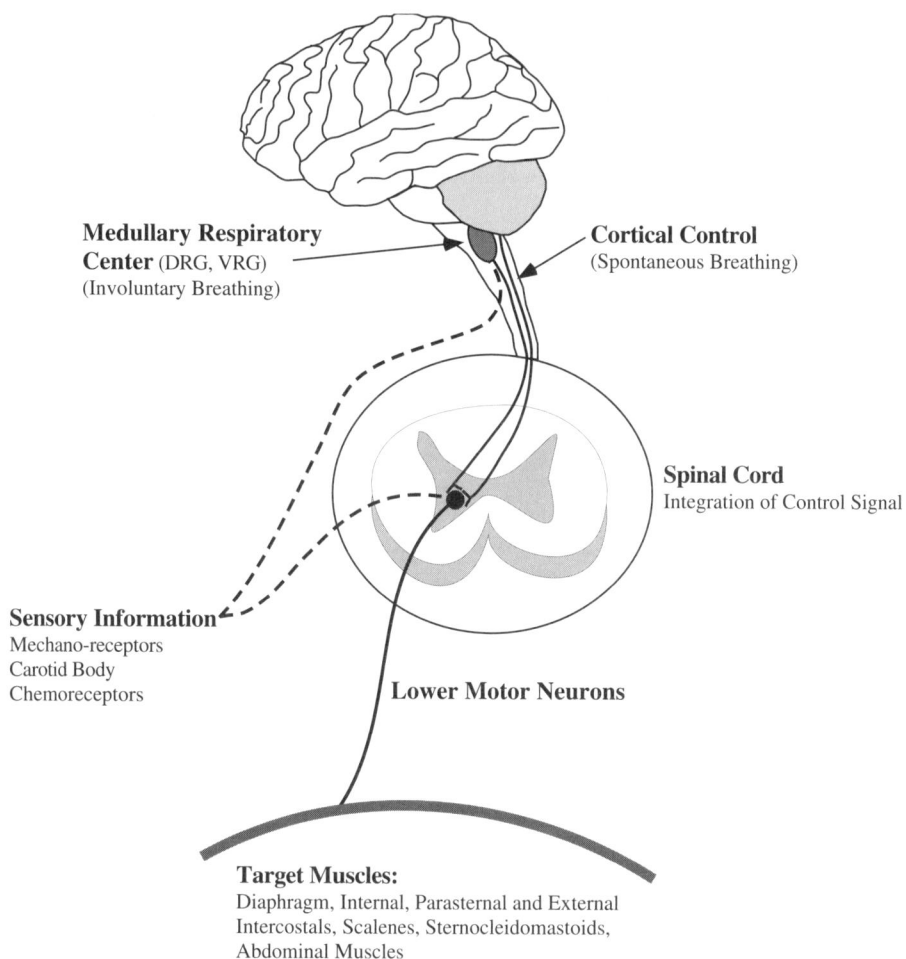

Figure 1. Neural control of respiration.

2.1. Primary muscles

Diaphragm

The diaphragm is the main inspiratory muscle. It is a muscular sheath that separates the thoracic and abdominal cavities. Its contraction accounts for nearly 70% to 80% of the air that inflates the lungs during quiet breathing [28]. The diaphragm can be divided structurally and functionally into two distinct parts: the costal and crural diaphragm. These two parts are essentially two separate muscles, with different actions, evolutionary and embryologic origins and segmental innervation [29, 30]. The contraction of the diaphragm increases the vertical dimensions of the thorax. How this occurs is the end result of the coordinated actions of the costal and crural diaphragm. The costal diaphragm consists of fibers that originate from the costal margin and the inner surfaces of the lower six ribs (sternum) and insert into the central tendon. Because its fibers are predominately aligned axially and apposed to the rib cage (the area of apposition), the costal part exerts its action on the rib cage and the abdominal cavity. As the fibers contract, they produce an upward force on the ribs while exerting a downward force on the central tendon and abdomen, forming the diaphragmatic dome, displacing the abdominal wall outward and increasing intra-abdominal pressure. This increase in pressure results in an expansion of the lower rib cage through the zone of apposition [28, 31]. The crural diaphragm consists of fibers that originate from the lumbar vertebrae and the medial and lateral arcuate ligaments and also insert on the central tendon. With no direct attachment to the ribs, it exerts its action primarily on the abdominal cavity by producing a downward force on the central tendon. As with the costal diaphragm, this downward force on the central tendon results in an increase in abdominal pressure thus moving the abdominal wall outward, and, through the area of apposition, acts to expand the lower rib cage. Simultaneously, through the expansion of the lower rib cage, costal and crural diaphragm muscle contraction causes a decrease in pleural pressure that results in an influx of air into the lungs. The fall in pleural pressure has an opposite effect on the surface of the upper rib cage. It opposes the action of the costal and crural diaphragm, resulting in a decrease in the diameter of the upper rib cage. Although the diaphragm is primarily an inspiratory muscle, this inward movement of the upper rib cage has an expiratory effect. The net result on the rib cage, abdomen and lungs depends on the sum of three forces: 1) the upward force on the lower rib cage by the costal diaphragm, 2) the downward force on the abdomen through the central tendon by the costal and crural diaphragm that results in an increase in lower rib cage expansion, and 3) the fall in pleural pressure caused by the change in abdominal pressure resulting in a deflating action on the upper rib cage [32-34].

The diaphragm muscle is unique in that it is a skeletal muscle that is required to function rythmically from birth until death. This is analogous to walking continuously without rest. The duty cycle (or ratio of active to inactive times) for the diaphragm muscle is between 40% to 45% [35]. The duty cycles for cat hindlimb skeletal muscles range from 1.9% for the extensor digitorum longus (predominantly fast twitch, Type II muscle) to 13.9% for the soleus muscle (predominantly slow twitch, Type I muscle) [36]. The intrinsic properties of the diaphragm muscle make this possible. The diaphragm is a composite of three types of muscle fibers: 55% of the fibers are Type I (slow twitch, fatigue resistant, high oxidative), 21% are Type IIA fibers (fast twitch, fatigue resistant, high oxidative) and 24% are

Type IIB fibers (fast twitch, fatigueable, low oxidative − glycolytic) [34, 37]. When activated, Type I fibers develop a slow rise in force whereas Type II fibers reach an optimal level of force rapidly, and, thus, are more prone to fatigue. During quiet breathing, the diaphragm is only working at 10% maximum force production capacity. Only a portion of the nerve fibers (thus muscle fibers) are activated − generally the Type I, slow twitch fibers. With increasing ventilatory demand, the Type I, IIA and IIB fibers are recruited sequentially [35]. The stimuli from the nerves are distributed among the fibers, allowing individual fibers a "rest" period between stimuli. This randomized recruitment along with the distribution of muscle fiber types allows the muscle to compensate for the varying metabolic demands placed on it by the body.

During normal, quiet breathing, the costal and crural diaphragms act in parallel. Thus, the forces produced by their contraction is additive. This is not the case at high lung volumes at which time the diaphragmatic dome is flattened [33, 38]. In this orientation, the fibers of the costal and crural diaphragm are directed perpendicular to the rib cage. As the fibers align themselves more radially rather than axially, the area of apposition decreases. This results in an increase in intra-abdominal pressure and an outward movement of the abdominal wall but, since the area of apposition has decreased, a decrease in the lower rib cage diameter. The absence of the outward motion of the lower rib cage and the decrease in upper rib cage diameter caused by the decrease in pleural pressure add to result in a net decrease in the rib cage diameter. In this manner, hyperinflation of the lungs may significantly affect diaphragm function. As the diaphragmatic dome descends, the muscle fibers become shorter and develop less force due to the force-length characteristics of the muscle. The force created by the diaphragm during contraction (inspiration) is measured through the transdiaphragmatic pressure gradient (P_{DI}) which is the difference between the abdominal pressure (P_{ab}) and the pleural pressure (P_{pl}) [39-41]. P_{DI} is generally measured through two balloon catheters: one placed in the esophagus (P_{pl}) and one in the stomach (P_{ab}). In normal persons, P_{DI} ranges from 10 to 20 cm H_2O during quiet breathing. In patients with severe obstructive pulmonary disease, where the functional residual capacity is increased mimicking the situation described, the P_{DI} is approximately 6 cm H_2O [42].

Neither the costal nor crural diaphragms play a major role in expiration. During quiet breathing, expiration is a passive process. As the muscles relax, the elastic recoil of the chest wall and lungs returns the abdominal and pleural pressures to their resting values.

Although it is primarily a respiratory muscle, the diaphragm does serve other functions. The rhythmic abdominal pressure changes corresponding to each breath (and muscle contraction) play a role in facilitating venous return to the heart. Under voluntary control, the muscle can be forcefully contracted to greatly increase intra-abdominal pressure to assist in the evacuation of pelvic organ contents (urine, feces, or a baby). The increased intra-abdominal pressure also serves to stabilize the trunk and spine to prevent flexion during the lifting of heavy weights.

The left and right phrenic nerves provide innervation for the left and right hemidiaphragms, respectively (see Figure 2). These nerves originate in the cervical plexus from the third, fourth and fifth cervical spinal roots. Studies have suggested that in as many as 76% of people, additional contributions to the nerve join the main nerve trunk in the chest several centimeters below the level of the clavicle [43]. The nerves descend bilaterally, crossing over the anterior surface of the anterior scalene muscle, through the thorax to activate the diaphragm. The nerves also play a role in transmitting sensory information from the muscle to the brain [44]. Just prior to entry into the diaphragm muscle, the nerves tri-furcate into three phrenico-abdominal branches (anterior, lateral and posterior), with each branch servicing a region of each hemidiaphragm [45]. An additional branch is sometimes present [46]. Neither the point(s) of entry nor the branches are visible from the abdominal side of the muscle. Although the distribution of the nerve fibers in the diaphragm muscle is not precisely known, the costal diaphragm is thought to be innervated by roots from C3 and C4, whereas the crural diaphragm is innervated by roots from C4 and C5 [28, 47]. During quiet breathing, there is incomplete activation of the phrenic nerves, and thus, the diaphragm. This allows for the muscle and nerve to recover between stimuli. Also, this "dormant" period serves as a reserve in the event of increased ventilatory demand. The motor neurons of the phrenic nerve can be divided into early and late firing units, depending on when they fire during inspiration. Evidence that supports this is that, in normal breathing, there is sequential activation of the crural diaphragm before the costal diaphragm [48-51]. Using the Henneman size principle, smaller diameter neurons are fired before larger diameter fibers [52, 53]. There may be more early firing units activating the crural part. As respiration increases, the frequency and number of firing units increases. The separate neural control over the costal and crural diaphragms is evidenced in other activities such as swallowing and vomiting where crural diaphragm activity is modulated [54]. However, when the phrenic nerves are activated through non-physiological means (e.g., electrical stimulation), both the costal and crural parts of the diaphragm contract [34, 35].

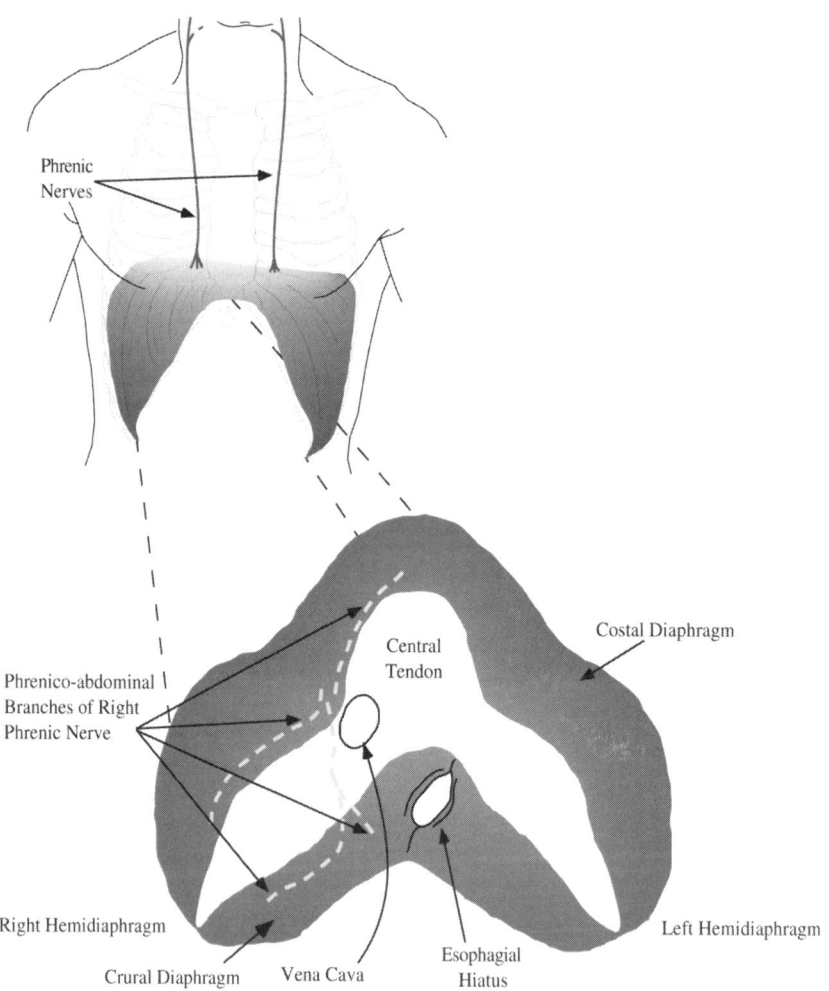

Figure 2. Inferior (abdominal) view of the diaphragm.

Internal, Parasternal and External Intercostals

The outer two layers of the anterolateral wall of the thorax are formed from a group of antagonistic muscles: the internal, parasternal and external intercostal muscles (see Figure 3). As these muscles contract, they draw the ribs together. The thoracic cage is composed of twelve pairs of ribs that attach to the thoracic vertebrae and, either directly or indirectly, to the sternum through costal cartilage. The 11 pairs of internal, parasternal and external intercostal muscles lie between the ribs, with their origins on the inferior border of the rib above and their insertion on the superior border of the rib below. The fibers of the external and parasternal intercostals are aligned obliquely from rib to rib (downward and forward). As these muscles contract, the ribs are pulled towards one another to elevate and increase the anterior-posterior dimension of the rib cage. Although the parasternal intercostal muscles are active during quiet breathing, there is debate over the role of the external intercostals in quiet breathing. This muscle group may play a more significant role with increased ventilatory demands. The fibers of the interosseus part of the internal intercostals run perpendicular to the external intercostals (downward and posteriorly). As they contract, the ribs are drawn together. However, because of their orientation, the internal intercostals act to depress the rib cage. The ventral rami of T2-T12 form the intercostal nerves that innervate the internal, parasternal and external intercostal muscles. These nerves run along the costal groove on the inferior border of each rib. Neural control over these nerves (and muscles) comes from the medullary respiratory center. This is complicated by the fact that the nerves supply the internal, parasternal and external muscles and these muscles have both inspiratory and expiratory actions [10, 28, 34, 51, 55].

Scalenes

The scalenes are a group of muscles that have their origins on the transverse processes of the lower five cervical vertebrae and insertions on the first two ribs (see Figure 3). Unlike many of the accessory respiratory muscles, the scalenes are active during quiet breathing. Control over these muscles is supplied through the cervical nerves originating from C2 to C7. Because of the orientation of both of these muscle groups, their contraction will result in the elevation and expansion of the upper rib cage and inspiration [28, 55].

2.2. Accessory muscles

Sternocleidomastoid

The sternocleidomastoids along with the scalenes are the major respiratory muscles of the neck (see Figure 3). The sternocleidomastoid is a two-headed muscle with its origin on the manubrium of the sternum and medial portion of the clavicle and its insertion on the mastoid process of the temporal bone. It is the primary head flexor. Cranial nerve XI innervates the muscles bilaterally. With increased ventilatory demands, these muscles tend to lift the sternum and increase the anterior-posterior diameter of the upper rib cage [10, 28].

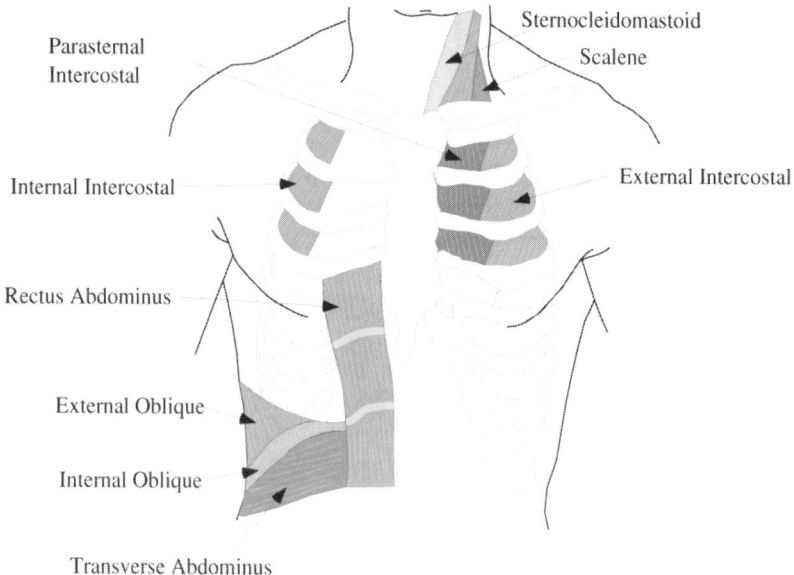

Figure 3. Accessory respiratory muscles.

Abdominal Muscles

The abdominal respiratory muscles include the external and internal obliques and the rectus and transverse abdominus (see Figure 3). Together, these muscles along with their aponeuroses form the anterolateral wall of the abdomen. These muscles are aligned in layers, with each adjacent layer at opposing angles. This orientation provides strength in contraction. The nerve supply to these muscles is from the thoracic nerves (T6-T12) with additional contributions from the lumbar nerves (L1) [10, 28, 51]. These muscles are mainly viewed as expiratory muscles that augment the passive recoil of the chest wall during deep and forceful breathing, but play a significant role in cough [56], in the evacuation of abdominal/pelvic organs and inspiration as well. Contraction of these muscles increases intra-abdominal pressure and, to an extent, fixes and depresses the lower ribs. As intra-abdominal pressure increases, the abdominal viscera are pushed cephalad. This decreases end-expiratory lung volume and increases end-expiratory diaphragm muscle length. The lengthened muscle is in a more favorable point in its length-tension curve allowing for a stronger contraction during the following inspiration. The resting tension of the abdominal muscles does play an inspiratory role in that it supports the abdominal viscera against the diaphragm muscle (thus maintaining the "dome" shape of the diaphragm) and facilitates an increase in abdominal pressure with each diaphragm contraction. Without this resting tension, the abdominal wall would tend to protrude outward instead of providing a fulcrum for diaphragm contraction during inspiration [28].

Upper Airway Muscles

The muscles of the upper airway that are involved in breathing include the posterior cricoarytenoid, the alae nasi, genioglossus and the muscles inserting on the hyoid bone. Contraction of the cricoarytenoid muscle opens the laryngeal aperture and decreases upper airway resistance. A similar effect is seen as the alae nasi, genioglossus and the muscles inserting on the hyoid contract. Contraction of these muscles dilates the upper airway passages [57]. Upper airway muscle activation is synchronized with respiration to provide an open passage for the movement of air to and from the lungs. The onset of neural activity to these muscles precedes activation of other respiratory muscles. This difference in onset of activation is believed to prevent airway obstruction. Further, inadequate activation of these muscles has been implicated in snoring and obstructive sleep apnea [58-60].

2.3. Inspiration and expiration

Even during quiet breathing, most of the respiratory muscles are active. Although the diaphragm is the primary muscle of inspiration, the accessory muscles play an important role in stabilizing the chest wall. This enables the system to run more efficiently. For instance, if the diaphragm alone is activated for inspiration, its contraction would decrease pleural pressure and increase abdominal pressure. Also, because no rib cage muscles are active, a paradoxic inward movement of the upper rib cage is seen which is an expiratory movement [33]. By adding accessory muscle activation, the rib cage is supported and the inward movement caused by the diaphragm contraction is counter-balanced by the contraction of the parasternal and external intercostals. Thus the paradoxical inward movement of the upper rib cage is no longer seen. As ventilatory demand increases, the diaphragm and the accessory muscles are activated to a greater extent.

3. Diaphragm pacing systems

Electrical activation of the nervous system has been used to restore and/or augment lost sensory and motor function in patients with central nervous system impairment or injury [61]. Systems for restoration of motor function include upper extremity prostheses for reaching and hand grasp [62], lower extremity prostheses for standing and stepping [63], and stimulation of the sacral anterior roots for bladder and bowl control [64]. Restoration of sensory functions includes stimulation of the auditory nerve for hearing [65] and electro-cutaneous stimulation for sensory feedback [66]. These systems have made a significant impact on and have improved the quality of life for many individuals.

With respect to respiration, the idea of stimulating the diaphragm muscle (or the nerves that supply the muscle – the phrenic nerves) has existed conceptually for centuries. Cavallo first proposed using electrical stimulation as a means of artificial respiration in 1777 [37, 67, 68]. In 1783, Hufeland proposed applying stimulation to the phrenic nerves of asphyxiated newborns. This technique was later used by Ure in 1818 to produce diaphragmatic contractions in a recently hanged criminal. In 1857, von Ziemssen demonstrated the first use of this technique for resuscitation in a patient who had been gas poisoned. Over the next 50 years, a number of groups including Boulogne, Remak, and Israel demonstrated the effectiveness of stimulation of the phrenic nerves/diaphragm in assisting or restoring respiration [37, 69].

Although phrenic stimulation was recognized as a means of treating respiratory insufficiency, the technique received little attention and use until the middle of the twentieth century. In 1948, Sarnoff and co-workers at Harvard coined the phrase "electrophrenic respiration" and began work on prolonged phrenic nerve stimulation (upwards of 52 hours with stimulation of one phrenic nerve) in both animals and humans. In these experiments, normal levels of gas exchange and tidal volumes were demonstrated [70-72].

The prospect of long-term stimulation of the phrenic nerves to support ventilation only became a clinical reality in the 1960s with the introduction of a radio frequency (RF) transmission system developed by Dr. William Glenn and colleagues at Yale University.

Since then, diaphragm activation through electrical stimulation of the phrenic nerves has been achieved through the use of nerve electrodes, intramuscular electrodes, and epimysial electrodes. Although nerve electrodes have a more widespread clinical use, there are important advantages to the use of other electrode configurations.

3.1. Prerequisites for diaphragm pacing

Regardless of the electrode configuration, phrenic pacing requires the availability of intact phrenic nerves, lungs, and diaphragm muscle. Functional assessment of each of these must be carried out prior to implementation of a pacing system. Phrenic pacing is not appropriate for primary neuromuscular disorders that affect the diaphragm, primary phrenic nerve injury, or severe pulmonary disease. Phrenic nerve viability can be determined through transcutaneous stimulation [73, 74]. Using landmarks such as the clavicular head of the sternocleidomastoid muscle as a guide, a thimble or needle electrode can be used to direct stimulation to the area where the nerve is presumed to be. If the nerve is intact, every stimulus will result in a "twitch" or contraction of the diaphragm muscle. Failure to elicit a response or inconsistent results may contraindicate pacing. Measuring phrenic nerve latency or conduction time can also provide insight into the viability of the nerves. This is done through stimulation of the phrenic nerves in the neck as described previously and measuring the diaphragmatic contraction with two surface electrodes (one placed near the xiphoid process and the other placed over the costal margin of the diaphragm in the 7th or 8th intercostal space on the anterior axillary line). The difference in time between the onset of stimulation and the corresponding muscle contraction is the phrenic nerve conduction time or latency. In normal adults, the latency is between 6 to 9 ms. A latency <15 ms may still indicate pacing [75-77]. Advantages to these two techniques are that they are non-invasive. However, they are not always accurate. In quadriplegics, the nerve may conduct properly but little or no diaphragm contraction may be seen. This may be due to post-deprivation diaphragm atrophy due to prolonged dependence on a mechanical ventilator [78]. The only true measure of nerve viability is through direct nerve stimulation. However, even with this approach, there has been a report of a case where the nerves could not be identified or found during a surgical procedure [79].

Besides the phrenic nerves, the chest wall, lungs, and diaphragm must be "intact." Diaphragm muscle function can be determined using fluoroscopy. A 4-5 cm descent should be seen with each hemidiaphragm on voluntary inspiration or, in the case of spinal cord injury, in response to a supra-maximal train of stimuli applied to the ipsilateral nerve. Disuse atrophy of the diaphragm muscle is not a contraindication for pacing. A sleep study and pulmonary function test may provide additional information (e.g., evidence of obstructive sleep apnea, CO_2 and O_2 saturation levels, respiratory rate, and heart rate) [37]. Additional considerations that should be evaluated in considering a patient as a candidate for a pacing system include a stable home environment and support system and an experienced health care team.

3.2. Nerve electrodes

Over the past 25 years, phrenic nerve or diaphragm pacing with nerve electrodes has been used to treat over a 1,000 patients worldwide with various types of chronic respiratory insufficiency, including high cervical quadriplegia, idiopathic central alveolar hypoventilation and lesions of the brain stem [1-7]. Much of this is attributable to the pioneering efforts of Dr. William Glenn and colleagues at Yale University. Since then, groups in Finland and Austria have developed pacing systems based on different electrode designs and stimulation techniques. All of these systems have both intracorporeal and extracorporeal components. Internal components include the implanted stimulating and indifferent electrode(s) and receiver/stimulator(s). An external, battery powered controller generates the power and control signal that is delivered to the implanted receiver through the skin via radio frequency (RF) pulses. An external antenna (connected to the controller) transmits the RF pulses that are received by an internal antenna (usually built into the implanted receiver/stimulator). The receiver converts the RF signal to an electrical signal that is then output to the electrodes. As such, there are no components piercing the skin. To date, three commercial systems are available for diaphragm pacing: Avery Laboratories (USA), Atrotech (Finland) and MedImplant (Austria).

Avery System

The systems developed by Glenn and co-workers and Avery Laboratories are widely used among the commercially available diaphragm pacing systems. The systems (Avery I-107A and I-110A) employ a "stimulating" nerve electrode, a remote "return" or indifferent electrode (Avery I-107A only) and an implantable receiver/stimulator that is controlled and powered by an external unit through a series of radio frequency transmitted pulses. One electrode and stimulator are required for each paced nerve, so, in order to achieve bilateral stimulation, two systems must be implanted. The latest system, Avery I-110A, replaced the well tested Avery I-107A in the early 1990's. The Avery I-107A experienced premature failure resulting from poor hermetic sealing and is no longer available. Stimulator failure was generally seen between 1.5 and 5 years post-implant [1, 78, 80]. The Avery I-110A which was adopted from a pain control application has overcome the sealing problems of its predecessor but has not been clinically tested to the extent of the I-107A [37, 80]. Preliminary data indicate that the Avery I-110A should last the lifetime of the patient [78].

The present system uses a half-cuff (180°, monopolar) electrode as the interface with the nerve. The half-cuff replaced the full-cuff (360°, bipolar) electrode used previously. The full-cuff electrode has been implicated in phrenic nerve injury, possibly by exerting abnormal pressures on the nerve and from circumferential scaring. Comparing the two electrode configurations, the half-cuff design exhibited the lowest risk of injury to the nerve [79]. However, there is some risk that the half-cuff electrode and nerve may be separated, which would require increased stimulation currents to achieve full nerve activation. The full-cuff design is indicated in cases where the patient has an implanted cardiac demand pacemaker [78].

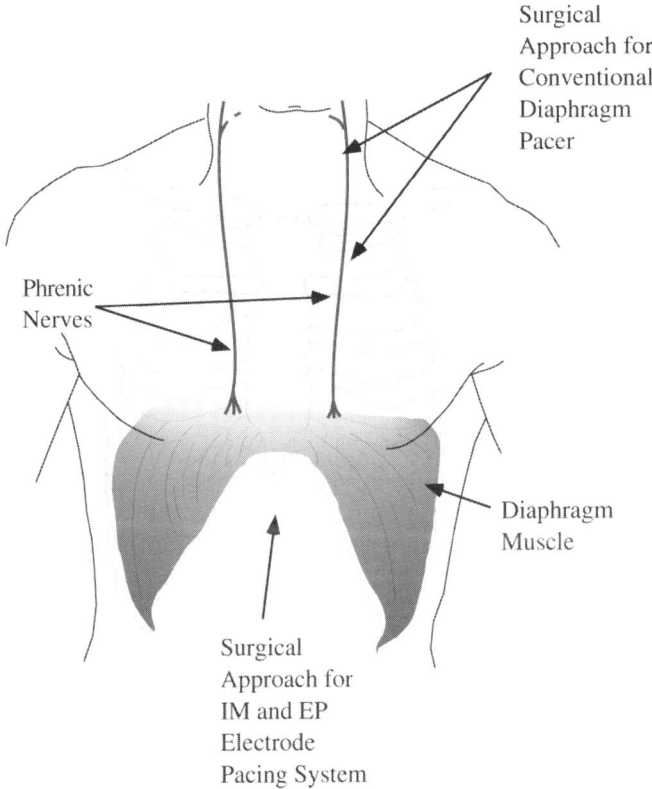

Figure 4. Surgical approach for implantation of diaphragm pacing systems. The conventional approach is in the neck or chest. An alternative approach is through a laparoscopy with intramuscular (IM) or epimysial (EP) electrodes.

The Avery electrodes are placed adjacent to the phrenic nerves in the neck or thorax, with the latter being the preferred approach (at least by the group at Yale) [37] (see Figure 4). Although the cervical approach avoids a thoracotomy, it is usually not used due to anatomic variations (e.g., the nerve maybe intramuscular in the scalenus anticus) [37], a higher incidence of infection (with its proximity to the tracheostomy), accidental activation of nearby nerves (with its proximity to the brachial plexus resulting in painful contractions of the upper limbs) [3] and failure to recruit all of the spinal contributions to the nerve [81]. For implantation in the chest, a three to four inch incision is made in the second or third intercostal space on the anterior chest wall. The phrenic nerve is visualized. A test probe is used to verify its identity (by watching for a diaphragm twitch in response to a stimulus). A section of the phrenic nerve overlying the mediastinum is exposed and mobilized. The electrode is placed behind the nerve so that the nerve rests in the half-cuff platinum contact of the electrode. Once in place, the silastic tabs on the electrode are sutured to the pleura to prevent migration. The lead wire from the electrode is tunneled subcutaneously to a flat region of the anterolateral lower rib cage where the implantable receiver and, for the Avery I-107A, an indifferent/return electrode are placed. The receiver for the Avery I-110A has an integrated return electrode that eliminates the need for an additional remote return electrode [78].

Atrotech System

The Atrotech system (Jukka Astrostim) also uses a nerve electrode that is connected to an implanted receiver/stimulator that is controlled and powered by an external unit [80, 82]. As with the Avery system, one electrode and stimulator are required for each paced nerve. Consequently, in order to achieve bilateral stimulation, two systems must be implanted. The Atrotech nerve electrode is a quadripolar design consisting of two connected strips of Teflon matrix, each containing two electrode contacts. One strip is placed in front of the nerve and the second behind the nerve. There is a 5 mm longitudinal separation between the two strips. Stimulation is directed longitudinally along the nerve between the four contacts so that one contact acts as the cathode with a contact 5 mm along the nerve and on the opposite strip as the anode. So, although all four contacts are used as cathodes, the sequential stimulation of only one contact at any given time is intended to mimic the natural activation of the phrenic nerve where only a portion of the nerve fibers are activated for each breath. This stimulation paradigm is thought to reduce or avoid diaphragmatic fatigue. Also, because the four contacts serve as cathodes and anodes, there is no need for a remote indifferent electrode.

The surgical placement of the Atrotech system is similar to that of the Avery system. The thoracic approach is preferred as it avoids potential complications of the cervical approach. Also, it affords more space for implantation (as the Atrotech electrode is larger than the Avery electrode). The main difference between the two is to place and fix the part of the electrode that lies on top of the nerve. The lead wires from the electrode are tunneled subcutaneously to an area on the lower rib cage where they are connected to the implanted receiver/stimulator.

MedImplant System

Similar to the Atrotech approach, the MedImplant system uses a group of electrodes/contacts to activate regions of the nerve [83, 84]. Unlike the Avery or Atrotech systems, the MedImplant system requires only one receiver/ stimulator for bilateral stimulation. The MedImplant system employs an epineural electrode with four loops (each 0.8 mm in diameter). The loops are sutured to the epineurium of the phrenic nerve with 8-0 Prolene suture through microsurgical techniques. Each loop or contact activates a region of the nerve. Also, the four contacts are activated sequentially by a technique called "carousel stimulation". Carousel stimulation changes the combination and sequence of contacts that are used as the stimulating and return elements with each breath (allowing for up to 16 combinations for each nerve). The resulting asynchronous recruitment of muscle fibers mimics natural neural activation and may reduce muscle fatigue [80].

Mayr and colleagues are developing a fully implantable pacing system similar to a cardiac pacemaker. This system would be similar to the present MedImplant system, but without the external controller [83].

Alternative Nerve Electrodes

Kimura and colleagues have developed an electrode and implant technique that would avoid the mobilization of the phrenic nerve, thus reducing the potential risk of nerve damage resulting from surgical manipulation. A carbon fiber electrode was developed that is attached to the nerve using fibrin glue. The surgical approach for implantation of this electrode is similar to the nerve electrodes described previously. The electrode is fixed on the nerve with moderate strength, allowing for removal if necessary. In studies in dogs, these electrodes demonstrated favorable properties for diaphragm pacing [85].

Diaphragm Pacing with Nerve Electrodes

Diaphragm pacing using nerve electrodes has made a significant contribution to the livelihood and quality of life of its users. Over the past 25 years, over 1,000 patients worldwide have been implanted with one of the three commercially available pacing systems. Twenty-five patients have been paced for at least 15 years [78]. The increased mobility, improved speech, and reduced hospital care afforded by the diaphragm pacing system(s) certainly make it an attractive and viable treatment option. Long-term follow-up of the pacing systems show that tidal volumes were maintained without decrement and that the stimulus parameters remained stable.

Comparing bilateral transvenous phrenic nerve pacing (using nerve electrodes) to positive pressure mechanical ventilation, Ishii et al. concluded that respiratory control by phrenic nerve pacing is hemodynamically superior to positive pressure ventilation [86].

Furthermore, phrenic nerve stimulation resulted in nearly a 20% increase in cardiac output (in both animals and humans). Because diaphragm pacing is a form of "negative pressure ventilation" and more closely resembles physiologic breathing, it poses less barotrauma danger to the lungs and may decrease pulmonary vascular resistance. In many cases, the tracheostomy, which is usually present in patients with a pacing system, may be plugged, at least temporarily, with a tracheal button. This may reduce potential complications including tracheal stenosis and malacia. Other advantages of diaphragm pacing include: improved speech, fewer secretions in the airway and therefore less risk of aspiration and no need for artificial humidification because the natural airway passages are no longer bypassed (when the tracheostomy is closed either surgically or with a button). In one study comparing artificial ventilation by way of a phrenic nerve pacer and a positive pressure mechanical ventilator, Esclarin et al. found fewer bronchial secretions and a lower incidence of respiratory complications (e.g., pneumonia and atelectasis) [87]. Diaphragm pacing is also less intrusive (both in space and sound) and results in quieter ventilation that appears more like normal breathing [81, 88].

Diaphragm pacing has afforded select patients who would otherwise be confined to a mechanical ventilator greater autonomy. With the proper supportive care, patients are able to live more independently, remain ambulatory during the day, attend college/school, maintain full- or part-time employment and travel. One review of outcomes of 165 patients at different medical centers showed that 64% lived at home, 23% lived in a hospital setting, 13% lived in a rehabilitation center and <5% lived in a nursing home. Of these patients, 42% were at least moderately active (e.g., working, in school), 16% were retired and 39% were inactive [79]. Pacing has had a significant impact on children and infants with central hypoventilation syndrome who require ventilatory support during wakefulness. As the children are not hindered by connection to a portable mechanical ventilator, they are more mobile and have more "normal" lifestyles and improved quality of life [25].

Although there has not been any study to determine whether diaphragm pacing improves life expectancy, with respect to high quadriplegia, Carter et al. reported a 63% survival at 9 years post-injury in patients treated with positive pressure ventilation [16, 17]. In one series of patients implanted at Yale University, 12 out of 12 patients were alive at 9 years post-implant [80].

When considering quality of life, phrenic pacers have made a significant positive impact on not only the patients but their families as well. The size and sound of the pacer, its aesthetic appearance and its portability all enable the patient to regain some semblance of a "normal" life. The overwhelming majority of patients implanted with phrenic pacers are satisfied with their decision and the system [16, 67, 80, 88-91].

Diaphragm Pacing with Nerve Electrodes - Disadvantages

Despite the clinical advantages associated with diaphragm pacing, it has seen relatively little use in only a carefully selected group of patients. Most patients with chronic respiratory insufficiency can be effectively treated by simpler techniques, e.g., positive pressure mechanical ventilation. There are a number of factors that play into this decision including risk of nerve injury, system components, risk of component/system failure, asynchronous stimulation, the required rehabilitation and risk of diaphragm muscle fatigue, obstructive sleep apnea and cost.

Because the implantation of any of the pacing systems involves mobilization of the phrenic nerve(s), there lies an inherent risk of damaging the nerve either by surgical manipulation or by the electrode. In one review by Glenn et al. of their experience with the Avery system, 7.2% of the nerves were judged to have sustained some sort of surgically related injury, with 4.9% sustaining some lasting damage [79]. In the same study, compromised nerve function was judged as probably electrode related in 7.8% (full-cuff) and 5.7% (half-cuff) of the nerves at risk. Although the cause of this injury was not known, the two main indications were abnormal pressures exerted on the nerve by the electrode and chemical irritation caused by the electrode (e.g., as a result of the ethylene oxide that had been used to sterilize the electrodes) [67, 79]. The lowest risk of injury as a result of the electrode was found to be with the half-cuff design implanted through a thoracic approach [79]. Using the half-cuff electrode (instead of the full-cuff design), the group at Yale has not seen any problems of this type in the last 10 years [90].

Unlike a cardiac pacemaker, present day phrenic pacers require extracorporeal components including a controller, power source and transmitting antenna to transmit both the power and control signal to an implanted receiver/stimulator. This is done through inductive coupling through the skin. If the coupling between the two antennae is lost (e.g., by the movement of the external antenna), the signal is no longer transmitted and stimulation is stopped. Much like disconnection from a ventilator, such an occurrence would have catastrophic consequences. The power supply is perhaps the biggest hurdle to overcome in order to eliminate the extra-corporeal components of present day diaphragm pacing systems. Unlike the heart that only requires a single twitch stimulus for complete contraction, the diaphragm muscle requires a train of pulses applied in rapid succession. This stimulus requirement and system use impact on the lifetime of the power supply. Present day diaphragm pacing systems use an *external* power source whose battery life is measured in hundreds of hours compared to cardiac pacemakers whose battery life may be well over 10 years [78]. Both improved battery technology and stimulus waveforms are necessary before any fully implantable diaphragm pacing system can be developed.

System component failure, both internal and external, is another complication associated with present pacing systems. This is of particular interest as these are life-sustaining devices. Although external components can be readily and easily replaced, internal component failure usually requires surgical intervention. Internal component failure is most likely either electrode lead wire breakage or stimulator/receiver failure. In one series of 34 pediatric patients, lead wire breakage was seen in 18% of the patients. Stimulator malfunction with the Avery I-107A was generally seen within the first five years post-implant. This generally was the result of poor hermetic sealing that resulted in the ingress of fluid [1].

At present, none of the systems have any feedback or timing mechanism to make them physiologically responsive or synchronized with the upper airway or accessory respiratory muscles. Attempts have been made to develop a demand phrenic pacemaker using end-tidal carbon dioxide as the "trigger" [92]. The ala nasi muscle has also been investigated as a potential trigger. The neural activity of the ala nasi, the muscle responsible for flaring the nostril, slightly precedes the onset of inspiration. Since patients with high cervical spinal cord injury still have control over this muscle, its activity could be used to "initiate" inspiration [59, 93, 94]. A diaphragm pacer with feedback control of the pacing rate has been developed and tested in animals [95]. This device used the animals' heart rate and body (arterial blood) temperature to vary the pacing rate to match changes in metabolic demands.

With prolonged disuse (e.g., following injury), the diaphragm as with any skeletal muscle undergoes atrophy. This change must be reversed in order for successful pacing to ensue. A gradual conditioning program is necessary to not only reverse diaphragm atrophy but to also "train" the muscle against fatigue. Muscle fatigue is generally defined to be a loss of force generating ability, which is reversible with rest [28]. The "normal" diaphragm muscle is a composite of three types of muscle fibers: 55% Type I slow twitch, 21% Type IIA fast twitch fatigue resistant and 24% Type IIB fast twitch fatigueable [34, 37]. With normal physiological activation (from the brain through the phrenic nerves to the muscle), Type I, IIA and IIB fibers are recruited sequentially based on ventilatory demand. Moreover, even with maximal contraction, not all of the fibers are recruited. This mechanism allows for fiber recovery following activation and avoids fatigue. However, with electrical activation (by way of a diaphragm pacer), the recruitment order is reversed. Thus, the muscle fibers that fatigue the fastest are activated first. Also, depending on the stimulus (electrode and stimulus waveform), all of the fibers may be recruited simultaneously. Without a recovery period and with prolonged stimulation, the muscle undergoes fatigue. Present pacing systems use various stimulus paradigms, electrode designs and conditioning protocols to both train the diaphragm and avoid muscle fatigue. In select patients, unilateral pacing may be sufficient. In these cases, pacing may be alternated from side to side, thus providing adequate ventilation while allowing for a muscle recovery. The electrode designs of the Atrotech and MedImplant systems attempt to circumvent the problem of muscle fatigue by applying the stimulus to a different region of the nerve with each breath. This approach attempts to mimic "normal" diaphragm activation [82, 84]. The diaphragm muscle is capable of adapting to changes in activation [35, 96]. Muscle conditioning relies on this adaptation mechanism to convert the muscle from a mixed fiber type composition to one with predominantly Type I slow twitch fatigue resistant fibers. The conditioning protocol usually involves assessing the strength and fatigue-resistance of the muscle periodically (every one to two weeks) to determine the appropriate stimulus parameters. Pacing is administered slowly at first (e.g., 15 minutes/hour). As the muscle adapts, the pacing time (minutes per hour and hours per day) is gradually increased until full-time pacing while avoiding fatigue is accomplished. This process may take anywhere from a couple of weeks to several months, depending on the degree of atrophy and the condition of the muscle prior to pacing [37, 67, 79, 97, 98].

A phenomenon seen with diaphragm pacing is obstructive sleep apnea (OSA). This results from the vigorous contraction of the muscle with each stimulus in the absence of upper airway or accessory muscle support (see Section 2). One approach to bypass OSA is to time the pacing stimulus with upper airway muscle activation. The presence of a tracheostomy avoids OSA by providing a patent, artificial airway. Thus, a tracheostomy, which is usually already present in individuals with CRI, is indicated with pacing and is used during sleep. Interestingly, there have been reports of individuals who use the pacer full-time and have had their tracheostomy closed permanently [78].

The cost of present pacing systems appears to be a deterrent to their use. Although the initial cost of the system, its implantation and associated rehabilitation costs have decreased (to nearly $100,000), it is still substantially higher than the alternative – a mechanical ventilator ($17,000). This initial cost should be recovered over the long run if institutional care (e.g., discharge from an intensive care unit to a less costly environment) and rehabilitation costs and cost of care (e.g., cost of disposable supplies for a mechanical ventilator) as well as indirect costs associated with increased productivity are factored in [78, 99]. The original high costs ($300,000 to $750,000) associated with the rehabilitative phase post-implant have decreased significantly. Much of this is due to reducing the post-implant hospitalization time and performing the necessary muscle conditioning at the patient's home [78].

3.3. Intramuscular electrodes

Nochomovitz et al. [93] demonstrated that the phrenic nerves could be electrically activated using intramuscular (IM) electrodes placed in the canine diaphragm muscle via the abdomen [100]. As with conventional phrenic pacing, viable phrenic nerves and diaphragm muscle are necessary for this approach. Although the electrode is placed in the muscle, the stimulus activates the nerve (nerve branches), which, in turn, distributes the electrically induced action potentials to many widely distributed muscle fibers. This approach via a celiotomy eliminates the surgical manipulation of the nerve as required with the previously described pacing systems' cervical or thoracic approaches (see Figure 4). These investigators demonstrated that single IM electrodes would evoke transdiaphragmatic pressures and tidal volumes comparable to those evoked by conventional phrenic nerve electrodes when the IM electrode was properly placed [93]. IM electrodes present an attractive alternative to phrenic nerve electrodes because they do not come in direct contact with the nerves, thus greatly reducing the possibility of nerve damage [93, 101-103].

In an effort to eliminate the celiotomy, Stellato et al. developed a laparoscopic surgical approach to place IM electrodes in the diaphragm [101]. The laparoscopy is a minimally invasive procedure resulting in decreased surgical trauma, thus requiring less time for implantation and patient recovery. Potentially, the electrodes could be implanted without general anesthesia. Because this approach stimulates the phrenic nerve branches in the diaphragm muscle, the proximity of the IM electrode to these branches directly relates to the force of muscle contraction. Their work showed that if an IM electrode was placed within 2.0 cm of the phrenic nerve motor points, full activation of the diaphragm muscle could be achieved. The IM electrode pacing system achieved 167% of the volume necessary to maintain basal metabolism while avoiding muscle fatigue. In chronic studies lasting up to 484 days, the IM electrodes demonstrated a favorable tissue response, stable recruitment over time and no mechanical or electrochemical electrode failures. In addition, Peterson et al. have shown that with muscle conditioning, there is nearly complete conversion of muscle fibers from fast-twitch oxidative and glycolytic to slow-twitch oxidative. With the appropriate stimulus, the potential for muscle fatigue may be reduced [97, 104].

The difficulties with the laparoscopic approach developed by Peterson and colleagues were accurately locating the points of phrenic nerve entry into the diaphragm and keeping the electrode insertion needle within the muscle during electrode placement. In their studies, anatomical landmarks on the peritoneal diaphragmatic surface (e.g., the indentations of the central tendon, the inferior vena cava, etc.) were used to estimate the location of the motor points. Although these landmarks were present, their location with respect to the motor points varied and did not guarantee accurate placement of the electrode. Once the optimal sites were found, a 17 gauge hypodermic needle, 30 cm in length, loaded with an IM electrode was passed into the abdomen through a cannula while under visualization through the laparoscope. The needle was inserted into the diaphragm for a distance of 1.5 to 2.0 cm and withdrawn, leaving the IM electrode anchored in place [101, 105, 106]. Although care was taken to keep the needle within the muscle, the perpendicular approach of the needle with respect to the plane of the muscle resulted in 12 of 32 electrodes implanted partially into the thorax [104].

An instrument has subsequently been developed that allows a surgeon to approach the implant site with the insertion needle parallel to the plane of the muscle and to accurately place IM electrodes in the diaphragm. Because the surgeon is able to control the angle of the needle insertion and the depth of needle penetration into the muscle, the risk of the needle passing through the muscle and entering the thorax is minimized. This instrument has been used to implant electrodes in animals for periods up to 14 months. These electrodes demonstrated full recruitment of the muscle with no degradation of the evoked response over the course of the study. On average, a single IM electrode (unilateral stimulation) achieved 108% of the volume necessary to maintain basal metabolism while avoiding muscle fatigue. Because the tidal volume contributions of the left and right hemidiaphragms are additive, the volume achieved using bilateral stimulation can be approximated to be 216% [107].

Dunn and coworkers have reported on using IM electrodes to affect diaphragm contraction [103]. Their electrode is sutured into place through a small abdominal incision. The suture electrode has a 5.5 cm deinsulated section that is placed within the muscle mass, thus providing for a large surface area for stimulation. In acute experiments in dogs, bilateral stimulation of the diaphragm through these electrodes produced tidal volumes between 104% and 180% of spontaneous breathing.

3.4. Epimysial electrodes

Schmit et al. developed an epimysial (EP) electrode that could be implanted through a laparoscopic procedure, thus retaining the advantages of the abdominal approach (e.g., reduced surgical and recovery time and reduced risk of phrenic nerve injury). An EP electrode system which included an electrode, a vacuum attachment device with an electrode carrier, a computer-assisted implant procedure and a delivery system was developed and tested in dogs [108-111]. Before permanent implant with staples, this electrode could be temporarily attached to the abdominal surface of the diaphragm, which provided the opportunity to vary its position for preliminary implant site testing to identify a site for maximal activation at a low stimulus amplitude. Analysis of the evoked muscle response data obtained using this vacuum attaching electrode enabled the surgeon to compare spatially different test locations, avoiding the guesswork involved in locating the implant site and the dependency on anatomical landmarks as indicators of the phrenic nerve motor point. Because the delivery system gave the surgeon precise control of the electrode position, because the electrode was always in sight and because the electrode was positioned on the surface of the muscle, the EP electrode based system eliminated the risk of inserting the electrode through the diaphragm and into the thorax.

Schmit and Mortimer found that even though there were no electrode failures and the device consistently evoked more than 100% of the tidal volume required to indefinitely sustain basal metabolism, the tissue adjacent to the stimulating surface of the electrode revealed an unexpected, chronic, inflammatory histological response. This response was the result of relative motion between the muscle as it shortened with each contraction and the non-compliant electrode assembly. The net potential effect of this response was an ever-increasing separation between the stimulating surface and the excitable tissue that could necessitate higher stimulus currents in the future as the separation between the electrode and excitable tissue increased [109].

Although the EP electrode may not be well suited for a long-term pacing system, the technique and methodology developed for its placement may prove invaluable in identifying the phrenic nerve motor point from an abdominal approach.

4. Alternatives to diaphragm pacing systems

Alternatives to diaphragmatic pacing include traditional mechanical ventilators and breathing aids, pharmacologic treatment, rehabilitative and surgical intervention and electrical activation of accessory respiratory muscles (see Section 2). Each approach has advantages and disadvantages compared to the diaphragm pacing systems.

4.1. Mechanical ventilation

Artificial ventilation by means of purely mechanical systems has existed for decades. These devices can be separated into two broad categories: negative and positive pressure systems. Within each category, invasive and non-invasive approaches exist including NPV (Negative Pressure Ventilation) by way of a body tank (e.g., iron lung), chest cuirass, or body wraps, PPV (Positive Pressure Ventilation) by way of a nasal mask, mouthpiece, face mask or tracheostomy and mechanical systems such as the rocking bed and intermittent abdominal pressure ventilator (IAPV) [112, 113].

Negative Pressure Ventilation

The negative pressure tank ventilator has existed conceptually since 1832 [114]. It, like other NPVs developed since then, intermittently applies sub-atmonpheric pressure to the thoracic and abdominal surfaces. Transpulmonary pressure is thus increased, and air is drawn into lungs. The efficiency of NPVs depends largely on the body surface area the pressure change is applied to and how airtight the enclosure is. There are three types of NPVs: body tanks (e.g., iron lung), chest shells and body wraps.

The body tank ventilator is the most efficient NPV with regards to tidal volume generation. Developed in the late 1920s, it was the mainstay for temporary and chronic ventilatory therapy until the 1950s [115, 116]. The apparatus includes a rigid, airtight enclosure or "tank" that surrounds the entire thorax and abdomen. Earlier models enclosed the entire body with the exception of the head and neck [114]. A negative pressure generator is connected to the tank, thus applying the sub-atmospheric pressure to the entire enclosed region. These systems, however, weigh well over 100 kg and are 3 m in length. Although portable, the lighter fiberglass enclosures are still bulky, weighing approximately 50 kg, not including the negative pressure generator that weighs between 10 and 20 kg. For all intensive purposes, ambulation is eliminated. Besides the weight and size, perhaps a bigger disadvantage with body tank ventilators is the reduced access they afford to the user for health care personnel. Problems associated with tank NPV's include leaky neck seals and upper airway obstruction during sleep (in the absence of a tracheostomy). Some pressure generators avoid this problem by maintaining a patent airway by creating continuous negative extrathoracic pressure (CNEP) or by applying continuous positive airway pressure (CPAP) [117].

A second type of NPV is the chest shell or cuirass. First described shortly after the development of the tank ventilator and similar to it in principal, the cuirass is a rigid shell that fits around the chest and abdomen [114]. In many cases, the shell is made to fit a cast of the user [67]. A generator is connected to the shell to provide the changes in pressure necessary for ventilation. Compared to the tank ventilator, the cuirass is portable, although the generator is still bulky. The shell is relatively easy to don and doff, but is less efficient than the tank NPV. This inefficiency is highlighted in patients with severely compromised respiratory function, chest wall deformities or back deformities in whom additional ventilatory support is usually mandated [117].

The body wrap ventilator is the most recently developed and, now, the most widely used NPV [114]. First described in 1955, it consists of a rigid chest piece that is covered by a wind-proof nylon or plastic jacket (the wrap). The jacket is sealed around the neck, torso and upper extremities to provide an airtight space. A generator produces the sub-atmospheric pressure environment in the jacket that enables ventilation. Wrap ventilators are more efficient than the cuirass but are more difficult to don and doff. Problems associated with the wrap NPV include air leaks and musculoskeletal pain.

Positive Pressure Ventilation

Positive pressure mechanical ventilation is the most common technique used to treat patients with respiratory failure. Unlike spontaneous breathing where airflow is generated by a decrease in pleural, alveolar and airway pressures, during positive pressure mechanical ventilation, air is forced into the lungs through positive pressure. The upper airway passages may or may not be bypassed. In the case of continuous pacing (e.g., with CRI resulting from high level spinal cord injury), ventilation via a tracheostomy is the preferred approach. In these cases, artificial humidification of the inspired air is required. If ventilatory assistance is required for only part of the day/night, a non-invasive interface such as a nasal mask, a mouthpiece or a face mask may be used.

Although these ventilators meet the daily metabolic gas exchange needs of the user, there are associated hazards. Positive pressure ventilation increases intrathoracic pressure, which can impede venous return to the heart. Barotrauma including pneumomediastinum and pneumothorax, hypotension and atelectasis are also seen. Other complications associated with this treatment method include alveolar over-distention resulting in alveolar rupture and crusting of the large airways (if the humidity of the ventilated air is insufficient). Gastric distention leading to an increased incidence of gastrointestinal bleeding as well as impaired hepatic and renal function may be seen. Furthermore, contamination of the system through respiratory tract secretions has been implicated as a source of pulmonary infection, including bronchitis and nosocomial pneumonia. In patients with a tracheostomy (the majority of those with chronic respiratory insufficiency), complications include tracheomalacia, granuloma formation and soft-tissue infection around the stoma site. Communication skills and swallowing may also suffer with prolonged use of an artificial airway. As the ventilator is a life-sustaining device, malfunction or disconnection will have devastating consequences. Thus, in the case of individuals who require ventilation for more than 20 hours/day, a back-up ventilator is mandated [117]. Finally, connection to a mechanical ventilator has the psychological disadvantages associated with the resulting losses of freedom, independence, self-reliance and mobility brought on by the size and unsightfulness of the apparatus [114, 115, 117-120].

Mechanical Aids for Ventilation

Positive and negative pressure mechanical ventilators achieve ventilation by forcing air through the airway, into the lungs. An alternative approach is to displace the abdominal viscera, thereby causing or augmenting diaphragm movement. Two examples of this type of system are the rocking bed [121, 122] and intermittent abdominal pressure respirator (e.g., pneumobelt) [117, 118, 123].

First used in 1932, the rocking bed is a bed that moves or "rocks" the head and feet through an arc of approximately 15° to 30° on an axis near the hip level [114, 117, 124]. This movement intermittently displaces the abdominal viscera, resulting in the back and forth movement of the diaphragm. As such, the system may not provide adequate ventilation in patients with severe chest wall deformities or in obese patients. Although it is well tolerated by most patients and is relatively simple to use, it is less efficient than NPVs, bulky and expensive.

The intermittent abdominal pressure ventilator (IAPV) consists of an inflatable rubber bladder that is worn around the abdomen. It is held in place by a nylon corset and is similar to the rocking bed in principal. The bladder is connected to a positive pressure ventilator. As the bladder is inflated, the diaphragm is moved upwards, resulting in a forceful expulsion of air. As the bladder deflates, the diaphragm and abdominal viscera return to their resting positions resulting in "passive" inspiration [114]. Because the system relies on gravity to return the diaphragm to its resting position, the IAPV works best in patients who are sitting upright. Advantages to this approach include the ease of donning and doffing and the fact that it does not use a nasal or oro-nasal mask, thus not interfering with eating or speech. IAPVs generally produce tidal volumes of 300 ml, but volumes as high as 1,200 ml have been reported [124]. Thus, the IAPV is best suited for temporary relief from more invasive or intrusive ventilators or to augment spontaneous activity.

In many cases, devices such as the rocking bed and IAPV only augment ventilatory function. Thus, the combination of NPV or PPV or other ventilatory assist devices with such mechanical aids may better suit some patients.

4.2. Pharmacologic

Pharmacologic agents have been used to treat chronic respiratory insufficiency. Most of these drugs aim to increase repiratory drive or improve pulmonary function. They include doxapram, protriptyline and other tricyclics, theophylline, caffeine, metaproterenol and ipratropium bromide [67, 99, 125-127]. Their use is not indicated in cases of high quadriplegia where the inherent respiratory drive still exists, but the neural pathway to elicit function has been damaged. These drugs have been used to treat patients with hypoventilation syndromes (including central alveolar hypoventilation and central sleep apnea where the central respiratory drive is diminished). At present, there does not appear to be an effective, long-term pharmacologic treatment option for CRI.

4.3. Rehabilitative

Although the diaphragm is the primary inspiratory muscle, the accessory muscles of the neck can be trained to augment or substitute for its function. Glossopharyngeal or "frog" breathing (GPB) is a totally non-invasive, relatively common technique used to assist alveolar ventilation [112, 113]. First observed in a patient with respiratory failure resulting from paralytic poliomyelitis who had learned the technique spontaneously, GPB uses the tongue and pharyngeal muscles to "swallow" or push air into the lungs [128]. The tongue seals against the palate with each swallow. This action is repeated 5 to 10 times to achieve tidal volumes of approximately 600 ml. The glottis is closed after each injection to retain the "inhaled" air. Exhalation is passive, relying on the recoil of the chest and lungs. The process can be repeated 10 to 12 times a minute to achieve normal or near normal minute volumes. Volumes as high as 2 to 2.5 L (with corresponding expiratory flow) can be achieved to aid in cough. The use of GPB allows for some free time from mechanical ventilation in patients with spinal cord injury or post-polio syndrome who suffer from chronic respiratory insufficiency [117]. GPB is relatively ineffective in the presence of a thracheostomy tube. Even when the tube is capped, the "swallowed" air tends to leak out around the tracheostomy site as the inspired volume (and pressure) increases [114]. GPB would certainly prove invaluable in the event of accidental disconnection from a mechanical ventilator by enabling the individual to maintain ventilation until mechanical ventilation is resumed.

4.4. Surgical intervention

In order for phrenic nerve pacing to be an option for a CRI patient, the phrenic nerves must be intact. Damage to the spinal cord in the C3-C6 region or to the peripheral nerve structure itself generally results in damage to the cell bodies of the nerves and subsequent axonal degeneration. Thus, the conduction pathway that the phrenic pacer relies on to deliver the stimulus to the target muscle is no longer patent. Considering spinal cord injury, incomplete and complete cervical injuries resulting in tetraplegia account for nearly 50% of this population [9, 11]. Cervical spinal cord injuries result in some degree of respiratory insufficiency as the accessory respiratory muscles (see Section 2) and the diaphragm (if the phrenic nerves are damaged) are no longer activated. As viable phrenic nerves are a prerequisite for diaphragmatic pacing, intermittent positive pressure ventilation is the predominant treatment option for these patients. With advances in microsurgical techniques and a better understanding of axonal degeneration/regeneration and neural anastomosis, the repair of damaged phrenic nerves and the subsequent reinnervation of the diaphragm may be a possibility [129-131]. With a viable nerve supply, diaphragmatic pacing may be a treatment option.

Surgical repair of this conduit by way of an anastomosis with a viable brachial nerve was performed in cats [132]. Following a recovery period (16 to 32 weeks) to allow for the growth of the axons from the brachial nerve onto the anastomosed phrenic nerve, stimulation resulted in diaphragm muscle contraction comparable to both spontaneous respiration and electrical stimulation of the intact contralateral phrenic nerve [132].

Following this initial study, Krieger and colleagues investigated using an intercostal nerve in place of the brachial nerve for the anastomosis [129]. The intercostal nerve was chosen as a potential donor due to its proximity to the phrenic nerve (thus reducing the course for axonal regeneration), its physiological function (activation of skeletal muscle for respiration) and its size (comparable to the phrenic nerve). This approach was carried out in a patient with diaphragm paralysis. Following a three month recovery period to allow for axonal growth, successful electrophrenic respiration was seen. Since then, two additional patients have undergone this procedure [133]. With this approach, individuals with an injury to the spinal cord in the C3-C6 region who would otherwise not be considered for phrenic pacing may now be potential candidates. However, long-term follow-up is necessary to determine if this approach is beneficial to the patient [129, 133, 134].

In cats, Baldissera and colleagues restored diaphragm muscle activity by way of laryngeal nerve to phrenic nerve anastomosis [131]. The choice of the laryngeal nerve for the anastomosis has some advantages and disadvantages. The laryngeal nerve originates in the brain stem. Thus, in the case of high tetraplegia, this nerve should still be intact allowing the potential for spontaneous control of the diaphragm. Disadvantages to using the laryngeal nerve for the anastomosis include possible vocal cord paralysis resulting from the diversion of the laryngeal nerve from the vocal cord to the phrenic nerve and the number of motor neurons in the laryngeal nerve compared to the phrenic nerve [131]. Also, obstructive apnea may be a consequence as a result of the lack of activation of the vocal cord from the diverted laryngeal nerve.

4.5. Magnetic stimulation

Over the past decade, stimulation of peripheral, spinal and cortical nerves by way of electromagnetic induction or magnetic stimulation has emerged as a useful, non-invasive approach to activate the nervous system [135-137]. Activation of the phrenic nerves and the diaphragm muscle by way of magnetic stimulation has been used in animals and humans [137-141]. Advantages to this approach include the ability to stimulate deep structures without discomfort to the patient, no risk of tissue damage due to electrochemical reactions at the electrode-electrolyte interface, and the non-invasive nature of the stimulation system. However, despite its advantages, there are a number of drawbacks to magnetic stimulation that hinder its widespread clinical use. These include inefficient energy transfer from the coil/stimulator to the excitable neural tissue thus increasing the stimulation threshold, limited duration for stimulation resulting from the coil heating and the stimulator itself which is bulky and expensive. With regards to respiratory insufficiency, a number of groups have demonstrated the ability to achieve significant inspired volumes and pressures with magnetic stimulation of the phrenic nerve trunks and roots [137, 139, 140]. Values comparable to those obtained with direct electrical stimulation are possible. With consideration of the limitations of magnetic stimulation, this technique may prove to be a valuable tool (and alternative to direct electrical stimulation) in assessing phrenic nerve function and diaphragm strength. At present, however, it does not seem to be an option for prolonged ventilatory support.

4.6. Electrical stimulation of the intercostal muscles

Electrical activation of the intercostal muscles is an attractive approach to treat respiratory insufficiency [142]. This technique bypasses two major prerequisites for diaphragm pacing: 1) viable phrenic nerves and 2) viable diaphragm muscle. The intercostal muscles of the rib cage account for up to 40% of the vital capacity. Although the intercostals perform both inspiratory and expiratory functions, the upper rib cage musculature is predominantly made up of the parasternal and external intercostals that are primarily inspiratory. Unlike the diaphragm, these muscles are innervated by a group of nerves (intercostal nerves originating from the ventral rami of T2-T12). However, by placing a single electrode in the epidural surface of the spinal cord through a dorsal laminectomy, this group of nerves/muscles can be activated. In animal studies, a single electrode placed at the T2 level achieved 35-40% of vital capacity. This value is comparable to the volumes achieved with combined stimulation of the four upper thoracic spinal roots [142].

Electrical activation of the intercostal muscles alone has been used for respiration in four patients. After a conditioning period, tidal volumes of up to 850 ml could be produced (range: 470 to 850 ml). However, the maximum duration of intercostal pacing (without mechanical ventilation or spontaneous breathing activity) remained relatively short (<3 hours) [143].

Based on this, a combined intercostal/diaphragm pacing system was investigated [80]. This system used the technique described previously to activate the intercostal muscles and added a commercially available diaphragm pacing system (activating only one phrenic nerve for unilateral pacing). By activating the intercostal muscles, the upper rib cage would be stabilized and supported. Individuals with only one intact phrenic nerve or moderate bilateral phrenic nerve function who would otherwise not meet the prerequisites for a traditional diaphragm pacing system may be potential candidates for this approach. The net result would be to augment and enhance the effect of both the diaphragm or intercostal pacer. This combined system has been tested in four patients yielding tidal volumes of up to 1200 ml (while unilateral diaphragm pacing alone yielded ≈600 ml) for periods up to 14 hours [144].

5. Conclusions and future direction

Individuals with lost or impaired ability for spontaneous ventilation require some sort of intervention to provide adequate alveolar ventilation. These individuals include those with injury to the spinal cord at or above the origin of the phrenic nerves or those with central hypoventilation syndromes secondary to an injury in the medullary respiratory center resulting from central nervous system infection, tumor, infarction, lesion or stroke. In treating a patient with chronic respiratory insufficiency, intermittent positive pressure ventilation (IPPV) delivered through a tracheostomy is the most common method of treatment. Although these systems do provide for adequate alveolar ventilation, there are associated complications including alveolar hypo- and hyperventilation, barotrauma, hypotension, atelectasis, impaired renal and hepatic function and gastric distention and bleeding. This does not include complications associated with the tracheostomy such as tracheomalacia and soft-tissue infection around the stoma or the psychological, social, quality of life, and financial implications these systems have on the patient, his/her family and the health care industry. As these systems are life-sustaining devices, accidental disconnection or failure would have catastrophic consequences. This mandates a back-up system with an alternate power source [117].

Over the past 25 years, electrical activation of the phrenic nerves has been used to provide artificial ventilation in patients with chronic respiratory insufficiency [1-7]. Despite their clinical effectiveness, their use has been limited to a carefully selected group of patients. Three commercial systems are in use today. These systems differ primarily in the electrode design and stimulus parameters. Phrenic pacers have been implanted in over 1,000 patients worldwide. Drawbacks to these systems include the risk of injury to the nerve either by surgical manipulation or by the electrode itself, system component failure and the high cost of the systems. Although the risk of injury to the nerve has decreased, it does exist as a section of the nerve must be mobilized for electrode placement. The incidence of component failure has declined as the systems have undergone revisions.

However, all three require some extracorporeal component. Unlike the cardiac pacemaker, phrenic pacers require an external transmitter and antenna to transmit both the power and control signal to an implanted receiver/stimulator. The development of a totally implantable system is feasible and under way [83]. It would be a significant advancement over presently available systems. Also, at present, none of the systems have any feedback or timing mechanism to make them physiologically responsive nor are they synchronized with the upper airway. Development of such a mechanism would be an added benefit to phrenic pacers over conventional mechanical ventilators. Cost is perhaps a larger hurdle to overcome. The pacing systems available today cost nearly $100,000 (for the system, implant and rehabilitation). Unlike cardiac pacemakers, because of the low number of potential candidates for these systems and the relatively low profit potential, there is little interest from major manufacturers of medical devices. This may explain the limited effort to develop improved pacing systems [80, 90].

Alternatives to mechanical ventilation and conventional phrenic pacing are being investigated by a number of groups [97, 103, 104, 107]. These approaches take advantage of advanced minimally invasive surgical techniques to implant the stimulating electrodes in the diaphragm muscle, thus avoiding manipulation of the nerve. In dogs, stimulation of the nerve through IM electrodes has been shown to achieve tidal volumes and pressures comparable to pacing via electrodes placed in direct contact with the nerve. The reduced risk of injury along with the less-invasive surgical approach may make diaphragm pacing an option to a wider patient population (e.g., patients who only require part-time ventilatory assistance or those who are unable to be weaned from mechanical ventilation post-surgery). Although the diaphragm is the primary respiratory muscle, including the accessory muscles in a pacing system has advantages. In patients with injury to the phrenic nerve, where conventional phrenic pacing is no longer an option, stimulation of the intercostal muscles has been shown to be a viable ventilatory therapy for a short duration of time (<3 hours) [143, 145]. If only one phrenic nerve is viable (or there is only moderate bilateral nerve function), a combined intercostal/diaphragm pacer may prove beneficial [80]. Another option for individuals with damage to the phrenic nerve may be repair of the damaged nerve through microsurgical neural anastomosis [129, 131].

With the increasing incidence of CRI comes the question of how to successfully medically manage the condition. An important component is knowing what technique best benefits the patient and is, at the same time, cost effective. A comparative study investigating the different treatment methods for CRI (e.g., positive pressure mechanical ventilation vs. diaphragm pacing) in terms of medical outcome, quality of life and cost would be invaluable. Along with this, increased awareness of the options available to both clinicians and patients is a necessity. The best approach to treat CRI may well be a combination of approaches from surgical repair, pharmacotherapy, mechanical support and diaphragmatic pacing. A combined approach that mimics natural breathing may potentially play a role in other activities of daily living that depend on the respiratory muscles including cough and bladder and bowel function.

Acknowledgments. This work was performed with the support of the Rehabilitation Research Service of the Department of Veterans Affairs.

References

[1] W. W. Glenn, M. L. Phelps, J. A. Elefteriades, B. Dentz, and J. F. Hogan, "Twenty years of experience in phrenic nerve stimulation to pace the diaphragm," *PACE*, vol. 9, pp. 780-784, 1986.

[2] M. N. Ilbawi, F. S. Idriss, C. E. Hunt, R. T. Brouillette, and S. Y. DeLeon, "Diaphragmatic Pacing in Infants: Techniques and Results," *Ann. Thor. Surg.*, vol. 40, pp. 323-329, 1985.

[3] H. Fodstad, "The Swedish experience in phrenic nerve stimulation," *PACE*, vol. 10, pp. 246-251, 1987.

[4] J. C. McMichan, D. G. Piepgras, D. R. Gracey, H. M. Marsh, and R. Sittipong, "Electrophrenic Respiration," *Mayo Clinic Proc.*, vol. 54, pp. 662-668, 1979.

[5] R. A. Langou, L. S. Cohen, D. Sheps, S. Wolfson, and W. W. Glenn, "Ondine's Curse: hemodynamic response to diaphragm pacing (electrophrenic respiration)," *Am. Heart J.*, vol. 95, pp. 295-300, 1978.

[6] C. E. Hunt, R. T. Brouillette, D. E. Weese-Mayer, A. Morrow, and M. N. Ilbawi, "Diaphragm Pacing in Infants and Children," *PACE*, vol. 11, pp. 2135-2141, 1988.

[7] L. L. Radecki and L. A. Tomatis, "Continuous Bilateral Electrophrenic Pacing in an Infant with Total Diaphragmatic Paralysis," *J. Pediatrics*, vol. 6, pp. 969-971, 1976.

[8] M. DeVivo, "Causes and costs of spinal cord injury in the United States," *Spinal Cord*, vol. 35, pp. 809-813, 1997.

[9] S. L. Stover, J. A. DeLisa, and G. G. Whiteneck, *Spinal Cord Injury: Clinical Outcomes from the Model Systems*, Aspen Publishing, Gaithersburg, MD, 1995.

[10] P. Williams, L. Bannister, M. Berry, P. Collins, M. Dyson, J. Dussek, and M. Ferguson, *Gray's Anatomy: The Anatomical Basis of Medicine & Surgery*, 38th ed., Churchill Livinstone, New York, 1995, p. 2092.

[11] "Spinal Cord Injury: Facts and Figures at a Glance," National Spinal Cord Injury Statistical Center (NSCISC), Birmingham, AL, Fact Sheet April 1999.

[12] P. Meyer and S. Heim, "Surgical Stabilization of the Cervical Spine," in *Surgery of Spine Trauma*, P. Meyer (Ed.), Churchill Livingstone, New York, 1989, pp. 397-523.

[13] D. Yashon, *Spinal Injury*, 2 ed., Appleton, Century, Crofts, Norwalk, CT, 1986.
[14] G. Whiteneck, "The High Costs of High-Level Quadriplegia," in *Management of High Quadriplegia*, G. Whiteneck, D. Lammertse, S. Manley, R. Mentor, C. Adler, C. Wilmot, R. Carter, and K. Wagner (Eds.), Demos Publications, New York, 1989.
[15] M. Berkowitz, C. Harvey, C. G. Greene, and S. E. Wilson (Eds.), *The Economic Consequences of Traumatic Spinal Cord Injury*, Demos Publications, New York, 1992.
[16] R. Carter, W. Donovan, L. Hasteald, and M. Wilkerson, "Comparative study of electrophrenic nerve stimulation and mechanical ventilatory support in traumatic spinal cord injury," *Paraplegia*, vol. 25, pp. 86-91, 1987.
[17] R. Carter, "Respiratory aspects of spinal cord injury management," *Paraplegia*, vol. 25, pp. 262-266, 1987.
[18] R. Waters, R. Adkins, J. Yakura, and I. Sie, "Motor and sensory recovery following complete tetraplegia," *Arch. Phys. Med. Rehabil.*, vol. 74, pp. 242-247, 1993.
[19] W. McKinley, "Late return of diaphragm function in a ventilator-dependant patient with a high cervical tetraplegia: a case report and interactive review," *Spinal Cord*, vol. 34, pp. 622-629, 1997.
[20] T. Oo, J. Watt, B. Soni, and P. Sett, "Delayed diaphragm recovery in 12 patients after high cervical spinal cord injury. A retrospective review of diaphragm status of 107 patients ventilated after acute spinal cord injury," *Spinal Cord*, vol. 37, pp. 117-122, 1999.
[21] T. J. Martin and M. H. Sanders, "Chronic Alveolar Hypoventilation: A Review for the Clinician," *Sleep*, vol. 18, pp. 617-634, 1995.
[22] D. Gozal, "Congenital central hypoventilation syndrome: an update," *Ped. Pulmonol.*, vol. 26, pp. 273-282, 1998.
[23] S. Thalhofer and P. Dorow, "Central Sleep Apnea," *Respiration*, vol. 64, pp. 2-9, 1997.
[24] S. Krachman and G. Criner, "Hypoventilation Syndromes," *Clin. Chest Med.*, vol. 19, pp. 139-155, 1998.
[25] C. E. Hunt and J. M. Silvestri, "Pediatric hypoventilation syndromes," *Curr. Opin. Pulm. Med.*, vol. 3, pp. 445-448, 1997.
[26] J. W. Kreit and W. L. Eschenbacher, "The Physiology of Spontaneous and Mechanical Ventilation," *Clin. Chest Med.*, vol. 9, pp. 11-21, 1988.
[27] N. Cherniack and A. Pack, "Control of Ventilation," in *Pulmonary Diseases and Disorders*, vol. 1, A. Fishman (Ed.), 2 ed., McGraw-Hill Book Company, New York, 1988, pp. 131-144.
[28] W. Reid and G. Dechman, "Considerations When Testing and Training the Respiratory Muscles," *Physical Therapy*, vol. 75, pp. 971-982, 1995.
[29] A. De Troyer, M. Sampson, S. Sigrist, and P. T. Macklem, "The Diaphragm: Two Muscles," *Science*, vol. 213, pp. 237-238, 1981.
[30] P. T. Macklem, "The diaphragm in health and disease," *J. Lab. Clin. Med.*, vol. 99, pp. 601-610, 1982.

[31] J. Mead, "Functional significance of the area of apposition of diaphragm to rib cage [proceedings]," *Am. Rev. Respir. Dis.*, vol. 119, pp. 31-32, 1979.

[32] P. Macklem, "The Mechanics of Breathing," *Am. J. Respir. Crit. Care Med.*, vol. 157, pp. S88-94, 1998.

[33] P. Macklem, "The Respiratory Muscles," in *Pulmonary Diseases and Disorders*, vol. 3, A. Fishman (Ed.), 2 ed., McGraw-Hill Book Company, New York, 1988, pp. 2269-2274.

[34] B. Celli, "The Diaphragm and Respiratory Muscles," *Chest Surg. Clin. N. Am.*, vol. 8, pp. 207-224, 1998.

[35] G. C. Sieck, "Physiological effects of diaphragm muscle denervation and disuse," *Clin. Chest Med.*, vol. 15, pp. 641-659, 1994.

[36] D. Kernell and E. Hensbergen, "Use and fibre type composition in limb muscles of cats," *Eur. J. Morphol.*, vol. 36, pp. 288-292, 1998.

[37] J. A. Elefteriades and J. A. Quin, "Diaphragm Pacing," *Chest Surg. Clin. N. Am.*, vol. 8, pp. 331-357, 1998.

[38] P. T. Macklem, D. M. Macklem, and A. De Troyer, "A model of inspiratory muscle mechanics," *J. Appl. Physiol.*, vol. 55, pp. 547-557, 1983.

[39] S. Yan, A. P. Gauthier, T. Similowski, P. T. Macklem, and F. Bellemare, "Evaluation of human diaphragm contractility using mouth pressure twitches," *Am. Rev. Respir. Dis.*, vol. 145, pp. 1064-1069, 1992.

[40] F. Bellemare, B. Bigland-Ritchie, and J. J. Woods, "Contractile properties of the human diaphragm in vivo," *J. Appl. Physiol.*, vol. 61, pp. 1153-1161, 1986.

[41] F. Bellemare and B. Bigland-Ritchie, "Assessment of human diaphragm strength and activation using phrenic nerve stimulation," *Respir. Physiol.*, vol. 58, pp. 263-277, 1984.

[42] M. Aubier, D. Murciano, Y. Menu, J. Boczkowski, H. Mal, and R. Pariente, "Dopamine Effects on Diaphragmatic Strength during Acute Respiratory Failure in Chronic Obstructive Pulmonary Disease," *Ann. Int. Med.*, vol. 110, pp. 17-23, 1989.

[43] W. Kelley, "Phrenic nerve paralysis. Special consideration of the accesory phrenic nerve," *J. Thor. Surg.*, vol. 19, pp. 923-928, 1950.

[44] J. Road, "Phrenic afferents and ventilatory control," *Lung*, vol. 168, pp. 137-149, 1990.

[45] R. Scott, "Innervation of the diaphragm and its practical aspects in surgery," *Thorax*, vol. 20, pp. 357-361, 1965.

[46] C. G. Hammond, D. C. Gordon, J. T. Fisher, and F. J. Richmond, "Motor unit territories supplied by primary branches of the phrenic nerve," *J. Appl. Physiol.*, vol. 66, pp. 61-71, 1989.

[47] A. De Troyer, M. Sampson, S. Sigrist, and P. T. Macklem, "Action of costal and crural parts of the diaphragm on the rib cage in dog," *J. Appl. Physiol.*, vol. 53, pp. 30-39, 1982.

[48] J. P. Derenne, P. T. Macklem, and C. Roussos, "The respiratory muscles: mechanics, control, and pathophysiology. Part III," *Am. Rev. Respir. Dis.*, vol. 118, pp. 581-601, 1978.

[49] J. P. Derenne, P. T. Macklem, and C. Roussos, "The respiratory muscles: mechanics, control, and pathophysiology. Part II," *Am. Rev. Respir. Dis.*, vol. 118, pp. 373-390, 1978.

[50] J. P. Derenne, P. T. Macklem, and C. Roussos, "The respiratory muscles: mechanics, control, and pathophysiology. Part I," *Am. Rev. Respir. Dis.*, vol. 118, pp. 119-133, 1978.

[51] C. Roussos and P. T. Macklem, "The respiratory muscles," *N. Engl. J. Med.*, vol. 307, pp. 786-797, 1982.

[52] M. C. Binder, P. Bawa, P. Ruenzel, and E. Henneman, "Does orderly recruitment of motoneurons depend on the existence of different types of motor units?," *Neurosci. Lett.*, vol. 36, pp. 55-58, 1983.

[53] H. R. Luscher, P. Ruenzel, and E. Henneman, "How the size of motoneurones determines their susceptibility to discharge," *Nature*, vol. 282, pp. 859-861, 1979.

[54] T. Abe, T. M. Kieser, T. Tomita, and P. A. Easton, "Respiratory muscle function during emesis in awake canines," *J. Appl. Physiol.*, vol. 76, pp. 2552-2560, 1994.

[55] A. De Troyer and M. Estenne, "Coordination between rib cage muscles and diaphragm during quite breathing in humans," *J. Appl. Physiol. Respir. Environ. Exerc. Physiol.*, vol. 57, pp. 899-906, 1984.

[56] S. Iscoe, "Control of abdominal muscles," *Prog. Neurobiol.*, vol. 56, pp. 433-506, 1998.

[57] E. Van Lunteren, W. B. Van de Graaff, D. M. Parker, K. P. Strohl, J. Mitra, J. Salamone, and N. S. Cherniack, "Activity of upper airway muscles during augmented breaths," *Respir. Physiol.*, vol. 53, pp. 87-98, 1983.

[58] A. Pack, L. Kline, J. Hendricks, and A. Morrison, "Control of Respiration during Sleep," in *Pulmonary Diseases and Disorders*, vol. 1, A. Fishman (Ed.), 2 ed., McGraw-Hill Book Company, New York, 1988, pp. 145-160.

[59] K. Strohl, M. Hensley, M. Hallett, et al., "Activation of upper airway muscles before the onset of inspiration in normal man," *J. Appl. Physiol.*, vol. 49, pp. 638-642, 1980.

[60] K. Strohl, "Control of the Upper Airway During Sleep," in *Breathing Disorders of Sleep*, N. Edelman and T. Santiago (Eds.), Churchill Livingstone, New York, 1986, pp. 115-137.

[61] R. B. Stein, P. H. Peckham, and D. B. Popovic (Eds.), *Neural Prostheses: Replacing Motor Function After Disease or Disability*, Oxford University Press, New York, 1992.

[62] P. H. Peckham and M. W. Keith, "Motor prostheses for restoration of upper extremity function," in *Neural Prostheses: Replacing Motor Function After Disease or Disability*, R. B. Stein, P. H. Peckham, and D. B. Popovic (Eds.), Oxford University Press, New York, 1992, pp. 162-190.

[63] R. Kobetic and E. B. Marsolais, "Synthesis of paraplegic gait with multichannel functional neuromuscular stimulation," *IEEE Trans. Rehab. Eng.*, vol. 2, pp. 66-79, 1994.

[64] G. H. Creasey, "Electrical stimulation of the sacral roots for micturition after spinal cord injury," *Urol. Clin. N. Amer.*, vol. 20, pp. 505-515, 1993.

[65] L. S. Eisenberg, A. A. Maltan, F. Portillo, J. P. Mobley, and W. F. House, "Electrical stimulation of the auditory brainstem in deafened adults," *J. Rehab. Res. Dev.*, vol. 24, pp. 9-22, 1987.

[66] L. L. Menia and C. L. Van Doren, "Independence of pitch and loudness of an electrocutaneous stimulus for sensory feedback," *IEEE Trans. Rehab. Eng.*, vol. 2, pp. 197-206, 1994.

[67] R. D. Chervin and C. Guilleminault, "Diaphragm Pacing: Review and Reassessment," *Sleep*, vol. 17, pp. 176-187, 1994.

[68] H. Fodstad, "Pacing of the diaphragm to control breathing in patients with paralysis of central nervous system origin," *Stereotact. Funct. Neurosurg.*, vol. 53, pp. 209-222, 1989.

[69] W. W. Glenn and M. L. Phelps, "Diaphragm pacing by electrical stimulation of the phrenic nerve," *Neurosurgery*, vol. 17, pp. 974-984, 1985.

[70] S. J. Sarnoff, E. Hardenbergh, and J. L. Wittenberger, "Electrophrenic respiration," *Am. J. Physiol.*, vol. 155, pp. 1-9, 1948.

[71] J. L. Whittenberger, S. J. Sarnoff, and E. Hardenbergh, "Electrophrenic respiration. II. Its use in man," *J. Clin. Invest.*, vol. 28, pp. 124-128, 1949.

[72] S. J. Sarnoff, L. C. Sarnoff, and J. L. Whittenberger, "Electrophrenic Respiration," *Science*, vol. 106, p. 482, 1948.

[73] M. Swenson and R. Rubenstein, "Phrenic Nerve Conduction Studies," *Muscle & Nerve*, vol. 15, pp. 597-603, 1992.

[74] R. Chen, S. Collins, H. Remtulla, A. Parkes, and C. Bolton, "Phrenic nerve conduction study in normal subjects," *Muscle & Nerve*, vol. 18, pp. 330-335, 1995.

[75] I. MacLean and T. Mattioni, "Phrenic nerve conduction studies: A new technique and its application in tetraplegic patients," *Arch. Phys. Rehabil.*, vol. 62, pp. 70-73, 1981.

[76] A. Moosa, "Phrenic nerve conduction in children," *Develop. Med. Child Neurol.*, vol. 23, pp. 434-438, 1981.

[77] D. K. McKenzie and S. C. Gandevia, "Phrenic nerve conduction times and twitch pressures of the human diaphragm," *J. Appl. Physiol.*, vol. 58, pp. 1496-1504, 1985.

[78] W. H. Dobelle, M. S. D'Angelo, B. F. Goetz, D. G. Kiefer, T. J. Lallier, J. I. Lamb, and J. S. Yazwinsky, "200 cases with a new breathing pacemaker dispel myths about diaphragm pacing," *ASAIO J.*, vol. 40, pp. M244-M252, 1994.

[79] W. W. Glenn, R. T. Brouillette, B. Dentz, H. Fodstad, C. E. Hunt, T. G. Keens, H. M. Marsh, S. Pande, D. G. Piepgras, and R. G. Vanderlinden, "Fundamental considerations in pacing of the diaphragm for chronic ventilatory insufficiency: a multi-center study," *PACE*, vol. 11, pp. 2121-2127, 1988.

[80] G. Creasey, J. Elefteriades, A. DiMarco, P. Talonen, M. Bijak, W. Girsch, and C. Kantor, "Electrical stimulation to restore respiration," *J. Rehabil. Res. Dev.*, vol. 33, pp. 123-132, 1996.

[81] J. Tibballs, "Diaphragmatic pacing: an alternative to long-term mechanical ventilation," *Anaesth. Intensive Care*, vol. 19, pp. 597-601, 1991.

[82] P. P. Talonen, G. A. Baer, V. Hakkinen, and J. K. Ojala, "Neurophysiological and technical considerations for the design of an implantable phrenic nerve stimulator," *Med. Biol. Eng. Comput.*, vol. 28, pp. 31-37, 1990.

[83] W. Mayr, M. Bijak, W. Girsch, J. Holle, H. Lanmuller, H. Thoma, and M. Zrunek, "Multichannel stimulation of phrenic nerves by epineural electrodes. Clinical experience and future developments," *ASAIO J.*, vol. 39, pp. M729-M735, 1993.

[84] H. Thoma, W. Girsch, J. Holle, and W. Mayr, "Technology and long-term application of an epineural electrode," *ASAIO Trans.*, vol. 35, pp. 490-494, 1989.

[85] M. Kimura, T. Sugiura, Y. Fukui, M. Togawa, and Y. Harada, "Glued Carbon Fiber Electrodes for Diaphragm Pacing," *Artificial Organs*, vol. 14, pp. 390-391, 1990.

[86] K. Ishii, H. Kurosawa, H. Koyanagi, K. Nakano, N. Sakakibara, I. Sato, M. Noshiro, and M. Ohsawa, "Effects of Bilateral Transvenous Diaphragm Pacing on Hemodynamic Function in Patients after Cardiac Operations," *J. Thor. Cardiovasc. Surg.*, vol. 100, pp. 108-114, 1990.

[87] A. Esclarin, P. Bravo, O. Arroyo, Mazaira, H. Garrido, and M. Alcaraz, "Tracheostomy ventilation versus diaphragmatic pacemaker ventilation in high spinal cord injury," *Paraplegia*, vol. 32, pp. 687-693, 1994.

[88] D. E. Weese-Mayer, A. S. Morrow, R. T. Brouillette, M. N. Ilbawi, and C. E. Hunt, "Diaphragm Pacing in Infants and Children - A Life-Table Analysis of Implanted Components," *Am. Rev. Respir. Dis.*, vol. 139, pp. 974-979, 1989.

[89] G. A. Baer and P. P. Talonen, "International Symposium on Implanted Phrenic Nerve Stimulators for Respiratory Insufficiency," *Ann. Clin. Res.*, vol. 19, pp. 399-402, 1987.

[90] J. Elefteriades, "Pacing of the Diaphragm," in *General Thoracic Surgery*, vol. 1, T. Shields (Ed.), 4 ed., Williams & Wilkins, Baltimore, 1994, pp. 613-627.

[91] J. Moxham and J. M. Shneerson, "Diaphragmatic pacing," *Am. Rev. Respir. Dis.*, vol. 148, pp. 533-536, 1993.

[92] I. Sato, J. F. Hogan, W. W. Glenn, and Y. Fujii, "A demand diaphragm pacemaker," *Trans. Am. Soc. Artif. Intern. Organs*, vol. 23, pp. 456-463, 1977.

[93] M. L. Nochomovitz, A. F. Dimarco, J. T. Mortimer, and N. S. Cherniack, "Diaphragm activation with intramuscular stimulation in dogs," *Am. Rev. Respir. Dis.*, vol. 127, pp. 325-329, 1983.

[94] M. L. Nochomovitz, B. D. Schmit, and J. T. Mortimer, "Electrical Activation of the Diaphragm," *Prob. Respir. Care*, vol. 3, pp. 507-533, 1990.

[95] M. Kimura, T. Sugiura, Y. Fukui, T. Kimura, and Y. Harada, "Heart rate and body temperature sensitive diaphragm pacing," *Med. Biol. Eng. Comput.*, vol. 30, pp. 155-161, 1992.

[96] S. Salmons, "The Importance of the Adaptive Properties of Skeletal Muscle in Long-term Electrophrenic Stimulation of the Diaphragm," in *Implanted Phrenic*

Nerve Stimulators for Respiratory Insufficiency, vol. 30, G. A. Baer, H. Frey, and P. P. Talonen (Eds.), Acta Univ Tamerensis, 1989 (ser. B), pp. 61-74.

[97] D. K. Peterson, M. L. Nochomovitz, T. A. Stellato, and J. T. Mortimer, "Long-Term Intramuscular Electrical Activation of Phrenic Nerve: Safety and Reliability," *IEEE Trans. Biomed. Eng.*, vol. 41, pp. 1115-1126, 1994.

[98] G. A. Baer, P. P. Talonen, V. Hakkinen, G. Exner, and H. Yrjola, "Phrenic nerve stimulation in tetraplegia. A new regimen to condition the diaphragm for full-time respiration," *Scand. J. Rehabil. Med.*, vol. 22, pp. 107-111, 1990.

[99] R. D. Chervin and C. Guilleminault, "Diaphragm pacing for respiratory insufficiency," *J. Clin. Neurophysiol.*, vol. 14, pp. 369-377, 1997.

[100] M. Nochomovitz, "Electrical activation of respiration," *IEEE Eng. Med. Biol.*, vol. 2, pp. 27-31, 1983.

[101] T. A. Stellato, D. Peterson, M. Nochomovitz, J. T. Mortimer, and R. Rhodes, "Diaphragm activation with laparoscopically placed intramuscular electrodes in dogs," *Proc. 71st Surg. Forum*, vol. XXXVL, pp. 297-299, 1985.

[102] D. K. Peterson, M. Nochomovitz, A. F. DiMarco, and J. T. Mortimer, "Intramuscular electrical activation of the phrenic nerve," *IEEE Trans. Biomed. Eng.*, vol. 33, pp. 342-351, 1986.

[103] R. B. Dunn, J. S. Walter, and J. Walsh, "Diaphragm and accessory respiratory muscle stimulation using intramuscular electrodes," *Arch. Phys. Med. Rehabil.*, vol. 76, pp. 266-271, 1995.

[104] D. K. Peterson, M. L. Nochomovitz, T. A. Stellato, and J. T. Mortimer, "Long-Term Intramuscular Electrical Activation of Phrenic Nerve: Efficacy as a Ventilatory Prosthesis," *IEEE Trans. Biomed. Eng.*, vol. 41, pp. 1127-1135, 1994.

[105] D. K. Peterson, T. Stellato, M. L. Nochomovitz, A. F. DiMarco, T. Abelson, and J. T. Mortimer, "Electrical activation of respiratory muscles by methods other than phrenic nerve cuff electrodes," *PACE*, vol. 12, pp. 854-860, 1989.

[106] T. A. Stellato, D. K. Peterson, P. Buehner, M. L. Nochomovitz, and J. T. Mortimer, "Taking the laparoscope to the laboratory for ventilatory research," *Am. Surg.*, vol. 56, pp. 131-133, 1990.

[107] H. Aiyar, T. A. Stellato, R. P. Onders, and J. T. Mortimer, "Laparoscopic Implant Instrument for the Placement of Intramuscular Electrodes in the Diaphragm," *IEEE Trans. Rehab. Eng.*, vol. 7, pp. 360-371, 1999.

[108] B. D. Schmit, T. A. Stellato, and J. T. Mortimer, "Staple Penetration and Staple Histological Response for Attaching an Epimysial Electrode onto the Abdominal Surface of the Diaphragm using a Laparoscopic Approach," *Surgical Endoscopy*, vol. 11, pp. 45-53, 1997.

[109] B. D. Schmit and J. T. Mortimer, "The Tissue Response to Epimysial Electrodes for Diaphragm Pacing in Dogs," *IEEE Trans. Biomed. Eng.*, vol. 44, pp. 921-930, 1997.

[110] B. D. Schmit, T. A. Stellato, M. E. Miller, and J. T. Mortimer, "Laparoscopic Placement of Electrodes for Diaphragm Pacing Using Stimulation to Locate the Phrenic Nerve Motor Points," *IEEE Trans. Rehab. Eng.*, vol. 6, pp. 382-390, 1998.

[111] B. D. Schmit and J. T. Mortimer, "Electrical Activation of the Diaphragm using Epimysial Electrodes," presented at 16th Int. Conf. IEEE-EMBS, 1994.
[112] M. Gilmartin, "Body ventilators. Equipment and techniques," *Respir. Care Clin. N. Am.*, vol. 2, pp. 195-222, 1996.
[113] J. Bach, "New approaches in the rehabilitation of the traumatic high level quadriplegic," *Am. J. Phys. Med. Rehabil.*, vol. 70, pp. 13-19, 1991.
[114] J. R. Bach, "Update and Perspectives on Noninvasive Respiratory Muscle Aids Part 1: The Inspiratory Aids," *Chest*, vol. 105, pp. 1230-1240, 1994.
[115] K. Chen, G. L. Sternbach, R. E. Fromm, and J. Varon, "Mechanical Ventilation: Past and Present," *J. Emer. Med.*, vol. 16, pp. 453-460, 1998.
[116] P. Drinker and L. A. Shaw, "An apparatus for the prolonged administration of artificial ventilation," *J. Clin. Invest.*, vol. 7, p. 229, 1929.
[117] B. J. Make, N. S. Hill, A. I. Goldberg, J. R. Bach, P. E. Dunne, J. E. Heffner, T. G. Keens, J. O'Donohue, W.J., E. A. Oppenheimer, and D. Robert, "Mechanical Ventilation Beyond the Intensive Care Unit," *Chest*, vol. 113 Supplement, pp. 289S-344S, 1998.
[118] P. A. Dettenmeier and N. C. Jackson, "Chronic hypoventilation syndrome: treatment with non-invasive mechanical ventilation," *AACN Clin. Issues Crit. Care Nurs.*, vol. 2, pp. 415-431, 1991.
[119] R. M. Streiter and J. P. Lynch, "Complications in the Ventilated Patient," *Clin. Chest Med.*, vol. 9, pp. 127-139, 1988.
[120] J. B. West, *Pulmonary Pathophysiology - The Essentials*, The Williams and Wilkins Company, Baltimore, 1977.
[121] P. Colville, C. Shugg, and J. Ferris, B.G., "Effects of body tilting on respiratory mechanics," *J. Appl. Physiol.*, vol. 9, pp. 19-24, 1956.
[122] F. Plum and G. D. Whedon, "The rapid-rocking bed: its effect on the ventilation of poliomyelitis patients with respiratory paralysis," *N. Engl. J. Med.*, vol. 245, pp. 235-241, 1951.
[123] H. J. Miller, E. Thomas, and C. B. Wilmot, "Pneumobelt use among high quadriplegic population," *Arch. Phys. Med. Rehabil.*, vol. 69, pp. 369-72, 1988.
[124] J. R. Bach and A. S. Alba, "Total ventilatory support by the intermittent abdominal pressure ventilator," *Chest*, vol. 99, pp. 630-636, 1991.
[125] D. Hudgel and S. Thanakitcharu, "Pharmacologic treatment of sleep-disordered breathing," *Am. J. Respir. Crit. Care Med.*, vol. 158, pp. 691-699, 1998.
[126] W. DeBacker, J. Verbraecken, M. Willemen, W. Wittesaele, W. DeCock, and P. Van deHeyning, "Central apnea index decreases after prolonged treatment with acetazolamide," *Am. J. Respir. Crit. Care Med.*, vol. 151, pp. 87-91, 1995.
[127] W. DeBacker, "Methods and clinical significance of studying chemical drives," *Respir. Physiol.*, vol. 114, pp. 75-81, 1998.
[128] C. W. Dail, J. E. Affeldt, and C. R. Collier, "Clinical aspects of glossopharyngeal breathing," *JAMA*, vol. 158, pp. 445-449, 1953.
[129] A. J. Krieger, M. R. Gropper, and R. J. Adler, "Electrophrenic respiration after intercostal to phrenic nerve anastomosis in a patient with anterior spinal artery

syndrome: technical case report," *Neurosurgery*, vol. 35, pp. 760-763; discussion 763-4, 1994.
[130] J. Terzis (Ed.), *Microreconstruction of Nerve Injuries*, Saunders, Philadelphia, 1987.
[131] F. Baldissera, P. Cavallari, G. Marini, and G. Tredici, "Diaphragm reinnervation by laryngeal motoneurons," *J. App. Physiol.*, vol. 75, pp. 639-647, 1993.
[132] A. Krieger, I. Danetz, S. Wu, M. Spatola, and H. Sapru, "Electrophrenic respiration following anastomosis of the phrenic nerve with brachial nerve in the cat," *J. Neurosurg.*, vol. 59, pp. 262-267, 1983.
[133] A. Krieger, "Electrophrenic respiration after intercostal to phrenic nerve anastomosis in a patient with anterior spinal artery syndrome: Technical case report," *Neurosurgery*, vol. 37, p. 553, 1995.
[134] H. Fodstad, "Electrophrenic respiration after intercostal to phrenic nerve anastomosis on a patient with anterior spinal artery syndrome: Technical case report," *Neurosurgery*, vol. 38, p. 420, 1996.
[135] A. T. Barker, R. Jalinous, and I. L. Freeston, "Noninvasive magnetic stimulation of human motor cortex," *Lancet*, vol. i, pp. 1106-1107, 1985.
[136] A. T. Barker, I. L. Freeston, R. Janilous, and J. A. Jarrat, "Magnetic stimulation of the human brain and peripheral nervous system: An introduction and the results of an initial clinical evaluation," *Neurosurgery*, vol. 20, pp. 100-109, 1987.
[137] S. Chokroverty, S. Shah, M. Chokroverty, A. Deutsch, and J. Belsh, "Percutaneous magnetic coil stimulation of the phrenic nerve roots and trunk," *Electroenceph. Clin. Neurophysiol.*, vol. 97, pp. 369-374, 1995.
[138] T. Similowski, B. Fleury, S. Launois, H. P. Cathala, P. Bouche, and J. P. Derenne, "Cervical magnetic stimulation: A new painless method for bilateral phrenic nerve stimulation in conscious humans," *J. Appl. Physiol.*, vol. 67, pp. 1311-1318, 1989.
[139] V. W. Lin, J. R. Romaniuk, and A. F. DiMarco, "Functional Magnetic Stimulation of the Respiratory Muscles in Dogs," *Muscle & Nerve*, vol. 21, pp. 1048-1057, 1998.
[140] S. Wragg, R. Aquilina, J. Moran, M. Ridding, C. Hamnegar, T. Fearn, M. Green, and J. Moxham, "Comparison of cervical magnetic stimulation and bilateral percutaneous electrical stimulation of the phrenic nerves in normal subjects," *Eur. Respir. J.*, vol. 7, pp. 1788-1792, 1994.
[141] G. Mills, D. Kyroussis, C. Hamnegard, S. Wragg, J. Moxham, and M. Green, "Unilateral magnetic stimulation of the phrenic nerve," *Thorax*, vol. 50, pp. 1162-1172, 1995.
[142] A. F. DiMarco, M. D. Altose, A. Cropp, and D. Durand, "Activation of the inspiratory intercostal muscles by electrical stimulation of the spinal cord," *Am. Rev. Respir. Dis.*, vol. 136, pp. 1385-1390, 1987.
[143] A. F. DiMarco, G. S. Supinski, J. A. Petro, and Y. Takaoka, "Evaluation of intercostal pacing to provide artificial ventilation in quadriplegics," *Am. J. Respir. Crit. Care Med.*, vol. 150, pp. 934-940, 1994.

[144] A. DiMarco, "Combined Intercostal/Diaphragm Pacing," Personal Communication, 1999.
[145] A. F. DiMarco, K. Budzinska, and G. S. Supinski, "Artificial ventilation by means of electrical activation of the intercostal/accessory muscles alone in anesthetized dogs," *Am. Rev. Respir. Dis.*, vol. 139, pp. 961-967, 1989.

Acronyms

CRI	Chronic Respiratory Insufficiency
IPPV	Intermittent Positive Pressure Ventilation
SCI	Spinal Cord Injury
CHS	Central Hypoventilation Syndrome
IM	Intramuscular
EP	Epimysial
NPV	Negative Pressure Ventilation
PPV	Positive Pressure Ventilation
IAPV	Intermittent Abdominal Pressure Ventilator
MPA	Medroxyprogesterone
GPB	Glossopharyngeal breathing
CNEP	Continuous Negative Extrathoracic Pressure
CPAP	Continuous Positive Airway Pressure
P_{DI}	Transdiaphragmatic Pressure
P_{pl}	Pleural Pressure
P_{ab}	Abdominal Pressure
DRG	Dorsal Respiratory Group
VRG	Ventral Respiratory Group
RF	Radio Frequency
OSA	Obstructive Sleep Apnea

Chapter 10

Intelligent systems in heart pacemakers

Rodica Strungaru and **Stefan Popescu**

The first section of this chapter is a brief review of different types of pacemakers and of the usual methods of adaptations to the demands of the body activity. A special emphasis is on the description of the state of the art in the field. In the second section, we present an overview of the intelligent systems proposed to improve the adaptability. In the subsequent section, we present the design of a fuzzy control system based on fuzzy logic. The controller is designed to work within an implanted cardiac pacemaker. The difficulties involved with the mathematical modeling of the nervous system of the heart are avoided by using a natural, linguistic description of the control rules. The behavior of the controller under various input conditions is analyzed. In the last section, we discuss the results and perspectives of the technology.

1. Pacemakers

1.1. Introduction

The modern technology can circumvent some biological impediments related to cardiac dysfunction. Many people may be subjected to a disability, whether by birth, or through illness or an accident, or have physical limitations that affect their activity, due to cardiac dysfunction. Advances in technology have helped to overcome such difficulties, and, as a result, people whose activity is restrained due to cardiac dysfunction are better reintegrating into normal life.

Delivering current to cardiac muscle in order to stimulate, defibrillate, or otherwise change the electric behavior of the heart is a common practice in clinical and experimental medicine.

The heart stimulators are used when the drug therapy is no longer efficient, that is, if the specialized conduction system cannot perform properly, but the contractile machinery of the heart is normal. The specialized conducting tracts from the atrium to the ventricle can be damaged or blocked. There are many situations when the specialized conducting tracts' deficiencies appear occasionally, for a short or a long time, and sometimes the AV-block can be complete. When the conduction is slow, all the depolarization pulses from the sinoatrial node pass to the ventricle, but the time intervals between atrial and ventricular systoles are longer (up to 0.5 s) versus the normal maximum limit (0.2 s).

When the conduction disturbances reach a certain degree, from time to time, the atrial depolarization pulse no longer arrives to the ventricle and thus a contraction is omitted. The atrial activity is normal. After the omitted contraction, the cardiac cycle duration is shorted again almost equal to the normal duration. In advanced disease, high degree block, the omitted contractions are more frequent. This disease is named partial heart block. In a more advanced block degree, the depolarization reaches the AV-node only after the every second, or third, or even fourth atrial contraction, that is, the ventricle responds only at three or four atrial contractions.

In the case of *first-degree heart block*, all atrial impulses reach the ventricle, the His bundle is not completely interrupted, but the P-R interval is abnormally prolonged because of an increase in transmission time through the affected region. In the *second-degree heart block*, one ventricular contraction follows every second atrial contraction.

When the AV-block is complete, the ventricles and the atria are contracting independently. The atrial contractions have their own rhythm of about 70 beats/min, which originate in the sinoatrial node, while the ventricle rhythm is approximately 30-45 beats/min, the *idioventricular rhythm*. Both ventricles are simultaneously contracting due to the fact that they are under the electrical control of a unique region with rhythmic activity. The ventricles' control center lies under the lesion part of the atrio-ventricular bundle. If a high automatism region is destroyed or isolated, the region with the closest automatism becomes a rhythm generator. When the sinoatrial conduction to AV-node is interrupted, the ventricles are commanded by the AV-node at a rate of 40-60 beats/min, and when the AV-node or the upper part of the His bundle is destroyed, the nearest lower region takes control of the ventricular rhythm at a rate of 20-40 beats/min. A ventricular rate of 30-40 beats/min is enough to keep the patient alive, but not in activity, due to the inability of the heart to maintain adequate body circulation.

A long break between contractions leads to a very low diastolic pressure and the brain blood flow is not satisfactory. If beside the complete AV-block the patient has the big vessels rigid or an aortic insufficiency, the diastolic blood pressure is even lower. If the cerebral blood circulation stops, the patient becomes unconscious, and often has a violent muscular activity like that from epileptic seizures (Adams-Stokes attack). If the cerebral blood circulation stops for a couple of minutes, the brain cells are damaged.

The cardiac block can be a result of occasional processes, usually in intensive efforts. It is only a cardiac electric conduction disease. A disordered atrial sinus mechanism, *sinus syndrome*, with or without an intact conduction pathway is another functional disturbance of the heart. In normal heart, the actions of both major branches of the autonomic nervous system, sympathetic and parasympathetic system, are integrated at the sinoatrial node, where normal heart rhythm is initiated. Changes in heart rate are related to the general levels of activity of these neural autonomic branches.

The arrhythmias, as abnormal heart beats and nonuniform timing between heart beats, are another heart disturbance. Some part of the heart, myocardial cells or specialized conducting cells, becomes self-depolarizing and appears as *ectopic focus*. The rate of ectopic depolarization can be sporadic, with the normal cycle transiently modified, or can be produced at a rhythm that exceeds the rate of the sinus node, when the tachycardia is set up.

Electrical stimulation of the heart muscle cells using an artificial pacemaker can restore the heart's normal pumping function. Many authors studied the effect of life prolongation by electrical heart stimulation. Details can be found in [1], and a comprehensive reference is [2].

1.2. Classification of pacemakers

The electrical stimulation of the heart was first introduced by Hyman [3], in 1932, as an emergency therapeutic procedure. Hyman used a large generator made with the technology of that time. In 1952, Zoll [4] tried to reintroduce the method, but without success. In 1958, Elmquist and Senning [5], after the invention of the transistor and the right ventricular catheter (by Furman [6]), implanted subcutaneously the first pacemaker at fixed pacing frequency with externally rechargeable batteries. This was the beginning for the development of one of the most widely accepted procedure to restore the heart's pumping function. The batteries' technological development offered soon the possibility to get an implantable cardiac pacemaker. The first and simplest pacemakers were those with frequency and stimulation impulse amplitude fixed before implantation.

In the case of the incomplete heart block, a competition appears between the pacemaker rate and the own rate of the patient's heart, when the specialized conducting tracts are working properly. The natural variation of the heart rate takes place depending on body activity, that is, depending on metabolic cell needs. By consequence, the pacemaker rate is only occasionally equal with the necessary body rhythm. If the pacemaker impulse is delivered during T wave, when the heart is spontaneously active, this could lead to ventricular fibrillation. As the energy of pacemaker stimulation impulse is low, the fibrillation probability is decreased. But these patients are generally under drug treatment, which increases the susceptibility of ventricular fibrillation.

The demand pacemaker is used by patients with incomplete or less frequent AV-block. The ventricle stimulating electrodes are connected to an amplifier. When the heart is spontaneously active, the R waves of the QRS complex are amplified and the pacemaker generates an impulse only when the spontaneous frequency is less then the preset frequency of the impulse generator. When the spontaneous activity is restored, the pacemaker is inhibited. The refractory period is introduced so that the impulse generator does not answer at this time when the amplifier detects an input signal. Thus, the circuit is able to reject the T waves, driven R waves and the decaying artifact of the impulse generator. The value of the refractory time is usually between 200 and 400 ms and is fixed by construction for each pacemaker or is adjusted at the programmable pacemakers. Thus, the artificial stimuli are used only if necessary and the competition between natural and artificial activity is removed.

This type of pacemaker is called a *negative demand pacemaker* or *negative synchronous (QRS)*, that is, a spontaneous QRS complex inhibits the impulse generator. When the waiting period of the spontaneous activity generator is equal to the period corresponding to the asynchronous stimulation frequency to which it was built, the pacemaker is considered to be without hysteresis. Instead, *hysteresis pacemakers* have been built in order to sustain the natural cardiac activity. They extend the time delay waiting for an R wave with almost 10-15% of the normal value of the corresponding stimulation frequency period.

The *positive demand pacemaker* (QRS_+ or $QRS_{TRIGGER}$) is working asynchronously when it does not detect a natural R wave and, when detecting a spontaneous ventricular activity, it generates instantly an impulse emphasizing the natural contraction.

The *double chamber pacemaker* or the combined atrio-ventricular pacemaker is used when atria cooperation is needed for the ventricular activity. In the cases presented above the ventricles are stimulated while the atria have their own natural beating rate. This is not bothersome because the ventricles are the power pumps, which supply the circulatory system. When a fully correlated cardiac activity is needed and there is no spontaneous atrial activity, two stimulating electrodes are used. One of them is in the right ventricle and the other one is in the right atrium. The pacemaker gives two impulses and the delay between them simulates the atrio-ventricular transmission time. Using combined stimulation, both atrial and ventricular, it can obtain an increase of almost 30% of the cardiac output.

An *atrial-controlled pacemaker* is indicated in the case with preserved sinus rhythm when implanting on active, young patients with normal atrial activity. It can be obtained with a self-acting frequency adjusting during physical effort. One electrode detects the atrial electric activity and the impulse to stimulate the ventricular muscle is delivered with a specified delay. This delay is equal to atrio-ventricular conduction time, 0.12 s, and is implemented as the sum of an electronically generated delay of 0.08 s, and the rest is represented by the ventricle muscular latency. If permanent or intermittent atrio-ventricular conduction disturbances exist, the use of the regular atrial action for P wave synchronized ventricular stimulation is physiologically the best solution. The pacemakers can have combined functions, i.e., demand pacemaker and atrial controlled.

If the atrial rhythm is too fast, a *coupled pacemaker* is used. This pacemaker provides a delayed impulse driven by the R wave detection. The impulse delay against the spontaneous R wave activity combined with ventricular muscle latency makes the impulse appear at the end of refractory period, that is, during the ST interval. This impulse modifies electrical activity but does not lead to a new ventricle contraction. The natural activity next P wave finds the ventricle's muscle still in the refractory time, forces it to be longer, and consequently, the muscle does not respond with a new contraction. Therefore, alternate ventricular contractions are omitted.

Pair pacemaker is used to obtain a more powerful ventricular contraction. It provides a pair of impulses: the first impulse stimulates the ventricles and causes contraction while the second is delayed so that it finds the ventricular muscle in the refractory period and improves the contraction. The critical parameter is the time between the two impulses.

In atrial pacing applications, sinus syndrome and an intact AV conduction pathway are indicated as *atrial inhibited, rate programmable pacemaker*. This type delivers the pacing stimulus when the patient's atrial rate falls below the programmed pacing rate of the pulse generator.

Pacemakers are classified based on a generic pacemaker code, derived from and compatible with the revised Inter-Society Commission for Heart Disease (ICHD) Code, proposed by the North American Society of Pacing and Electrophysiology (NASPE) Mode Code Committee and the British Pacing and Electrophysiology Group (BPEG). The NASPE Board of Trustees [7] adopted the code. It is abbreviated as the NGB Code. This pacemaker code and details on it are at http://www.sjm.com/stjude/clinit/htm/pg2.htm.

Cardiac rhythm management by a pacemaker can be expressed using from three to five capital letters, depending on the functional complexity:
- The first letter stands for the stimulated heart chamber initial letter: **0** means no heart chamber is paced, **A** means that the atrium is paced, **V**

means the ventricle is stimulated, **D** means the double chambers are paced, and **S** means that a single chamber is paced.
- The second letter stands for the supervised heart chamber initial letter (the chamber in which the spontaneous activity is measured); that is, the second letter can be **0**, **A**, **V**, or **D**.
- The third letter stands for the initial letter of the way the electrical generator is working. **0** means that the pacemaker works asynchronously; that is, the electrical generator is not controlled (for instance, **VOO** is the simplest pacemaker, with fixed frequency and with no measurement of the cardiac activity). **T** denotes the triggered mode, i.e., the generator provides an electrical impulse when detecting a signal. The letter **I** denotes the inhibited mode, i.e., the generator is blocked by a detected signal; **D** means dual function mode, **T** and **I**.
- The fourth letter is added only when one or more parameters of the pacemaker can be programmed: **P** – simple programmable and **M** – multiprogrammable, or **C** – communicating, the presence of data analyzing, storing and transmission capability. **R** means that the pacemaker delivers pacing stimulus with rate modulation (adaptive-rate pacing).
- The fifth letters indicates if the pacemaker performs an anti-tachyarrhythmia, cardioversion, or defibrillation function. **0** means that no function is performed. In case of anti-tachyarrhythmia pacing function, denoted by **P**, the pulse amplitude is high, to dominate the spontaneous high rate. The shock function, denoted by **S**, means an electric shock strong enough, above the upper limit of vulnerability, is delivered to successfully end ventricular fibrillation. Lower potential shock fails because it stimulates some portions of the myocardium during their vulnerable period, and thus reinitiates fibrillation. Finally, the dual function **D** means both **P** and **S** functions are available.

At the beginning of the evolution of this technology, implantable pacemakers were developed to save lives from episodes of bradycardia or complete heart block. Today, they help improve the quality of life by performing numerous various functions automatically performed and documented. Modern pacemakers offer extensive diagnostic functions to help diagnose patient symptoms and pacemaker system-related problems. They offer high flexibility to permit easy programming of extensive diagnostic functions and of available therapies [8-12].

1.3. Methods of adaptations to the demands of the body activity

For a heart with normal sinus node function, any conduction problem is solved with an atrial controlled pacemaker, which simulates the normal course of cardiac excitation in a physiological manner, i.e., the ventricular pacing rate follows atrial rate, which increases with body activity.

For a heart with atrial conduction abnormalities or sinus node dysfunction such as total or partial sinus node block, sinus bradycardia, absolute bradyarrhythmia, atrial fibrillation, flutter, tachycardia or progredient bifascicular blocks, an implanted pacemaker should provides an appropriate pacing rate which is not dependent on the atrial activity. The electrical impulse must be delivered to the ventricle at a rate in order to increase cardiac output to a level in accordance with the patient's routine daily tasks. Cardiac output is defined as the volume of blood ejected by one ventricle in one minute and it equals the product of heart rate and stroke volume. In everyday life, the cardiac output must be continually changing. To achieve appropriately varying pacing rates, an exercise responsive pacemaker must have information about body activity and this information must control the pacemaker.

In the past twenty years different exercise responsive parameters have been studied in order to determine their appropriateness for increasing ventricular pacing rate with workload. An optimal pacemaker controller must perform a heart pacing rate adapted to the body activity. This pacing rate should simulate the intact heart rate functioning in a human body with normal life [13].

In the normal human being, the heart rate control mechanisms according to performance of body activity are due to the adaptation of the cardiovascular system to changes in the energy equilibrium by the efferent innervation. Mainly, modification of the myocardial contractility, heart muscular strength, and the heart rate perform the efferent innervating control. In exercise, the rate and stroke volume both increase.

At the beginning of workload, the amount of blood returned to the heart is increased due to vasoconstriction of the capillaries. Stroke volume is controlled primarily by filling pressure via the Frank-Starling mechanism [14] and by myocardial contractility, and it is opposed by arterial pressure [15]. The filling pressure is referred to as the central venous pressure, which is the pressure in the great veins at their point of entry into the right atrium. The pressure distending the right ventricle, namely the right ventricular end-diastolic pressure, is almost equal to the central venous pressure. At the left heart, pulmonary vein pressure is almost equal to the left ventricular end-diastolic pressure. Therefore, the central venous pressure plays a key role in regulating stroke volume. The following factors act on central venous pressure. Because about two-thirds of the entire blood volume is located in the venous system, the greater the blood volume is, the greater the average venous pressure. Gravity, venous tone, and the muscle pump determine the distribution of venous blood between peripheral veins and thoracic veins. Sympathetic nerves that excite venoconstriction innervate the veins of the skin, kidneys, and splanchnic system. During inspiration, intrathoracic pressure becomes more negative and intraabdominal pressure more positive and this increases the venous pressure gradient from abdomen to thorax and promotes filling of the central veins. Central venous pressure also depends on cardiac output, because the pumping action of the heart transfers blood from the venous system into the arterial system, and this raises arterial pressure and lowers the central venous pressure. The central venous pressure has a great role on the cardiac output control, as is pointed out by the circulation analysis [16].

Besides, if workload is performed, oxygen consumption of the muscle increases, the pH of the blood decreases, and erythrocytes easily release oxygen. In the acid environment, capillaries of the muscle dilate. In consequence, arterial pressure decreases. This results in an increase of the heart rate. Nevertheless, vasodilatation in the exercising skeletal reduces the peripheral vascular resistance, and arterial pressure can fall at the start of light exercise. Based on these cardiac output control mechanisms related to the increased metabolic demand, many models were elaborated in order to investigate the dynamic behavior of the heart and to find the best variable responding to the tasks [16-19]. The exercise related physiological parameters investigated are briefly presented subsequently. The pacemakers with *stimulus-to-T wave* interval control have been proven effective for exercise and emotional stress [20]. In the normal heart, the time interval between the Q wave and the end of the T wave decreases when the heart rate increases. Following this correlation, the measuring parameter used to control pacing rate was the time interval from the pacing stimulus to the peak of the T wave.

Physical and emotional activity increases the central venous blood temperature. Temperature of right ventricular blood [21] was measured, and proportional and two step controllers [22] have been used for pacemaker rate control. However, an intelligent controller must be used, because an increased portion of the total blood supplies cooler peripheral tissues at the beginning of exercise and may cause a transient decrease in central blood temperature [23]. This controller has to make allowance for the errors introduced by the effects of fever or some environmental temperature influences. The muscle contraction and the body movement, generated during body activity, were also used as a control parameter [24]. Although the parameter is not related to workload or metabolism, this kind of pacemaker was widely accepted in spite of its sensitivity to mechanical sources of vibration from environment.

Hydrogen-ion concentration of the blood increases when workload is performed. A sensor on the pacing lead in the atrium was used to measure the blood pH which decrease according to the increase of exercise [53]. Long-term stability problem of the pH sensor limited the use of this pacemaker type.

An increase in respiration rate and minute volume takes place during exercise due to rapid increase of oxygen consumption and carbon dioxide production [26]. These parameters are estimated by impedance measurements. In spite of significant undesired changes of the respiration during speech, hyperventilation and even during arm movement, this type of rate responsive pacemaker was easily accepted.

The change rate of the right ventricular blood pressure, dP/dt, is another indicator for contractile force. According to the Frank-Starling law, the more the venous return increases, the more the ventricle distends, and the myocardial fibers contract with greater force. However, because dP/dt is affected by the dynamics of contraction, a competition between spontaneous rate and paced rate appears [27]. The oxygen saturation level in the venous blood decreases as oxygen consumption increases. Moreover, the effect of workload on the oxygen saturation is increased by the Frank-Starling mechanism and entails a short time response of the oxygen saturation decreasing to the onset of exercise [28]. Its high sensitivity at low load levels is a great advantage [29]. The stroke volume, ejection rate, and pre-ejection interval are significant hemodynamic parameters related to cardiac output. These parameters are estimated from four- or two-electrode impedance measurements in the right ventricle [30-32]. Intracardiac impedance is influenced by kinetics of contraction, but also by electrode location and catheter movement.

Intelligent controllers must be able to adapt themselves to changes in patient conditions occurring during their activity. In fact, the several factors affecting stroke volume and heart rate act to change simultaneously in a coordinated fashion to produce a regulation of the cardiac output. If in a patient with an artificial pacemaker only the heart rate increased to adapt the cardiac output to exercise, then the fitting is not obtained because stroke volume falls. One reason for the decrease in stroke volume is that any increase in pacing rate shortens diastole duration, not systole ones, and the ventricular filling time becomes shorter. The other reason is that any increase in pumping transfers faster venous blood from the heart input to the arterial output, lowering end-diastolic pressure and raising arterial pressure, both of which impair stroke volume. The effect is that at a high pacing rate the cardiac output decreases. Thus, a coordinated cooperative algorithm in all the controlling factors must be developed to adapt the cardiac output during body activity. Patients with even fixed rate pacemakers benefit from the moderate increase of cardiac output, due to increase in stroke volume by increased muscle pumping, peripheral vasodilatation and adrenaline enhanced contractility during moderate body activity. The increased cardiac output during exercise and emotional stress thus involves a coordinated interaction between changes *within* the heart – rate and contractility — and *outside* it — central venous pressure and systemic vascular resistance.

2. System requirements and design consideration for implementation of intelligent cardiac pacemakers

The complexity of pacing the human heart, as presented above, as well as the aim to completely recover for a large palette of heart diseases by giving patients the chance to have a normal life impose stringent requirements on cardiac pacemaker design. However, it is not easy and it is indeed a challenging task to fully understand how the human body works to accomplish the daily tasks and, as a byproduct, how to teach machines to replace parts of the body. Complex pacemakers that are able to adapt themselves to changes in patient conditions occurring during their activity have to incorporate a lot of intelligence or automatism similar to the one naturally provided by the nervous system of the healthy heart. Increasingly adding intelligence to machines seems to be the force that pushed ahead the technologies during the last 30 years and will probably do the same at the dawn of the next millenium. Unfortunately, the initial enthusiasm revealed by the large number of published papers on different artificial intelligence subjects found much less concrete applications in the industry fields. This is of no doubt explainable by the huge computing resources demand that most of the artificial intelligent approaches require. In the past, manufacturers of medical equipment have contended with performance versus cost tradeoffs, with no apparent fulfillment of both. Nevertheless, the design of an intelligent heart controller must additionally deal with drastic limitations in size and power needs that are hard to achieve when using powerful computing engines.

Fortunately, a simple and innovative concept called Fuzzy Logic was introduced earlier in the middle of the 1960s. It provided a simple way to close up the gap between human reasoning and computers. This concept has repeatedly proven that for artificial intelligence applications a low-power, low-cost microcontroller can equal or exceed the performance of a more expensive and power-hungry number crunching DSP (digital signal processor).

2.1. Short introduction to fuzzy logic

In this section, we briefly review some basic concepts on fuzzy logic. Readers who are familiar with fuzzy logic may consider skipping this section.

A difficulty of communication between human and computers and of knowledge transferring to machines is the human communication language. Human natural language is imprecise and ambiguous; however, it is understood and used in everyday life. Humans make an extensive use of attributes to classify objects that belong to any universe of discourse. Today computers dealing with classical Boolean logic are very good for understanding well-behaved, crisp attributes and categories such as odd or even; but they have difficulties in dealing with vague terms such as "young" or "old." This is because today's machines are based on binary logic, which relates any universe of discourse to a binary representation (based on 0 and 1). A classical example will better illustrate this problem. In order to define the adjective young the classical logic will define a threshold value, say 30 years, so that a person less than 30 is young and one more than 30 is old. The unreasonable result is that in a matter of seconds someone who is just about to become 30 would change status from young to old.

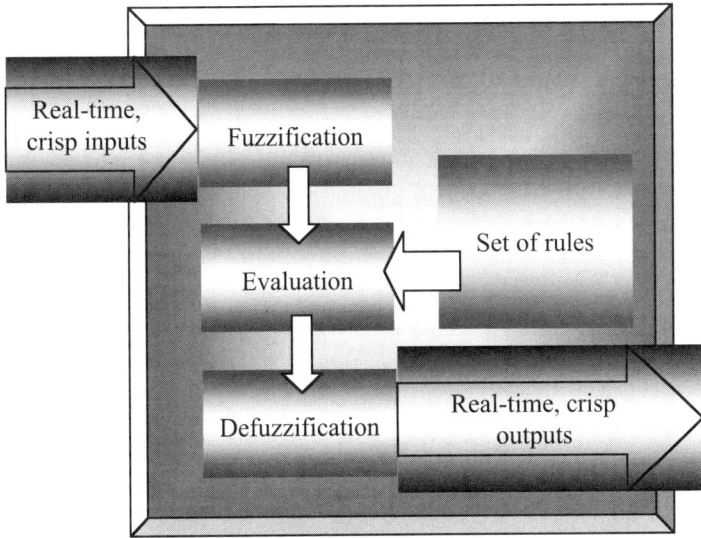

Figure 1. Architectural diagram of a fuzzy system.

Fuzzy logic provides a way to deal with uncertainty and imprecision commonly handled by human reasoning. Fuzzy methods allow us to express knowledge by linguistic sentences rather than mathematical equations, as humans do in order to communicate their knowledge on various systems. Applied to controllers, this methodology assigns predefined *degrees of truth* to the entire range of inputs of the controlled system and processes inputs through a set of rules to derive a weighted system output. The fuzzy inference consists of three basic steps, namely the *fuzzification* of the crisp input variables, linguistic rule evaluation, and *defuzzification*.

Fuzzy logic allows us to design a control system for those processes normally described by complex equations, affected by nonlinearity or governed by vague or ambiguous rules [34], [35], [38]. In the beginning of the 1990s, the Japanese engineers recognized the superiority of the fuzzy approach compared to the conventional control design in the case of complex systems. They have published many papers on successful industrial applications based on fuzzy logic in fields such as control and scheduling of the subway trains, elevator control, car antilock and brake control, engine and transmission control, and active suspension control. Shortly thereafter it became evident that the fuzzy design is often superior to an alternate approach in three main areas:

- design of controllers for systems where an adequate model is difficult to define;
- design of nonlinear controllers for model or model-less systems;

- systems governed by imprecision such as economic systems, natural sciences or behavior sciences.

Based on the popular analogy with the probability theory, the fuzzy logic found for the first time its way in the biomedical applications as knowledge-based automatic diagnose systems [39]. The uncertainly always-presented in medical information can be easily expressed in terms of fuzzy sets, whereas the human expertise or observation can be converted into linguistic rules [36], [41]. Nevertheless, it seems not to be a good idea to teach machines the human language, before using machines to replace parts of the human body.

2.2. Hardware and software for fuzzy logic in medical applications

2.2.1. Generalities

Although for many years fuzzy logic was an attractive approach for designers of industrial, consumer and automotive products, the balance between cost + space + power consumption and performance + reliability has not always been easy to trade in medical applications. Generally, the fuzzy algorithms were implemented on low-cost general-purpose microcontrollers. When the real-time performance is an important issue, the software overhead involved by implementing fuzzy methods on the Neumann architectures of conventional microprocessors often makes the resulted performance unacceptable. Dedicated fuzzy chips designed specially to handle fuzzy logic can meet the time performance required by demanding application. A few years ago semiconductor leaders such as former SGS-THOMSON Microelectronics and Motorola recognized the need and power of fuzzy logic and developed specialized fuzzy kernels and support tools for a number of their micro-controllers.

SGS-THOMSON realized a dedicated high-speed fuzzy logic coprocessor to implement high-level control in sensitive applications. Called *Weight Associative Rule Processor* –WARP, it exploits the benefits of the fuzzy logic approach by implementing high-level control without requiring specialized digital signal processors. This device targeted performance demanding, time-critical applications where an external fuzzy coprocessor boosts the processing performance by providing an external unit that can be connected to the most general-purpose controllers. It requires only a minimal number of external passive components, leading to simpler design, reduced size, and better reliability in a variety of fuzzy controls especially in medical control.

The fuzzy logic section of this controller includes input fuzzification and output defuzzification stages, a high-speed inferencing unit, memory for storing rules, antecedents and consequents, and control logic to handle the downloading of rules and variables. The chip is able to handle up to 8 inputs, 4 outputs, and 256 rules and to complete a fuzzy iteration in about 200 microseconds by storing the membership functions into dedicated on-chip memory. The device is supported by a development system providing graphical software development and the neuro-fuzzy modeling. Unfortunately for space, cost, and power sensitive applications, this approach is not suitable and a separate microprocessor is often required to handle the interface with sensors, actuators, and other crisp (non-fuzzy) system components.

2.2.2. A fuzzy microcontroller

The world of embedded controllers is currently experiencing a push into the realm of fuzzy logic. This fact was recognized also by Motorola (http://www.mot.com), which created software fuzzy kernels for several of their microcontrollers, including the Neuron Chips. The Neuron Chip is a communication and control processor implementing an embedded protocol in which received network inputs on the processor's communication port are used to control processor outputs on its I/O port. Related to this design is an important concept, the *intelligent distributed control*, that distributes control among several Neuron processors called nodes. The individual nodes share the input data and output port within one network imitating the way the human brain processes the information. This architecture is especially useful in fuzzy applications where the input data is sent to a fuzzy node within the network, which runs a fuzzy engine and set its outputs accordingly. Motorola's approach is mainly a software one, where the fuzzy kernel is simply a skeleton of programming code, which performs the three basic fuzzy steps: fuzzification, inference and defuzzification. A specialized programming language called Neuron C supports it but the limiting factor is the resulted slow inference time.

Opposed or complementary to this approach, ST Microelectronics (http://www.st.com) introduced a fuzzy device aimed to fill the gap between the logic and fuzzy approaches providing a combined architecture within a single chip that meets the needs of a wide range of control applications. The family ST52×301 DuaLogic™ microcontroller combines a dedicated hardware fuzzy processor with an Arithmetic/Logic Unit for Boolean operations and a comprehensive set of peripheral functions optimized for real-world interfaces.

The new fuzzy logic device exploits the benefits of fuzzy logic without sacrificing the convenience advantages of traditional microcontrollers. The fuzzy processor handles four fuzzy inputs, two outputs and up to 300 rules. For maximum flexibility the architecture supports multiple sets of fuzzy rules within the same program, allowing independent fuzzy algorithms such as control, monitoring and sensing to be implemented on the same device. The hardware fuzzy processor provides significantly higher performance than the performance achieved by the software approach (i.e., by running the fuzzy algorithms on a conventional microcontroller).

A development kit supports the design. It includes graphical software development tools and the neuro-fuzzy modeling tools, which allow the user to automatically extract fuzzy parameters and rules from a set of input/output values. Nevertheless, the dual core architecture also supports the conventional microcontroller operations required by most fuzzy logic applications, providing a set of arithmetic and program control instructions. Coupled with the on-board peripheral functions, this allows the device to meet all the control needs of a wide range of medical applications.

2.2.3. The fuzzy logic language

Fuzzy Logic Language (Fu.L.L.) is a description language oriented to the definition of fuzzy control systems and allowing data exchange between the various Fuzzy Logic software tools. A fuzzy system in Fu.L.L., besides being generated automatically by the above tools, can also be generated by using a normal text editor. A Fu.L.L. program consists of two main sections: the declarations part that defines the fuzzy variables term set (name universe) and the procedural part that defines the control rules.

To define the term set, the language provides the following actions:
- Associates a label to a universe of discourse.
- Defines templates and modifiers for the membership functions.
- Defines a variable specifying the name, the associated universe, and the membership functions.
- It composes the term set.

The set of rules, having the general format *IF – THEN*, defines the knowledge base to determine the values of output variables, starting from the input variable values. The antecedent part of the rules consists of a logic expression based on the fuzzy operators AND, OR, and NOT. Each premise is defined by an IS relation between a variable and one of its membership function. The consequent part of the rules is a linguistic expression, composed by elementary consequence terms joint by the connective AND.

2.3. Implementing a fuzzy controller for pacemakers

Suffering from various heart pathologies, especially those irreversible affecting the autonomous nervous system of the heart, some patients must undergo surgical intervention to survive. As described before, the strategy is to implant into the patient's body a pacemaker that will be responsible for controlling the heart contraction. The major problem for the design of this controller is to regulate the heart rate by imitating the normal functionality of the sino-atrial node normally responsible for the heart rate control. As usual for biomedical systems, the dynamic evolution of the cardiac rate is a very complex process and thus it is difficult to model. Even for healthy humans, accurate studies have revealed a chaotic component in heart rate behavior that will be impossible to express in crisp, precise mathematical equations. Moreover, the chaotic component becomes dominant in case of heart diseases

The prediction of the cardiac rhythm behavior was only partially possible using the methods of deterministic chaos [40]. Herein after, we present the design of a fuzzy controller included within a cardiac pacemaker used to pace an ill human heart. It takes control over the nervous system of the heart and adapts the cardiac rate to the actual physical effort and to the fatigue of the cardiac muscle. The system performs the functions of the sino-atrial node and is implanted through surgery into the thorax of the patients suffering from major heart damage. The pacemaker uses stimulation electrodes implanted into the upper-left side of the myocardial wall and applies current pulses that initiate the heart contractions. It also uses special sensors to build a closed-loop (feedback based) control of the heart rate.

The difficulties involved with the precise mathematical modeling of the nervous system of the heart and its control are avoided by using a natural, linguistic description of the control rules. The simulation and analysis of the state diagram helps establish the behavior of the controller under various input conditions. The design of the fuzzy controller followed the methodology suggested by Brubaker [34], [35]:

a) Identify the system inputs; establish the fuzzy ranges and the shape of the membership functions at input.

b) Identify the system outputs; establish the fuzzy ranges and the shape of the membership function at output.

c) Specify the rules that map the inputs to the output.

d) Determine the method of combining fuzzy rule actions into executable output.

Details are subsequently presented.

a) *Specialized sensors supply the inputs to the controller*:
1. EXERCISE is the actual effort (momentary level of physical exercise) performed by the patient carrying the device; it is obtained by analyzing the partial oxygen concentration (*oxygen saturation level - O2Sat*) in the blood returning from the body [28], [29], [45], [46].
2. TIREDNESS is the fatigue of the heart and muscles obtained by measuring the accumulation of residual components (increasing of blood acidosis) produced by the oxidation process within the muscle fibers as a result of mechanical contractions [53-55].
3. PULSE is the actual heart rate in beats-per-minute (bpm), obtained by monitoring the R wave of the ventricular electrogram.

The fuzzy linguistic input variables EXERCISE and TIREDNESS may have three possible fuzzy values, denoted by the tokens LOW, MEDIUM, and HIGH. For simplicity of the simulation, we normalized the output voltage of the respective transducers to span the range 0...1000 mV (e.g., 0 mV = 100% O2Sat and 1000 mV = 0% O2Sat). Concurrently, the shapes of the membership functions are the same for both variables. The linguistic variable PULSE is defined to have the following possible values: VERY LOW, LOW, MEDIUM, HIGH, VERY HIGH.

The membership functions used for the input are shown in Figure 2. The shaping of the membership functions at input and output is part of the design process of the controller. The membership function shapes significantly influence the global performance and are subject to a refinement procedure that tune-up the controller's behavior under various input conditions.

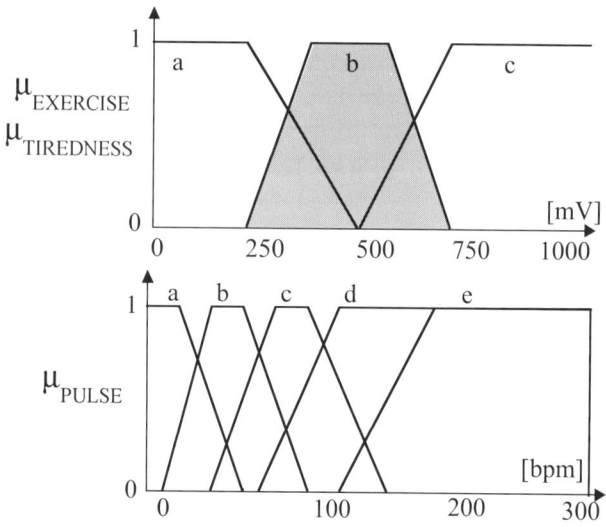

Figure 2. Membership functions for variables EXERCISE and TIREDNESS — upper diagram (a-LOW, b-MEDIUM, c-HIGH) — and for PULSE — lower diagram (a-VERY LOW, b-LOW, c-MEDIUM, d-HIGH, e-VERY HIGH).

b) *The fuzzy variable COMMAND* denotes the output of the controller. It adjusts the frequency of stimuli applied to the heart that are provided by a frequency controlled oscillator. We normalized the control variable to span the range between –50% and +50%. For negative input the oscillator will lower its current frequency (pacing rate), for positive input the oscillator increases its actual rate and for zero input it holds its current rate. For relative input values of +50%, the oscillator doubles the instant rate, while for input value of –50%, it reduces the rate to half of its current value. The membership functions at output in this case are depicted in Figure 3.

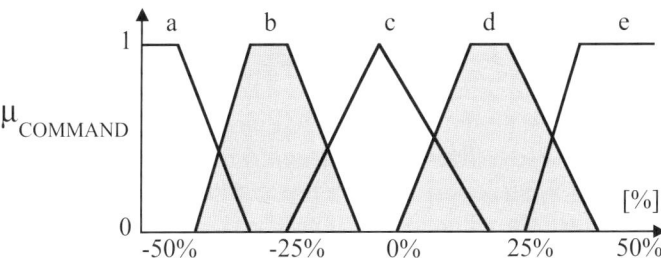

Figure 3. Membership functions for the output variable COMMAND (a-DECREASE FAST, b-DECREASE, c-HOLD, d-INCREASE, e-INCREASE FAST).

c) *Expressing the initial knowledge into the fuzzy rules.* Many fuzzy controllers are based on intuitive logic. For example, it is difficult to express by formulas the dependencies between the muscle's tiredness and the heart rate, or between the exercise level and the body's need of oxygen. However, it is easy to express such dependencies using ambiguous words, and to describe which is the behavior of the controller in various situations. The dynamic heart behavior is expressed in this case using simple rules that handle the system's complexity and avoids the necessity to derive mathematical expressions that are difficult to refine. A common template to write the base of rules is to use the matrix format (Table 1).

Table 1. Matrix representation of the Exercise-Pulse subset of linguistic rules (upper half) and Tiredness-Pulse subset of linguistic rules (lower half)

PULSE EXERCISE	VERY LOW	LOW	MEDIUM	HIGH	VERY HIGH
LOW	Increase	* Hold	Decrease	Decrease Fast	Decrease Fast
MEDIUM	Increase Fast	Increase	Hold	Decrease	Decrease Fast
HIGH	Increase Fast	Increase Fast	Increase	Hold	Decrease
TIREDNESS					
LOW	Increase Fast	Increase Fast	Hold	Hold	Decrease
MEDIUM	Increase Fast	Increase	Hold	Decrease	Decrease Fast
HIGH	Increase	Hold	Hold	Decrease Fast	Decrease Fast

The table on the previous page covers 30 rules. Each rule can be also expressed using fuzzy sentences. By example the cell marked with a star (*) can be expressed as:

if (EXERCISE is LOW and PULSE is LOW) then (COMMAND is HOLD)

The common logical background of the above rules is to adjust the heart rate according to the exercise and tiredness levels by avoiding that the heart rate goes extremely low or extremely high. The table presented above contains two subsections of the global rule base that were only artificially separated to simplify the presentation. The complete controller's rule base can be globally expressed as a 3-D matrix (difficult to present here but simple to describe in software) having the following general template:

if (PULSE is P_VAL) & (EXERCISE is E_VAL) & (TIREDNESS is T_VAL)
    then COMMAND is C_VAL

Figure 4 represents the block structure of the fuzzy heart controller. It consists of a crisp→fuzzy converter for the input signals, a fuzzy inference engine functioning as rule driven system and a fuzzy→crisp converter to transform the fuzzy output value into a defined (crisp) output signal.

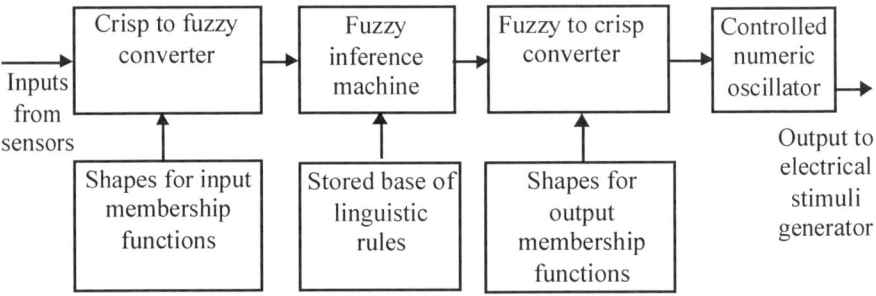

Figure 4. Block diagram of the fuzzy controller.

Because the linguistic rules work in the fuzzy space, the input variables must be converted from crisp values into fuzzy values. Data processing takes place within the fuzzy space. An inference engine elaborates decisions by sampling the controller's inputs at regular intervals and applying the rules to determine the output value.

d) *Calculating the crisp output of the fuzzy controller*. The result of the logical inference performed by the controller is expressed by one or more fuzzy values. Depending on the input values, several rules from the rule base may fire simultaneously and predict different output values. To obtain a crisp output value, the fuzzy system uses a converter that is a part of the design and transforms the fuzzy output values into a single crisp value. The major difference to other knowledge-based systems is that for fuzzy system the degree of execution for fired rule depends on the degree of confidence in the clause of the rule. Consequentially, we need a method to combine the output of the fired rules into a single output value based on confidence in the rule's clause. The defuzzification is performed by several methods [35], [38]. We used the centroid method that is more accurate than other simpler but faster defuzzifications methods as mean-of-maxima or weighted average. The centroid method finds the equivalent center of gravity of the fired rules in the plane of the membership functions. The output in this case is the horizontal coordinate of the gravity center. In order for the output value to continue it is necessary to have at least two rules firing each time. Overlapping the membership functions avoids discontinuities in the output.

2.4. Simulation of a fuzzy pacemaker

The fuzzy approach greatly simplified the design of the initially complex heart rate controller. The design of the fuzzy control system was only concentrated in shaping the membership functions and elaboration of the rule base. The inference engine and the converters were reused from other projects. The base system can be ported as C source code and cross-compiled for a different target platform. Actually, most of the work was put in the simulation of controller's operation. Because the fuzzy controller handles an extremely complex and nonlinear system such as the human heart, it is impossible to analyze mathematically its correct operation. To predict the behavior of the controller we turn to simulation by constructing the 3D-diagram of state transition [37]. This allowed us to find the answer to different input conditions and to predict the response to other practical conditions.

Figure 5 depicts the behavior of the open-loop controller system when the exercise input increases from null to maximum for different possible heart rate values. The simulations where performed by programming the controller within the MATLAB environment. The value of the crisp output Command was evaluated for 11×11 Exercise-Pulse discrete pairs uniformly covering the defined input range for the two crisp inputs with the third input TIREDNESS set to MEDIUM.

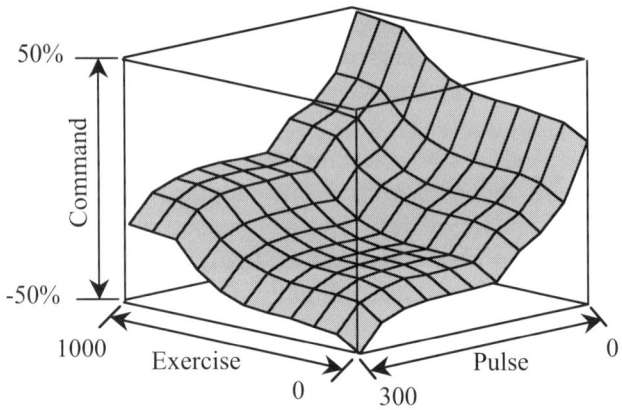

Figure 5. The state diagram for output variable Command when Exercise increases from 0 to max for different Pulse values when TIREDNESS is MEDIUM.

The controller acts as expected, reducing the rate at high pulse, or increasing the rate for high exercise. The above presented state diagram generated for different values of TIREDNESS provides complete information regarding the controller behavior.

2.5. Experimental results

We tested the controller behavior off-line in *in vitro* conditions on animal heart artificially maintained in ringer solution. Various parts of the heart's nervous system are damaged by cardiac ablation and later paced using our controller. Feature tests are performed in vivo also on animal heart using the experimental set-up illustrated in Figure 6.

A separate simulator controlled by the master PC is used to induce leg movements and to simulate various exercise levels. The input signals are converted to digital values using the analog inputs of the fuzzy controller. The pacemaker is able to adjust the amplitude of the output pulse using the pulse width modulated output (DIF) and an integration amplifier (IntA).

The first motivation of building our experimental set-up described above was to acquire the practical knowledge about the functionality rules that govern the healthy heart automatism. Studies carried out on healthy animals provided the data about the behavior of the instant heart rate under various workload conditions such as high effort followed by longer repose sequences or moderate effort at a high repetition rate. The goal of this research stage was to gather the necessary information in order to describe the heart response in natural language sentences, rather than the more complex usual way of fitting complex math equations through extensive data sets. The preliminary work resulted in the set of fuzzy variables, their names and universe of values (adjectives) as well as the preliminary shape for the membership functions.

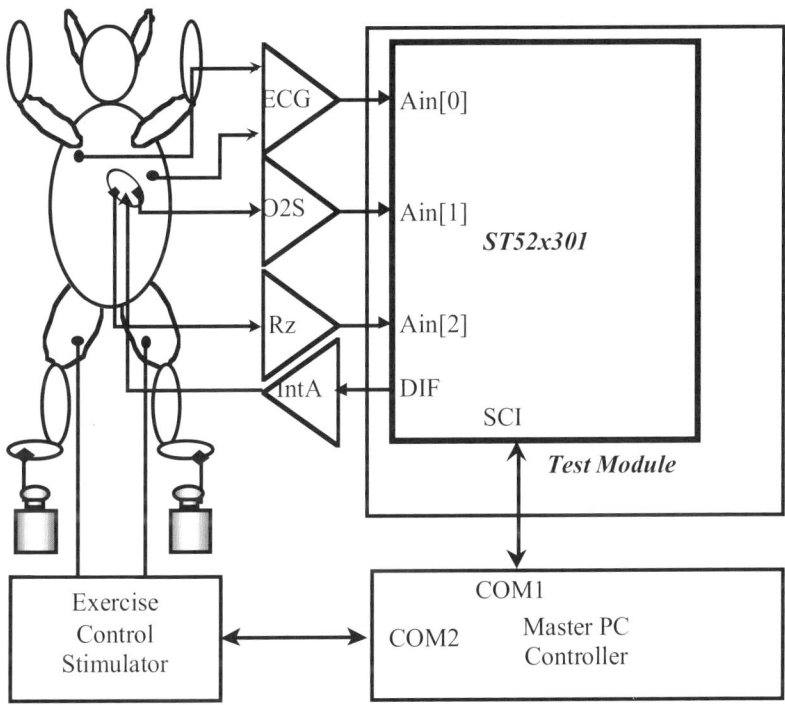

Figure 6. Experimental set-up used to test the heart controller.

In the second stage of the experimental investigation, we have built the rule base and we proceed to refine the membership function. We compared the response of the fuzzy controller against the response of the natural one under the same experimental conditions (workload sequences) that we used to acquire the initial knowledge. We found that the best innovation of the experimental set-up described above was that we could compare the artificial and the fuzzy controller under almost identical experimental conditions on the same animal. Initially, with the animal in healthy state, we measured and stored the typical response to every workload sequence. Later on the animal heart was put in ill condition by the effect of drogues or surgery, i.e., inhibiting or killing the natural heart controller, and the heart was paced by the closed feedback loop of our artificial one. The purpose of this test was to check that the intelligence and knowledge that we transferred into the machine could perform as similar as the natural controller could. We tuned off-line the shape of the membership function to achieve similar behavior.

As many investigators agree, the normal sinus rhythm is the gold standard to compare the rate response of a rate adaptive pacemaker [51]. The aim of this study was to assess the rate of the fuzzy controller by continuous comparison of the normal sinus rate (NR) and controller paced rates (PR). The operation of the controller was tested in a mongrel dog with induced complete atrio-ventricular block. The test exercise workload has imitated the exercise workload required by Kaltenbach's step test (defining a 6-minute submaximal exercise and a 6 minute recovery period). The pacing rate was increased from about 180 beats/minute (bpm) before exercise to more than 220 bpm during the workload. Cardiac output was increased from 2.02+/-0.08 liters/minute(l/pm) at the beginning to 2.33+/-0.12 l/pm at maximum. The natural and paced rate in bpm over the 12 minute test period results are shown in Figure 7.

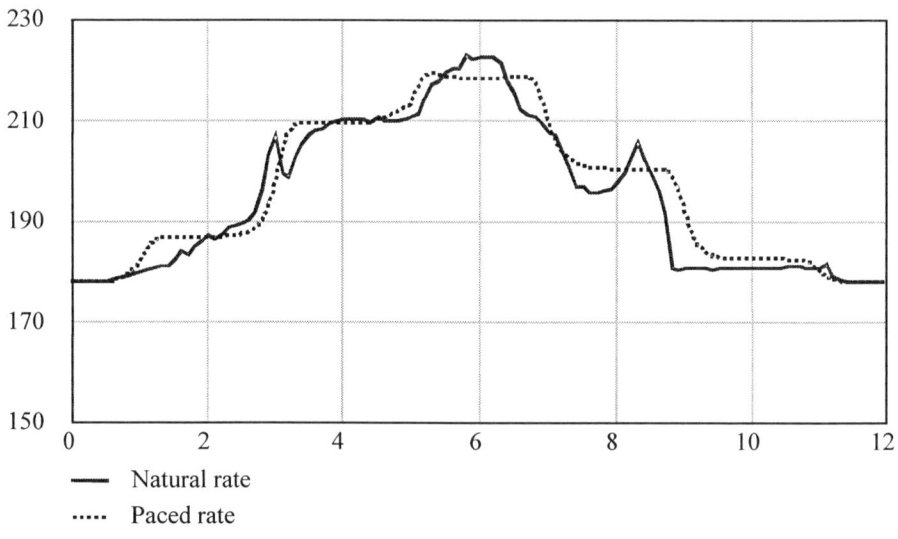

Figure 7. Test result on tuning data — moderate exercise workload.

The third stage of testing the fuzzy controller was inspired by the methodology used to train and test the artificial neural networks. We compared the response of the natural and artificial controller to a second set of workload sequences that was different from the one that we used to acquire and refine the initial knowledge and that we never used before.

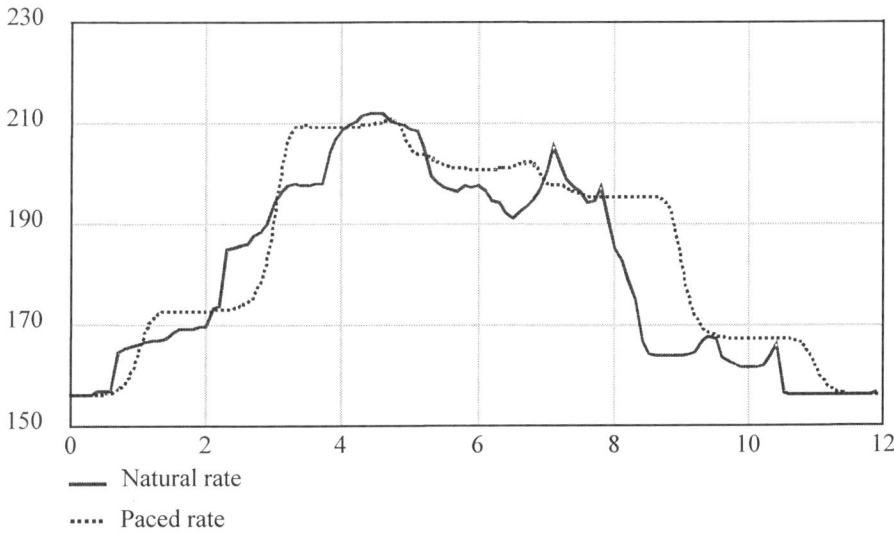

Figure 8. Test result with moderate-maximal exercise workload.

PR was less accurate for a more vigorous workload, but most of the PR was within the normal NR variation within 30 bpm, remembering that the best sensor is the sinus node and that synchronous pacemakers are only second best.

2.6. Conclusions

The three-stage procedure described above revealed interesting results that we didn't expected in the beginning. The construction and elaboration of the base of rules as well as the dictionary of adjectives was a simpler task. More difficult than estimating initially was the task of optimizing the shape of the membership functions, especially as we have no theoretical background to deal with. Our goal to get a controller that very closely resembles the natural one, in what is concerning the response to various workload sequences, proved to be a very difficult task. Advances in the field of tuning the membership functions, as the self-tuning method of Sugiura et al. [25], helped to refine the performance of our system.

Without substantial effort, the first iteration of the controller performed as expected, adjusting the heart rate according to the load intensity and duration. Future experiments under stage 3 described above revealed that the artificial controller slightly departs from the natural one in the response latency, or in the recovering sequence after heavy loading. Many factors explain this departure, for example, the nonaccounting for the efferent innervating control of the natural heart, which we ignored in our model. Moreover, the chaotic component of heart activity, revealed by Liebert in 1991 [40], that becomes dominant in the case of a heart disease may have been influenced our results.

3. Discussion

A new potential indication for cardiac pacing is chronotropic incompetence, that is, an inadequate cardiac rate response to exercise and other metabolic demands [47]. Many patients being paced for indications such as complete heart block, sick sinus syndrome or nodal diseases also have chronotropic incompetence. Such patients are not adequately treated with a constant-rate pacemaker. Adaptive-rate pacemakers increase the pacing rate in proportion to signals derived from body. The term "synchronous pacemaker (SPM)" is also frequently used to describe all pacemakers of which the frequency can be accelerated by means of a sensor other than the sinus node. Possible sensors include atrial rate, Q-T interval, pH, venous oxygen saturation, respiratory rate, cardiac output, body motion, and blood temperature. However, no single sensor/algorithm is ideal and improvement has been sought by introducing new sensors, adjusting the algorithms by which biosensor signals are converted to the most appropriate pacing rate.

The development of implantable pacemakers in the clinical setting mirrors the implementation of advanced technical possibilities. In the United States, 83% of all pacemakers implanted in 1996 had the rate response as a programmable option [49]. A variety of sensors have been used for rate control. Rate-adaptive pacemakers are increasingly becoming part of clinical routine, the most widespread systems being activity-controlled pacemakers that detect low-frequency acceleration, vibration, gravitation, movement, and pressure for controlling the rate adaptation. Among these concepts, accelerometer-controlled pacing is the most widely used rate-adaptive principle.

However, due to the considerable difference in signal amplitude for different types of exercise of the same intensity, an activity-controlled pacemaker system cannot entirely meet metabolic conditions and requirements [42], [43], [52]. The body vibration is not closely related to physiological needs and it has similar limitations in rate response as the body activity directed (Activitrax) pacemakers. Although these pacemakers respond to an increase in walking speed, neither one appropriately responds to walking up different gradients. In both cases, ascending and descending of stairs resulted in similar pacing rates [44].

Central venous oxygen saturation (SvO2) closely reflects cardiac output and tissue oxygen consumption. In the absence of an adequate chronotropic response during exercise, SvO2 will decrease and the extent of desaturation may be used as a parameter for rate-adaptive cardiac pacing [45]. The SvO2 sensor demonstrated a more physiological response to activities of daily living compared with the activity sensor. For humans patients during bicycle exercise testing the O2Sat decreased on average from 61% +/- 4% at rest to 36% +/- 4% ($P < 0.0001$) at peak exercise, at the maximum pacing rate of 122 +/- 5 beats/min. The time delay until the O2Sat had dropped 10%, 65%, and 90% of the total reduction during exercise was 4.8 +/-0.9 seconds, 39.8 +/- 3.8 seconds, and 71.3 +/- 7.5 seconds, respectively [46].

Many types of sensors have been developed and applied clinically during recent years. Technical improvements can be achieved through greater sensitivity and especially through more specificity for various physical or preferably physiologic signals. However, to date no single sensor properly reflects metabolic demands under all circumstances, no single sensor is ideal for all potential applications.

Actual investigations use two or more sensors or combine sensors in such a way that a composite bio-signal is derived to provide a linear relationship with the appropriate heart rate. A successful new algorithm is the rate augmentation algorithm for use with minute ventilation, which provides a better initial pacing rate response. A combination of minute ventilation sensed by impedance changes and movement sensed with piezoelectric crystals maintains the rapid response from the piezoelectric crystal and overcomes its lack of proportionality. Another successful new combination of sensors is QT sensing from the evoked ventricular potential and motion sensing with a piezoelectric crystal. Yet, these innovations have not been extensively tested. They have been shown to confer some clinical benefit, and the improvements so far obtained justify the expectance of further improvements.

In a manner analogous to the normal sinus node, the input from several sources will have to be considered. This leads to the development of eventually multi-sensor pacemakers, in which the rate is computed based on information on the various parameters [50]. Several pacemakers that use multiple sensors with different but complementary operating characteristics are already commercially available. Although preliminary findings are encouraging, additional clinical experience with these pacemakers is needed to determine their ultimate role in clinical practice. Simultaneous use of multiple complementary artificial sensors may permit development of cardiac pacemakers that operate more physiologically yet require less specialized medical follow-up [48].

Although the use of a second sensor is currently of proven benefit for a limited number of patients, the concept of closed-loop pacing, implementing a negative feedback between pacing rate and some control signal derived from the body to avoid over-pacing is subject to further investigation. The maximum heart rate of the normal sinus node is approximated by the formula: HRmax = (220-age) with a variance of approximately 15%. However, the nominal upper rate of most permanent pacemakers is 120 beats/min, a value that remains unchanged for many patients. As this nominal setting falls well below the maximum predicted heart rate for most patients, the chronotropic response of rate adaptive pacemakers during moderate and maximal exercise workloads is less than optimal [56]. This is of special importance in defibrillator patients whose myocardial contractility is generally limited. These patients are most sensitive to pacing rates that are too high for a given metabolic situation. This is the reason we chose to add a rate-limiting input to our fuzzy controller. Experimental in vitro testing coupled with clinical studies have shown that in humans a pH sensor will sense acute changes in pH occurring in response to exercise [54]. A cardiac pacemaker capable of responding to blood acidosis by change in its stimulation rate allows adjustment to a patient's metabolic needs. An iridium oxide electrode in the right atrium senses the blood pH. During exercise the venous pH decreases. As the paced ventricular rate increases, the acidosis should return to initial values. Yet if the acidosis persists, the paced rate must gradually return to baseline [53]. Previous authors have selected the variations of blood pH to drive the pacing rate according to the new biological balance created by exercise. The clinical tests performed on the patients who have had a pH-triggered pacemaker implanted one year previously demonstrated that during physical exercise there is an increase of cardiac rate triggered by the pacemaker, comparable with that noted when sinus rhythm is present [55]. Contrary to this approach we used the increased and persistent detected blood acidosis as an indication to temperate the paced rate in order to avoid heart over-pacing.

The use of combined sensors and advanced algorithms can improve the rate performance over a single sensor system. Combinations of sensors and algorithms that are more sophisticated, however, invariably increase the complexity of pacemaker programming. The work developed in the frame of this study as well as the results published by other authors (see for instance [25], [57]) demonstrated that the fuzzy approach might be an optimum compromise to implement complex pacemakers within the physical limitations of implantable devices. Several technological constraints have to be carefully considered for such critical applications of fuzzy logic; for a discussion on safety and hardware requirements for fuzzy processors in pacemakers, see [57]. Nevertheless, advances in cardiac pacing continue at an astounding rate and occasionally, technologic capabilities are developed almost faster than they can be implemented and tested clinically.

Appendix – Fu.L.L. program for the heart controller

```
UNIVERSES
    sensor = [0,1000];
    heartrate = [0, 300];
VARIABLES
exercise, tiredness = sensor .
    {
    low = POLYLINE { 0/1, 250/1, 500/0 };
    medium = POLYLINE { 250/0, 400/1, 600/1, 750/0 };
    high = POLYLINE { 500/0, 750/1, 1000/1 };
    }
```

puls = heartrate .
   {
   verylow = POLYLINE { 0/1, 20/1, 60/0 };
   low = POLYLINE { 10/0, 40/1, 50/1, 100/0 };
   medium = POLYLINE { 40/0, 75/1, 90/1, 150/0 };
   high = POLYLINE { 70/0, 115/1, 300/1 };
   veryhigh = POLYLINE { 115/0, 180/1, 300/1 };
   }

command = [-50,50] .
   {
   decreasefast = POLYLINE { -50/1, -40/1, -30/0 };
   decrease = POLYLINE { -40/0, -30/1, -20/1, -10/0 };
   hold = POLYLINE { -20/0, 0/1, 20/0 };
   increase = POLYLINE { 10/0, 20/1, 30/1, 40/0 };
   increasefast = POLYLINE { 30/0, 40/1, 50/1 };
   }

BEGIN
   "The rules of exercise"
   IF pulse IS verylow AND exercise IS low THEN command IS increase;
   IF pulse IS verylow AND (exercise IS medium OR high) THEN command IS increasefast;
   IF pulse IS low AND exercise IS low THEN command IS hold;
   IF pulse IS low AND exercise IS medium THEN command IS increase;
   IF pulse IS low AND exercise IS high THEN command IS increasefast;
   IF pulse IS medium AND exercise IS low THEN command IS decrease;
   IF pulse IS medium AND exercise IS medium THEN command IS hold;
   IF pulse IS medium AND exercise IS high THEN command IS increase;
   IF pulse IS high AND exercise IS low THEN command IS decreasefast;
   IF pulse IS high AND exercise IS medium THEN command IS decrease;
   IF pulse IS high AND exercise IS high THEN command IS hold;
   IF pulse IS very high AND (exercise IS low OR medium) THEN command IS decreasefast;
   IF pulse IS very high AND exercise IS high THEN command IS decrease;

   "The rules of tiredness"
   IF pulse IS verylow AND tiredness IS NOT high THEN command IS increasefast;
   IF pulse IS verylow AND tiredness IS high THEN command IS increase;
   IF pulse IS low AND tiredness IS low THEN command IS increasefast;
   IF pulse IS low AND tiredness IS medium THEN command IS increase;
   IF pulse IS low AND tiredness IS high THEN command IS hold;
   IF pulse IS medium THEN command IS hold;
   IF pulse IS high AND tiredness IS low THEN command IS hold;
   IF pulse IS high AND tiredness IS medium THEN command IS decrease;

IF pulse IS high AND tiredness IS high THEN command IS decreasefast;
IF pulse IS very high AND tiredness IS low THEN command IS decrease;
IF pulse IS very high AND tiredness IS NOT low THEN command IS decreasefast;
END

References

[1] Seipel, L., G. Pietrek, R. Koerfer and F. Loogen: Prognosis following pacemaker implantation, *Internist*, vol. 18, no. 1, pp. 21-24, 1977
[2] Stangl, K. and A. Wirtzfeld: Antibradykarde Stimulation: Prognose, Haemodynamik, Indikationen. In: Stangl, K., H. Heuer and A. Wirtzfeld (Eds.), *Frequenzadaptive Herzschrittmacher. Physiologie, Technologie, klinische Ergebnisse*. Steinkopff Verlag, Darmstadt, 1990
[3] Hyman, A.S.: Resuscitation of the stopped heart by intracardial therapy, *Arch. Int. Med.*, vol. 50, pp. 289-308, 1932
[4] Zoll, P.M.: Resuscitation of heart in ventricular standstill by external electric stimulation, *New Eng. J. Med.*, vol. 247, pp. 768-771, 1952
[5] Elmquist, R. and A. Senning: An implantable pacemaker for the heart. In: Smyth, C.N. (Ed.), *Medical Electronics*. Proc. 2nd Int. Conf. Med. Electr., London, Hiffe & Sons, 1960
[6] Furman, S. and G. Robinson: The use of an intracardiac pacemaker in the correction of total heart block, *Surg. Forum*, vol. 9, 1958
[7] Bernstein, A.D., A.J. Camm, R.D. Fletcher, R.D. Gold, A.F. Rickards, N.P. Smyth, S.R. Spielman and R. Sutton: The NASPE/BPEG generic pacemaker code for antibradyarrhythmia and adaptive-rate pacing and antitachyarrhythmia devices, *Pacing Clin. Electrophysiol.*, vol. 10, pp. 794-799, 1987
[8] Saoudi, N., U. Appl, F. Anselme, M. Voglimacci and A. Cribier: How smart should pacemakers be?, *J. Cardiol.*, vol. 83, no. 5B, pp. 180D-186D, 1999
[9] Provenier, F. et al.: Quality of life in patients with complete heart block and paroxysmal atrial tachyarrhythmias: a comparison of permanent DDIR versus DDDR pacing with mode switch to DDIR, *Pacing Clin. Electrophysiol.*, vol. 22, no. 3, pp. 462-468, 1999
[10] Marshall, H.J., Z.I. Harris, M.J. Griffith and M.D. Gammage: Atrioventricular nodal ablation and implantation of mode switching dual chamber pacemakers: effective treatment for drug refractory paroxysmal atrial fibrillation, *Heart*, vol. 79, no. 6, pp. 543-547, 1998
[11] Schuchert, A. and T. Meinertz: Pacemaker therapy in patients with atrial fibrillation, *Herz*, vol. 23, no. 4, pp. 260-268, 1998
[12] Saxon, L.A., J.P. Boehmer, J. Hummel, S. Kacet, T. De Marco, G. Naccarelli and E. Daoud: Biventricular pacing in patients with congestive heart failure: two prospective randomized trials. The VIGOR CHF and VENTAK CHF investigators, *Am. J. Cardiol.*, vol. 83, no. 5B, pp. 120D-123D, 1999

[13] Strungaru, R.: Influence of the cardiovascular system on the heart rate. Report Grant no. ERB-CIPA-CT-92-10200, Bucharest, 1992
[14] Keurs, H. E. D. J. and M. I. M. Noble: *Starling's Law of the Heart Revisited.* Kluwer Academic Publishers, 1988
[15] Levick, J.R.: *An Introduction to Cardiovascular Physiology.* Butterworth, 1991.
[16] Guyton, A.C., C.E. Jones and T.G. Coleman: *Circulatory Physiology: Cardiac Output and Its Regulation.* Saunders, 1973
[17] Moeller, D.: Simulation of a closed loop nonlinear average model of the cardiovascular system. In: Kenner, T., R. Busse and H. Hinghofer-Szalkay (Eds.), *Cardiovascular System Dynamics.* Plenum Press, 1982
[18] Smith, J.M. and R.J. Cohen: Simple finite-element model accounts for wide range of cardiac dysrhythmias, *Science*, vol. 81, pp. 233-237, 1984
[19] Clancy, E.A., J.M. Smith and R.J. Cohen: A simple electrical-mechanical model of the heart applied to the study of electrical-mechanical alternans, *IEEE Trans. Biomed. Eng.*, vol. 38, no. 6, pp. 551-559, 1991
[20] Rickards, A.F. and R.M. Donaldson: Rate responsive pacing, *Clin. Prog. Pacing Electrphysiol.*, vol. 1, pp. 12-19, 1983
[21] Adler, S., P. Cahill, R. Atkins and R. Martin: Appropriateness of temperature as a metabolic sensor for rate control of an implantable pacemaker, *Proc. 8th Annual Internat. Conf. of the IEEE Engineering in Medicine & Biology Society*, vol. 8, pp. 84-88, 1986
[22] Sugiura, T., Y. Itoh, S. Mizushina, T. Hasegawa, K. Yoshimura and Y. Harada: Microcomputer-based cardiac pacemaker control system through blood temperature, *J. Med. Eng. Technol.*, vol. 8, pp. 267-269, 1984
[23] Sellers, T.D., N.E. Fearnot and H.J. Smith: Right ventricular blood temperature profiles for rate responsive pacing, *Pace*, vol. 10 (Part I), pp. 467-479, 1987
[24] Anderson, K., D. Humen and G.J. Klein: A rate variable pacemaker which automatically adjusts for physical activity, *Pace*, vol. 6, Part II, pp. A-12, 1983
[25] Sugiura T., N. Sugiura, T. Kazui and Y. Harada: A self-tuning effect of membership functions in a fuzzy-logic-based cardiac pacing system. *J. Med. Eng. Technol.* 22(3), pp. 137-143, 1998
[26] Lau, C.P., A. Antoniou, D.F. Ward and A.J. Camm: Reliability of minute ventilation as a parameter for rate responsive pacing, *Pace*, vol. 12, p. 321, 1989
[27] Sutton, R., A.D. Sharma and A. Ingram: First derivative of right ventricular pressure as a sensor for an implantable rate responsive VVI pacemaker, *Pace*, vol. 11, p. 800, 1988
[28] Wirtzfeld, A., R. Heinze, K. Stangl, K.N. Hoekstein, E. Alt and H.D. Liess: Regulation of pacing rate by variations of mixed venous oxygen saturation, *Pace*, vol. 7, pp. 1257-1262, 1984
[29] Inbar, G.F., R. Heinye, K.N. Hoekstein, H.D. Liess, K. Stangl and A. Wirtzfeld: Development of a closed-loop pacemaker controller regulating mixed venous oxygen saturation level, *IEEE Trans. Biomed. Eng.*, vol. 35, no. 9, pp. 679-690, 1988
[30] Boheim, G. and M. Schaldach: Intrakardiale Impedanzplethysmographie, *Biomedizinische Technik*, Band 33, Ergaenzungsband 2, pp. 305-306, 1988

[31] Chirife, R., R. Pesce, E. Valero de Pesce and M. Favoloro: Initial studies on a new adaptive-rate pacemaker controlled by pre-ejection interval or stroke volume. Circulatory and pharmacologic challenges, *Pace*, vol. 12, p. 1568, 1989

[32] Hoekstein, K.N.: *Cardiac stroke volume estimation from two-electrode electrical impedance measurement*. Dissertation Thesis. Universitaet der Bundeswehr, Muenchen, 1990

[33] Popescu, S.: Fuzzy Controller takes Over an Ill Heart. *Proceedings of The 16th European Congress on Intelligent Techniques and Soft Computing EUFIT'98*, Aachen, Germany, vol. 3, pp. 1863-1866, 1998

[34] Brubaker, I.D.: Fuzzy-logic basics: intuitive rules replace complex math, *Electronic Design News*, vol. 13, pp. 111-116, 1992

[35] Brubaker, I.D.: Fuzzy-logic system solves control problem, *Electronic Design News*, vol. 13, pp. 121-128, 1992

[36] Brubaker, I.D.: Designing a fuzzy-logic control system, *Electronic Design News*, vol. 7, pp. 76-88, 1993

[37] Brubaker, I.D.: Everything you always wanted to know about fuzzy-logic, *Electronic Design News*, vol. 7, pp. 103-106, 1993

[38] Bühler, H.: *Réglaje par logique floue*. Présses Polytechniques et Universitaire Romandes, Lausanne, Lausanne, CH 1994

[39] Cios, J.K. et al.: Using Fuzzy Sets to Diagnose Coronary Artery Stenosis, *Computer*, vol. 24, no. 3, pp. 57-63, 1991

[40] Liebert, W.: *Chaos und Herzdynamik*. Verlag Harri Deutsch, Frankfurt am Main, Germany, 1991

[41] Negoita, C.V.: *Expert Systems and Fuzzy Systems*. The Benjamin/Cumming Publishing Comp. Inc., Menlo Park/CA, USA, 1985

[42] Alt, E., M. Matula, H. Theres, M. Heinz and R. Baker: The basis for activity controlled rate variable cardiac pacemakers: an analysis of mechanical forces on the human body induced by exercise and environment, *Pacing Clin. Electrophysiol.*, vol. 12, 10, pp. 1667-1680, 1989

[43] Alt, E., M. Matula and K. Hölzer: Behavior of different activity-based pacemakers during treadmill exercise testing with variable slopes: a comparison of three activity-based pacing systems, *Pacing Clin. Electrophysiol.*, vol. 17, 11 Pt. 1, pp. 1761-1770, 1994

[44] Lau, C.P., W.S. Tse and A.J. Camm: Clinical experience with Sensolog 703: a new activity sensing rate responsive pacemaker, *Pacing Clin. Electrophysiol.*, Oct. 11(10), pp. 1444-1455, 1988

[45] Lau, C.P., Y.T. Tai, W.H. Leung, S.K. Leung, J.P. Li, C.K. Wong, I.S. Lee, C. Yerich and M. Erickson: Rate adaptive cardiac pacing using right ventricular venous oxygen saturation: quantification of chronotropic behavior during daily activities and maximal exercise, *Pacing Clin. Electrophysiol.*, vol. 17(12 Pt. 1), pp. 2236-2246, 1994

[46] Faerestrand, S., O.J. Ohm, L. Stangeland, H. Heynen and A. Moore: Long-term clinical performance of a central venous oxygen saturation sensor for rate adaptive cardiac pacing, *Pacing Clin. Electrophysiol.*, vol. 17(8), pp. 1355-1372, 1994

[47] Katritsis, D., C.F. Shakespeare and A.J. Camm: New and combined sensors for adaptive-rate pacing, *Clin Cardiol.*, vol. 16 (3), pp. 240-248, 1993
[48] Benditt, D.G., M. Mianulli, K. Lurie, S. Sakaguchi and S. Adler: Multiple-sensor systems for physiologic cardiac pacing, *Ann. Intern. Med.*, vol. 121(12), pp. 960-968, 1994
[49] Alt, E.: What is the ideal rate-adaptive sensor for patients with implantable cardioverter defibrillators: lessons from cardiac pacing, *Am. J. Cardiol.*, vol. 83(5B), pp. 17D-23D, 1999
[50] Kappenberger, L.J.: Technical improvements in sensors for rate adaptive pacemakers, *Am. Heart J.*, vol. 127 (4 Pt 2), pp. 1022-1026, 1994
[51] Lau, C.P., S.K. Leung, M. Guerola and H.J. Crijns: Comparison of continuously recorded sensor and sinus rates during daily life activities and standardized exercise testing: efficacy of automatically optimized rate adaptive dual sensor pacing to simulate sinus rhythm, *Pacing Clin. Electrophysiol.*, vol. 19(11 Pt 2), pp. 1672-1677, 1996
[52] Candinas, R., M. Jakob, T.A. Buckingham, H. Mattmann and F.W. Amann: Vibration, acceleration, gravitation, and movement: activity controlled rate adaptive pacing during treadmill exercise testing and daily life activities, *Pacing Clin. Electrophysiol.*, vol. (7), pp. 1777-1786, 1997
[53] Cammilli, L., L. Alcidi, G. Papeschi, V. Wiechmann, L. Padeletti and G. Grassi: Preliminary experience with the pH-triggered pacemaker, *Pacing Clin. Electrophysiol.*, vol. 1(4), pp. 448-457, 1978
[54] Cammilli, L., L. Alcidi, E. Shapland and S. Obino: Results, problems and perspectives with the autoregulating pacemaker, *Pacing Clin. Electrophysiol.*, vol. 6(2 Pt 2), pp. 488-493, 1983
[55] Cammilli, L., L. Alcidi, G. Papeschi, L. Padeletti and G. Grassi: Clinical and biological aspects in patient with pH-triggered implanted pacemaker (article in Italian), *G. Ital. Cardiol.*, vol. 8 Suppl 1, pp. 252-258, 1978
[56] Carmouche, D.G., R.S. Bubien, G.N. Kay: The effect of maximum heart rate on oxygen kinetics and exercise performance at low and highworkloads, *Pacing Clin. Electrophysiol.*, vol. 21(4 Pt 1), pp. 679-686, 1998
[57] Teodorescu, H.N., A. Kandel and D. Mlynek: System requirements for fuzzy and neuro-fuzzy hardware in medical equipment. In: Teodorescu H.N., Kandel A., Jain L.C. (Eds.), *Fuzzy and Neuro-Fuzzy Systems in Medicine*, CRC Press, Boca Raton, Fl., USA, 1999

Part 5.

Robotic systems and advanced mechanics

Chapter 11

Service robots for rehabilitation and assistance

Mitch Wilkes, Anthony Alford, Todd Pack, Tamara Rogers, Edward Brown, Jr., Alan Peters, II, and **Kazuhiko Kawamura**

To reduce the health care expenses, new and cost-effective rehabilitation technologies are needed to help people who have limited control over their limbs. They require improved mobility, dexterity, and control to facilitate everyday tasks. We present the development of service robots for persons with physical disabilities. One of our key developments has been a software architecture for building intelligent service robots, including high-level software agents: the Human Agent and the Self Agent.

1. Introduction

Breakthroughs and improvements in modern day medical technologies have had the unsurprising effect of producing a healthier population. People are living longer than their parents and grandparents. Unfortunately, living longer is not necessarily living better. Physical ailments accrue over time for the elderly making simple, everyday tasks (such as feeding oneself) difficult and cumbersome. The same is true for people having life-long physical disabilities resulting from disease or unfortunate accidents. As health care costs rise, it is paramount that new and cost-effective developments in rehabilitation technologies emerge to serve the commercial market. This is particularly necessary for people who have had strokes, spinal cord injuries, or muscular atrophying diseases (such as muscular dystrophy) and have limited control over their limbs. They require improved mobility, dexterity, and control to facilitate everyday tasks.

1.1. Service robotics

In Vanderbilt University's Intelligent Robotics Laboratory (IRL), we specialize in service robotics for the person with a physical disability [22,24,25,26,27,28,31]. As the name describes, these robots assist the human user in the home, the workplace, and anywhere there is a repetitive task that requires unsupervised attention. Our emphasis is on human-robot interaction and machine intelligence. We use vision, voice, gesture, touch, sonar, infrared (IR), and other sensory inputs to study and improve collaboration and symbiosis between users and service robots. We also employ flexible biomimetic actuators (McKibben artificial muscles) and various nonlinear control and modeling techniques, including fuzzy logic and sliding mode control in our robot systems [20,21]. Our continuous research in service robots for assisting persons with a physical disability contains several unstructured and general problems (e.g., human-robot interfaces, interactivity, object recognition, navigation, system integration, and control).

In the early stages of our research we departed from traditional industrial robots and began to consider service robots for the persons with physical disabilities [18,22]. The close interaction with humans opened up an entirely new range of problems for research, such as reflex control [13,23]. The complexity of the problem at hand was just beginning to reveal itself, and therefore we began considering software architectures for robotics [4,6,7,18], intelligent user interfaces [22,24], and other topics relevant to the problem [17,21].

1.2. Human-machine interfacing and system integration

The human-machine interface and system integration are extremely important in the development of service robots. In the Intelligent Robotics Laboratory (IRL), we seek to develop service robots with sufficient local autonomy and human interactivity to enhance the lives of the human users. A primary goal of the IRL is to develop robots that are not only intelligent, but are also socially adaptable. We want these robots to cooperate with the user as well as each other to provide a powerful and robust system centered on the human user.

The idea of robots communicating and collaborating with their human user is a desirable one, indeed, but research reveals that this is not a trivial problem.

The IRL uses a variety of sensory inputs to study and improve collaboration and symbiosis between service robots and their users. To achieve a high level of collaboration, it is necessary that the various systems within the robot utilize some mechanism for communicating effectively with one another. The robot is ineffective if information about its environment is not successfully disseminated to the robot's higher level, decision-making functions. An intelligent mechanism for interaction is also needed to improve the symbiotic relationship necessary between the service robot and the user. This mechanism should place the human user at the center of the interactive system where the interfaces between the human and the robot are natural and comfortable. Natural and efficient interfaces enable the human and the robot to work together successfully to achieve common goals. This type of interface is mandatory in the study of rehabilitation robots [32].

1.3. System integration using agents

Agents can be described as software objects that perform specific tasks. Agents are intelligent and autonomous, and can be compared to having a personal secretary or advisor at one's fingertips. They can assist a user through a variety of means. This includes seeking and filtering information, personalizing a web environment, automating tasks, optimizing complex systems, and collaborating and negotiating services among other agents to achieve a common goal [19]. We believe that an agent-oriented architecture will facilitate proper negotiation and collaboration among the various hardware systems within a robot. Successful integration of these systems for performing desired tasks is entirely dependent on how well they are able to share knowledge with each other. For example, if we want our humanoid robot, ISAC (which stands for Intelligent Soft Arm Control), to feed a user with a physical disability, ISAC's vision, manipulation, and force sensing systems must work together and perform in coordination with one another to safely achieve this task. These systems can be considered to be individual primitive agents. As agents, they must collaborate effectively or the human is at immediate risk of being indefinitely hungry!

The above example also demonstrates how agents working together can assure communication between the robot and the human user. Rich and Sidner [46] discuss the value in having autonomous agents interact with people. Agents can become very powerful tools for system integration if they learn how to communicate and interact under the same principles and guidelines implicit during regular human collaboration. The obvious assumption is that if the agent uses a familiar, more "human" method of communication, it will ultimately be simpler for people to understand and to use. Collaborative agent architectures should also provide data structures and algorithms for representing and manipulating goals, actions, and shared plans. A shared plan is a formal representation of the data structures or mental states obtained from the participants of the collaboration. For successful collaboration, the participants need to have common mutual beliefs about the capabilities, intentions, and commitments of each participant. Thus, collaborating agent architectures can indeed prove useful for increasing the intelligence of a robot system.

1.4. Software architectures

Within the IRL we have developed a software architecture for building intelligent service robots, the Intelligent Machine Architecture (IMA) [40]. Three software architectures that have greatly influenced our agent architecture are Brooks' subsumption architecture [9], Arkin's hybrid deliberative/reactive AuRA architecture [10], and Albus's Real-time Control System (RCS) [1,2,3]. All three philosophies have been taken into consideration in the development of our architecture. Subsumption, reactivity, and deliberation provide a means for dealing with robot systems that must integrate sensors and various robot hardware apparatus in an organized manner. Robustness is the focus of these architectures.

Brooks' subsumption architecture promotes task-achieving behavior for a mobile robot system. It is a multi-level architecture in which the various hardware systems of the robot work in parallel. This contrasts to the traditional architectures where the hardware systems are arranged in a series decomposition of the functional unit modules. Each level or layer of control in the architecture has a certain amount of competence (i.e., desired class of behavior) associated with it. The higher the level, the greater the competence. Each layer can examine the layer directly beneath it. Upper layers can also suppress or inhibit data flow of lower layers. Thus, a higher layer can subsume a lower one, and as a result, complex behavior can be induced for a robot system.

Arkin's approach is characterized by a tight coupling between sensing and action without the use of any intervening global representations. Motor schemas are the basic units of motor behavior in his system. Each schema functions as a concurrent and independent agent contributing to the global success of the robot's task. The behaviors formed in Arkin's system include the following: move-to-goal, move-ahead, avoid-static-obstacle, escape and dodge, noise (move randomly), move-up, move-down, maintain-altitude, docking (move in a particular pattern towards a goal), avoid-past (avoid where the robot has been recently), and probe (seek out new areas).

Another influential architecture is Albus's Real-time Control System from the National Institute of Standards and Technology (NIST). In contrast to the above architectures, RCS emphasizes deliberative reasoning and world modeling. The architecture is composed of a hierarchy of computational units which provides a gradient between slower, deliberative planning at the higher layers, to faster, reactive behaviors at the lower layers. Sensors and actuators for interacting with the world reside at the lowest layer and provide information which the other layers use to construct a world model. By making a tradeoff between long term planning with coarse resolution at higher levels and short term planning with fine resolution at lower levels, the architecture keeps the computational burden of each unit manageable. This architecture has been applied to a wide range of applications including manufacturing applications such as machining, and navigation applications for autonomous ground and undersea vehicles.

1.5. Intelligent machine architecture (IMA)

The Intelligent Machine Architecture provides an integrated approach for designing control software for intelligent machines. It uses a system model that is agent based. Agents, as described above, are intelligent software modules that perform a desired task and can be combined to imitate and induce human-like reactive behavior. The IMA also uses an agent level model based on COM (Component Object Model) and DCOM (Distributed Component Object Model). COM and DCOM are software technologies developed by Microsoft and form the basis for many of their products.

The IMA offers a solution to complex software design for intelligent machines. It addresses software engineering issues such as reuse, extensibility, and management of complexity as well as system engineering issues including parallelism, scalability, reactivity, and robustness. IMA is well suited to the development of human centered systems, such as a service robot [52]. IMA is implemented under Windows NT 4.0 using Microsoft Visual C++, Microsoft Visual Basic, COM, and DCOM. Using this approach insures that IMA will run on a wide variety of standard PC hardware, and that programming is performed within a sophisticated development environment.

1.6. Human directed local autonomy (HuDL)

In creating technologies for the persons with physical disabilities, we follow the Human Directed Local Autonomy (HuDL) paradigm. HuDL is IRL's design philosophy of having robots that interact closely with the user and each other. It suggests a "user in the loop" strategy. If a service robot gets trapped or confused, it will require help from the user. Having the user in the loop makes the human-robot system more intelligent overall. However, there should be a definite balance between local robot autonomy and user intervention. The human should not have to concern himself too much with the operations of the robot. This defeats the point of developing intelligent robots.

Thus, we wish to avoid teleoperation, but take advantage of the human's considerably superior object recognition, planning, and reasoning abilities.

HuDL is based on exploiting the symbiotic relationship between the human user and the robot. In essence, the idea is to make maximum use of the things that humans do well and the things that robots do well. A good example is a robot to aid a person with a physical disability, perhaps suffering from some degree of paralysis. The human is intelligent, but has physical limitations in mobility and dexterity. The robot is mobile and/or able to manipulate objects, but may lack the intelligence to solve many real-world problems. A symbiotic combination of human and robot can improve the ability of the human to control his environment and enhances the usefulness of the robot by significantly augmenting its intelligence with that of the user. One key feature is flexible human integration. The background for this is clear: human intelligence is superior whenever unexpected or complicated situations are met. Roles and methods for integrating humans into different types of activities must be defined and developed.

For example, the user may request the robot to go into the kitchen and bring him a drink (see Figure 1). The robot may have sufficient intelligence to navigate to the kitchen, but the planning and object recognition problems may prove too difficult. If appropriate visual feedback is supplied to the user (perhaps a monitor lets him "see" what the robot sees), he/she can narrow the search space for the robot by giving high-level instructions. One way to do this is through a speech recognition system that provides a natural and convenient interface, and facilitates high-level commands such as "Pick up the red glass on the counter to your right." The robot may see several red objects that could be the glass in question, moves forward, points to the most likely object, and sends a message to the user, "Do you mean this one?" The user responds "No, that is a bottle of catsup, the glass is further to your right." In this way, the user guides the robot through the difficult object recognition task, greatly enhancing the likelihood of success. Similarly, the robot has enabled the human to have more control over his environment.

We are using HuDL to guide the development of a cooperative service robot team consisting of a dual-armed stationary humanoid, called ISAC (see Figure 2), and a modified Yaskawa Helpmate mobile robot, simply called Helpmate (see Figure 3). The user interfaces currently under development include speech recognition (for verbal input), text to speech (for verbal output), vision (for tracking of faces and hands as well as many other tasks), gesture (a vision based interface), force, touch, and sound localization. These interfaces are being used to make the overall interaction with ISAC and Helpmate into a natural "multimedia" experience that is comfortable for nontechnical users. ISAC is even able to play an electronic musical instrument, a theremin, with perfect pitch. Indeed, this may be one of the most interesting social skills of a service robot to date.

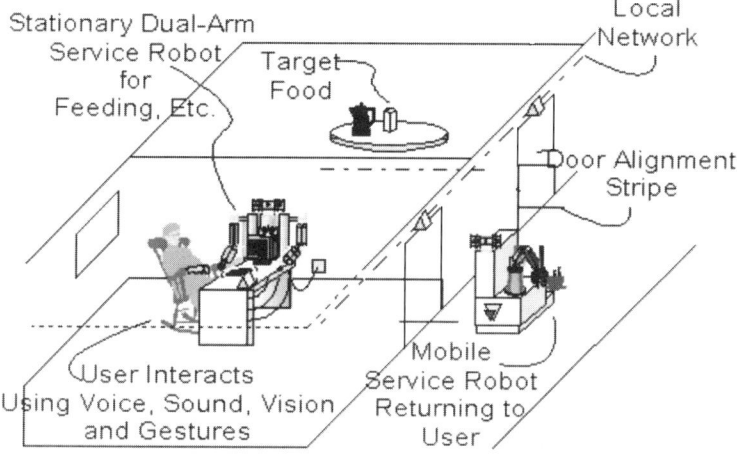

Figure 1. Service robot system testbed.

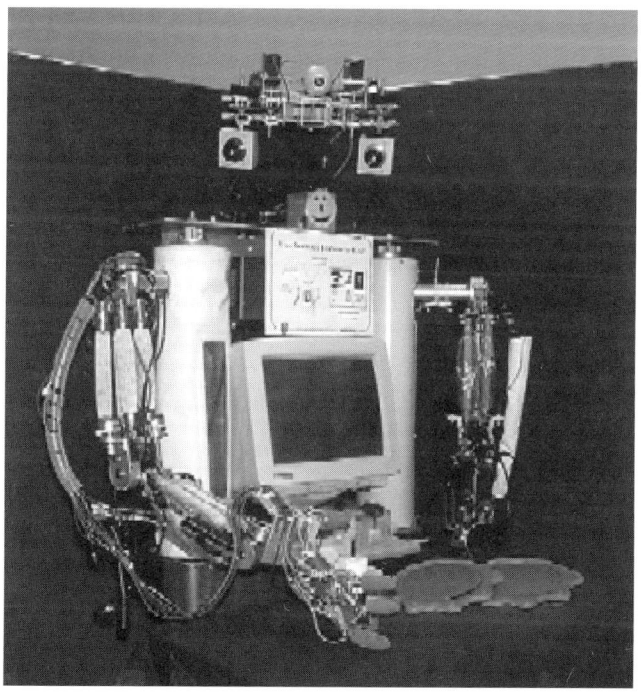

Figure 2. The humanoid robot ISAC.

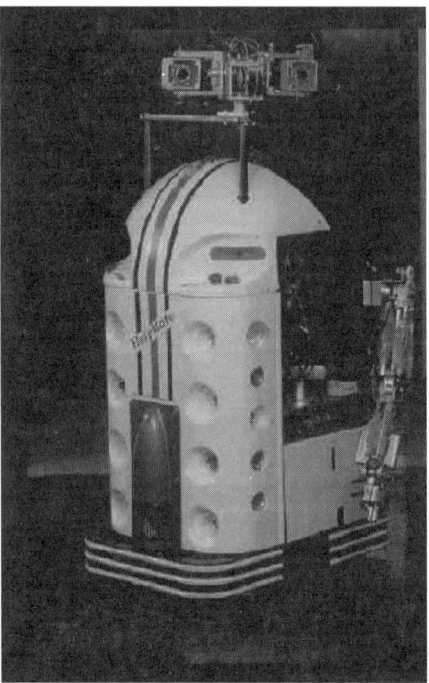

Figure 3. The mobile robot, Helpmate.

The remainder of this chapter is organized as follows. Section 2 describes the historical perspective that led to the IMA, while Section 3 describes the IMA itself. Section 4 explains the HuDL paradigm as well as two high level intelligent agents, the Human Agent and the Self Agent. Section 5 describes some of our results. The chapter ends with a section on conclusions and future work.

2. Historical background: software architectures in the IRL

In order to understand the need for IMA, we will place its development into an historical context.

2.1. The previous architecture

Before we developed our current software architecture, our robot ISAC used a distributed control architecture based on a "blackboard" [6]. In this system, the ISAC/Distributed Objects architecture, several independent software modules communicated via a shared resource, the blackboard. Modules requiring the services of other modules posted requests on the blackboard. Each module monitored the blackboard for requests it could perform. Most of the system software ran on Sun workstations. A parallel controller based on Transputers controlled the robot's arm hardware. A PC served as the host for both communication and software development. Image processing was performed on dedicated image processing hardware. The software modules accessed the blackboard and the arm controller host using TCP/IP streams over an Ethernet LAN.

2.2. Shortcomings of the previous approach

In our exploration into which properties would be desirable in a software architecture we considered ideas from many different areas including:
- real-time operating systems,
- behavior-based control systems [35],
- the ISAC/Distributed Objects system [5,7],
- parallel processing systems,
- architecture documents from other robotics research groups [38,47]
- control systems,
- software engineering, and
- personal experience with various aspects of system development.

We wanted to combine ideas from all these sources. The resulting architecture would not be guaranteed to be optimal in any sense. It would be a practical compromise of methods intended to maximize the capability and productivity of our research group in developing service robotic systems with the hardware currently available, or which will soon become available in the next few years.

2.2.1. Motivations
The architecture is a set of organizing principles and core components that are used to build the basis for the system. We desired an architecture that defined a working paradigm for highly interactive service robot systems.

2.2.2. Pitfalls of the past
There are assumptions made in any system and the ISAC/Distributed Objects [7] system had worked rather well. However, there were a number of problematic assumptions that were in that system that greatly reduced our productivity and the potential for ISAC. The following is a description of these problems.

2.2.3. The problem of interfaces

When the interface to a module becomes more complex than the module itself there is a serious interface problem from the software perspective. In fact, our previous system had entire modules that translated between equivalent but incompatible interfaces for modules. These modules were nothing but interfaces. They didn't contribute to the operation of the system at all.

From software engineering, we know that interfaces support encapsulation and help hide details to make modules more independent. However, it only applies to properly chosen interfaces. If a "low level" module hides too much from the upper layers, you must continuously modify that module to incorporate an increasingly complex interface and then modify all other "high level" software to take advantage of this new interface feature.

Thus the type of encapsulation used and the interfaces between modules must be carefully selected so that new capabilities can be added to the system by adding modules with new capabilities, not by modifying all the modules in the system.

2.2.4. The problem of streams

The core communication paradigm upon which ISAC/Distributed Objects was based was TCP/IP Streams. The assumption of this paradigm is that two programs will create a fixed connection between each other and the socket will act like a bi-directional FIFO between the system elements. The problem with this paradigm is that there is no delimiter in the communication. Neither program can control when the data that it writes to the socket is communicated to the other program. There are no message boundaries in streams. This paradigm is fine for data transfer, but not at all suited for control. Note that this is not implementation dependent, it is an explicit assumption of the protocol that neither program knows or cares when the other program gets the data that they exchange.

2.2.5. The problem of the blackboard

At the most basic level, the Blackboard paradigm implied two things about our system. First, it was a central point of communication and all relevant communication had to go through the blackboard. Second, it implied that there was one single universal internal "language" that was spoken by all components that connected to the blackboard and each module must learn that language or at least part of it. Most discussions of blackboard architectures focus on modules "sharing knowledge" or "goals" on the blackboard. This implies a very highly centralized representation for all aspects of the system. There was no real specification for this representation [7]. It was built by word of mouth within our laboratory community and had no formal basis. There was little documentation of this language, which compounded the problem. To phrase this problem differently, any new capability in the system required a new language element to describe the capability, and other modules had to be modified to use this new element to access the capability.

In the ISAC/Distributed Objects system, the idea was that the modules would be loosely coupled by having them share information through the blackboard. However, in practice it turned out that this created such tight interdependency between modules that it was extremely difficult to modify or update a module without changing and recompiling all the other modules in the system as well. Thus, for our system the blackboard was self-defeating. It decoupled the modules so much that they could not cooperate effectively or deal with time explicitly, but made all the modules critically dependent on the complex "Blackboard Language" that they shared.

2.2.6. Desirable properties of a new architecture

We now describe the properties that we believe a new architecture should have. This is a list of specifications for our new core software components.

Multiple Granularity — Modules in the system correspond to differing levels of granularity in terms of processing time and data flow. This granularity is a way to differentiate between high- and low-level modules in the system; nevertheless, high- and low-level modules share control of the system as equals.

Direct Composition — Modules plug together naturally to build up the functionality of the system. Adding a module means adding new or improved functionality. Furthermore, some modules are really "composed" of simpler modules. Thus there is a hierarchical way to describe the relationships between modules.

Reconfigurable/Reusable Modules — Modules can be combined in new ways or combined with one or two new modules to change the system. If we desire a new capability for the system, we build a module to give the system that capability, without modifying all the other modules.

Inherently Parallel — All modules are concurrent processes and there is no single link or central point that can choke the entire system. This is commonly desired for fault tolerance.

Event Driven — The most important thing in the world of a robot is an event. Without external events it does nothing. However, it must respond rapidly to external events. The passage of time is itself an event so an event-driven paradigm provides a natural and uniform way to deal with time and other "data" type events.

Explicit Representations — All relevant sensory information in the system should be made explicit within the system and not encapsulated within a module. Otherwise, this module will have to be continually modified to change its interface to export more information. This does not mean that everything broadcasts to everything else. But it does imply that sensory modules will largely be transparent to other modules in the system.

Flat Connectivity — All modules in the system are equal with respect to sensory information access and actuation command generation. The information might have various granularities, but any module can access it. This type of connectivity is not just a logical construct in the case of our system. It is a property of the most basic communication protocol.

Asynchronous — All modules execute asynchronously as quickly as they can [47]. There is no attempt to maintain a single global clock since the complexity of implementing it would overwhelm the complexity of the system. Synchronization happens primarily through sensory input or through explicit messaging between modules. Modules that are directly tied to hardware can synchronize with that hardware.

Incremental Commands — All modules that produce commands for the hardware work in an incremental mode. This implies that these actuation modules always try to go in the best current direction. This has the effect of greatly reducing the need for global representations in the system by simplifying low-level module interfaces.

3. A new architecture

The high degree of human-robot interaction we desire to achieve has implications for the system integration process, i.e., both the robot software and hardware must exhibit certain characteristics. For safety reasons, the robot software must be reactive, responding quickly to the presence and actions of a human. The software must provide support for a variety of human interaction modes, such as speech and gestures, and must be able to interpret human input. The robot hardware must also be designed with safety in mind, thus care must be taken in choosing the actuators. In this regard, we use flexible pneumatic actuators (specifically, McKibben artificial muscles) in our robot arms [29,32,39]. These flexible, compliant, lightweight actuators provide safe but useful robot arms. Another concern is sensing; the robot should be capable of sensing a human presence.

Intelligent service robot software in general is complex, because the robot must exhibit a large number of diverse skills or competencies to make it useful. Thus, development of a service robot involves difficult software problems. There are several design issues involved in developing the software for the robot: the choice of computing platform for the robot, the degree of modularity and extensibility desired, and the division of labor among programmers. As our laboratory has focused on service robot development [6,29,32,39], we have found that a key issue is software system integration. Others have made similar observations. An International Conference on Robotics and Automation

(ICRA) '96 panel identified system integration as one of the grand challenges for the robotics research community [12].

Development of robot skills requires knowledge of many domains (e.g., artificial intelligence, control systems, image processing, software engineering, computer science and engineering). Service robot software development is therefore a team effort. Integration of software produced by many programmers imposes additional complexity. It is also desirable that the robot software run on a system of distributed processors. This has many advantages: parallelism, scalability, redundancy, cost. However, the software must be written to take advantage of distributed processing. In particular, communication among the distributed modules becomes critical.

Our solution to the problems of system integration has been to develop a software architecture, the Intelligent Machine Architecture [30]. In the IMA, the system is designed as a collection of primitive agents. We use the term "primitive agent" to mean a software module that has the following properties:

Autonomy — Primitive agents own their components. They are separate and distinct concepts or objects in the domain for which the software is written. Thus, they have a strong conceptual encapsulation boundary at the system level.

Proactivity — Primitive agents act locally based on their own internal state, the available resources, and the observations of other agents through specific relationships. The core of the primitive agent's operation is a decision or action selection process.

Reactivity — Primitive agents are reactive because they respond to changes in their external environment.

Connectivity — Primitive agents are cooperative because they give and receive information from other primitive agents to achieve their tasks.

Resource Bounded — Primitive agents are resource driven and may be competitive because they represent only a single conceptual element and depend on other primitive agents as their resources. In a properly structured system, the competition between primitive agents for a resource should represent a natural property of the system, not a bottleneck in the software architecture. In these cases, arbitration between various actions becomes important.

In the IMA, a primitive agent models some element of the system: a task, a skill, a robot resource, or even a physical object such as a table or a human. This decomposition has the following advantages:

Distributed processing — Primitive agents need not all be on the same computer.

Parallelism — Primitive agents can work in parallel across a network.

Encapsulation — Component object technology enables primitive agents to have strong encapsulation boundaries, thus enforcing proper access of the agents.

Scalability — The object decomposition approach provides flexibility for a system that grows in complexity over time.

Robustness — Distributed communicating agents provide graceful degradation if a subset of the system fails.

In addition to the system-level decomposition into primitive agents, each primitive agent is designed as a collection of components. In IMA, components are software objects created using the COM and DCOM. Currently, we develop components using Microsoft Visual C++ version 6.0 and Visual Basic 6.0.

A component's methods and data can be accessed only through well-defined interfaces. Because of this, components created by different programmers can be easily integrated. Components encapsulate reusable and distinct attributes of a primitive agent, such as functionality or data. For example, a component may represent an image, or a vector, or an algorithm, such as a PID controller, a visual servoing algorithm, a speech recognition module, etc. This component model offers several advantages. For one, component reuse is high. For example, a primitive agent is typically composed of four or five components. Of these, usually only one or two need to be developed as new components. The others are reused, i.e., they are previously developed components. Primitive agents are also easily configured and extended. New algorithms or data representations are easily integrated into the system. Also, since a component is limited in scope, code development and debugging are easier (e.g., no monolithic programs).

4. Intelligent agents for human-robot interaction

4.1. HuDL, humans and robots working together

For the past ten years, our research has focused on service robotics research. We have continually observed that a key research issue in service robotics is the integration of humans into the system. This has led to our development of guiding principles for service robot system design [29]. Our paradigm for human/robot interaction is HuDL, initially introduced in [32].

In traditional industrial robotics settings, a human presence is highly undesirable and can be dangerous. In a service robotics setting, however, a human presence is not only possible, it can be highly desirable. Why should humans and robots interact? Obviously if a service robot is to be of use to the human, it must be able to communicate with the human. The human needs some way of telling the robot what service to perform, or to stop what it is doing, or even provide an evaluation of how well the robot is performing.

Pook and Ballard [44] have shown that both full robot autonomy and human teleoperation of robots have disadvantages. In their deictic teleassistance model, a human uses hand signals to initiate and situate a robot's autonomous behaviors. This deictic strategy has also been used to control a wheelchair robot used as an aid for persons with physical disabilities [11]. HuDL also maintains the concept of autonomous robot behaviors directed by a human user. The philosophy of HuDL is that the human is "in the loop." The human does not teleoperate the robot, but rather commands and guides the robot at a higher level. The role of the human in controlling the robot can be described by a spectrum [44]. At the extremes of the spectrum are teleoperation and full autonomy. These extremes have both advantages and disadvantages. Teleoperation is tiring and tedious for the user while full autonomy is very difficult to achieve and is often fragile. The middle of the spectrum tries to balance robot autonomy and human control in order to keep the advantages of the extremes, while avoiding their disadvantages.

Integrating humans into a robot system in this way has several advantages. First is the use of the human's intelligence and decision-making abilities. For example, the human can interpret the robot's sensor data (e.g., indicating a target object in a camera scene), thereby simultaneously reducing the computational burden on the robot and increasing the robustness of the overall system. The human can also detect an exceptional or error situation, and assist the robot in recovering [16]. However, the human is not directly or explicitly driving the robot's actuators. This relieves the human of the often tedious and frustrating, or in the case of users with physical disabilities, impossible task of manual teleoperation.

HuDL allows the achievement today of a service robot of useful but limited intelligence and ability. Over time the system will be improved by the addition of better user interfaces, object recognition, reasoning, planning, navigation, etc. as well as improved hardware such as better manipulators, cameras, sensors, computers, etc. In this way, a "glide path" toward much greater autonomy will be established in the near future. In particular, newer user interfaces need to be developed that enable the robot to detect and understand the users feelings and emotional state such as joy, anger, fatigue, etc., and to act in an appropriate manner for that emotional state. Thus, the new field of affective computing plays a significant role in the development of socially intelligent service robots [42]. Also, the robot should have a learning capability to allow it to adapt its behavior to the particular needs and personality of the user. Therefore, over time the service robot becomes suited to a particular individual or group of individuals.

HuDL is dialog-based, rhythmic, and adaptive. Dialog-based human-robot interaction has been explored in areas such as robot programming [14] and as an interface to a mobile manipulator [33]. A dialog-based interaction provides an active mechanism for the robot to receive information from the human; that is, the robot can direct the human's input in order to satisfy the robot's information requirements. For example, as described in the scenario of the introduction, the robot may be unsure of which possible item is correct and request assistance. Or perhaps more generally, upon entering a room the robot may ask the human to direct it to that portion of the room containing the desired object, thus significantly reducing the search space and increasing both the speed and the robustness of the overall task.

The iterative nature of the dialog leads us to the idea of rhythmic interaction. Rhythmic responses from computer systems have become important indicators of correct function: animated cursors for windowing systems, animated icons for web browsers, even the sound of disk access—all these things let us know that our computers are working. As an example, if the computer ceases to give some type of rhythmic response, i.e., the cursor stops moving, the disk access stops, etc., the human knows that it has "locked up" and should take corrective action. The same idea can apply to a robot. As long as it can provide a rhythmic response, the human is more confident that it is functioning. If the human-robot interaction is rhythmic, exceptional or error states can be detected by the simple technique of the timeout. The human expects the robot to respond within a certain time interval. If it does not, the human may suspect the robot has failed in some way. Likewise, the robot also expects some input from the human. If the human does not provide it, the robot may ask if the human is busy, confused, or perhaps even in need of medical attention.

As the human becomes more familiar with the robot, and proficient in interaction, his interaction patterns will change. Consider the user of a word processor. At first, as the user discovers the capabilities of the software, he probably does things "the hard way," by searching through menus, etc. As he becomes more familiar with the program, he begins to learn shortcuts. Likewise, the user of a robot is likely to desire shortcuts in using the robot. Besides the obvious customizations of shortcuts, macros and preferences, the adaptive aspect of the human-robot interaction provides richer avenues for "personalizing" the robot. For example, through the use of an appropriate learning mechanism, the robot may learn to anticipate what the human will request next. Although it would be annoying and possibly dangerous to have the robot execute tasks before it is asked, the robot could prepare to execute the task by, for example, searching for target objects or positioning its manipulators.

Since service robots are specifically intended to perform tasks for and around humans, special consideration must be given to the modalities of interaction between robots and people. To make the interaction more "normal" for the human user, communication should go far beyond human keyboard input and flashing lights on the robot. We want the human and robot to interact using as many different media as possible. Ideally, these media include those natural to human interaction, such as speech [16,51], gestures [41,44], and touch [37]. The motivation for using these natural modes is that they are familiar, are more comfortable, and require less training for the user. Computer-based GUIs with pointing devices can also be used effectively [11], and because of our robot control hardware and software architecture, are also "natural" interfaces for our robots.

As an example, imagine again that a robot is requested by the user to retrieve a certain item, but the robot's visual object classification system is not robust enough to identify correctly the object in the current environment. The robot can indicate its best estimate of what it "thinks" is the object to the user. The user responds either by saying "Yes, that is the item," or "No, the item I want is the large item to the right." Use of symbolic natural language terms such as "to the right" is more natural and convenient for human-robot interaction. Using natural language for describing spatial relationships is explored further in [51] and [34].

4.1.1. Speech

Speech is often regarded as one of the most natural forms of communication between humans. Robots that relate to humans should, then, be able to incorporate that type of communication. Speech recognition is a maturing technology that allows a machine to understand not just that something was spoken, but also which words and phrases were spoken. As a result of the advances in this area, there are several commercial products currently available that are cost-effective and have appropriately large vocabularies.

Text-to-speech technology allows the robot to speak text rather than just display it on a screen. The advances in this aspect of speech technology likewise have generated an available market of products. The current products have a variety of properties used to customize the characteristics of the voice, including gender and speed.

4.1.2. Gesture

Gesture is also very prevalent in human interaction, often resorted to in expressing emphasis. Since gestures are used to communicate many things, an important design decision is to investigate what kinds of gestures will be useful in service robotics. Although many researchers have investigated the understanding of finger spelling or American Sign Language, those types of gestures are not the most natural for communicating with a service robot. Gestures that are more applicable are those that do not have a formal syntax or perform as formal language. Designing the robot to understand gestures that supplement language and more compactly convey basic information will enhance other interaction modalities, and not merely duplicate effort. Some basic gestures convey commands to come, or stop, or to indicate selection or direction. All of these are related to action, place, or movement, which are physical and spatial, rather than abstract verbal concepts.

4.1.3. Human detection and localization

Service robots are expected, by definition, to provide services to human users. It is, therefore, critically important that service robots be aware of humans. The sensing group report from the recent International Workshop on Biorobotics: Human-Robot Symbiosis clearly identified this capability as one of the foremost abilities required for service robots [48]. The report then went on to say, "Traditionally, humans are treated as obstacles for the robot. That is, in a human-robot symbiotic system where humans and robots act in close association, each must be aware of the other in the sense that they must be capable of understanding each other's behaviors and, to some extent, predict each other's intentions."

If the robot is to interact with humans, it is important for the robot to know when a human is present. This awareness of presence may indicate to the robot that it is being observed or that the user desires to give input. In addition to simply knowing that a human is present, a well-designed service robot will benefit from knowing where this human is in relation to itself. It is clear to see that human localization is essential for a service robot, both to avoid harming users and bystanders, as well as to enhance communication with humans. The requirement of human detection and localization is quite possibly unique to service robotics. Most other fields of robotics are not so closely coupled with humans.

Human detection is a higher-level capability that employs several input modalities. We choose to list it here as a modality itself in order to emphasize it as a capability of central importance. Various technologies, such as the ones described below, must be integrated into the overall system and their results fused to robustly determine the presence of a human.

4.1.4. Face detection and tracking

One feature of humans that robots can be trained to recognize is the face. Face detection and tracking involve determining if a face is represented in the visual system of the robot [43,45,49,50]. Once a face is detected, the robot's attention may be directed toward that person. Tracking allows the robot to continue to focus attention on the user while moving.

4.1.5. Skin detection and tracking

The color of human skin is another feature that a robot can be trained to recognize. Identifying skin color usually indicates that a user is present. Skin detection and tracking can be used in ways similar to that of face detection and tracking. However, skin tracking is not limited to tracking faces, but can also be used for tracking hands, feet, or whatever may be useful for the specific application.

4.1.6. Sound localization

Detection of humans is not limited to the visual system of service robots. The auditory system may also be used. One feature of binaural hearing is sound localization, the ability to determine the direction from which a sound has come. Sound localization may be used to direct the robot's attention toward the location of the sound.

4.1.7. Identification of users

Combining the above technologies gives the robot an awareness that a human is in its presence, provided that the user is visible, or has spoken to the robot. This information may then be further combined to produce some confidence measure of the detection. Additionally, the robot may combine face, skin tone, and speech characteristics to identify and distinguish frequent users from one another.

4.1.8. Physical interaction

A major distinction of service robots from many other socially intelligent agents is that service robots engage in physical interaction. These robots must be aware of their surroundings and other actors in the environment. This knowledge is key to the safe and successful execution of physical manipulations, which may include touching a human, handing off an object, moving an object, or moving toward an object. Physical interaction is directly concerned with the sensors and actuators of the robot.

Sensors are the components of a robot that are used to detect what is in the robot's surroundings. A CCD camera is a very common sensor in robotics for acquiring visual information. Infrared sensors are also helpful in determining the presence of humans. Force and touch sensors are used to let the robot know that it is touching another object and how hard. These sensors can also be used in control algorithms to achieve the desired motion performance. Actuators are the components of a robot that enable physical manipulation. These include arms, hands, legs, wheels, motors, etc. The robot controls the actuators to achieve its goals.

4.2. The human agent

We are developing our human/robot software for a dual-armed humanoid robot called ISAC. ISAC has two SoftArm manipulators, a stereo color camera head, and an anthropomorphic 4-fingered hand. Some desired properties of our system are as follows:

- The robot should be "user-friendly," with not only a humanoid appearance but also the ability to have conversation (albeit limited) with the user.
- The user can discover the robot's abilities through conversation.
- The user can invoke the robot's abilities.
- The robot can detect failures and inform the user of failure.
- The user and robot can converse about the robot's internal state, including diagnostic conversation about failures.

To achieve these goals, we have proposed developing two high-level agents: the Human Agent and the Self Agent (Figure 5).

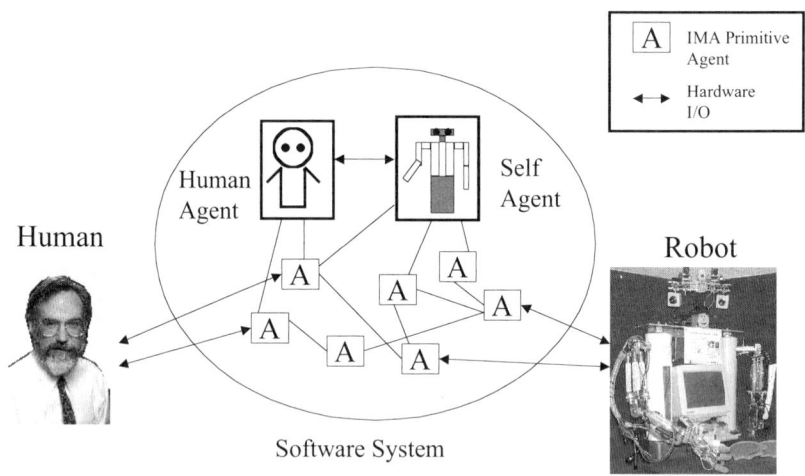

Figure 5. Human-Robot System.

The role of the Human Agent is to encapsulate what the robot knows about the human; for example, the human's identity, his location, and any information the human is trying to communicate through speech or gestures. The Self Agent's role is to represent the robot in interactions with the human. The goal of this human interaction is to allow the human to command the robot and to detect and diagnose failures. The Self Agent maintains knowledge about the internal state of the robot and can communicate this to the human. In addition, the Self Agent can affect the state of the primitive agents in the system to change the overall behavior of the robot in the context of the human interaction.

In service robotics in general, and especially in the case of robots for persons with physical disabilities, human-robot interaction is of great importance. Indeed, the usefulness and acceptance of such a robot may completely rely on the quality of the interaction. The desire for human-robot interaction to be natural and comfortable is the motivating factor for the development of the Human Agent. Interaction with a human, an inherent component of a service robotic system, is complex and must be described for the robot. The nature of the complexity lies in the fact that humans are not just objects to be detected, but also are often authorized to change the robot's task. The Human Agent allows the human the ability to communicate information to the robot, even the need for control, without taking the direct role of operator.

The primitive agents used to implement the Human Agent's abilities are shown in Figure 6. The Human Agent has three major capabilities that are responsible for providing the information about the human: detection, monitoring, and identification. Each capability of the Human Agent allows the human to have a more natural interaction with the robot.

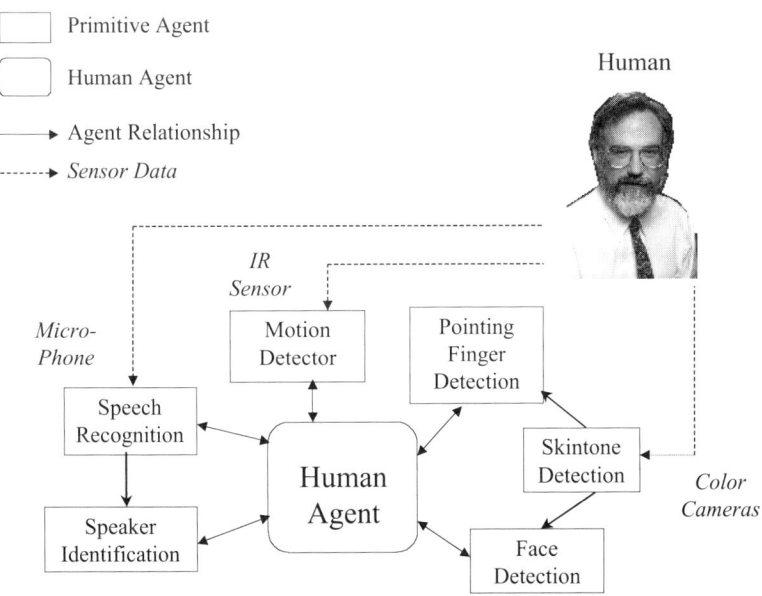

Figure 6. Interaction with the Human Agent.

Detection: Detection allows the robot to detect that humans are in its environment, integrating several technologies that are tuned to features of humans. Primitive agents connected to sensors provide raw data for detecting and interacting with people, e.g., the motion detector uses the IR sensors, and speech recognition uses the microphone. Skintone detection uses color images from the camera head. Other primitive agents use the data from these. For example, speaker identification uses data from speech recognition. Likewise, face detection and pointing finger detection are each based on the results of skintone detection. Each of these technologies is tuned to particular features of people. The weaknesses of one sensing mode can be strengthened by the support of another sensor. The detection module is responsible for activating or deactivating these primitive agents depending on the current interaction. It also integrates and interprets their responses to indicate if a human has been detected and with what level of certainty.

Monitoring Module: Once the robot is aware of the presence of a human being in its environment, the monitoring module is responsible for keeping up with the human and all that is known about the human. This includes monitoring physical characteristics as well as information inferred from the human. Localization and tracking algorithms allow the robot to keep up with the human's place in space. "Watching" the human includes tracking visual characteristics of humans, such as hands and faces. Monitoring also includes detecting changes in position through infrared motion sensing. The monitoring module is responsible for scheduling and monitoring the data from the tracking and localization primitive agents used for the current task.

The monitoring module also monitors human communication and interprets input from the human to determine if there is important information being conveyed. Two key modes of communication that are monitored are speech and the gesture of a pointing finger. Speech recognition (SR) is used to process the human vocal patterns to determine the words spoken to the robot. Using key words or phrases, the robot can be trained for interaction in certain environments. Speech recognition also can be sensitive to particular words and phrases to be used as emergency commands. The ability to override is essential when machines are working closely with humans.

Pointing finger detection gives the robot the ability to find and interpret a pointing finger on a human hand and can be used to supplement speech input. This is particularly useful in a situation where a selection is needed to eliminate ambiguity in a statement. For example, pointing to a particular object while giving a general command, "pick that up," can allow clarification to the robot. In this way, the pointing finger acts as another input device that allows for interaction with a robot in a way that is natural for the human.

Identification module: Identification requires the ability to distinguish detected humans from others. Features that can be quantified distinctly can be combined to form a feature set. If the feature field is chosen wisely, then the identification can be thought of as projecting features of the currently detected human onto this space. The identification module is responsible both for determining the identity of the current user and personalizing the robot's interaction based on experience with that particular person. Identification is based on prior and currently monitored information. This module is responsible for combining the results of several detection schemes to obtain an identity, as well as an indication of certainty. At present, the only mode that performs identification is speaker identification. Speaker identification identifies a user based on the vocal patterns in an utterance. It returns the identity found for the current speaker and the confidence measure.

It is also the responsibility of the identification module to maintain the information it knows about the humans it encounters. Once the person's identity has been determined, either through identification techniques, or by simply asking, personalized settings are considered. Based on prior interactions, the robot may know a person's preference for tasks, or the quickest way to beat them in a game. It is the purpose of the identification module to encapsulate information the robot has learned through personal interaction in a form that is useful and retrievable upon future interaction.

4.3. The self agent

The Self Agent has several aspects: human interaction, action selection, and robot status evaluation. The purpose of the human interaction aspect is to map the human's goals into robot action, particularly into task and environment primitive agents. This aspect works with the Human Agent, using communication data from the human to determine the human's goals. This aspect also generates the robot's communication to the human, including speech and facial expressions (similar to [8]).

The action selection aspect interfaces with primitive agents in the system and activates them based on information from the human interaction component. This aspect also alters robot behavior based on information about the human's identity or emotional state, and based on the status of the robot.

The robot status evaluation aspect detects failure in primitive agents and maintains information about the overall state of the robot. This information is used by the action selection aspect, and by the human interaction aspect.

A prototype Self Agent has been developed. The current design of the Self Agent consists of four modules: Emotion Module, Description Module, Activator Module, and Conversation Module. Figure 7 shows the modules of the Self Agent and their constituent components.

Emotion Module: The Emotion Module (EM) is an artificial emotional model used to describe the current state of the robot and provide internal feedback to the robot's software agents, similar to that described in [8]. Artificial emotions are modeled by numerical variables stored in IMA representation components. The value of each variable is controlled by an IMA relationship component. This relationship component arbitrates among the numerical contributions of the primitive agents that participate in the relationship. Each emotional variable has its own relationship. A fuzzy evaluator (FE) component is used to provide a textual description for each emotion.

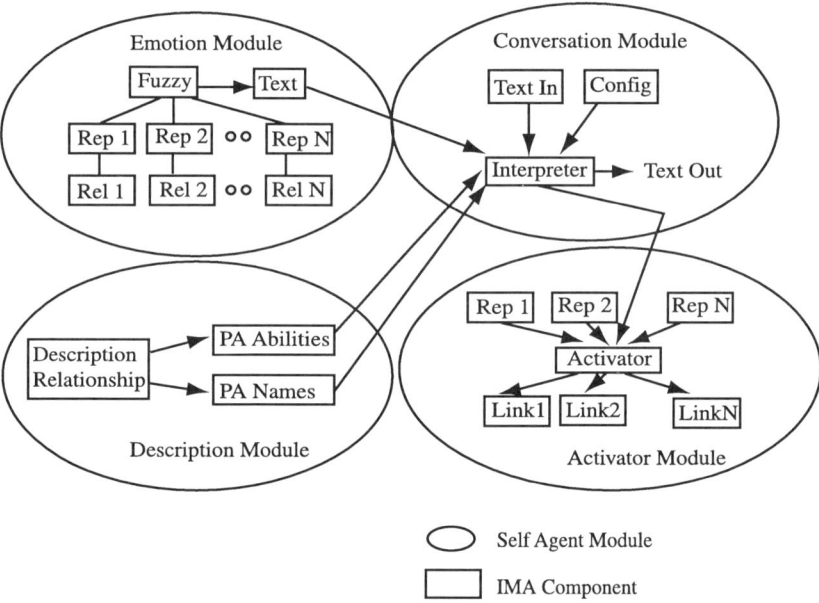

Figure 7. The Self Agent.

Description Module: The Description Module (DM) provides descriptions of the primitive agents available in the system. An IMA relationship component allows agents to contribute text strings containing their names and a description of their purpose. The primitive agents also provide information about their status: whether they are active or inactive, and whether they are achieving their goals or not. The DM then has text representations containing the names and descriptions of all primitive agents, all active primitive agents, all successful primitive agents, and all failed primitive agents. These text strings can be used to provide feedback to the human.

Activator Module: The Activator Module (AM) controls the activation state of primitive agents. An IMA component called the Activator maintains a list of primitive agent names. Each primitive agent also has an associated agent link and a representation component. The representation component stores a numerical value that is the primitive agent's activation level. When the activation level passes a threshold, the Activator component sends a signal to the primitive agent via the agent link component, causing the primitive agent to become active. The Activator component automatically decreases each primitive agent's activation level over time, and deactivates any whose activation falls below the threshold. The Activator also exposes an interface method that allows other components to add to or subtract from a primitive agent's activation level.

Conversation Module: The Conversation Module (CM) interprets the human's input and generates responses to the human. Currently, the CM operates only on text, but the principles could be extended to other modes of input, such as pointing. An IMA component called the Interpreter handles the human's text input. The Interpreter is based upon the Maas-Neotek robots developed by Mauldin [15,36]. A configuration file defines a series of blocks. Each block contains a "pass-band" filter, a "stop-band" filter, a set of textual response templates, and a list of primitive agent names and activation deltas.

The pass-band filter consists of a list of pattern strings. The input text is matched against the input using a "wild card" scheme using asterisks that match against any number of characters in the input. The stop-band is a list of strings against which the input text is matched exactly; that is, asterisks are not allowed. If an input string matches the pass-band, and does not match the stop-band, then the Interpreter generates a textual response. The block has a set of response templates. These templates can contain constant strings, the characters matched by an asterisk in the pass-band, and text from data representation components. The Interpreter chooses a template randomly and uses it to generate a response. In addition to generating a text response, the Conversation Module can also increase or decrease the activation level of a primitive agent in the Activator Module.

5. Results

An initial demonstration of the human/robot interaction capabilities of the prototype Self Agent used the software agents illustrated in Figure 8. Along with the Self Agent, the following primitive agents were used in the demonstration:

Hardware Primitive Agents
Arm. Controls the robot's arm hardware. Accepts position and velocity commands and reports current position.

Head. Controls the robot's head hardware. Accepts position and velocity commands and reports current position.

Hand. Controls the robot's hand hardware. Accepts commands to open, close, and "auto-close" (close when the proximity sensors fire) and reports the state of proximity sensors in the palm.

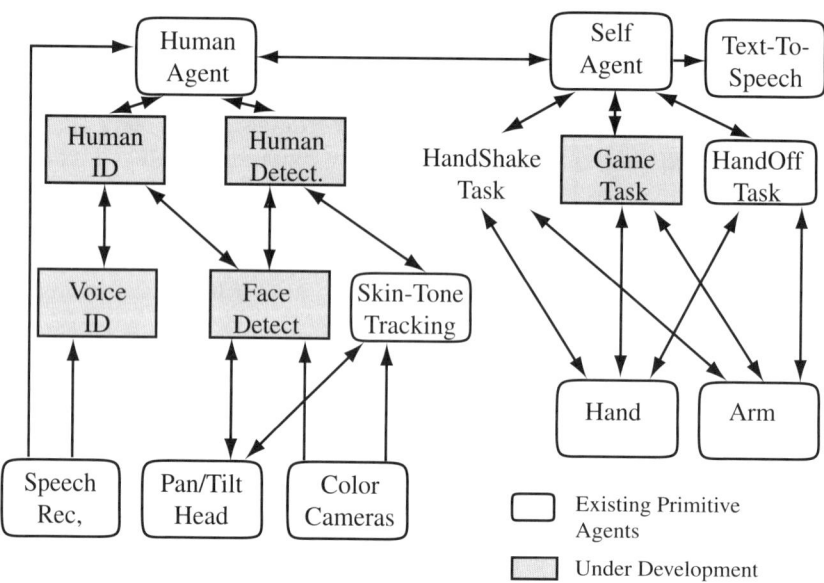

Figure 8. Self Agent Testbed System.

Color Image. Snaps color images and makes them available to other agents. Skill and Behavior Primitive Agents

Color Tracking. Segments color images using a skintone model, computes a track point, and sends commands to the Head agent, which tends to move the track point to the center of the image.

Task Primitive Agents
HandShake. Self explanatory.
HandOff. Self explanatory.

The task primitive agents are simple sequencing scripts. For example, HandShake works as follows:
1. Send Arm command to extend the robot's manipulator.
2. Send Hand command to open the fingers.
3. Send Hand command to "auto-close."
4. Wait for Hand to report proximity sensors fired.

5. Send Arm commands to "shake" (i.e., a pre-computed sinusoidal trajectory).
6. Send Hand command to open the fingers.

During the demonstration, ISAC could understand and respond to simple phrases spoken into a microphone. For example, phrases such as "Hello, ISAC," "It's nice to meet you," or "My name is Anthony," caused ISAC to welcome the human and shake hands. Another phrase, "Take this," caused ISAC to verbally acknowledge the request and invoke its handoff task primitive agent, accepting an object from the human and placing it in a box.

ISAC could also answer simple questions. Phrases such as "How are you?" were answered by reporting the fuzzy description of its emotional state. "What can you do?" caused ISAC to list the descriptions of the task primitive agents in the system: "Shake hands with people, put things in a box."

6. Conclusions and future work

Our laboratory has focused on developing service robots for persons with physical disabilities. Our robot systems have been featured in the magazine *Discover* (vol. 18, no. 9, September 1997) as well as on several local television news stations. One of our key developments has been a software architecture for building intelligent service robots, the Intelligent Machine Architecture (IMA). In creating technologies for persons with physical disabilities, we follow the Human Directed Local Autonomy (HuDL) paradigm. HuDL is our design philosophy of having robots that interact closely with the user and each other. To achieve these goals, we have proposed developing two high-level software agents: the Human Agent and the Self Agent.

The Human Agent is presently under development. Currently, the Human Agent's detection module is working using the IR motion detectors. Other technologies, such as speech recognition and face detection, will soon be integrated into the module. Skintone tracking, pointing finger detection, and speech recognition are all working technologies that await integration with the monitoring module. The identification module works with speaker identification. Also under investigation is determining what information about a human user is worth "remembering."

The Self Agent is also under development. Currently, the Self Agent is limited to responding to simple phrases spoken into a microphone and answering simple questions about the state of the robot. Development efforts are focused on increasing the robot's ability to evaluate the status of its software modules.

It is upon the completion and full integration of these two high-level agents that we will be able to speed our move to physical interaction with people. Giving our robots the ability to participate in robust interaction with people will be the springboard for developing applications. Our robots will better serve people by effectively interpreting their desires and giving feedback to them. The fundamental property of this system is that it requires minimal teaching and physical manipulation by the human user. This is a desirable feature for all people that a robot may serve, but it is essential to persons with physical disabilities.

We would also like to investigate further the use of *affective computing* [42] in our robots. Specifically, we want the robot to be aware of, and respond to, changes in the human user's emotional state. Other areas of interest are the development of a model for robot intelligence, based on the structure of vertebrate brains.

References

[1] Albus, J.S.: Outline for a theory of intelligence, *IEEE Transactions on Systems, Man and Cybernetics*, vol. 21, No. 3, May/June 1991.

[2] Albus, J.S.: A reference model architecture for intelligent hybrid control systems, *Proceedings of the 1996 Triennial World Congress, International Federation of Automatic Control (IFAC)*, San Francisco, CA, July 1996.

[3] Albus, J.S.: The NIST real-time control system (RCS) an approach to intelligent systems research, Special Issue of the *Journal of Experimental and Theoretical Artificial Intelligence*, vol. 9, pp. 157-174, 1997.

[4] Bagchi, S., Biswas, G., and Kawamura, K.: Generating plans to succeed in uncertain environments, *Second International Conference on AI Planning Systems*, Chicago, IL, AAAI Press, 1994.

[5] Bagchi, S., Biswas, G., and Kawamura, K.: A spreading activation mechanism for decision-theoretic planning, *AAAI Spring Symposium on Decision-Theoretic Planning*, March, 1994.

[6] Bagchi, S. and Kawamura, K.: ISAC: a robotic aid system for feeding the disabled, *Proceedings of the AAAI Spring Symposium on Physical Interaction and Manipulation*, Stanford University, 1994.

[7] Bagchi, S. and Kawamura, K.: An architecture for a distributed object-oriented robotic system, *1992 IEEE/RSJ International Conference on Intelligent Robots and Systems*, vol. 2, pp. 711-716, July, 1992.

[8] Breazeal (Ferrell), C.: Regulating human-robot interaction using 'emotions', 'drives' and facial expressions, *Autonomous Agents 1998 Workshop "Agents in Interaction - Acquiring Competence through Imitation."*

[9] Brooks, R.A.: A robust layered control system for a mobile robot, *IEEE Transactions on Robotics Automation*, vol. RA-2, No. 1, pp. 14-23, 1986.

[10] Cameron, J., MacKenzie, D., Ward, K., Arkin, R.C., Book, W.: Reactive control for mobile manipulation, *Proceedings of the 1993 IEEE International Conference on Robotics and Automation*, Atlanta, GA, pp. 228-235, May 1993, Vol. 3.

[11] Cleary, M.E. and Crisman, J.: Canonical targets for mobile robot control by deictic visual servoing, *IEEE 1996 International Conference on Robotics and Automation*, pp. 3093-3098, 1996.

[12] Crisman, J.D. and Bekey, G.: Grand challenges for robotics and automation: the 1996 ICRA panel discussion, *IEEE Robotics and Automation Magazine*, 3(4):10-16.

[13] El-Gamal, M., Kara, A., Kawamura, K., and Fashoro, M.: Reflex control for an intelligent robotic system, *1992 IEEE/RSJ International Conference on Intelligent Robots and Systems*, vol. 2, pp. 1347-1354, July, 1992.

[14] Friedrich, H. and Dillmann, R.: Robot programming based on a single demonstration and user intentions, *Proceedings of the 3rd European Workshop on Learning Robots at ECML'95*, Heraklion, Greece.

[15] Foner, L.: Entertaining agents: a sociological case study, *The Proceedings of the First International Conference on Autonomous Agents (AA '97)*, Marina del Rey, CA, 1997.

[16] Fröhlich, J. and Dillmann, R.: Interactive robot control system for teleoperation, *Proceedings of the International Symposium on Industrial Robots (ISIR '93)*, Tokyo, Japan.

[17] Fujiwara, K., Peters, R. A., and Kawamura, K.: Color-object detection for a mobile robot, *Proceedings of the SPIE Conference on Applications of Digital Image Processing XVII*, vol. 2298, pp. 457-470, July, 1994.

[18] Gan, W., Sharma, S., and Kawamura, K.: Development of an intelligent robotic aid to the physically handicapped, *Proceedings of the 22nd Southeastern Symposium on System Theory*, Cookville, TN, March, 1990.

[19] Gilbert, D. and Apparicio, M.: Intelligent agents, *IBM Intelligent Agent Center*, http://www.networking.ibm.com/iag/iaghome.html, February 1998.

[20] Iskarous, M. and Kawamura, K.: A fault-tolerant transputer-based parallel controller for the soft arm robot, *The Sixth Conference of the North American Transputer User Group*, Vancouver, Canada, pp. 239-246, May, 1993.

[21] Iskarous, M., Pack, R. T., and Kawamura, K.: A parallel fuzzy controller for a manipulator with flexible joints, *Proceedings of the First Asian Control Conference (ASCC)*, Tokyo, Japan, July, 1994.

[22] Kara, A., Bagchi, S., Chawla, S., Iskarous, M., and Kawamura, K.: Intelligent control of a robotic aid system for the physically disabled, *Proceedings of the IEEE International Symposium on Intelligent Control*, Arlington, VA, August, 1991.

[23] Kara, A., Kawamura, K., Bagchi, S., and El-Gamal, M.: Reflex control of a robotic aid system for the physically disabled, *IEEE Control Systems Magazine*, vol. 12, pp. 71-77, June, 1992.

[24] Kawamura, K.: Trends in rehabilitation and medical robots, *Journal of Robotics Society of Japan*, vol. 11, no. 1, pp. 71-75, 1993.

[25] Kawamura, K., Bagchi, S., Iskarous, M., Pack, R., and Saad, A.: An intelligent robotic aid system for human services, *Proceedings of the Conference on Intelligent Robots in Field, Factory, Service, and Space (CIRFFSS 94)*, Houston, TX, vol. 1, pp. 413-419, 1994.

[26] Kawamura, K., Bishay, M., Bagchi, S., Saad, A., Iskarous, M., and Fumoto, M.: Intelligent user interface for a rehabilitation robot, *Fourth International Conference on Rehabilitation Robotics*, Wilmington, DE, 1994.

[27] Kawamura, K., Cambron, M., Fujiwara, K., and Barile, J.: A cooperative robotic aid system, *Proceedings of the Virtual Reality Systems Fall '93, Teleoperation '93, & Beyond Speech Recognition Conference*, New York, NY, 1993.

[28] Kawamura, K. and Iskarous, M.: Trends in service robots for the disabled and the elderly, *International Conference on Intelligent Robots and Systems (IROS 94)*, Munich, Germany, 1994.

[29] Kawamura, K., Pack, R., Bishay, M., and Iskarous, M.: Design philosophy for service robots, *Robotics and Autonomous Systems*, 18:109-116.

[30] Kawamura, K. and Pack, R. T.: Object-based software architecture for service robot development. *Proceedings of the International Conference on Advanced Robotics*, 1997.

[31] Kawamura, K., Peters, R.A., Bagchi, S., Iskarous, M., and Bishay, M.: Intelligent robotic systems in service of the disabled, *IEEE Transactions on Rehabilitation Engineering*, vol. 3, no. 1, pp. 14-21, March, 1995.

[32] Kawamura, K., Wilkes, D.M., Pack, T., Bishay, M., and Barile, J.: Humanoids: future robots for home and factory. *Proceedings of the International Symposium on Humanoid Robots*, Waseda University, Tokyo, Japan, pp. 53-62, 1996.

[33] Lueth, T. C., Laengle, T., Herzog, G., Stopp, E., and Rembold, U.: KANTRA - human-machine interaction for intelligent robots using natural language, *Proceedings of the ROMAN '94*.

[34] Maaß, W.: How spatial information connects visual perception and natural language generation in dynamic environments: towards a computational model, *Spatial Information Theory: A Theoretical Basis for GIS. Proc. of the Int. Conference COSIT '95*, Semmering, Austria, pp. 223-240.

[35] Maes, P.: Modeling adaptive autonomous agents. *Artificial Life*, vol. 1, pp. 135-162, 1994.

[36] Mauldin, M.: Chatterbots, tinymuds, and the turing test: entering the Loebner Prize competition, *AAAI-94*, 1994.

[37] Muench, S. and Dillmann, R.: Haptic output in multimodal user interfaces, *Proceedings of the 1997 International Conference On Intelligent User Interfaces (IUI97)*, Orlando, FL, pp. 105-112.

[38] Musliner, D.: CIRCA: cooperative intelligent real-time control architecture, Ph.D. Thesis, University of Michigan, 1993.

[39] Pack, R.T. and Iskarous, M.: The use of the soft arm for rehabilitation and prosthetics, *Proceedings of the RESNA 1994 Annual Conference*, Nashville, TN, pp. 472-475.

[40] Pack, R. T., Wilkes, D. M., and Kawamura, K.: A software architecture for integrated service robot development, *1997 IEEE Conf. On Systems, Man, and Cybernetics*, Orlando, FL, pp. 3774-3779, September 1997.

[41] Penny, S.: Embodied cultural agents: at the intersection of art, robotics, and cognitive science, *Working Notes of the AAAI Fall Symposium on Socially Intelligent Agents*, 1997.

[42] Picard, R.: *Affective Computing*. Cambridge, MA: MIT Press, 1997.

[43] Podilchuk, C. and Zhang, X.: Face recognition using DCT-based feature vectors, *Proc. Int. Conf. Acoust., Speech, and Sig. Proc.*, Atlanta, 1995.
[44] Pook, P.K. and Ballard, D.H.: Deictic human/robot interaction, *Proceedings of the International Workshop on Biorobotics: Human-Robot Symbiosis*, Tsukuba, Japan, pp. 259-269.
[45] Qiu, B.: Face and facial feature detection in a complex scene, M.S. Thesis, Vanderbilt University, 1997.
[46] Rich, C. and Sidner, C. L.: COLLAGEN: when agents collaborate with people, *Agents*, pp. 284-291, 1997.
[47] Rosenblatt, J.: DAMN: a distributed architecture for mobile navigation, *AAAI Spring Symposium: Lessons Learned from Implemented Software Architectures for Physical Agents*, 1995.
[48] Sandini, G., Yamada, Y., Wilkes, D.M., and Bishay, M.: Sensing group report, *International Workshop on Biorobotics: Human-Robot Symbiosis, Robotics, and Autonomous Systems*, vol. 18, pp. 207-211, 1996.
[49] Sinha, P.: Object recognition via image invariants: a case study, *Investigative Ophthalmology and Visual Science*, vol. 35, pp. 1735-1740, 1994.
[50] Sinha, P.: Qualitative image-based representations for object recognition, A.I. Memo No. 1505, Dept. of Brain and Cognitive Sciences, MIT, 1994.
[51] Stopp, E., Gapp, K. P., Herzog, G., Laengle, T., and Lueth, T.: Utilizing spatial relations for natural language access to an autonomous mobile robot, *Deutsche Jahrestagung für Künstliche Intelligenz (KI '94)*, 1994.
[52] Woods, D. and Winograd, T.: Breakout group 3 report, *Human-Centered Design, NSF Workshop on Human-Centered Systems*, Arlington, VA.

Chapter 12

Computerized obstacle avoidance systems for the blind and visually impaired

Shraga Shoval, Iwan Ulrich, and **Johann Borenstein**

This chapter gives an overview of existing devices for the guidance of visually impaired pedestrians and discusses the properties of the white cane and of conventional electronic travel aids. Also described are the disadvantages of using a standard mobile robot for this purpose. Next follows a description of the NavBelt, a computerized travel aid for the blind that is based on advanced mobile robot obstacle avoidance technology. The NavBelt is worn by the user like a belt and, via a set of stereo earphones, provides acoustic signals that guide the user around obstacles. One limitation of the NavBelt is that it is exceedingly difficult for the user to comprehend the guidance signals in time to allow fast walking.

This problem is effectively overcome by a newer device, called the GuideCane. The GuideCane uses the same mobile robotics technology as the NavBelt but it is a wheeled device pushed ahead of the user via an attached cane. When the GuideCane detects an obstacle, it steers around it. The user immediately feels this steering action and can follow the GuideCane's new path easily and without any conscious effort. This chapter describes the GuideCane system, including the mechanical, electronic, and software components, followed by a description of the intuitive user-machine interface.

The chapter ends with a discussion of the GuideCane's novel information transfer approach and its advantages and disadvantages in practical terms.

1. Introduction

There are about two million visually impaired or blind persons in the United States alone [15]. Many of these persons use the white cane – the most successful and widely used travel aid for the blind. This purely mechanical device is used to detect obstacles on the ground, uneven surfaces, holes, steps, and other hazards. The inexpensive white cane is so lightweight and small that it can be folded and slipped into a pocket.

The main problem with the white cane is that users must be trained in its use for more than one hundred hours – a substantial "hidden" cost. In addition, this device is rather inconvenient, as it requires the user to actively scan the small area ahead of him/her. In addition, the white cane cannot detect obstacles beyond its reach (3 to 6 feet), and therefore the traveler perceives only limited information about the environment. Another drawback of the white cane is that obstacles can be detected only by contact. This can become inconvenient to the traveler and the surroundings, for example, when traveling in a crowded street. Travel can even become unsafe through improper use of the white cane. The white cane is also not well suited for detecting potentially dangerous obstacles at head level.

Guide dogs are very capable guides for the blind, but they require extensive training. Fully trained guide dogs cost between $12,000 to $20,000 [15], and their useful life is typically on the order of only five years. Furthermore, many blind and visually impaired people are elderly and find it difficult to care appropriately for another living being. As a result, only 1% of the estimated two million blind and visually impaired people in the U.S. have guide dogs.

2. Conventional electronic travel aids

With the development of radar and ultrasonic technologies, a new series of devices, known as *electronic travel aids* (ETAs), was developed for blind travelers during the past 30 years. In terms of operational principles, most ETAs are similar to radar systems. Namely, a laser or ultrasonic "beam" is emitted in a certain direction in space; the beam is reflected from objects that it confronts on its way; a matching sensor detects the reflected beam and the distance to the object is calculated according to the time difference between emitting and receiving the beam. Existing ETAs can detect objects in the range of up to 15 feet away from the user, but require continuous scanning of the environment in the desired direction (with the exception of the *Binaural Sonic Aid* and the *Pathsounder,* which depend on head or torso movements).

The best known ETA is the *C5 Laser Cane* [1], which is based on optical triangulation with three transmitters and three photodiodes as receivers. An UP channel detects obstacles at head-height, the FORWARD channel detects obstacles from the tip of the can forward, (in the range of 1.5-3.5 m) and the DOWN channel detects drop-offs in front of the user.

The *Mowat Sensor* [23] and the Sona [17] are hand-held devices that inform the user of the distance to detected objects by means of tactile vibrations, where the frequency of the vibrations is inversely proportional to the distance between the sensor and the object. The *Mowat* sensor is a secondary aid for use in conjunction with a *long cane* or a guide dog. The *Mowat* sensor has been found helpful, and users feel they benefit from it [4].

The Russell Pathsounder [25] is one of the earliest ultrasonic travel aids. Two ultrasonic transducers are mounted on a board that the user wears around the neck, at chest height. This unit provides only three discrete levels of feedback (series of clicks), roughly indicating distances to objects. The *Pathsounder* does not require active manual scanning of the environment by the user, but torso movement is the only search strategy potential [19].

The Binaural Sonic Aid (Sonicguide) [16] comes in the form of a pair of spectacle frames, with one ultrasonic wide-beam transmitter (55° cone) mounted between the spectacle lenses and one receiver on each side of the transmitter. Signals from the receivers are shifted and presented separately to the left and right ear. The resulting interaural amplitude difference allows the user to determine the direction of the reflected echo and thus of the obstacle. The distance to an object is encoded in the frequency of the demodulated low-frequency tone, which together with the wearer's head orientation provides clear information about the object's location. As the *Sonicguide* does not require active manual scanning, it can serve as a secondary device, in conjunction with an additional hand-held device or a guide dog.

In spite of the large variety of ETAs, only a small percentage of the blind population regularly use these devices. The National Research Council [21] identifies three fundamental shortcomings in all ETAs discussed in the foregoing sections:

1. The user must *actively* scan the environment to detect obstacles (no scanning is needed with the *Sonicguide*, but that device does not detect obstacles at floor level). This procedure is time-consuming and requires the traveler's constant activity and conscious effort.
2. The traveler must perform additional measurements when an obstacle is detected in order to determine the dimensions and shape of the object. The user must then plan a path around the obstacle. Again, a time-consuming, conscious effort that reduces the walking speed.

3. Another problem with all ETAs based on acoustic feedback is their interference (called *masking*) with sound cues from the environment, reducing the blind person's ability to hear these essential cues [9, 16, 18].

3. Mobile robotics technologies for the visually impaired

Visually impaired people and mobile robots face several common problems when performing navigation. Hence, it seems only natural to apply mobile robotics technologies to assist the visually impaired. *Obstacle avoidance systems* (OASs), originally developed for mobile robots, lend themselves well for incorporation in travel aids for the visually impaired [26]. An obstacle avoidance system has to detect obstacles through its sensors and has to plan a path around them. Travel aids equipped with mobile robotics technologies have the potential of overcoming the fundamental shortcomings of existing travel aids, and can thus provide several advantages to the blind traveler.

3.1. Mobile robot obstacle avoidance sensors

Most mobile robots use ultrasonic sensors (also called "sonars" in the remainder of this chapter) to detect obstacles and to measure the distance between the sensor and the obstacle. By far the most widely used ultrasonic sensor in mobile robot applications is the one manufactured by [22] and shown in Figure 1.

The Polaroid sonar emits a short burst of ultrasound when it is "fired." If an object is located in front of the sensor, then some of the ultrasound waves will be reflected back to the sonar, which switches into a microphone mode immediately after firing. Once the echo from the object is received at the sonar, its associated electronics (see Figure 1) send an electrical signal to the computer that controls the sonar(s). The computer measures the time that elapsed between firing the sonar and receiving the echo. Because the velocity of ultrasound traveling through air is almost constant, the computer can easily compute the distance between the object and the sonar from the measured time-of-flight. Polaroid sonars have a maximum range of 10 meters (33 ft) and an accuracy of about 0.5% of the distance measured.

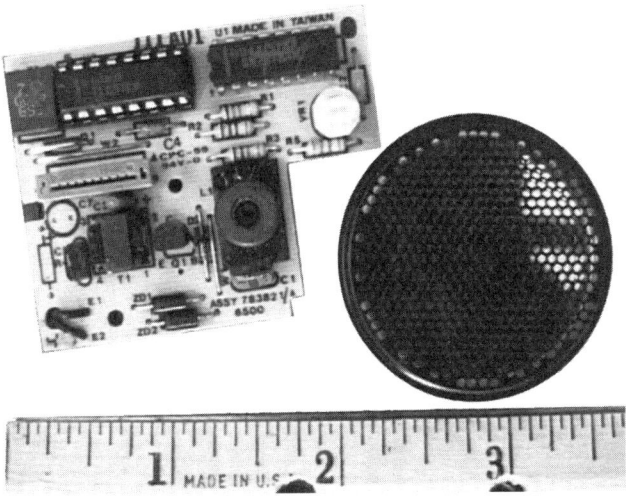

Figure 1. The Polaroid ultrasonic range sensor is widely used for mobile robot obstacle avoidance.

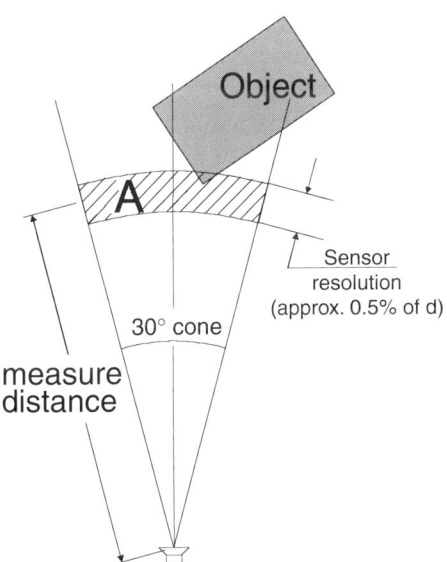

Figure 2. Ultrasound propagates from the sonar in a 30° cone-shaped profile.

Ultrasound waves propagate from the sonar in a cone-shaped propagation profile, in which the opening angle of the cone is about 30° (see Figure 2). This property is exploited in most mobile robots by mounting the sonars on a semi-circular ring on the periphery of the robot at 15-degree intervals. This arrangement assures complete coverage of the area in front of the sonars. One major difficulty in the use of multiple ultrasonic sensors is the fact that these sensors cause mutual interference, called crosstalk. Crosstalk is a phenomenon in which the wave front emitted by one sonar specularly reflects off smooth surfaces and is subsequently detected by another sonar. In the past, researchers had to employ slow firing schemes to allow each sensor's signal to dissipate before the next sensor was fired.

This problem was resolved by the Error Eliminating Rapid Ultrasonic Firing (EERUF) method, developed at the University of Michigan's Mobile Robotics Lab [7]. EERUF detects and rejects crosstalk so that there is no need to wait for echoes to dissipate. Consequently, it is possible to fire sonars at a rate of up to 60 ms (i.e., each sensor fires once every 60 ms). This fast firing technique allows faster sensor acquisition, and thus faster travel. The EERUF algorithm also rejects environmental ultrasonic noise, and filters out erroneous readings.

3.2. Mobile robot obstacle avoidance

A mobile robot obstacle avoidance system is comprised of a set of sensors and, typically, some rather complex computer algorithms that use the sensor data to compute a path that would lead the robot safely around the object. There are as many different obstacle avoidance methods as there are research labs around the world. However, in both the NavBelt and the GuideCane an algorithm known as the Vector Field Histogram (VFH) method is used, which was developed at the University of Michigan's Mobile Robotics Lab. The VFH method is explained in the following section.

3.2.1. The vector field histogram method for obstacle avoidance

The Vector Field Histogram (VFH) method builds a local map of its immediate surroundings based on the recent sonar data history. This local map allows the robot[1] to take into account not only the current sonar readings, but also previous readings. This results in significantly better performance than that produced by simpler systems.

In the VFH method the map is represented by a two-dimensional array, called a *histogram grid* [6], which is based on the earlier *certainty grid* [20] and *occupancy grid* [10] approaches. Each cell contains a *certainty value* that indicates the measure of confidence that an obstacle exists within the cell area. This representation is especially suited for sensor fusion, as well as for the

---

[1] The term "robot" is used here because the VFH method was originally developed for mobile robots. However, the discussion is true for both the NavBelt and the GuideCane, as described later.

accommodation of inaccurate sensor data such as range measurements from ultrasonic sensors. In both the NavBelt and GuideCane a cell size of 10 × 10 cm is used. Figure 3, which was created in an actual experiment, illustrates how a typical experimental environment translates into the histogram grid representation.

The local map is updated through *histogramic in-motion mapping* (HIMM), a real-time map building method developed by Borenstein and Koren [5]. HIMM increases the certainty value of only one cell in the histogram grid for each sonar reading, and decreases the certainty values of cells located between the sonar and the incremented cell. While this approach may seem like an oversimplification, a probability distribution is actually obtained by continuous and rapid sampling of each sensor while the robot is moving. In addition, to compensate for the adverse scattering effects caused by in-motion sampling, a *growth rate operator* (GRO) is added. The GRO increases the value of a cell faster if its immediate neighbors hold high certainty values. As a result, HIMM produces high certainty values for cells with high probability of existence of obstacles in them and keeps low certainty values for cells that were increased because of misreadings or moving objects. Any range reading is immediately represented in the map and can thus immediately influence the obstacle avoidance output.

EERUF and HIMM are an effective combination for building good representations of a robot's immediate surroundings based on ultrasonic sensors. The resulting histogram grid is then used by the local obstacle avoidance algorithm as its world model to determine an appropriate instantaneous direction of motion.

Next, the two-dimensional histogram grid is reduced to a one-dimensional *polar histogram* that is constructed around the robot's momentary location (the mathematical process is beyond the scope of this text and is omitted here). The polar histogram provides an instantaneous 360-degree panoramic view of the immediate environment, in which elevations suggest the presence of obstacles and valleys suggest that the corresponding directions are free of obstacles. The polar histogram has 72 sectors that are each 5° wide. The numerical values associated with each sector are called "*obstacle density*" values. High obstacle density values suggest a high likelihood for either a small object nearby or a larger object further away in the direction of that sector. Figure 4 shows the polar histogram for the environment of Figure 3 and it was also created from an actual experiment. High obstacle density values are shown as taller bars in the bar chart-type representation of Figure 4a. Note that Figure 4b represents the same polar histogram as that of Figure 4a, except that it has been overlaid onto the histogram grid for better illustration.

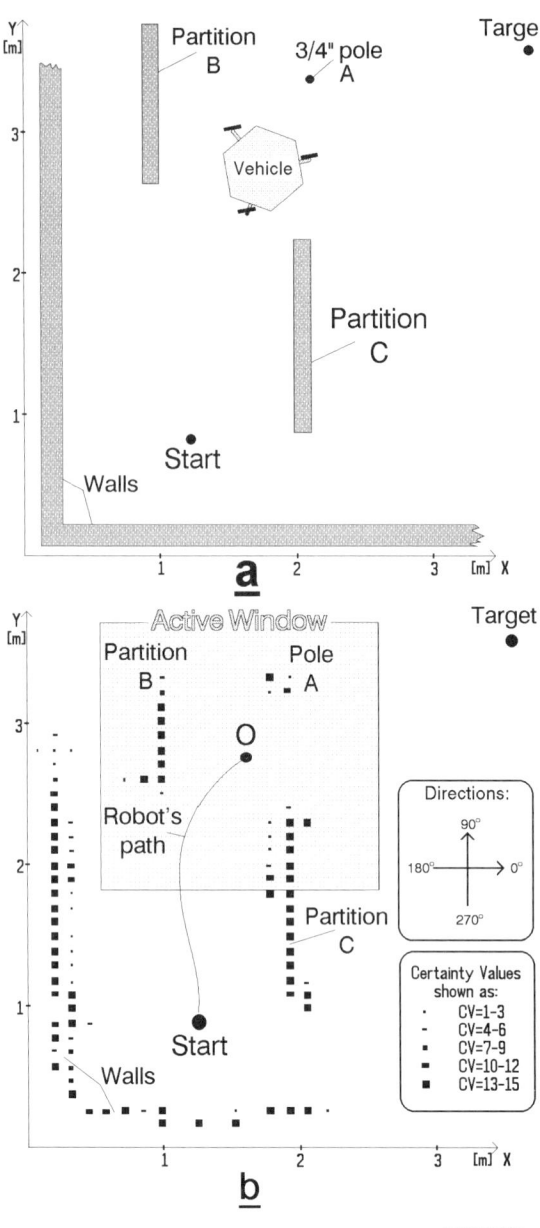

Figure 3. (a) A typical experimental environment. A vehicle is shown traversing the environment at some instant t. (b) The histogram grid, built from the sonar data, is comprised of cells, each holding a value that expresses the certainty for the existence of an obstacle at that cell's location.

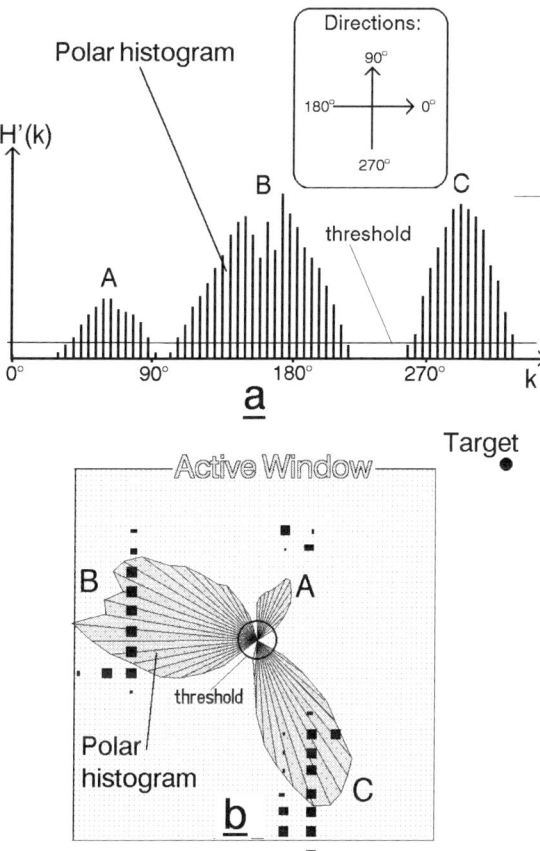

Figure 4. Two ways of visualizing the same polar histogram generated at instant t for the environment of Figure 3. The 360-degree panoramic view is divided into 72 sectors, each 5° wide. The numerical values associated with each sector represent the likelihood for either a small object nearby or a larger object further away in the direction of that sector.

Although the description in this section is fairly complex, the necessary computations are performed in just a few milliseconds. Indeed, during motion a new polar histogram is recomputed every 10 ms.

It is evident from Figure 4b that the polar histogram provides comprehensive information about the environment (with regard to obstacles), yet the amount of numeric information is quite small. Exactly how the information of the polar histogram is used in a robotic device differs from application to application, and will be discussed separately for the NavBelt and the GuideCane in the respective sections below.

3.2.2. Limitations of mobile robots as guides for the blind

In general terms, one could argue that any mobile robot with obstacle avoidance can be used as a guiding device for the blind. However, conventional mobile robots with powered wheels are inherently unsuited to the task of guiding a blind person. Actively driven wheels require motors and thus more powerful batteries, making a standard mobile robot larger and heavier than the NavBelt and the GuideCane. The added weight and size are a considerable inconvenience for a user whenever he/she encounters situations like stairs or raised sidewalks.

Another problem with powered wheels is that the speed of the robot could make the user feel uncomfortable by either pulling a cautious user forward or by slowing a confident user down unnecessarily. An additional interface would be required so that the user could indicate the desired speed to the robot. However, with both the NavBelt and the GuideCane configuration, the user is in direct control of the speed, allowing for the most intuitive and easiest use possible.

Another concept is to have a visually impaired person sit in a powered semi-autonomous wheelchair equipped with sensors and obstacle avoidance technology. The main problem of this approach is that a visually impaired user with healthy legs would unnecessarily be burdened with the additional handicap of limited mobility.

4. The NavBelt

For more than 10 years, the University of Michigan Mobile Robotics Laboratory has been active in applying its technologies to travel aids for the visually impaired. The major results are two novel devices: the NavBelt and the GuideCane, whose concepts originated in 1989 and 1995, respectively. Both devices rely on advanced obstacle avoidance systems that were originally developed for conventional mobile robots. This section describes the NavBelt, which overcomes the first two shortcomings of existing travel aids by employing multiple sensors that free the user from scanning the surroundings manually.

4.1. Concept

The NavBelt consists of a belt, a small computer worn as a backpack, and an array of ultrasonic sensors. The computer processes the signals arriving from the sensors, applies the obstacle avoidance algorithms, and relays them to the user via stereophonic headphones, using so-called stereo imaging techniques.

The NavBelt system does not use a mobile robot, but it applies mobile robot technology in a portable device. This technology transfer is illustrated in Figure 5. The main difference is that the electrical signals, which originally guided a robot around obstacles, are replaced by acoustic signals aimed at guiding the user around obstacles. However, the computation of an obstacle-free path and the sensing techniques are similar in both applications.

The NavBelt is equipped with an obstacle avoidance system (OAS) that scans the environment with eight sonars simultaneously. The OAS employs a unique real-time signal-processing algorithm to produce active guidance signals.

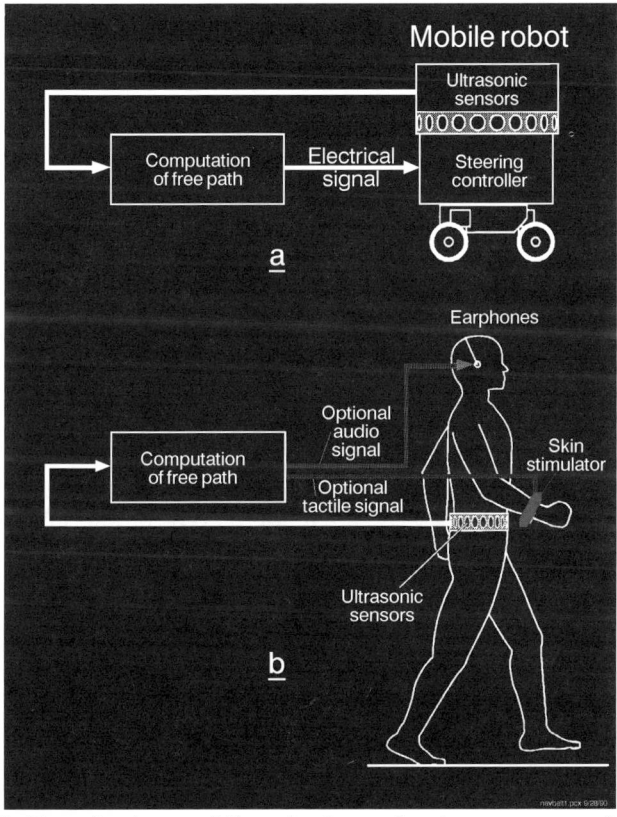

Figure 5. Transferring mobile robotics technology to a portable navigation aid for the blind: the concept of the NavBelt.

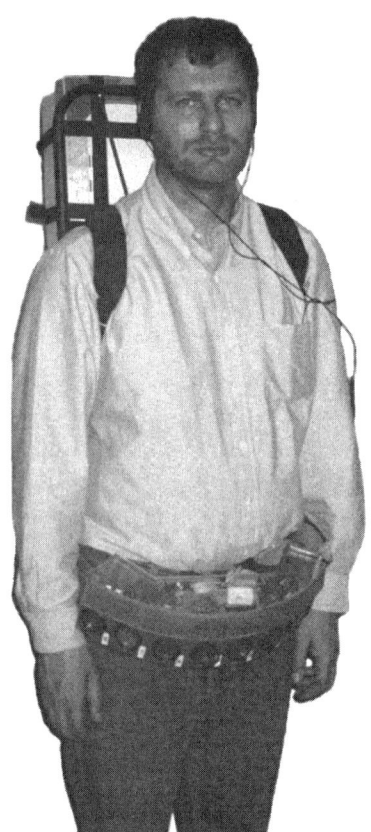

Figure 6. The experimental prototype of the NavBelt.

The OAS computes the recommended traveling direction according to the user's current position, target location, and the obstacles in the surroundings by using a method called the *Vector Field Histogram* (VFH) [6]. In the absence of obstacles, the recommended direction is simply the direction toward the target. If, however, obstacles block the user's path, then the OAS computes an alternative path, which safely guides the user around the obstacles.

The user wears the NavBelt around the waist like a "fanny pack" (see Figure 6), and carries a portable computer as a backpack. Eight ultrasonic sensors, each covering a sector of 15° are mounted on the front pack, providing a total scan sector of 120°. Small stereophonic headphones provide the user with the auditory data. A binaural feedback system (BFS) based on internal time difference (phase difference between the left and right ears) and amplitude difference (volume difference between the two ears) creates a *virtual direction* (i.e., an impression of directionality of virtual sound sources).

The NavBelt is designed for three basic operational modes, each offering a different type of assistance to the user:

Panel: Auditory Displays

The use of auditory displays in travel aids for the blind has been investigated by several researchers:

- Tachi et al. [29] developed a method to quantitatively compare various auditory display schemes for tracking with an electronic travel aid. The performance of the traveler was evaluated by calculating the transfer function of the human in terms of effective gain and reciprocal time delay. It was found that monaural displays with varying loudness and binaural displays with varying position and loudness are superior to other types of auditory displays. Fish [12] suggested using a two-dimensional coding system, which produces a series of tone bursts representing distances to objects. Although laboratory experiments showed that subjects were able to avoid obstacles using the two-dimensional auditory display, the information complexity and size did not allow the traveler to walk at a reasonable speed.

- Ifukube et al. [14] devised an interesting method for information transfer in a travel aid for the blind, which was based on the principle of echolocation of bats. In this method, frequency modulated ultrasonic waves were transmitted to detect objects, and the reflected waves were picked up by a two-channel receiver. The waves were then converted to acoustic signals with a simple proportional converter. The acoustic signals were presented to the blind traveler binaurally by headphones. Experiments showed that the method was very effective at detecting small objects, but no practical experiments were reported for implementing it in a travel aid.

- Kay's [16] Binaural Sensory Aid, also known as Sonicguide, relays information to the user by two sound sources to the left and right ears, using special tubes for minimal occlusion of external auditory cues. The interaural differences between the two sound sources provide the user with directional information about objects, as well as the object's shape and even a rough estimate about the surface texture.

---

1) **Guidance Mode** — The acoustic signals actively guide the user around obstacles in pursuit of the target direction. The signals carry information regarding the recommended travel direction as well as the speed and proximity to obstacles. The signals consists of a single stereophonic tone, the direction of which determines the travel direction, while the frequency determines the recommended travel speed (higher frequencies for slower speeds). The speed is inversely proportional to the proximity to the nearest object. Using a keyboard (which can eventually be replaced by an acoustic coding system using another input device suitable for blind users), the user inputs the desired target position. The target can be selected as relative coordinates (i.e., 500 ft forward, turn right, etc.), or, when traveling in a known environment and the computer is equipped with a navigation map, the user can specify the target name (i.e., street corners, specific buildings etc). One problem with the *Guidance Mode* is that it requires knowledge about the user's momentary position at all times. In the current NavBelt prototype, there is no sensor to provide this information. However, developments in positioning method, such as satellite-based systems (GPS) for outdoor environments, may provide solution to this problem. Golledge et al. [13] developed a navigation aid based on GPS technology, which provides the user with updated information about the topographical features of the surroundings.

2) **Image Mode** — This mode presents the user with a panoramic *acoustic image* of the environment. A sweep of stereophonic sounds appears to "travel" through the user's head from the right to the left ear. The direction to an object is indicated by the spatial direction of the signal, and the distance is represented by the signal's pitch and volume (higher pitch and volume for shorter distances). As the information in this mode is more detailed than the information in the *Guidance Mode*, subjects found it more difficult to interpret the signals and to react to them quickly. To reduce the amount of information transferred, unnecessary information is suppressed and only the most important sections of the environment are transmitted to the user. The selection of these relevant sections from the panoramic map is performed by the computer based on proximity of objects in the direction of travel. For example, when traveling in a crowded street or when entering a narrow passage, the computer transmits information about the sectors containing the closest objects to the user while ignoring all other, more distant objects.

3) **Directional Guidance Mode** — This mode allows the user to control the global navigation, while the obstacle avoidance is performed by the NavBelt. The system actively guides the user toward a temporary target, the location of which is determined by the user via a joystick. The joystick used for this purpose during the development of the Navbelt may not be ideal for this purpose in a final product. A special auditory coding system or a speech control device may conceivably be better suited. The target position is selected according to the direction the joystick is pointing to. When the joystick is not pushed, the system selects a default target five meters ahead of the user. If the traveler wishes to turn sideways, he or she deflects the joystick in the desired direction and a momentary target is selected five meters ahead of the user in that direction. In case an obstacle is detected, the NavBelt provides the user with the relevant information to avoid the obstacle with minimal deviation from the target direction.

The variety of operational modes allows for different levels of assistance to the user, and different information formats. The *Guidance* mode is the most "automated" mode as the majority of the perception and cognition tasks are performed by the computer. This mode is efficient when the user is traveling in an unknown cluttered environment and the NavBelt serves as the primary aid. In the *Image* mode the computer tasks are limited to scanning the surroundings and informing the user about the position of obstacles, while the global path planning and navigation tasks are performed by the user.

The NavBelt's acoustic imaging technique can produce several informative parameters:

- **Direction of the audio signal's source:** In the *Image* mode the signal produces a virtual source that represents the direction of the object. In the *Guidance* and *Directional Guidance* modes the virtual sound source represents the recommended travel direction.
- **Volume:** This parameter represents the proximity of the object to the user (*Image* mode) or the recommended traveling speed (*Guidance* modes).
- **Pitch:** In the *Guidance* modes, the pitch is proportional to the complexity of the travel in that direction. This complexity depends on the distance to the nearest obstacle, number of obstacles, and the width between them (i.e., traveling through a narrow passage or among several small objects is more demanding than traveling in an uncluttered environment).
- **Transmission rate:** The signals' transmission rate is proportional to the conscious effort required from the user. When the NavBelt detects a potential hazard (a nearby obstacle, for example), the frequency at which the signals are transmitted (in all operation modes) is increased, thereby alerting the traveler.

The use of stereophonic displays in travel aid for the blind has already been implemented (i.e., the Sonicguide [16]), and many researches deal with the problem known as auditory localization [3], [11]. However, there are two major differences between the use of auditory localization in the Navbelt and the Sonicguide:

1. In the *Guidance mode*, the auditory cue signals the recommended travel direction, rather the location of an obstacle.
2. In the *Image mode*, the stereophonic sweep provides a full panoramic virtual image of the surrounding, thanks to the 120-degree wide coverage by the array of sensors. Furthermore, when traveling in a cluttered environment the sensors can detect several objects simultaneously, providing sufficient information for traveling through doorways, narrow passages, etc.

4.2. Implementation of the guidance mode

In the *guidance* mode, the computer provides the user only with the recommended travel speed and direction, based on the VFH obstacle avoidance algorithm (see Section 3.2.1). The VFH method calculates the travel direction from the polar histogram by searching for sectors with a low so-called "obstacle density" value. In practice, the VFH determines a threshold level, and all sectors with a lower obstacle density than that level become candidate sections. Next, the VFH searches for the candidate sector that is closest to the direction of the target. The travel speed is determined by the VFH method according to the proximity of the robot (or human in the Navbelt) to the nearest object. The speed is determined inversely proportional to the minimal distance, with maximum speed of 1.2 m/sec attained when the distance between the traveler and the closest object is larger than 3 m.

The recommended travel speed and direction are relayed to the user by a single stereophonic signal. The virtual direction of the signal is the direction the obstacle avoidance system has selected for travel. The pitch and amplitude are proportional to the recommended travel speed. Higher pitch and amplitude attract more human attention [2], thereby motivating the traveler to reduce the walking speed and to concentrate on the stereophonic signal. A special low pitch signal (250 Hz) is transmitted when the direction of motion coincides (within ±5°) with the required direction. This special tone is a simple feedback signal for the user, indicating that the travel direction is correct. Furthermore, low pitch tones occlude external sound from the environment less than medium and high pitch tones do [2]. The higher pitch tone is transmitted only when the traveler needs to change the travel direction, and as soon as that direction coincides with the recommended direction the low pitch returns.

Another important parameter involved in the guidance mode is the rate at which signals are transmitted. Although a low transmission rate causes less occlusion of external sounds, it may also be too slow to alert the traveler to hazards. An adaptive information transfer system adjusts the transmission rate according to changes in the process and the user's requirements, similar to the way the information flow is adjusted in the *Image* mode. When the user is traveling in an unfamiliar environment cluttered with a large number of obstacles, the transmission rate increases, and may reach up to 10 signals per second. On the other hand, when traveling in an environment with little or no obstacles, the transmission rate is reduced to one signal every three seconds.

4.3. Implementation of the image mode

As previously mentioned, the *image* mode provides the user with a panoramic auditory image of the surroundings. The principle is similar to the operation of radar systems used in air traffic control, submarines, etc. An imaginary beam travels from the right side of the user to the left through the sectors covered by the NavBelt's sonars (a range of 120° and 5 m radius). A binaural feedback system invokes the impression of a virtual sound source moving with the beam from the right to the left ear in what we call a sweep. This is done in several discrete steps, corresponding to the discrete virtual direction steps. The angular displacement of the virtual sound source is obtained by a combination of the interaural phase and amplitude shift of the left and right signals. The phase shift is based on the different perception time of an auditory signal due to the difference in travel distance of the sound wave. The phase shift ($i \times N$ terms of time difference between left and right ears) is given by Eq. 1:

$$\Delta t = K \cos \theta \tag{1}$$

where $K = 0.000666$ sec is the time phase constant, and θ is the angular position of the virtual source from the median plane in front of the user (see Figure 7). The interaural amplitude difference of a sound source due to angular shift is given by:

$$\theta = K \log \left[\frac{A_R}{A_L} \right] + \theta_0 \tag{2}$$

where A_R and A_L are the amplitudes to the right and left ears, K is the sensitivity factor and θ_0 is a constant offset. Rowel [24] showed that for most of the range of audible frequencies the sensitivity constant is 2. For the NavBelt we therefore assume $K = 2$ and $\theta_0 = 0$. The amplitude of the dominant channel – the channel closest to the object – is set according to the proximity to the object in that direction. For example, for the configuration shown in Figure 7, the amplitude of right channel, A_R, is set proportionally to the distance d and the amplitude of the left channel is therefore:

$$A_R = A_L \cdot e^{\frac{\theta}{K}} \tag{3}$$

At each step, the amplitude of the signal is set proportionally to the distance to the object in that virtual direction. If no obstacles are detected by the beam, the virtual sound source is of a low amplitude and barely audible. If, on the other hand, obstacles are present, then the amplitude of the virtual sound source is louder.

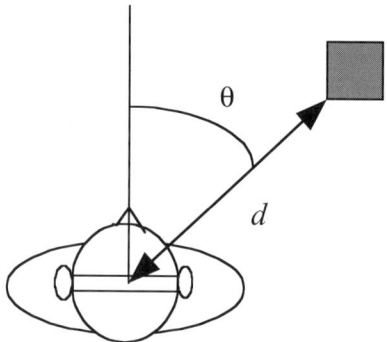

Figure 7. Angular displacement of auditory source.

Figure 8 demonstrates the principle of the *image* mode. Obstacles are detected by the ultrasonic sensors (Figure 8a), and are projected onto a so-called polar histogram,[2] as shown in Figure 8b. Based on the polar histogram, the binaural feedback system generates the sweep, which comprises 12 steps (Figure 8c). Each step "covers" a sector of 15°, so that the whole sweep covers a panorama of 180°. Each of the eight sectors in the center of the panorama (covering the sectors between 30° and 150°) is directly proportional to the corresponding sensor. The remaining four sectors (two at each side of the panorama) represent sectors which are not covered by the sonars. The value of these sectors is extrapolated based on the averaged values of adjoining sectors. For example, if the third and fourth sectors (representing the first and second sonar) contain an object, than the first and second sectors are automatically assigned the averaged value.

Each signal is modulated by an amplitude A (indicating the distance to the obstacle in that direction), the duration T_s for which the square wave signal is audible, and the pitch f of the square wave. The *spacing time* T_n is the length of the interval between consecutive signals during a sweep. After each sweep, there is a pause of duration T_c, to allow the user to comprehend the conveyed image. Many meaningful combinations of these parameters are possible. For example, because of the short-term memory capability of the human ear, a sweep may be as short as 0.5 sec. Given enough cognition time T_c, the user will comprehend the image. Alternatively, the sweep time may be as long as one second, combined with a very short cognition time. Notice that each sweep starts with an anchor signal. This signal has a unique pitch, which provides the user with a convenient marker of the start of a sweep.

---

[2] How this is done is explained in greater detail in Section 5.5.

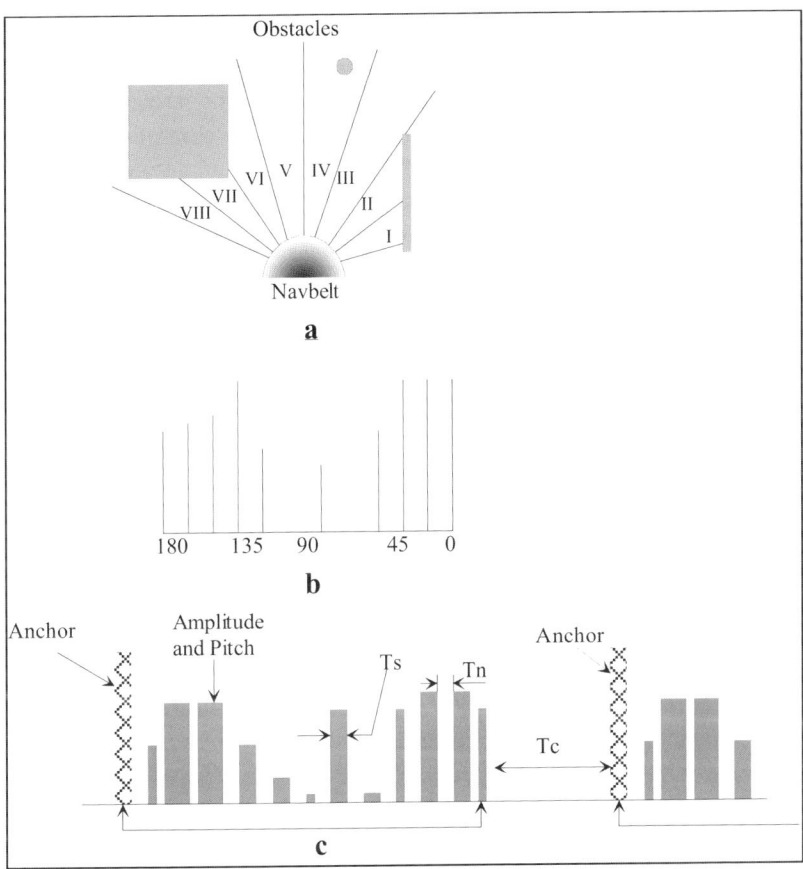

Figure 8. The image mode. (a) Obstacle are detected by the ultrasonic sensors. (b) Sonar range readings are projected onto the polar histogram. (c) An acoustic sweep is generated from the polar histogram.

One of the important features of the *image* mode is the acoustic directional intensity (ADI), which is directly derived from the polar histogram. The virtual direction of the ADI provides information about the source of the auditory signal in space, indicating the location of an object. The intensity of the signals is proportional to the size of the object and its distance from the person as directly derived from the polar histogram.

The directional intensity is a combination of the signal duration T_s, the amplitude A, and the pitch. Experiments with human auditory perception show [2] that the perceived intensity increases with the signal's amplitude, pitch, and duration. Adjusting the acoustic directional intensity according to the location of obstacles in the surroundings attracts the user's attention to the most relevant sections in the environment, while suppressing irrelevant data.

The information adjustment is based on updating the sweep intensity according to the human and environment models. For example, if the human reaction is not satisfactory, then the sweep transmission rate and the ADI are increased. Similarly, the transmission rate and intensity are reduced when the expected performance (calculated from the user and environment models) shows that few obstacles are ahead.

4.4. Experimental results

The NavBelt was extensively tested during its five-year long development. Some of the key experimental results are presented in this section.

4.4.1. Experiments with real obstacles

In this experiment, subjects walked through laboratory obstacle courses comprising various types of obstacles and using the various operation modes of the NavBelt. In the first experiment, several vertical poles with different diameters were positioned along the travel path. It was found that the NavBelt can detect objects as narrow as 10 mm. However, this can be done only if the objects are stationary and the subject is walking slowly (less than 0.4 m/sec). It was also found that the NavBelt can reliably detect objects with a diameter of 10 cm or bigger, regardless of the travel speed. Other tests were conducted inside an office building where subjects traveled along corridors, located doors and curves, and detected and avoided furniture.

In other experiments, subjects traveled outside buildings, detecting and avoiding common objects such as trees and large bushes, parked cars, walls, bicycles, and other pedestrians. One major concern of users was that the current prototype NavBelt lacked the ability to detect overhanging objects, up- and down-steps, sidewalk edges, etc. Future improvements to the NavBelt will require the addition of sonars pointing up and down to detect these type of obstacles.

4.4.2. Experiments with different walking patterns

The next experiment tested the NavBelt in terms of walking patterns. It was found that uneven walking patterns cause the sonars to move along the vertical plane (sonars swinging up and down), which reduces the reliability of the sonar data. In addition, it was found that the relative angle between the sonars and the vertical orientation of the NavBelt (the angle of the sonars with the horizon) affects object detection. For example, if the NavBelt is tilted by

±5° from the horizon, the sonar reading can be off by more than 9%. Swinging the arms during the normal walking pattern did not interfere with the sonar performance as no sonars are directed to the sides. However, using the white cane (the most common device used by blind travelers) can cause interference to the sonar performance, mainly when it is used to detect objects above ground level (higher than 0.5 m). However, since the cane is used mainly to detect objects at ground level, while the NavBelt is designed to detect objects above ground level, this interference is not critical to the general performance.

The experiments with the NavBelt prototype showed the importance of training. Subjects with more experience traveled faster and generally were more comfortable. After 20 hours of practice with a NavBelt simulator and 40 hours of practice with the experimental prototype NavBelt, subjects traveled at 0.8 m/sec in the *Guidance* mode and at 0.4 m/sec in the *Image* mode. Subjects with less experience (10 hours with the simulator and 10 hours with the prototype) traveled at an average speed of 0.6 m/sec in the *Guidance* mode and 0.3 m/sec in the *Image* mode.

4.5. Conclusions on the NavBelt

In this section, we discussed the concept, implementation, and experimental results of the NavBelt, a portable navigation aid for the blind. The NavBelt offers three modes of operation: (1) Guidance Mode, (2) Directional Guidance Mode, and (3) Image Mode.

Both Guidance modes were found effective, allowing reasonably high walking speeds after a relatively small amount of practice (in the order of 40+ hours). The problem with both Guidance modes, however, is the fact that they require accurate feedback about the user's momentary position and heading. With the current state of technology, this feedback is not available, and thus the two Guidance modes cannot be implemented for practical purposes.

The Image mode provides the user with more detailed information about obstacles in the environment – a feature found to be desirable by some of the blind subjects that were interviewed in the course of the development. However, the "cost" of the increased information is that it takes substantially longer to comprehend the acoustic images provided by the NavBelt. It also took substantially longer to become practiced in the interpretation of the acoustic images. After 100 hours of practice in the Image mode a user could walk through a moderately dense obstacle course at walking speeds of about 0.3 – 0.4 m/sec.

We concluded that the Image mode is too slow to be practical for most users, although we believe that performance would further improve with much additional practice. We also concluded that advances in position estimation technology for pedestrians might make the NavBelt's Guidance modes more practical. Some recent developments have been made in this direction and have resulted in a commercially availability device called PointMan™ Navigator II, which combines GPS and personal dead reckoning. However, we haven't tested this device at our lab.

5. The GuideCane

The foremost problem with the NavBelt, as concluded above, is the difficulty of conveying information (in Image mode) to the user to allow him/her to react in time to obstacles ahead. Even if the NavBelt's Guidance modes could be implemented in practice, they would still require the user to concentrate on the acoustic guidance signals and to react to them quickly and efficiently.

A new invention made at the University of Michigan's Mobile Robotics Lab in 1995 aimed at overcoming these problems. This invention, called *GuideCane*, can be thought of as a robotic guide-dog, but it does not have the disadvantages of mobile robot guide-dogs.

Figure 9 shows a schematic view of the GuideCane and its functional components. Much like the widely used white cane, a user holds the GuideCane in front of himself/herself while walking. The GuideCane is considerably heavier than the white cane, but it rolls on wheels that support the GuideCane's weight during regular operation. A servomotor, operating under the control of the GuideCane's built-in computer, can steer the wheels left and right relative to the cane. Both wheels are equipped with encoders to determine their relative motion. For obstacle detection, the GuideCane is equipped with ten ultrasonic sensors. To specify a desired direction of motion, the user operates a mini joystick located at the handle. Based on the user input and the sensor data from its sonars and encoders, the built-in computer decides where to head next and turns the wheels accordingly. Similar to the NavBelt, the GuideCane is equipped with an array of ultrasonic sensors and an obstacle avoidance system.

5.1. Functional description

During operation, the user pushes the GuideCane forward. Using the thumb-operated mini joystick, the user can prescribe a desired direction of motion. This directional command is understood to be relative to the GuideCane's current direction of motion. For example, if the user presses the button forward, then the system considers the current direction of travel to be the desired direction. If the user presses the button to the left, then the computer adds 90° to the current direction of travel and, as soon as this direction is free of obstacles, steers the wheels to the left until the 90° left turn is completed.

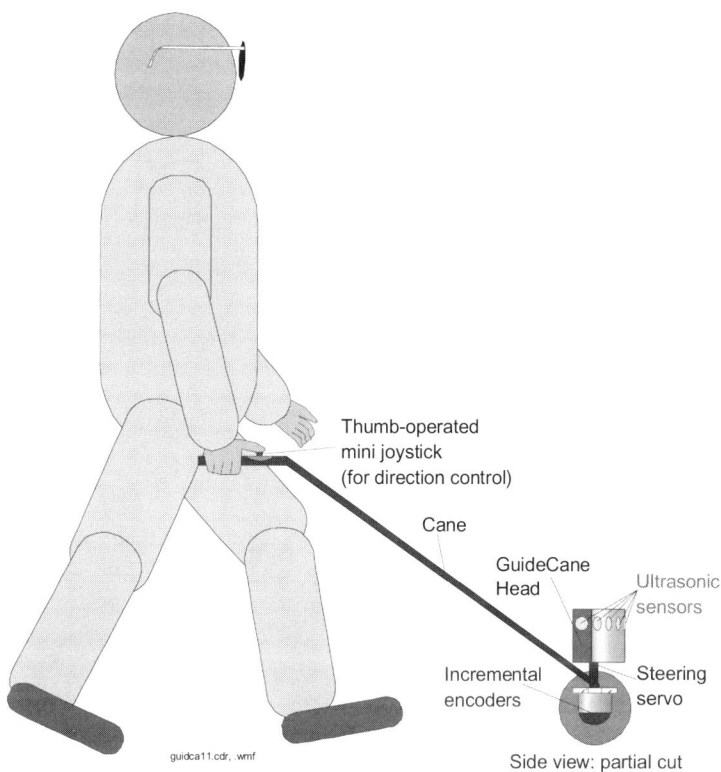

It is important to note that the user can usually indicate a new direction well before the change of direction should occur. In the case of a corridor, if the user presses the button to the left, then the GuideCane will continue down the corridor until it reaches an intersection where it can turn to the left. The ability to indicate a desired direction of motion in advance significantly enhances the GuideCane's ease-of-use.

While traveling, the ultrasonic sensors detect any obstacle in a 120° wide sector ahead of the user (see Step 1 in Figure 10). The built-in computer uses the sensor data to instantaneously determine an appropriate direction of travel, even among densely cluttered obstacles. If an obstacle blocks the desired travel direction, then the obstacle avoidance algorithm prescribes an alternative direction that clears the obstacle and then resumes in the desired direction (see Step 2 in Figure 10).

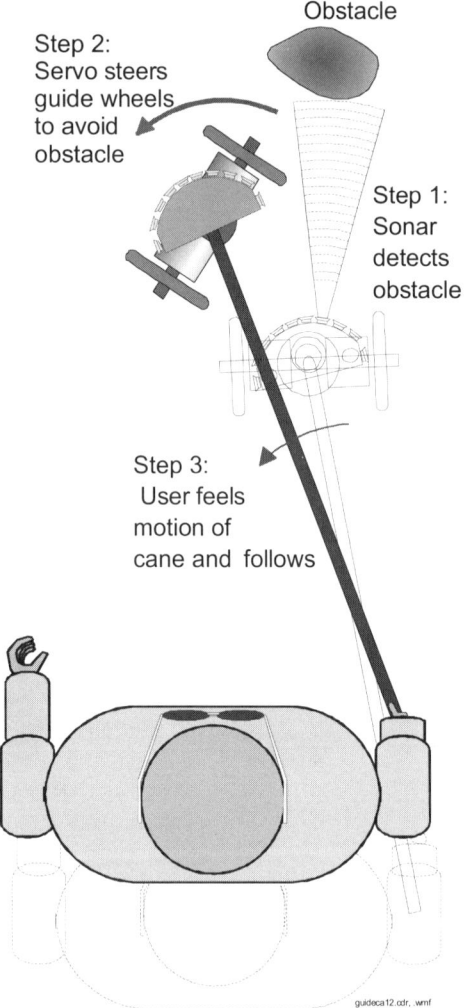

Figure 10. How the GuideCane avoids obstacles.

Once the wheels begin to steer sideways to avoid the obstacle, the user feels the resulting horizontal rotation of the cane (see Step 3 in Figure 10). In a fully intuitive response, requiring virtually no training time, the traveler changes his/her orientation to align himself/herself with the cane at the "nominal" angle. In practice, the user's walking trajectory follows the trajectory of the GuideCane similar to the way a trailer follows a truck. Because of the short handle length, the user's trajectory is very close to the GuideCane's trajectory. Once the obstacle is cleared, the wheels steer back to the original desired direction of travel. The new line of travel will be offset from the original line of travel. Depending on the circumstances, the traveler may wish to continue walking along this new line of travel, or the system can be programmed to return to the original line of travel. This latter option is made possible by the GuideCane's dead-reckoning capability.

A particular problem is the detection of stairs. The GuideCane offers separate solutions for down-steps and up-steps. Down-steps are detected in a fail-safe manner: when a down-step is encountered, the wheels of the GuideCane drop off the edge until the shock-absorbing bottom hits the step – without a doubt a signal that the user can not miss. Because the user walks behind the GuideCane, he/she has sufficient time to stop. Up-steps can be detected by additional front-facing sonars as described in [8]; however, this method is not yet implemented in the GuideCane.

5.2. Guidance signals versus obstacle information

Existing ETAs are designed to notify the user of obstacles, usually requiring him/her to perform some sort of scanning action. The user must evaluate all of the obstacle information, which comprises the size and proximity of each obstacle, and then decide on a suitable travel direction. In sighted people, such relatively high bandwidth information is processed almost reflexively, usually without the need for conscious decisions. Nature had millions of years of evolution to perfect this skill. However, the evaluation of obstacle information presented acoustically is a new skill that must be acquired over hundreds of hours of learning, as we concluded in the introductory section and in [27]. Even then, exercising such a skill requires a great deal of conscious effort, and thus processing time. The required effort further increases with the number of detected obstacles.

The GuideCane is fundamentally different from other devices in that it first analyzes the environment and then computes the momentary optimal direction of travel. The resulting guidance signal is a single piece of information – a direction – which means that the bandwidth of the information is much smaller. The consequence is that it is far easier and safer to follow the low-bandwidth guidance signal of the GuideCane than to follow the high-bandwidth information of other existing systems. However, reducing the high-bandwidth obstacle information to a momentary optimal direction of travel requires the use of advanced mobile robot technologies.

5.3. Information transfer

In prior research with the NavBelt, different methods were tested that use binaural (stereophonic) signals to guide the user around obstacles as described in Section 4. Subjects found it difficult to recognize and react to such signals at walking speed [28]. By contrast, our tests have shown that untrained subjects could *immediately* follow the GuideCane at walking speed, even among densely cluttered obstacles.

This advantage can be credited to another unique feature of the GuideCane: information transfer through direct physical force. This process is completely intuitive so that everybody can use the system right away without learning how to interpret artificially defined acoustic or tactile signals, as with existing ETAs. Yielding to external forces is a reflexive process that does not require a conscious effort. Moreover, many blind persons are accustomed to being guided by sighted people in a similar fashion.

Even though the GuideCane's wheels are unpowered, the GuideCane can apply a substantial amount of physical force on the user. The sideways motion of the wheels results in a rotation of the handle of the cane, which is clearly noticeable. A second force, immediately felt after the wheels change their orientation (but even before the user feels the rotation of the cane), is the increased reaction force that is opposed to pushing the cane forward. When walking while the cane and the wheels are aligned, the user must only overcome the reactive force F_r resulting from the friction in the bearings and the roll resistance of the wheels. If the wheels steer an angle θ in either direction of the cane, then the user has to push the cane with an increased force equal to $F_r/\cos\theta$ to overcome the reactive force of the wheels. This change in reactive force is immediately felt by the user and prepares him/her for an upcoming steering maneuver.

5.4. Hardware implementation

The GuideCane must be as compact and as lightweight as possible so that the user can easily lift it, e.g., for coping with stairs and access to public transportation. For the same reason, the electronic components should require minimal power in order to minimize the weight of the batteries. In addition, both the mechanical and electronic hardware must be designed to facilitate the software's task: allowing real-time performance with limited on-board processing power.

5.4.1. Mechanical hardware

The GuideCane consists of three main modules: housing, wheelbase, and handle. The housing contains and protects most of the electronic components. The current prototype is equipped with ten Polaroid ultrasonic sensors that are located around the housing. Eight of the sonars are located in the front in a semi-circular fashion with an angular spacing of 15°, covering the area ahead of the GuideCane with a total angular spacing of 120°. The other two sonars face the sides and are particularly useful for following walls and for going through narrow openings, such as doorways.

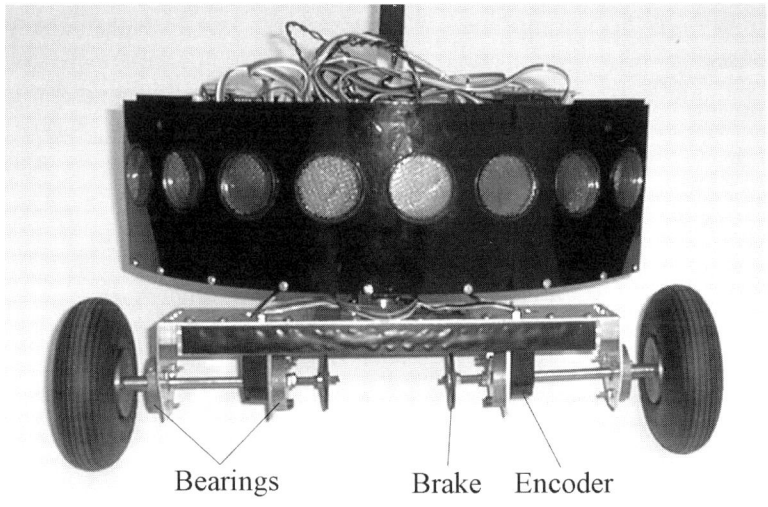

Figure 11. The GuideCane housing and wheelbase.

The wheelbase can be rotated by a small servomotor. As shown in Figure 11, the wheelbase uses ball bearings to support two unpowered wheels. To perform odometry, both wheels are equipped with lightweight quadrature encoders. Using full quadrature decoding, the resolution of the encoders is 2,000 pulses per revolution, resulting in more than 5 pulses for a wheel advancement of 1 mm. The GuideCane's odometry equations are the same as for a differential drive mobile robot. However, because the wheels are unpowered, there is considerably less risk of wheel slippage.

The handle serves as the main physical interface between the user and the GuideCane. The angle of the handle can be adjusted to accommodate users of different heights. At the level of the user's hand, a joystick-like pointing device is fixed to the handle. The pointer consists of a mouse button (similar to the pointing devices used on some notebook computers) that the user can press with his/her thumb in any direction. The selected direction indicates the desired direction of travel relative to the current orientation of the cane. In the current implementation, this direction is discretized into eight directions.

5.4.2. Electronic hardware

The electronic system architecture of the GuideCane is shown in Figure 12. The main brain of the GuideCane is an embedded PC/104 computer, equipped with a 486 microprocessor that is clocked at 33 MHz. The PC/104 stack consists of four layers. Three of the modules are commercially available boards, including the motherboard, the VGA utility module, and a miniature 125-MB hard disk. The fourth board, which was custom built, serves as the *main interface* between the PC and the sensors (encoders, sonars, and potentiometer) and actuators (main servo and brakes).

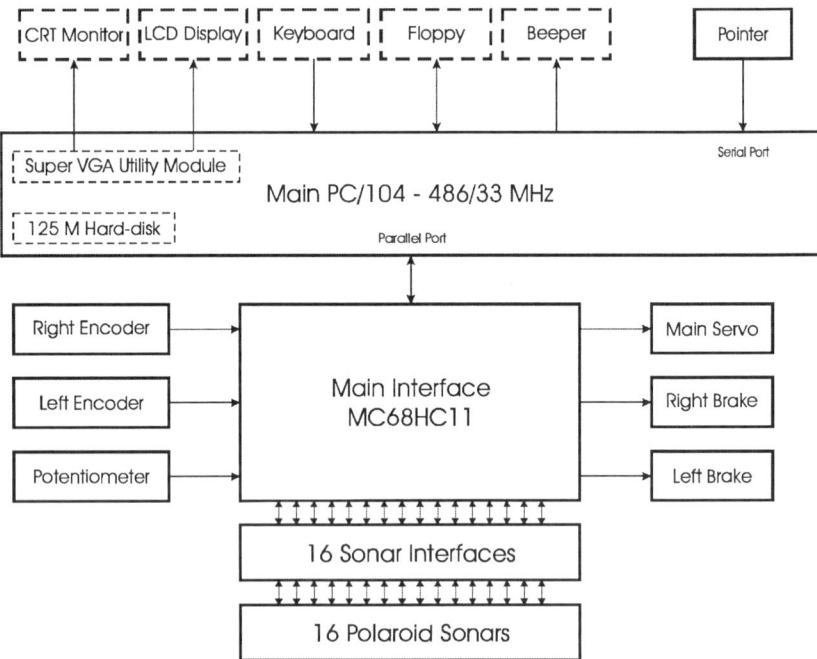

Figure 12. The GuideCane system. Dashed lines indicate components that are only required during the development stage.

The main interface executes many time-critical tasks, such as firing the sonars at specific times, constantly checking the sonars for an echo, generating the PWM (Pulse Width Modulation) signals for the servos, and decoding the encoder outputs. The main interface also acts as an asynchronous buffer for the sonar data. Although the GuideCane currently uses only 10 sonars, the main interface provides hardware and software support for up to 16 sonars.

The PC is connected to the main interface through its bi-directional parallel port. The interface preprocesses most of the sensor data before the data is read by the PC. In addition, all communications are buffered. The preprocessing and buffering not only minimizes the communications between the PC and the interface, but also minimizes the computational burden on the PC to control the sensors and actuators. Because the main interface completes all the low-level tasks, almost all of the PC's computational power can be dedicated to medium- and high-level tasks. The interface consists of three MC68HC11E2 microcontrollers, two quadrature decoders, a FIFO buffer, and a decoder. Thus, the GuideCane can be described as an embedded system equipped with four processors.

The embedded PC/104 computer provides a convenient development environment. For stationary development, the system is connected to a regular keyboard and a CRT monitor. For mobile tests, the computer is connected to a smaller keyboard and a color LCD screen that is fixed to the handle a little below the developer's hand. The entire system is powered by rechargeable NiMH batteries, allowing mobile testing for several hours. Even during development, the GuideCane was a truly autonomous system in the sense of power and computational resources.

Although the current prototype consists of four PC/104-sized modules, only two of them are required during operation. One module that provides the VGA display interface is very useful for visual feedback during development, but it is not needed during operation. Another module that houses the hard-disk can also be eliminated in a final product. The final software will be stored in an EPROM that can be added to the motherboard. This solid-state solution will also eliminate potential problems with the moving parts of the hard-disk, which is sensitive to shocks and vibrations. All components that can be eliminated in a final product version of the GuideCane was indicated in Figure 12 by boxes drawn with dashed lines.

5.5. Software implementation

The GuideCane is a semi-autonomous system, providing full autonomy for *local* navigation (obstacle avoidance), but relying on the skills of the user for *global* navigation (path planning and localization). Combining the skills of a mobile robot with the existing skills of a visually impaired user is the key idea behind the NavBelt and the GuideCane. This combination of skills is what makes this particular application feasible at the current stage of mobile robotics research. While reliable global navigation algorithms might be available in the future, they are not essential for the GuideCane. Although visually impaired people have difficulties performing fast local navigation without a travel aid, they are in most cases perfectly capable of performing global navigation.

The main task of the GuideCane is to steer around obstacles and to proceed toward the desired direction of travel. The GuideCane's performance is thus directly related to the performance of its obstacle avoidance algorithm. To achieve safe traveling at fast walking speeds through cluttered and unknown environments, the GuideCane employs mobile robot obstacle avoidance methods that were developed earlier at the University of Michigan's Mobile Robotics Lab.

Local map building

Like the NavBelt, the GuideCane also uses EERUF to control the ultrasonic sensors to achieve a fast firing rate [7]. Each of the ten sonars is fired at a rate of 10 Hz, so that the GuideCane receives 100 sonar readings per second. EERUF's fast firing rate is a key factor for the reliability and robustness of the GuideCane's obstacle avoidance performance and is necessary for allowing safe travel at fast walking speeds. And, also as in the NavBelt, the GuideCane employs the VFH obstacle avoidance method described in Section 3.2.1. However, several improvements over the original VFH method were implemented in the GuideCane. The improved method, called VFH+, is discussed next.

One of the improvements of VFH+ is that the polar histogram is modified to rule out those obstacle-free directions that cannot be taken because of the kinematic and dynamic constraints of the GuideCane (see [30] for details). The modified polar histogram is called the *masked polar histogram.* A threshold applied to the masked polar histogram determines which directions are actual *candidates* for travel. A hysteresis is applied to the threshold to provide smoother and less oscillatory motion.

The VFH+ algorithm selects the most suitable direction (out of all candidate directions) of motion based on a so-called *cost function*. The cost function includes three terms: the angular deviation from the desired direction, the angular deviation from the current orientation of the wheelbase, and the angular deviation from the previously selected direction of motion. For each candidate direction the cost of choosing this direction is computed, using the fixed, preprogrammed cost function. Selecting the most suitable direction therefore means simply selecting the candidate direction with the lowest cost.

Although the performance of the VFH+ method is adequate in most situations, it sometimes directs the GuideCane into local dead-ends (e.g., concave obstacles) that were detected as such by its sensors, and thus could have been avoided. To avoid steering into such dead-ends, the VFH+ method was combined with the A* search algorithm, and includes an appropriate cost, a heuristic function, and a discounting factor [31]. The A* search algorithm is used to find an optimal path of a short length, using the VFH+ method to determine suitable directions of motion at a given position (state).

5.6. Experimental results

The actual GuideCane prototype, shown in Figure 13, was extensively tested at the University of Michigan's Mobile Robotics Laboratory.

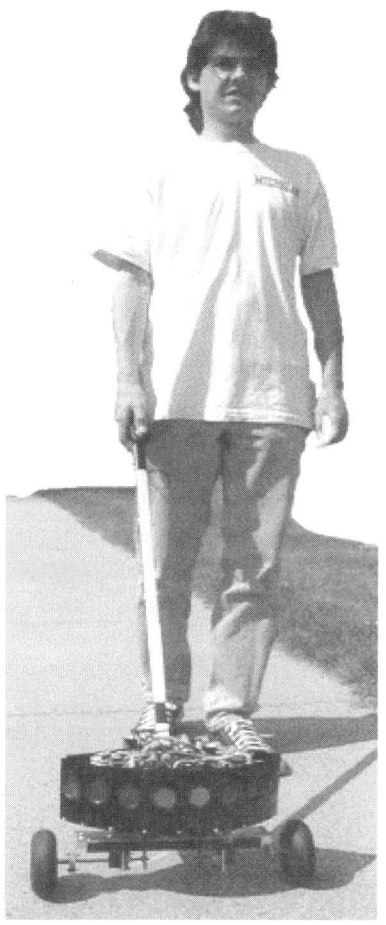

Figure 13. The actual GuideCane prototype.

A performance analysis of the experimental GuideCane prototype can be divided into two categories: 1) the usefulness of the concept, and 2) the performance of the obstacle avoidance system. The GuideCane concept fulfilled all our expectations and confirmed our initial hypothesis that following the GuideCane is a completely intuitive process. All subjects were able to follow the GuideCane easily, at fast walking speeds of up to 1 m/sec, while completing complex maneuvers through cluttered environments.

Subjects rarely needed more than a few minutes to get used to the GuideCane. Actually, blind subjects needed a few minutes to understand the GuideCane concept, as they could not visually observe how the device was working. Blindfolded subjects, on the other hand, needed some time to simply become accustomed to walking around without sight. Nonetheless, blind and blindfolded subjects alike noticed that walking with the GuideCane was completely intuitive and did not require any conscious effort.

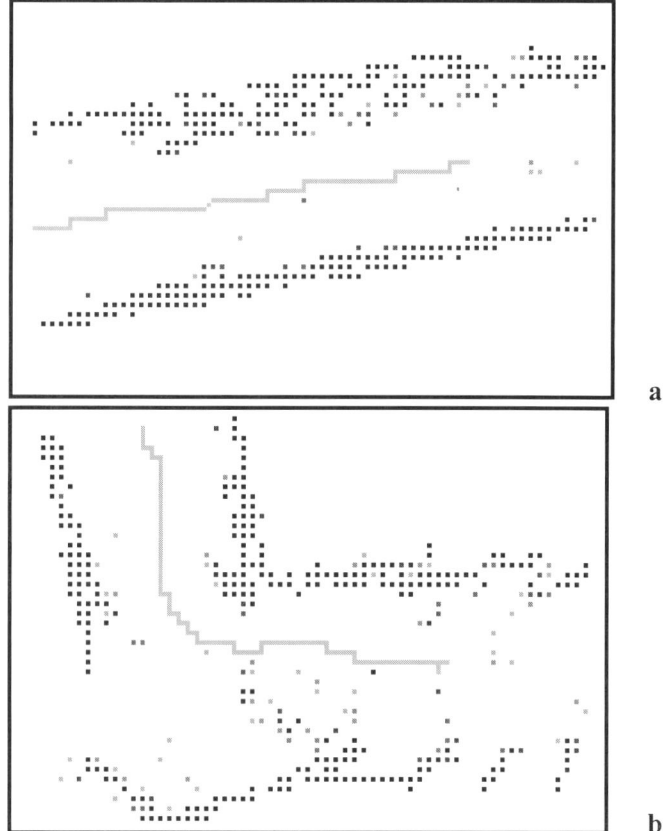

Figure 14. Two screen captures showing the path of the actual GuideCane through corridors. In both experiments, the target direction is towards the right. The intensity of a histogram grid cell indicates its certainty value. The gray line indicates the robot's trajectory, based on its odometry. a) The GuideCane continues down a corridor. b) The GuideCane makes a left turn at a T-shaped intersection.

The second category, the obstacle avoidance performance, is adequate in many indoor environments. The performance of the combined

EERUF/HIMM/VFH+ system is excellent as long as the obstacles are indeed detected by the sonars. Screen captures of two test runs with the actual GuideCane are shown in Figure 14, demonstrating the processes of the local map building and the obstacle avoidance algorithms.

Failures of the obstacle avoidance system were in most cases caused by obstacles that were not detected by the sonars. For example, the GuideCane is currently not able to detect overhanging obstacles like tabletops. However, these obstacles should easily be detected with the additional upward-looking sonars of the next prototype version. The addition of these sonars is expected to improve the GuideCane's performance to a level where a visually impaired person could effectively use the device indoors. Outdoors, however, the implementation of an additional type of sensor will be required to allow the GuideCane to detect important features, such as sidewalk borders. In order for the GuideCane to become a truly useful tool for a visually impaired person, it will be essential to develop a real-time method for the detection of these features.

6. Discussion

Both the NavBelt and the GuideCane successfully overcome the first two fundamental shortcomings of existing ETAs, as identified in Section 2. The first shortcoming is overcome by using multiple sensors that face in different directions, thus covering a large area regardless of the user's orientation. Therefore, the user no longer needs to actively scan the surroundings manually.

The second shortcoming is overcome by the use of obstacle avoidance technology. Due to the multi-sensor system and the accumulation of sensor data, no additional measurements are required for the obstacle avoidance algorithm to determine a path that guides the blind traveler around the obstacles. In the case of the GuideCane, the obstacle avoidance algorithm provides full autonomy for local navigation, thus allowing the user to fully concentrate on the less time-constrained tasks of global path planning and localization. As a consequence, faster walking speeds can be achieved even with a smaller conscious effort on the user's part.

The NavBelt does not overcome the third shortcoming, as it relies on acoustic feedback and thus masks acoustic cues that are important for the user. The GuideCane successfully overcomes this shortcoming by using a much simpler and more direct interface that is based on physical force instead of acoustic feedback.

The GuideCane offers two additional advantages over the NavBelt. (1) The GuideCane is much more intuitive to use, and thus requires very little training time. (2) Because the GuideCane rolls on wheels that are in contact with the ground, it can get an estimate of its position through odometry. The position estimation not only allows for the easier guidance mode, but it also allows for a better obstacle avoidance performance. On the other hand, the NavBelt could be used together with the white cane, which is not the case for the GuideCane.

References

[1] Benjamin, J. M., Ali, N. A., and Schepis, A. F., 1973, "A Laser Cane for the Blind," *Proceedings of the San Diego Biomedical Symposium,* Vol. 12, pp. 53-57.
[2] Benson, K. B., 1986, "Audio Engineering Handbook," *McGraw-Hill Book Company,* New York.
[3] Bissitt, D. and Heyes, A. D., 1980, "An Application of Biofeedback in the Rehabilitation of the Blind," *Applied Ergonomics,* Vol. 11, No. 1, pp. 31-33.
[4] Blasch, B. B., Long, R. G., and Griffin-Shirley, N., 1989, "National Evaluation of Electronic Travel Aids for Blind and Visually Impaired Individuals: Implications for Design," *RESNA 12th Annual Conference*, New Orleans, Louisiana, pp. 133-134.
[5] Borenstein, J. and Koren, Y., 1991, "Histogramic In-Motion Mapping for Mobile Robot Obstacle Avoidance," *IEEE Transactions on Robotics and Automation,* August, pp. 535-539.
[6] Borenstein, J. and Koren, Y., 1991, "The Vector Field Histogram - Fast Obstacle-Avoidance for Mobile Robots," *IEEE Journal of Robotics and Automation,* Vol. 7, No. 3, June, pp. 278-288.
[7] Borenstein, J. and Koren, Y., 1995, "Error Eliminating Rapid Ultrasonic Firing for Mobile Robot Obstacle Avoidance," *IEEE Transactions on Robotics and Automation,* February, Vol. 11, No. 1, pp. 132-138.
[8] Borenstein, J. and Ulrich, I., 1997, "The GuideCane - A Computerized Travel Aid for the Active Guidance of Blind Pedestrians," *IEEE International Conference on Robotics and Automation*, Albuquerque, NM, April, pp. 1283-1288.
[9] Brabyn, J. A., 1982, "New Developments in Mobility and Orientation Aids for the Blind," *IEEE Transactions on Biomedical Engineering,* Vol. BAM-29, No. 4, pp. 285-290.
[10] Elfes, A., 1989, "Using occupancy grids for mobile robot perception and navigation," *Computer Magazine*, June, pp. 46-57.
[11] Ericson, M. A. and Mckinley, R. L., 1989, "Auditory Localization Cue Synthesis and Human Performance," *IEEE Proceedings of the National Aerospace and Electronics Conference,* V2, pp. 718-725, NASEA9.
[12] Fish, R. M., "An Audio Display for the Blind," *IEEE Transactions on Biomedical Engineering,* Vol. BME-23, No. 2, March, pp. 144-153.
[13] Golledge, R. G., Loomis, J. M., Klatzky, R. L., Flury, A., and Yang, X. L., 1991, "Designing a personal guidance system to aid navigation without sight: progress on GIS component," *International Journal of Geographical Information Systems,* Vol. 5, No. 4, pp. 373-395.

[14] Ifukube, T., Sasaki, T., and Peng, C., 1991, "A Blind Mobility Aid Modeled After Echolocation of Bats," *IEEE Transactions on Biomedical Engineering,* Vol. 38, No. 5, May, pp. 461-465.
[15] Jackson, C., 1995, Correspondence with Carroll L. Jackson, Executive Director of the Upshaw Institute for the Blind, August 11, available at ftp://ftp.eecs.umich.edu/people/johannb/Carroll_Jackson_Letter.pdf.
[16] Kay, L., 1974, "A Sonar Aid to Enhance Spatial Perception of the Blind: Engineering Design and Evaluation," *Radio and Electronic Engineer,* Vol. 44, No. 11, pp. 605-627.
[17] Kelly, G. W. and Ackerman, T., 1982, "Sona, The Sonic Orientation and Navigational Aid for the Visually Impaired," *Fifth Annual Conference on Rehabilitation Engineering,* Houston, Texas, p. 72.
[18] Lebedev, V. V. and Sheiman, V. L., 1980, "Assessment of the Possibilities of Building an Echo Locator for the Blind," *Telecommunications and Radio Engineering,* Vol. 34-35, No. 3, pp. 97-100.
[19] Mann, R. W., 1974, "Technology and Human Rehabilitation: Prostheses for Sensory Rehabilitation and/or Sensory Substitution," *Advances in Biomedical Engineering,* Vol. 4, Academic Press, Inc. pp. 209-353.
[20] Moravec, H. P., 1988, "Sensor fusion in certainty grids for mobile robots," *AI Magazine,* Summer, pp. 61-74.
[21] National Research Council, 1986, "Working Group on Mobility Aids for the Visually Impaired and Blind", National Academy Press, Washington D.C.
[22] POLAROID Corp, "Ultrasonic Ranging System – Description, operation and use information for conduction tests and experiments with Polaroid's Ultrasonic Ranging System," Ultrasonic Components Group, 119 Windsor Street, Cambridge, MA.
[23] Pressey, N., 1977, "Mowat Sensor," *Focus,* Vol. 11, No. 3, pp. 35-39.
[24] Rowel, D., 1970, "Auditory Factors in the Design of a Binaural Sensory Aid for the Blind," Ph.D. Thesis, University of Canterbury, New Zealand.
[25] Russell, L., 1965, "Travel Path Sounder," *Proceedings of Rotterdam Mobility Res. Conference,* New York: American Foundation for the Blind.
[26] Shoval, S., Borenstein, J., and Koren, Y., 1994, "Mobile Robot Obstacle Avoidance in a Computerized Travel Aid for the Blind," *IEEE International Conference on Robotics and Automation,* San Diego, CA, May 8-13, pp. 2023-2029.
[27] Shoval, S., Borenstein, J., and Koren, Y., 1998, "The NavBelt - A Computerized Travel Aid For The Blind Based On Mobile Robotics Technology," *IEEE Transactions on Biomedical Engineering,* Vol. 45, No. 11, November, pp. 1376-1386.
[28] Shoval, S., Borenstein, J., and Koren, Y., 1998, "Auditory Guidance with the NavBelt - A Computerized Travel Aid for the Blind," *IEEE Transactions on Systems, Man, and Cybernetics,* Vol. 28, No. 3, August, pp. 459-467.
[29] Tachi, S., Mann, R. W., and Rowel, D., 1983, "Quantitative Comparison of Alternative Sensory Displays for Mobility Aids for the Blind," *IEEE Transactions on Biomedical Engineering,* Vol. BME-30, No. 9, September, pp. 571-577.

[30] Ulrich, I. and Borenstein, J., 1998, "VFH+: Reliable Obstacle Avoidance for Fast Mobile Robots," *IEEE International Conference on Robotics and Automation*, Leuven, Belgium, May, pp. 1572-1577.
[31] Ulrich, I., 1997, "The GuideCane - A Computerized Travel Aid for the Active Guidance of Blind Pedestrians," Master Thesis, University of Michigan, MEAM, Ann Arbor, August.

Chapter 13

Advanced design concepts for a knee-ankle-foot orthosis

Kenton R. Kaufman, Steven E. Irby, Jeffrey R. Basford, and **David H. Sutherland**

Conventional knee-ankle-foot orthoses (KAFOs) are used for stability during stance. KAFOs with a drop lock provide stance phase stability but prevent knee motion during swing. Alternatively, KAFOs with an eccentric knee joint allow knee motion during swing but provide limited stability during stance. Either design results in an inefficient gait. A knee joint which automatically unlocks at the end of the stance phase and automatically locks at the start of the stance phase results in a significant improvement of the gait and stability of a KAFO user. This gait is much smoother than the gait with a conventional KAFO where the knee remains locked throughout the gait cycle.

An orthosis utilizing the design goal of free knee motion during swing and locked knee position during stance is superior to conventional KAFOs. Work is currently underway by several groups to achieve these design goals. However, field trials of these devices have not been conducted yet. Although the preliminary results are quite promising, objective performance data, and long-term durability trials are still needed. Continued engineering development and creativity will be required for the transformation of these conceptual designs into a viable product, which can be used by patients with knee instability during stance.

1. Introduction

More than 1.5 million people in the United States have partial or complete paralysis of the extremities [1]. The prevalence of paralysis increases with age (Figure 1) and it is not surprising that the mobility of individuals with neuromuscular disorders is one of the most common and complicated issues treated by rehabilitation professionals. Many of these individuals require assistive technology (AT) in the form of an orthosis to enhance mobility. In fact, it is estimated that 989,000 people use a knee orthosis, 596,000 people use a leg orthosis, and 282,000 people use a foot orthosis [2]. In addition to people who require an orthosis for ambulation, there are 173,000 individuals who use a leg or foot prosthesis [2]. Thus, more than 2 million people need some form of lower extremity AT (Table 1). It is important to note that, although there is a greater need for assistive technology as age increases (Figure 1), the use of AT actually decreases with age [3] (Figure 2). The prevalence of a foot or leg orthosis is higher among younger individuals, and artificial limb usage is highest among people in the 45- to 64-year range (Figure 2). Typically, lower extremity orthoses are extremely simple and often have none or only two moving parts. This simplicity is accompanied by ease of donning and durability, but leaves functional abilities only partially improved. The following sections discuss how an intelligent KAFO can be used to restore function in individuals with paralysis of the lower extremity beyond the level possible with traditional orthoses.

Table 1. U.S. population requirements for assistive technology for the lower extremity, 1994.

Device	Population
Knee orthosis	989,000
Leg orthosis	596,000
Foot orthosis	282,000
Leg or foot prosthesis	173,000
Total	2,040,000

Source [2].

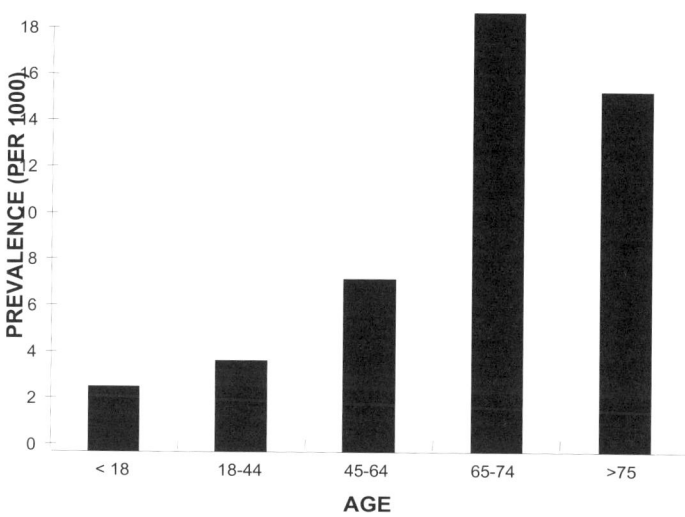

Figure 1. Prevalence of people in the United States with partial or complete paralysis of the extremities. There is a greater need for assistive technology as age increases. Source [1].

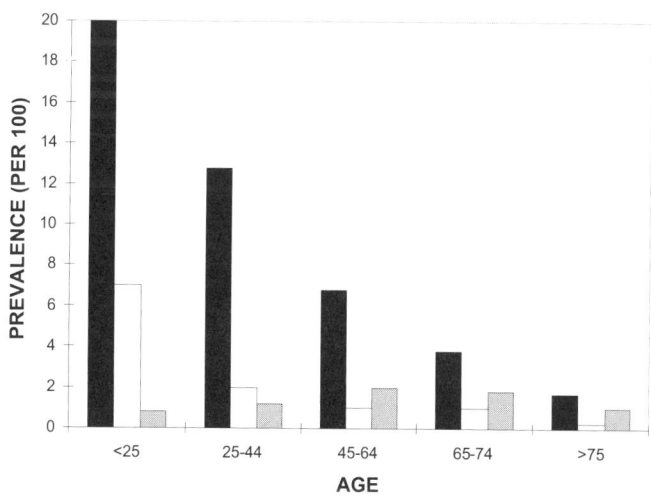

Figure 2. Prevalence of people in the United Stated who use some form of assistive technology for the lower extremity. The prevalence of usage decreases with increasing age (■leg; ☐foot; ▨artificial limb). Source [3].

2. History

People with partial or complete paralysis of the lower extremity require bracing for stability during stance. Individuals with proximal weakness are often prescribed knee-ankle-foot orthoses (KAFOs), also known as long leg braces, to compensate for severe weakness of the lower-limb muscles. Many engineering efforts have been made to produce a dynamic brace to address the conflicting needs for knee stability, freedom, and minimized weight. Previous dynamic knee joint designs fall into four broad categories: (1) interference, (2) extension assist, (3) friction, and (4) hydropneumatic cylinders. The simplest designs are those that rely upon mechanical interference to counteract flexion moments about the knee. These designs primarily offer a single locked conformation at full extension [4-11]. Some designs include eccentric or polycentric hinges to augment joint locking [5,8,12]. Multiple locking positions are possible in designs using a ratchet and pawl assembly [13,14]. An additional benefit of the latter design is that joint extension is possible after the joint is engaged. Some investigators have suggested using elastic bands to resist knee flexion, but not lock the joint [15-18]. These designs fail to offer the complete stability during weight bearing that severely disabled individuals require. One design has incorporated this technique with a locking mechanism that engages at full extension [10]. Friction based devices offer the possibility of an infinite number of stable positions. Several forms of friction brakes have been proposed as solutions for knee joint control: a caliper brake, band brake, wrap spring clutch, multiple leaf disc brake, and pivoting wedge and clevis [19-23]. Hydraulic knee joint systems allow an infinite number of locked positions, but are awkward and require more space than any other joint control approaches. Advances in manufacturing technology have made the size and dynamic properties of hydraulic cylinders more compatible with the constraints of orthotic design [24]. Few of these designs have been reduced to working models. Furthermore, scientific reports are lacking on the benefits of these orthosis systems.

3. Current knee-ankle-foot orthosis design

Currently, two types of KAFOs are generally prescribed: eccentric (or free) knee joint or locked (or fixed) knee joint. Eccentric knee orthoses are stable in extension as long as the ground reaction force vector passes anterior to the knee hinge axis. The eccentric hinge orthosis design, thus, provides limited stance stability and allows flexion and extension at all times. However, the individual must maintain the force vector anterior to the knee hinge axis during stance for stability. The locked KAFO achieves maximum stability through the use of drop or pawl locks. These locks keep the knee joint locked at all times except when disengaged manually or with a bail lock to permit knee flexion during sitting. This design allows stance-phase stability but does not allow any swing-phase knee flexibility.

Unfortunately, KAFOs are heavy, rigid and frustrating devices. In practice, people who require KAFOs typically accept them for a very short period following injury or disease but soon reject them at rates of from 60% to nearly 100% [25,26], presumably because walking with locked knees is so energy inefficient. Cerny, Waters, Hislop, and Perry [27] showed that walking with KAFOs is more inefficient than wheelchair propulsion in individuals with paraplegia who require KAFOs to walk, even for those who customarily use orthoses for locomotion. (Walking with KAFOs is much less energy efficient than typical walking, whereas values for wheelchair propulsion approximate values for typical walking.) These data suggest that wheelchair propulsion is selected as the primary mode of locomotion because walking with KAFOs is more taxing.

Design engineers face fewer technical problems in developing a prosthetic limb replacement as compared with the development of an orthotic brace system. As a result, most of the research and development efforts aimed at improving impaired gait have been directed at prosthetic systems. The difficulties of an orthotic device include the existing (rather than absent) weight and volume of the lower extremity requiring an orthosis, which limit the size and weight of any practical device. Other than the application of modern plastics to orthotic designs, there have been no real changes in the function of conventional long leg braces for decades [28].

4. Advanced concepts in orthosis design

An ideal knee orthosis should provide complete stability in the stance phase of gait, yet permit unhampered knee movements during the swing phase of gait. Efforts are currently underway by several groups to achieve this ideal design.

4.1. Logic-controlled electromechanical free-knee orthosis

The logic-controlled free-knee orthosis is composed of two major parts (Figure 3): mechanical hardware and an electronic control system [29-32]. The mechanical hardware consists of a polypropylene long leg brace, a mechanical knee flexion restraint mechanism, and a knee release actuator solenoid. To incorporate the electromechanical components into a standard orthosis, the medial knee hinge struts are left intact and the lateral hinge is removed.

Specially fabricated stainless steel brackets connect the clutch mechanism to the lateral thigh and shank struts.

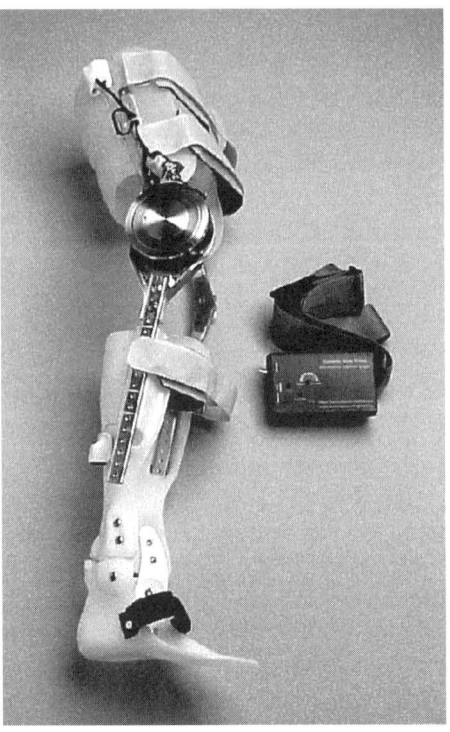

Figure 3. Logical Controlled Electromechanical Free-Knee Long-Leg Orthosis. The control mechanism is attached to the lateral strut of the KAFO at the knee. The electronic control system is in the small box.

The knee hinge clutch mechanism is a wrap-spring clutch, which is a special class of overrunning clutch, a mechanism that allows torque to be transmitted from one shaft to another in one direction of rotation but not in the other (Figure 4). A wrap-spring clutch was selected because it offers unidirectional rotation without any intrinsic control input, silent engagement at any position, low disengagement force, free bidirectional rotation when disengaged, and fail-safe operation. A typical wrap-spring clutch uses a close-wound helical spring to transmit torque across a pair of mating, concentric clutch hubs (Figure 4). Torque is transmitted when the relative rotation of the input and output hubs causes the spring to wrap down on (or grip) both the input and output hubs. Overrunning occurs when the relative rotation of the input and output hubs causes the spring to unwind. The wrap-spring clutch is mounted on the KAFO so that knee extension is not restricted at any time. To release the clutch, allowing rotation in either direction, a linear solenoid is used to unwind the wrap spring slightly (3°-5°). It is held in this expanded position until joint flexion is no longer needed. When the solenoid is de-energized the spring is released and the clutch reverts back to its flexion-resisting configuration.

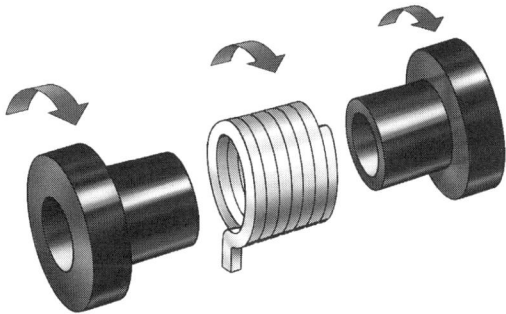

Figure 4. An overrunning wrap-spring clutch is comprised of three principal components: an input hub, an output hub, and a helical spring. If the input hub is rotated so as to unwind the spring, minimal torque is transmitted to the output hub. Conversely, if the input hub is rotated so as to wind the spring down on the hub (as indicated by arrow), maximum torque is transmitted. The radial projecting spring tang is used to unwind the spring so that the output hub is free to rotate in either direction. (Illustration courtesy of Warner Electric, South Beloit, IL.)

The inputs to the control circuitry are signals generated by strategically located foot contact sensors. The control inputs correspond with naturally occurring gait events. The timing and repeatability of these events are critical to a successful application. The chronology of foot contact events, as they relate to gait kinematics and kinetics, was used to guide the control system design. Knee joint engagement must occur after peak knee flexion is attained during swing phase, but no later than foot strike. (Figure 5a). The clutch can be engaged any time after peak knee flexion in swing because extension is possible at all times due to the overrunning capability of the wrap-spring clutch. The high rate of loading at the onset of stance creates an inviolable constraint lest the knee collapse into flexion. (Figure 5b). Disengagement must occur after sufficient weight transfer to the opposite leg has taken place (after opposite foot strike) (Figure 5b), but soon enough to allow the knee to flex before toe-off (Figure 5a). Thus there is a narrow time window in which the clutch must be activated.

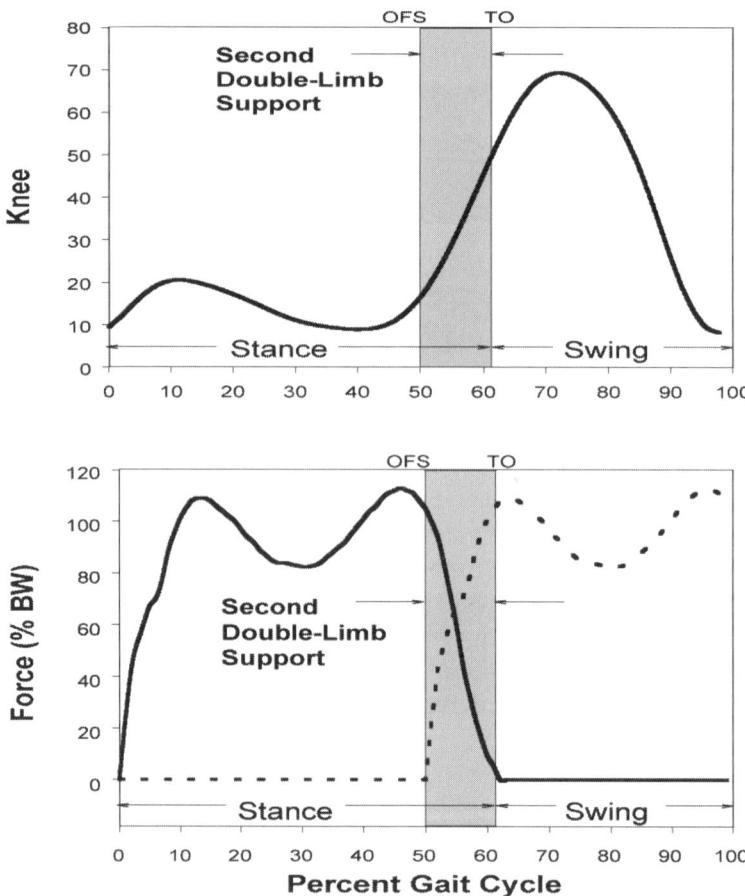

Figure 5. (a) Normal sagittal knee motion and (b) normal foot-floor contact forces perpendicular to floor plane (normalized to percent of body weight). The dashed line represents opposite limb forces. Normal timing of opposite foot strike (OFS) and toe-off (TO) establish boundaries around the critical time period for knee joint control. The knee control mechanism must be released after sufficient weight transfer has occurred. That is, after OFS but prior to TO, in order for sufficient knee flexion to occur and to obtain foot clearance during the swing phase of gait. Source [32].

The electronic control system is composed of digital logic integrated circuits. The inputs to the control circuitry are signals generated by strategically located foot contact sensors. A combinatorial logic network monitors input data and produces electrical output commands based on the input states. The finite state approach [33] to control system design was selected because of the ease in which a simple circuit could be fabricated that would meet the control needs (Figure 6). Each foot had a heel and a forefoot sensor connected, via ribbon cable, to the control system. Sensor input are passed to an electronically programmable read-only memory (EPROM) which has been programmed to output the appropriate control signals for all 16 possible input combinations (i.e., four sensors with two states each yields $2^4 = 16$ combinations, see Table 2). Based on the input, the controller algorithm generates an actuation signal that is sent to the solenoid for release of the electromechanical knee joint mechanism during the swing phase of gait.

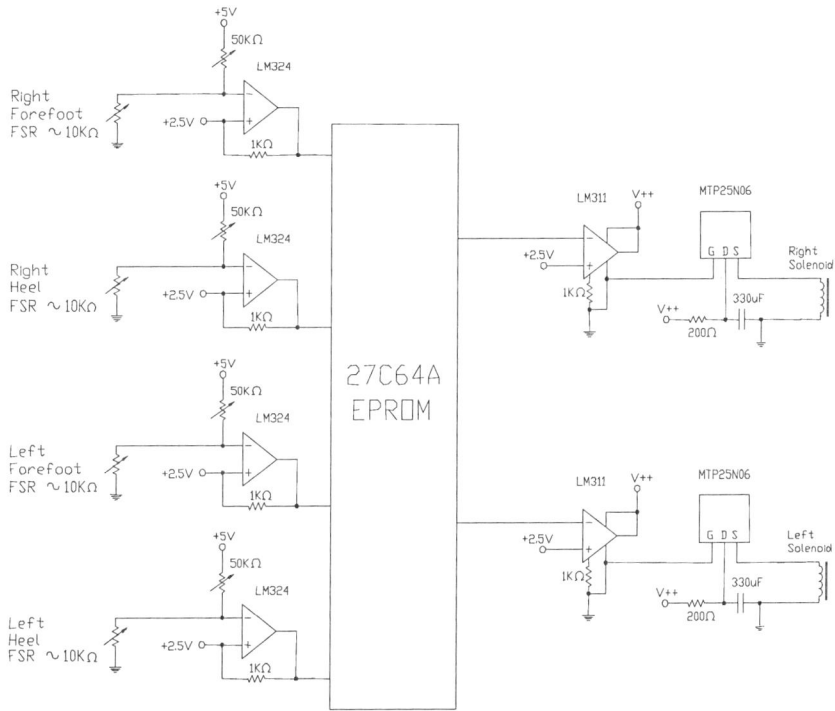

Figure 6. Control circuit schematic. A comparator circuit based on an LM324 operational amplifier conditions analog output from each footswitch sensor. The foot switch signals are input to a programmable read-only memory (EPROM, type 27C64A). Output from the EPROM controls high-voltage comparators (type LM311), which in turn control field effect power transistors (type MTP25N06). An initial energizing surge of current is provided to each solenoid by a 330-μF capacitor. The holding current was limited by a 200-Ω resistor, which limits battery drain rate. Source [32].

Table 2. EPROM truth table. All possible foot switch combinations have been assigned a corresponding set of solenoid control signals. Note that this system is designed for bilateral application.

State No.	Footswitch Input				Control Output	
	Right Heel	Right Forefoot	Left Heel	Left Forefoot	Right	Left
1	0	0	0	0	0	0
2	0	0	0	1	1	0
3	0	0	1	0	1	0
4	0	0	1	1	1	0
5	0	1	0	0	0	1
6	0	1	0	1	0	0
7	0	1	1	0	0	0
8	0	1	1	1	0	0
9	1	0	0	0	0	1
10	1	0	0	1	0	0
11	1	0	1	0	0	0
12	1	0	1	1	0	0
13	1	1	0	0	0	1
14	1	1	0	1	0	0
15	1	1	1	0	0	0
16	1	1	1	1	0	0

0 = No Ground Contact, Switch Open	0 = Solenoid NOT Energized, Knee Flexion Locked
1 = Ground Contact, Switch Closed	1 = Solenoid Energized, Knee Free to Flex

Source [33].

Dynamic gait analysis shows clear improvements in the knee motion pattern of patients with lower extremity weakness while using this new KAFO [29] (Figure 7). When the brace was tested in the locked configuration to simulate a standard locked KAFO, the knee motion (as expected) did not change during stance or swing. Significant improvement in swing-phase knee flexion was recorded when the brace was switched to free-knee operation. When the knee control algorithm was actuated, the knee maintained a stable, locked configuration during stance, yet the knee swing-phase motion pattern approximated the motion of typical walking.

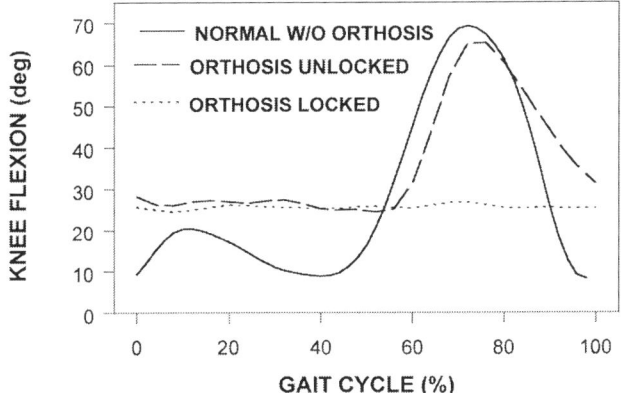

Figure 7. Knee motion when walking with stiff-knee gait (i.e., orthosis locked) and free-knee gait (i.e., orthosis free). Both bracing conditions provided a locked, stable knee during stance. The orthosis-locked condition did not allow knee motion during swing, whereas the orthosis-unlocked condition allowed normal knee swing-phase motion. (— normal; - - - orthosis free; ••• orthosis locked.) Source [29].

The energy consumption in a subject with poliomyelitis while using the new KAFO design was compared with conventional bracing [29]. The subject walked on a treadmill at speeds ranging from 15 to 80 meters per minute. The oxygen consumption rate increased in a linear manner with speed for both brace-locked and brace-unlocked conditions (Figure 8). The increase in the oxygen consumption rate was significant for both the brace-locked ($r^2 = .96$, $p = .001$) and the brace-unlocked ($r^2 = .96$, $p = .001$) conditions on level ground (0% slope). A similar pattern was true for the 5% incline with the increase in the oxygen consumption rate again significant for the brace-locked ($r^2 = .99$, $p = .027$) and brace-unlocked ($r^2 = .98$, $p = .099$) conditions. For each slope condition, the oxygen consumption rate was always greater for the brace-locked configuration. Comparison of the regression lines at 0% slope revealed that the intercepts were not significantly different ($p>.05$) yet the slopes of the two lines were not the same ($p<.025$). Comparison of the regression lines for the 5% incline showed that the slopes were parallel ($p<.05$) but the lines were not coincident ($p = .07$). Thus, the brace-unlocked configuration reduced energy requirements for ambulation. Nevertheless, the energy requirements for the participant were higher than those of individuals without mobility impairments (Figure 8).

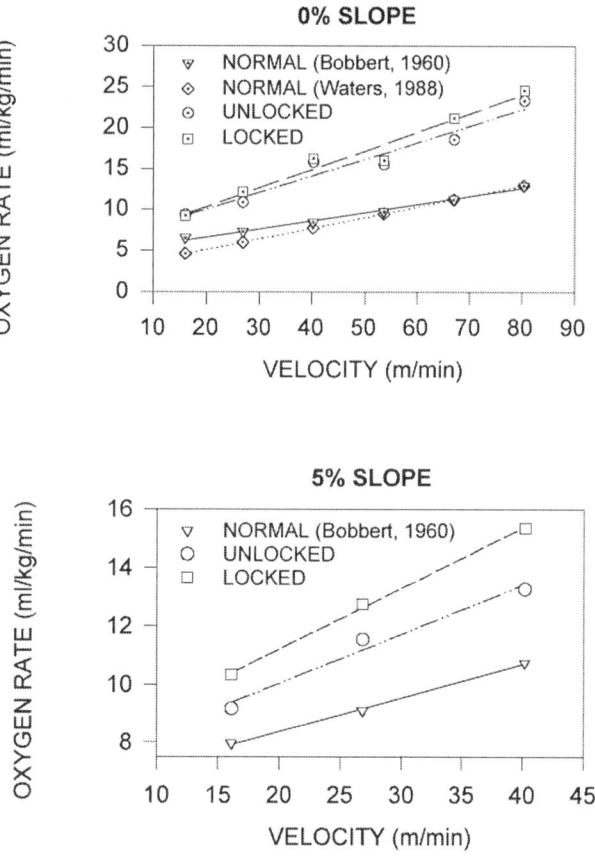

Figure 8. Oxygen consumption rates. (a) Walking on level ground (0% slope). (∇ normal [38]; ◊ normal [39]; ☉ unlocked; ❑ locked.) (b) Walking on a 5% slope. (∇ normal [38]; O unlocked; ❑ locked.) Data are presented for stiff-knee gait (i.e., orthosis locked) and free-knee gait (i.e., orthosis free). The oxygen consumption rate increased linearly for both conditions. The energy consumption was significantly less for the orthosis-free condition. Source [29].

Continued development efforts are underway. Concentration is being given to component size and weight reduction, durability, and patient testing.

4.2. UTX® - swing orthosis

The UTX is short for UTIKS, an abbreviation for University of Twente Intelligent Knee Stabilization. The UTX orthosis is a single sided, lateral orthosis (Figure 9). The orthosis has a knee joint that automatically unlocks during the swing phase of walking and a stable or locked knee joint during stance phase and standing. The orthosis is recommended for patients with single sided supple paralysis or paresis, e.g., caused by poliomyelitis. The device is acceptable for use in patients up to 120 kg body weight. The patient must have ankle joint mobility of at least 10° and sufficient control of hip muscles for advancement of the limb. The device is contraindicated in patients with spasticity (especially in the ankle region), medial-lateral knee instability, significant contractures of the knee and/or ankle, and severe medial-lateral ankle instability. The orthosis is lightweight, between 0.8 and 1.0 kg.

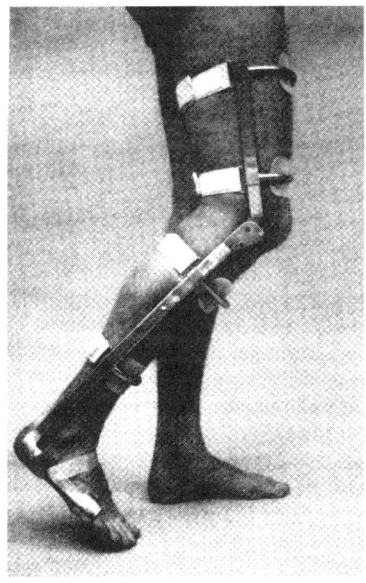

Figure 9. UTX orthosis. A single sided, lateral orthosis with an automatically unlocking knee joint. Source [34].

Van Leerdam and Kunst [34,35] describe the biomechanical fundamentals of the UTX knee-ankle-foot orthosis. The UTX knee joint consists of a ratchet and several springs that are activated by a cable (Figure 10). Two torsion springs are used. The locking spring pushes the ratchet in the locked position, and the buffer spring stores the detection signal, generated by the ankle joint, until an extending knee moment exists. The control strategy of the orthosis is based on detection of events during the gait cycle. During the swing phase the knee is unlocked. Detection of the end of the swing phase occurs when the knee angle reaches sufficient extension at the end of the swing phase. If sufficient extension of the joint has been realized, the locking spring of the ratchet automatically pushes the ratchet into its locked position and assures knee joint stability. The ratchet of the UTX knee joint is positioned at 8° of flexion. This is the only knee joint angle at which the orthosis stabilizes the leg.

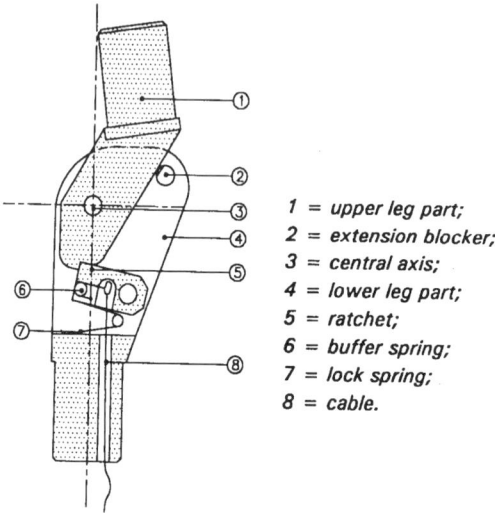

1 = upper leg part;
2 = extension blocker;
3 = central axis;
4 = lower leg part;
5 = ratchet;
6 = buffer spring;
7 = lock spring;
8 = cable.

Figure 10. The UTX knee joint, second prototype. Source [34].

During the stance phase, the knee remains locked. The end of stance phase has to be detected in order for the knee joint to unlock and enable knee flexion during the swing phase. Two parameters need to be detected to signal the end of the stance phase. First, an external dorsiflexing ankle moment needs to exceed a certain threshold. Second, in addition to the dorsiflexing ankle moment, an external extending knee moment must be present. Otherwise, if the external knee joint moment is a flexion moment, unlocking the knee in that situation would lead to immediate collapse of the patient. So, the detection signal (dorsiflexing ankle moment or ankle angle) and the signal that indicates an external knee extension moment must both be present before the knee joint is unlocked (Figure 11). Detection of the ankle moment or the ankle angle is obtained by a simple lever mechanism integrated in the ankle, which responds to the dorsiflexing ankle moment. The dorsiflexing ankle moment causes a dorsiflexion of the ankle resulting in a displacement of the cable and the buffer spring. The detection signal is stored in the buffer spring, and the spring exerts an unlocking force on the ratchet. This force, however, is very small compared to the forces exerted on the ratchet by the knee joint, due to an external knee flexion moment. This spring will unlock the ratchet when the knee joint moment changes to an external knee extension moment, and thus it is safe to unlock the knee joint.

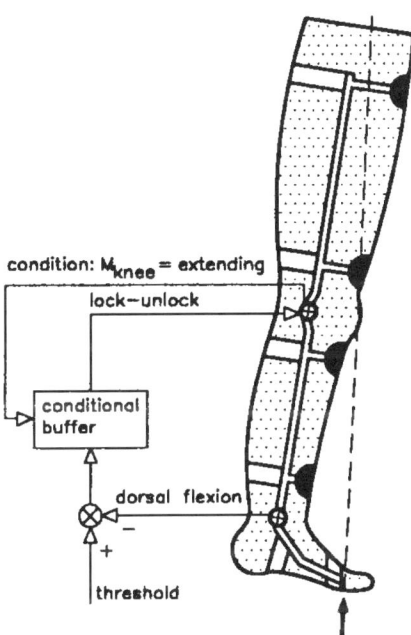

Figure 11. Schematic representation of the detection procedure. A dorsiflexing external ankle moment exceeding a certain threshold results in a detection signal that will be buffered until an extending external knee moment exists. Then, and only then, will the knee joint be unlocked. Source [34].

The orthosis has been tested in three patients with complete paralysis of the leg. All three patients managed to walk well after only limited training. Walking speeds equal to those obtained with their conventional KAFOs were reached within 15 hours of training. No limitations in the use of the knee stabilization system were found with respect to the more difficult walking tasks such as ramps and uneven surfaces. The knee kinematics of a patient while using the UTX orthosis was measured and compared to a conventional orthosis (Figure 12). Considerable knee flexion was obtained during the swing phase with the UTX orthosis.

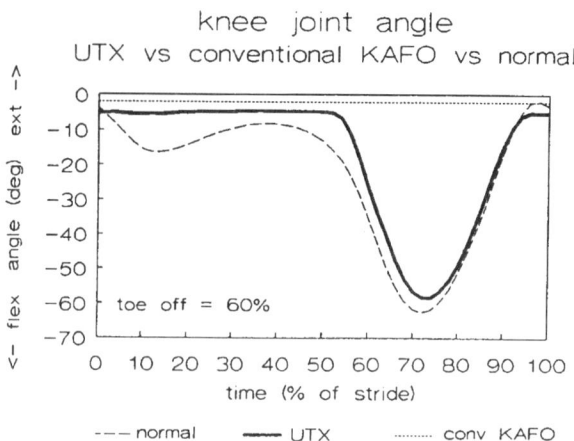

Figure 12. The knee joint angle during walking with the UTX orthosis compared to walking with a conventional KAFO and normal walking. When using the UTX orthosis, the knee flexion movement during the swing phase of walking is within the normal range. Source [34].

After extended training (maximum 3 months) all three patients managed to equal or increase both their freely chosen comfortable walking speed and their maximum walking speed with the UTX orthosis, compared to their conventional KAFO. One patient used the orthosis full time for a period of about two years. In general, the users were very satisfied with the increased functionality of the device and the superior kinematic features. Nonetheless, problems were encountered with the prototypes, which centered around the detection system, knee joint wear, and the plastic shell. Based on the experience gained, the UTX orthosis has been revised and further testing is planned.

4.3. Selectively lockable knee brace

A four-person National Aeronautics and Space Administration (NASA) team at the Marshall Space Flight Center in Huntsville, Alabama has developed the selectively lockable knee brace [36]. The knee brace includes right and left assemblies that contain identical joint mechanisms but are orientated slightly differently to accommodate the configuration of the knee (Figure 13a). The knee orthosis is strapped above the knee with hook and pile (Velcro or equivalent) straps. Below the knee, bars extend from the knee joint to a heel strike mechanism, which is used to activate unlocking of the knee brace [37] (Figure 13b). The heel strike mechanism consists of a small plate located under the heel that is depressed whenever the heel is in contact with the ground, and pushes a strike bar up against the strike bar guide plates. This action pushes the tube and plunger assemblies upward, causing pivoting of the levers, and thereby pushing the forward ends of the levers downward and pulling on the cables. Longitudinal sliding of the plungers inside the tubes is resisted by overload springs, which regulate the tension applied to the cables. Resulting forces are transmitted to the locking mechanism at the knee via a $1/16^{th}$-inch (1.59 mm) diameter cable that runs up each side of the lower leg brace.

The clutch for the selectively lockable knee brace is referred to as a releasable, conical roller clutch (Figure 14). Needle bearings join the upper and lower sections of the brace at the knee. These bearings permit free rotation of the joint while supporting the loads carried by the brace. Locking of the joint is accomplished with the clutch design. Depressing the heel strike plate pulls downward on the cables (Figure 13b), which in turn pulls the actuation rods in the knee joint. Each actuation rod, via a cam mechanism, engages a clutch on either side of the knee joint mechanism. When the activation rod is pulled down with respect to the lower housing, the actuation rod return spring is compressed causing the cam to rotate counterclockwise about the pin. When the cam rotates, it forces the back plate and the upper housing to the left, causing the cone clutch (coated with a fluoroelastomer such as Viton, or its equivalent) surfaces to engage. This locks the knee joint. When the heel strike mechanism releases tension on the cable, the return spring causes the activation rod to retract. This rotates the cam clockwise, back to its original position. In doing so, the right hand nose of the cam contacts the upper housing, forcing it to the right and thus disengaging the cone clutch. This allows the joint to rotate freely again. The releasable conical roller clutch provides positive locking with little wear. It is a compact design that will free wheel in both directions but, when engaged, will limit rotation to just one direction. When activated, the conical surface of the clutch comes in contact with a set of rollers that reside in tapered pockets in the mating housing. Any attempt at rotating in the direction of the taper causes the rollers to pinch the cone. Rotation in the opposite direction is still possible because the rollers tend to move away from the taper. If weight is applied while the foot is raised, such as when climbing stairs, the joint will lock in one direction, providing support, but can still be straightened.

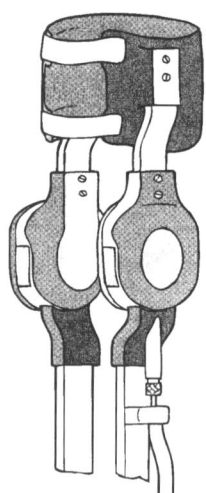

Figure 13a. Selectively Lockable Knee Brace. This *Knee Brace* is strapped at its upper end to the leg above the knee, and anchored at the lower end (not shown) by a stirrup under the foot. Source [36].

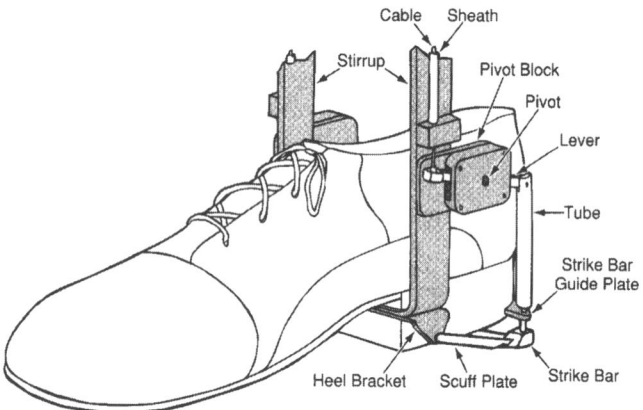

Figure 13b. The Heel-Strike Mechanism pulls the cable when weight is placed on the heel. Source [37].

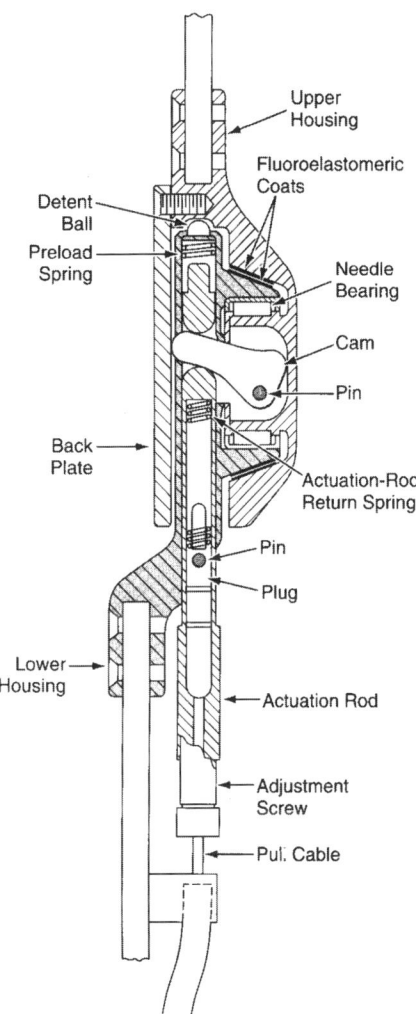

Figure 14. Clutch for selectively lockable knee brace. This *Joint Mechanism* (ideal mechanisms would be used in the left and right assemblies) allows the knee joint to flex freely except when weight is applied to the heel. Source [36].

With completion of the prototype development, the invention was patented by NASA and advertised to American industry in a period of open solicitation. An exclusive license to manufacture the brace was granted. The orthosis is currently undergoing clinical trials to prove its effectiveness and reliability. No data has been published to date regarding the performance of the selectively lockable knee brace.

5. Design critique

The logic-controlled electromechanical free-knee orthosis will probably be the easiest of all three designs to adapt to differing ground conditions because it uses a digital logic circuit and foot sensors to determine when the knee should be unlocked. Yet if the power fails, the knee will remain locked and the brace will function like a conventional KAFO. Further, when the clutch is locked, the knee can always be extended. Thus, knee stability is provided at any flexion angle. However, this flexibility is achieved by the largest increase in weight as compared to the other two designs. The UTX-Swing Orthosis is the lightest of the three designs, but offers the least amount of restraint to the limb in all three planes and is restricted in its clinical patient population application. Further, this orthoses only locks at one knee flexion angle. If this knee joint angle is not obtained at the end of swing, the patient will not have stance-phase stability. Both the UTX orthosis and the selectively lockable knee brace use heel movement to unlock the knee joint. It is important to note that heel rise occurs before opposite foot strike during normal gait. Thus, if the knee is unlocked at heel rise, the patient will fall. The UTX orthosis has made a provision to assure that the external knee moment is extending the knee before the knee is unlocked. The selectively lockable knee brace does not state how this condition is handled. Nevertheless, the selectively lockable knee brace utilizes an elegant and compact clutch design which can be placed on both the medial and lateral struts. This clutch placement will minimize any twisting of the brace. Further, the clutch is capable of locking at any knee joint angle and still allows the brace to extend at any time during stance. Thus, all three design approaches have relative strengths and weaknesses which must be considered.

Acknowledgment. This work was partially supported by NIH Grant RO1-HD30150. Appreciation is expressed to Barbara Iverson-Literski for careful manuscript preparation.

References

[1] Benson, V., Marano, M.A., Current estimates from the National Health Interview Survey, 1995. National Center for Health Statistics. *Vital Health Statistics*, 10, 77, 1998.

[2] Russell, J.N., Hendershot, G.E, LeClere, F., Howie, L.J., *Trends and differential use of assistive technology devices: United States, 1994*. Hyattsville, MD: National Center for Health Statistics, No. 292, 1, November 13, 1997.

[3] Persons using devices and/or features to assist with impairments, by age: 1990 *Statistical Abstract of the United States*. Washington, DC: U.S. Department of Commerce, 1994.
[4] Heimlich, M.P., *Brace for the Infirm Leg*. French Patent No. 948.372, 1949.
[5] Rainey, F.E., *Leg Brace*. US Patent No. 2883982, 1959.
[6] Tarte, M.C., *Artificial Leg*. US Patent No. 3546712, 1970.
[7] Williams, A.C., *Artificial Leg*. US Patent No. 4578083, 1983.
[8] Harris, A.I., *Automatically Releasing Knee Brace*. US Patent No. 4632096, 1986.
[9] Chen, D.Y.H., *An Automatic Electrically Controlled Leg Brace for Knee Joint Instability*. Department of Electrical Engineering. Columbus, Ohio: Ohio State University, PhD Dissertation, 1972.
[10] Taylor, B.M., *Support for Normal Body Locomotion*. US Patent No. 2267848, 1941.
[11] Boulanger, J., *Appareil orthopédique pour membre inférieur*. French Patent No. 1230323, 1960.
[12] Allard, P.L., *Knee Joint Orthosis*. US Patent No. 4457003, 1984.
[13] Liberson, W.T., *Electromechanical Prosthetic Devices for the control of Movements in Handicapped Individuals*. US Patent No. 3553738, 1971.
[14] Pansiera, T.T., *Hinge Means for Orthopedic Brace*. US Patent No. 4502472, 1985.
[15] Joyce, R.D., *Strap Device for Assisting in Hip, Knee, and Foot Movement*. US Patent No. 4252112, 1981.
[16] Salort, G.J., *External Apparatus for Vertical Stance and Walking for Those with Handicapped Motor Systems of the Lower Limbs*. US Patent No. 4422453, 1983.
[17] Spahn, E., *Knee and Ankle Brace*. US Patent No. 1072369, 1913.
[18] Vito, R.P., Boehm, H.R., *Cable Controlled Orthopedic Leg Brace*. US Patent No. 4602627, 1986.
[19] Blatchford, B.G., *Artificial Leg with Stabilized Knee Mechanism*. US Patent No. 4351070, 1982.
[20] Moissonnier, G., *Device Permitting the Control of the Flexion of a Defective Limb of a Handicapped Person Which is Fitted with an Orthopaedic Appliance for its Support and Articulation*. US Patent No. 4489717, 1984.
[21] Malcolm, L.L., Sutherland, D.H., Cooper, L., Wyatt, M., A digital logic-controlled electromechanical orthosis for free-knee gait in muscular dystrophy children. *Orthopaedic Transactions*, 5, 90, 1980.
[22] Hunt, N.L., *Design of an Electrical Orthosis Joint Brake*. Boston, MA: Massachusetts Institute of Technology, Masters Thesis, 1985.
[23] Weddendorf, B.C., *Automatic Locking Orthotic Knee Device*. US Patent No. 5267950, 1993.
[24] Yang, P.Y., *A Study of Electronically Controlled Orthotic Knee Joint Systems*. Columbus, OH: Ohio State University, PhD Dissertation, 1975.
[25] Kaplan, L.K., Grynbaum, B.B., Rusk, H.A., Anastasia, T., Gassler, S., A reappraisal of braces and other mechanical aids in patients with spinal cord dysfunction: Results of a follow-up study. *Archives of Physical Medicine and Rehabilitation*, 47, 393, 1996.

[26] Phillips, B., Zaho, H., Predictors of assistive technology abandonment. *Assistive Technology*, 5, 36, 1993.
[27] Cerny, K., Waters, R., Hislop, H., Perry, J., Walking and wheelchair energetics in persons with paraplegia. *Physical Therapy*, 60, 1133, 1980.
[28] Lehnis, H.R., Orthotics: The state of the art. *Journal of Rehabilitation Research and Development*, 30, vii, 1993.
[29] Kaufman, K.R., Irby, S.E., Wirta, R.W., Sutherland, D.H., Energy efficient knee-ankle-foot orthosis: A case study. *Journal of Prosthetics and Orthotics*, 8, 79, 1996.
[30] Irby, S.E., *A Digital Logic Controlled Electromechanical Free-Knee Brace*. San Diego: San Diego State University, Masters Thesis, 1994.
[31] Irby, S.E., Kaufman, K.R., Wirta, R.W., Sutherland, D.H., Optimization and application of a wrap spring clutch to a dynamic knee-ankle-foot orthosis. *IEEE Trans Rehabilitation Engineering*, 7, 130, 1999.
[32] Irby, S.E., Kaufman, K.R., Mathewson, J.W., Sutherland, D.H., Automatic Control Design for a Dynamic Knee Brace System *IEEE Trans Rehabilitation Engineering*, 7, 135, 1999.
[33] Tomovic, R., McGhee, R.B., A finite state approach to the synthesis of bioengineering control systems. *IEEE Trans Human Factors Engr*, 7, 65, 1966.
[34] van Leerdam, N.G.A., *The Swinging UTX Orthosis: Biomechanical Fundamentals and Conceptual Design*. Utrecht, The Netherlands: University of Twente, PhD Dissertation, 1993.
[35] van Leerdam, N.G.A., Kunst, E.E., Die neue Beinorthese UTX-Swing: Normales Gehen, kombiniert mit sicherem Stehen. *Orthopädie-Technik*, 6, 506, 1999.
[36] Myers, N., Forbes, J., Shadoan, M., Baker, K., Knee brace would lock and unlock automatically. *NASA Technical Briefs*, 28, December 1995.
[37] Myers, N., Shadoan, M., Forbes, J., Baker, K., Heel-strike mechanism for rehabilitative knee brace. *NASA Technical Briefs*, 72, November 1996.
[38] Bobbert, A.C., Energy expenditure in level and grade walking. *Journal of Applied Physiology*, 5, 1015, 1960.
[39] Waters, R.L., Barnes, G., Husserl, T., Silver, L., Liss, R., Comparable energy expenditure after arthrodesis of the hip and ankle. *Journal of Bone & Joint Surgery*, 70A, 1032, 1988.

Index of acronyms and abbreviations

AC	Alternative Current
A/D	Analog to Digital (converter, conversion)
AGC	Automatic Gain Control
AP	Arterial Pressure
ASK	Amplitude Shift Key
ARMA	Auto Regressive Moving Average (time series)
AT	Assistive Technology
BFS	Binaural Feedback System
bmp	beats per minute
BODH2O	body water
CA	Communication Assistant
CLK	clock
CM	Center of Mass
CMAC	Cerebellar Model Articulation Controller
CMOS	Complementary MOS circuit (technology)
CNS	Central Nervous System
CO2A	arterial CO2 content
CP	Center of Pressure
CRT	Cathode Ray Tube (display)
CV	Cyclic Voltammetry
DAC	Digital to Analogue Converter
DC	Direct Current
DC/DC	Direct Current to Direct Current (converter, conversion)
DLL	Delay Locked Loop
DSP	Digital Signal / Speech Processor
EMG	ElectroMyoGraphic
ETA	Electronic Travel Aid
EERUF	Error Eliminating Rapid Ultrasonic Firing
FIFO	First In First Out (memory)
FSR	Force Sensing Resistor
FuLL	Fuzzy Logic Language
GA	genetic Algorithm(s)
GFR	glomerular filtration rate (ml/Min)
GRO	Growth Rate Operator

ISM	Interpretive Structural Modeling
KAFO	Knee-Ankle-Foot Orthosis
KCMASS	cellular protein mass
LCD	Liquid Crystal Device (display)
LED	Light Emitting Diode
LSB, lsb	least significant bit
MARC	Multiple-unit Artificial Retinal Chipset
MAV	Mean Absolute Value
MCA	Microprocessor Controlled Arm
MES	Myoelectric Signal
MLP	Multi-Layer Perceptron
MOS	Metal-Oxide-Semiconductor transistor (technology)
MUSFLO	muscle blood flow (ml/Min)
NAMASS	extracellular sodium mass
NMOS	n-type MOS (transistor, circuit)
NN	neural networks
OAS	Obstacle Avoidance System
PFD	Phase Frequency Detector
PHEO	pheochromocytomia
PHOXYN	alpha-blocker multiplier
PVC	plastics in the family of Poly-Vinyl-Chlorides
PWM	Pulse Width Modulation
RF	Radio Frequency
RSYMPS	relative strength of sympathetic activity
SMD	Surface Mounted Device (technology)
SME	Small and Medium Enterprises
SYT	sympathetic total neuro-component
TDD	Telephonic Device for the Deaf
VFH	Vector Field Histogram
VGA	Video Graphic Adapter
VR	Virtual Reality
ZC	Zero Crossings

Compiled by Horia-Nicolai Teodorescu

Index of terms

A

acid/base balance 281
activation pattern 226
actuator 244, 283, 382
actuator control 247
actuator equation 283
adaptation 353
adaptation to demands 353
afferent activity 215
agent 383
agent-oriented architecture 383
age-related macular degeneration 31
amputee 129, 219
ankle joint 214
antenna 318
apnea 306
artificial heart 273
artificial limb 450
artificial retina 31
atrophy 317
auditory analysis 94
auditory feedback 142
auditory logogen 94
auditory pathways 93
auditory system 93
automatic gain control 101
automatic grip 251
autonomous wheelchair 422
autonomy 382
autoregressive model 176

B

balance 130
barotrauma 322
basal metabolism 326
below-elbow amputee 157
binaural feedback system 424
biocompatibility 36, 211
biofeedback 129

biphasic stimulus 219
bipolar electrode 179
bladder 210
blindness 32
blood flow 275
blood pressure 273
blood viscosity 276
blood volume 281
bonding 63

C

camera 36
carbon dioxide balance 281
cardiac function 281
cardiac pacemaker 321, 347
cathodic pulse 227
cellular automata 274
center of mass 136
center of pressure 136
central sleep apnea 306
centrifugal blood pump 273
chaos theory 5
chemoreceptor 307
chip 31
chipset 32
chronic respiratory insufficiency 302
circulatory model 274
circulatory physiology 274
closed loop control 215
cochlea 93
cochlear implant 93
cognition 116
complex behavior 221
computer-aided support system 275
connectivity 391
context-sensitive network 194
control 381
control of exercise 281
control of ventilation 281
control system 154

controlled activation 214
controller 318, 347
conversation 399
coordinated control 167
cophosis 95
cornea 36
correlation matrix 277
corrosion 214
Corti's organ 105
cosmetic glove 245
cosmetic hand 245
cuff electrode 214, 318

D

data acquisition 137
deafness 93
degree of freedom 245
degree of selectivity 217
demodulator 53
diagnosis of a circulatory system 273
diaphragm 301
differential pressure 276
digital speech processor 106
distributed processing 393
double helix electrode 213
dynamic knee joint 452
dynamic model 274
dynamic performances 274

E

electrical stimulation 32, 143, 311
electrochemical evaluation 84
electrochemical reaction 211
electrode 31, 106, 316
electrode array 31
electrode corrosion 229
electrode design 318
electrode failure 179
electronic control 453
electronic travel aid 413
EMG signal 246
emotion 395
encoder 440
energy consumption 459
environment model 432

epimysial electrode 316
epineural electrode 218
estimation technique 276
evoked potential 116
evoked response 223
expert system 5
extracellular stimulation 221
extracorporeal pressure transducer 275
eye 37

F

face detection 398
feedback signal 215
filter 51
filtering 248
flexible electrode 50
flicker 38
flow calculation 273
fluid infusion and loss 281
focus ion beam technique 69
foot orthosis 450
forceplate 137
force sensing resistor 144, 250
force sensor 250
frequency shift 100
functional evaluation 181
fuzzy control 347
fuzzy expert system 262
fuzzy logic 5, 173, 347, 356
fuzzy logic controller 265
fuzzy logic inference 274
fuzzy microcontroller 359
fuzzy rule 360

G

gait 449
gait analysis 137, 458
gait events 455
gait kinematics 455
gait kinetics 455
gas exchange 281
genetic algorithms 5
general circulation 281
gesture 382
glossopharyngeal respiration 312

granularity 391
graphical expression 275
graphical interface 263
grasp force 230
grasping 246
grip strength 246
groove electrode 219
guidance 413
guidance mode 425

H

Hall effect 260
hearing aid 95
hearing impairment 95
hearing mechanism 98
heart block 348
heart-reflex interaction 281
heat dissipation 44
hierarchical control 174
hierarchy graph 273
histogram 418
    polar ~ 419
Human model 274
humanoid robot 383
human-robot interaction 382
hybrid device 231
hydraulic knee joint 452
hyperventilation 335
hypotension 330
hypoventilation 301

I

image processing 389
implant 213, 318
implantable prosthesis 32
implantable transducer 275
implantation 37
indirect measurement technique 273
inference engine 364
information 414
infrared sensor 399
intelligent orthosis 450
intelligent support system 273
intercostal muscle 303
internal model 129

interoceptive system 133
interpretive structural modeling 275, 278
intrafascicular stimulation 217
intramuscular electrode 213, 316
intraneural electrode 215
intraneural microstimulation 216
intraocular chip 45
intraocular prosthesis 36
intraspinal electrical stimulation 222
involuntary feedback 246
iridium 37
iridium oxide 79

J

Jacobian controller 193

K

Kapton 79
knee-ankle-foot orthosis 450
knee brace 464
knee kinematics 463
knee orthosis 450

L

Lagrangian equations 170
language 93, 390
laparoscopy 319
large circulatory model 273
leg orthosis 450
life-sustaining device 324
linear estimation 273
locking mechanism 452
locomotor control 222
logogen 95
lower limb prostheses 130

M

machine intelligence 382
macular degeneration 31
magnetic stimulation 324
manipulator 395
mechanical aid 331
mechanical impedance 219

mechanical properties 211
mechanoreceptor 134
mechatronic device 5
Meissner corpuscle 134
membership function 264, 359
membrane dynamics 227
Merkel receptor 134
metalization 85
microcontroller 247, 359
microelectrode array 226
micromachining 79
microstimulation 216
micturition 220
micturition assist 220
middle ear 99
middle ear aid 104
mock circulatory loop 284
model 219
model reduction 276
motion detection 252
motor control 129
motor evoked response 225
motor neuron 210
motor prosthesis 210
motor system 212
multi-channel autoregressive model 178
multielectrode 106
multi-focal electrical stimulation 37
multifunction control 154
multilayer perceptron 184
multirate stimulation 112
muscle-based electrode 210
muscle fatigue 220, 321
muscular atrophying disease 381
muscular dystrophy 381
myoelectric control 153
myoelectric prosthesis 243
myoelectric signal 154

N

natural language 397
navigation 382, 423
nerve electrode 316
nerve stimulation 209
neural damage 215
neural network 5, 184

neural prosthesis 219
neural stimulation 209
neurological disorder 209
neuronal activation 227
neuronal tracing 222
nonlinear control 382
nonlinear equation 287

O

object recognition 382
obstacle avoidance 413
obstacle information 437
odometry 439
optical sensor 252
orthotic device 167
orthosis 450
oxygen balance 281
oxygen consumption 459
oxygen saturation level 355

P

pacemaker 347
    coupled ~ 351
    demand ~ 350
    double chamber ~ 350
    negative demand ~ 350
    pair ~ 351
    positive demand ~ 350
pacing 301
Pacini corpuscle 134
packaging 45
pain suppression 220
paralysis 450
paraplegia 304
pattern 154
pattern recognition 5, 154
peripheral nerve 215
peripheral receptor 131
pharmacology 281
photonic device 33
photoreceptor 31
photosensor 253
phrenic nerve 218
phrenic stimulation 316
piezoelectric cell (device) 137

pitch 111
platinum 37
platinum oxide 79
polyimide 36
potassium balance 281
pressure transducer 275
proactivity 393
programmable prosthesis 101
proprioception 134
proprioceptive sensation 133
prosthesis 130, 155
protein balance 281
psychoacoustical experiment 95
pulsatile blood pump 275

Q

quadripolar electrode 320
quality of life 316

R

radio frequency 316
reactivity 384
red cell mass 281
reduced correlation matrix 277
reflex 281
reflex control 222
reflex function 231
rehabilitation 129
rehabilitation robot 383
renal hormone 281
renal excretion 281
respiration 302
respiratory insufficiency 302
respiratory muscle 303
retinal prosthesis 31
robot 381, 413
    mobile ~384
    humanoid ~383
    wheelchair ~ 394
robotic hand 244
Ruffini corpuscle 134

S

scalability 385

sealing 319
selective activation 209
selective stimulation 209
self-organizing control 173
sensitive matrix 253
sensor 414, 455
    contact ~ 455
    distance ~ 414
sensorial system 244
sensorized insole 137
sensory control 243
sensory input 382
sensory substitution 129
sensory system
service robotics 382
silicone electrode arrays 79
silicone rubber 36
silicon substrate 231
skin detection 398
sliding mode control 382
slip signal 230
slipping sensor 246
sodium balance 281
software architecture 382
sonar 382, 416
sonogram 97
sound localization 386
sound processor 108
speaker identification 402
speech 386
speech input 402
speech processor 106
speech recognition 386
speech technology 397
sphincter 223
spinal cord injury 303, 381
spinal motor neuron 228
spinal neuron 222
stability 449, 452
stainless steel 229
statistical decision 166
status of kidney 281
stimulation rate 112
stimulator 318
stimulator telemeter 230
stimulus 212
stimulator circuit 59

strain gauge sensor 261
strength sensor 246
stress (mechanical) 51
stroke 381
stroke volume 353
structural analysis 276
substrate 40
surface electrode 248
symbiotic system 398
synaptic excitation 227
synchronization 53
synchronization circuit 53
synergy 131
system integration 382

T

tactile corpuscles 134
tactile feedback 129
tactile sensation 133
tele-assistance 267
telemetry 31, 115, 138
telemetry protocol 36
teleoperation 385
temperature regulation 281
testbed 387
tetraplegia 303
text-to-speech 397
thoracotomy 319
timing generator 53
tolerance 74
topographic organization 216
touch 385
tracheostomy 306
transducer 273
transient burst 182
travel aid 413
tuning 262
    automatic ~ 262
    manual ~ 266

U

ultrasonic sensor 434
upper-extremity amputee 157
upper limb prosthesis 245
urea balance 281
urethral sphincter 223

V

vectormyogram 172
ventilation 301
ventilatory support 302
vibration 144
vibrator 103
    bone-integrated ~ 103
video camera 31
video board 72
video processing chip 31
virtual arm simulation 185
virtual sound source 424
virtual reality 5, 15
vision 33, 382
visual feedback 141, 246
visual prosthesis 32
visually impaired 413
vocal tract 97
voice 382
voice production 96
voltammetry 84
volume distribution 281

W

walking pattern 432
water balance 281
waveform 324
wavelets 117
wheelchair 394
wirebond 78

Compiled by Horia-Nicolai Teodorescu